SCHOOL NEUROPSYCHOLOGY

Also Available

Traumatic Brain Injury in Children and Adolescents:
Assessment and Intervention
Margaret Semrud-Clikeman

School NEUROPSYCHOLOGY

A Practitioner's Handbook

SECOND EDITION

Margaret Semrud-Clikeman
Catherine A. Fiorello
James B. Hale

Foreword by Elaine Fletcher-Janzen

gp

THE GUILFORD PRESS
New York   London

Library of Congress Cataloging-in-Publication Data

Names: Hale, James B., 1961–2023 author. | Semrud-Clikeman, Margaret, author. | Fiorello, Catherine A., author.
Title: School neuropsychology : a practitioner's handbook / Margaret Semrud-Clikeman, Catherine A. Fiorello, James B. Hale.
Description: Second edition. | New York : The Guilford Press, [2026] | Revised edition of: School neuropsychology / James B. Hale, Catherine A. Fiorello. 2004. | Includes bibliographical references and index. |
Identifiers: LCCN 2025033432 | ISBN 9781462555185 (paperback) | ISBN 9781462559367 (cloth)
Subjects: LCSH: Pediatric neuropsychology. | School psychology. | School children—Mental health services. | Behavioral assessment of children.
Classification: LCC RJ486.5.H235 2025
LC record available at *https://lccn.loc.gov/2025033432*

*To the hundreds of children and parents I was privileged to work with
at Mequon-Thiensville schools when I was a school psychologist there
in the 1970s and '80s, and to the children I saw in my practice at the
University of Washington, The University of Texas at Austin,
and the University of Minnesota Medical School.*

*To my many graduate students who taught me as much as I taught
them. I am thankful for the mentorship I received from Dr. George
Hynd, Dr. Anne Ellison, and Dr. Dennis Norman.*

*Finally, I thank my parents, Margaret and Ray Semrud,
as well as my late husband, John Clikeman, for their support
and cheerleading, which I needed when things got tough.*

—MS-C

*To my family, who always support my academic
and professional pursuits.*

*And to the children and students, from whom I learn
as much as I teach.*

—CAF

About the Authors

Margaret Semrud-Clikeman, PhD, is Professor Emerita in the Division of Clinical Behavioral Neuroscience at the University of Minnesota Medical School. A board-certified pediatric neuropsychologist, she formerly served on the faculties of The University of Texas at Austin and Michigan State University and practiced as a school psychologist in Wisconsin. Dr. Semrud-Clikeman's research interests include neuroimaging in children with nonverbal learning disability and autism spectrum disorder, as well as neuropsychological studies of cerebral malaria in Malawi and Uganda. She has published over 100 peer-reviewed articles, 75 chapters, and several books; has presented her work internationally; and has been an invited professor in Singapore, Italy, New Zealand, and Finland.

Catherine A. Fiorello, PhD, is Professor of School and Counseling Psychology at Temple University. She is an elected Fellow of Division 16 (School Psychology) of the American Psychological Association and of the American Academy of School Psychology, and is a board-certified school psychologist. Dr. Fiorello's research focuses on cognitive and neuropsychological assessment, with an emphasis on ensuring the fairness of assessment measures for students who are culturally and linguistically diverse and those growing up in poverty. She also has publications and clinical experience in the areas of learning and behavior disorders, health-related disorders, low-incidence disabilities, intellectual giftedness, and school neuropsychology.

James B. Hale, PhD, until his death in 2023, was an internationally respected expert in the field of pediatric neuropsychology. He served on the faculties of several universities and, after retiring from academia, opened a clinical practice serving children and families of the Pacific Northwest. Additionally, he was founding director of the Center for Teaching Brain Literacy in Bellingham, Washington. A board-certified pediatric neuropsychologist, Dr. Hale was also a licensed school psychologist and certified special education teacher. He conducted research to make neuropsychological assessment relevant for school intervention for children with high-incidence learning and behavior problems. A frequent conference presenter, Dr. Hale was author or coauthor of numerous scholarly publications.

Foreword

This is the second time that *School Neuropsychology* is going to make a unique contribution to the fields of school psychology, special education, clinical psychology, and neuropsychology. The first edition, published in 2004, was the first powerful message by experts that neuropsychology should be incorporated into school psychology practice. Hale and Fiorello blazed a path for school psychologists to understand the basics of pediatric neuropsychological assessment and its practical implementation. By doing so, they also set the standard for this translational work in the field.

Over the years, the first edition of *School Neuropsychology* held a very popular and exemplary place for delivering a wealth of information in a concise and focused manner. The breadth and depth of information was carefully balanced and the translation of neuroscience from the "research-bench to the school-desk" was a natural result. The book not only incorporated the basic history and neuroscience needed for neuropsychological assessment, but also provided a model for learning disabilities assessment, case studies, focused chapters on specialty areas such as brain injury, and an overall detailed map of how to apply the content directly into practice. Herein lies the essential and unique value of the book, as it seamlessly translates the relationship between pediatric neuropsychology and everyday school psychology practice.

The second edition of *School Neuropsychology* continues this essential work, but also offers unique contributions that bring us up to the cutting edge of practice. The new edition includes updated and research-based chapters that delve into the latest neuroscience and challenge established theories of brain localization and organization; brand new chapters about genetic conditions and chronic illness; and new case studies with notes that relate to what we see on the ground in school psychology every day.

At the time work began on the second edition of *School Neuropsychology*, Dr. Semrud-Clikeman was added to the authorial team. Her inclusion not only brought added editorial expertise but also ended up providing support for adjustments that had to be made. Importantly and poignantly, Dr. Hale passed away in 2023. His passing made his contributions to this volume all the more profound and enduring. A board-certified pediatric neuropsychologist, scholar, and clinician, Dr. Hale had committed his career to bridging neuropsychological insight with the tangible needs of children and schools. His legacy imbues this second edition with both deep expertise and heartfelt purpose.

In addition, during this period of time, we were all worried about how to bring translational pediatric neuropsychology into what was the most complicated and difficult sentinel event in our health history of the past century. SARS-CoV-2 (COVID-19) was raging unrestrained through the infant, child, and adolescent populations around the world, and at that time we knew very little about its long-term physical and neurological sequelae. For some children it was mortal, and for others the virus left a set of symptoms that ranged from medical trauma to memory and learning issues, many of which interfered with meeting the demands of everyday life. Research was just beginning on pediatric "long-haul" effects, and fledgling studies were plagued by confounding issues such as small sample sizes, lack of randomized/controlled study designs, lack of premorbid data, diversity of severity of symptoms, and so on. Some years later this is still the case, but at least we are all now on notice that our practice must become more sophisticated and defensible. Only neuropsychologically informed, comprehensive assessments can deliver the necessary sensitivity and specificity for this task. Therefore, the second edition of this seminal work is needed by school psychologists more than ever.

One particular virtue of *School Neuropsychology* is that any school psychologist, from graduate student to highly experienced veteran, can use this book to learn about the history and evolution of neuroscience, up-to-date knowledge of brain development, how to conduct a comprehensive neuropsychological assessment, and specialized knowledge of all kinds of disorders and disabilities. All school psychologists can use this book to develop an internal roadmap that will guide differential diagnosis, intervention, and good outcomes.

It is a rare book that can take on the entire history of neuropsychology, theoretical models of brain function, functional neuroanatomy, neuropsychological assessment instruments, models of differential diagnosis, report writing, special neurodevelopmental conditions, and interventions in an accurate, detailed, and practical manner. The worth of this book is well established, not solely by its outstanding content, but also by the context in which we find ourselves at its publication. We will need the best training, the best advice, and our best sense of advocacy to go forward and serve children well in the coming years, and Dr. Semrud-Clikeman, Dr. Fiorello, and Dr. Hale have packed the second edition of *School Neuropsychology* with all of the tools that we will need to be successful.

ELAINE FLETCHER-JANZEN, EdD, NCSP, ABPdN
Past President, American Academy of Pediatric Neuropsychology

Contents

Introduction

Recognizing and Applying Neuropsychological Principles

Studying Brain–Behavior Relationships

At a time when societal norms are being challenged, civil rights are being reconsidered, public health crises threaten our lives, and online learning has been the norm, it is even more important to understand brain–behavior relationships. There are also children who now survive medical conditions that are being served in schools. In the past these children would not have survived their diseases. New interventions and new techniques for diagnosis provide a window into disorders that children, in the past, did not survive or that were largely unrecognized. These viruses cross the blood–brain barrier and cause difficulties for a substantial minority of children in the areas of memory and attention as well as learning. For many children who survive cancer and other diseases, there are long-term effects not only for neuropsychological processes but also for the effects of having lost out on school experiences due to lockdowns or to the need to protect these vulnerable children from possible infection. In addition, given the limited opportunity offered during online instruction for these children, who really require hands-on teaching, these students are even more likely to be behind normative expectations. For this reason, it becomes more and more important for school personnel to have information about the long-term effects of treatments/instruction (or lack of treatments/instruction) and psychologists serve as important conduits who can provide such information to multidisciplinary teams.

This second edition of *School Neuropsychology: A Practitioner's Handbook* provides a basic primer of brain–behavior relationships and applies this knowledge to commonly experienced learning problems in reading, writing, and written language. These chapters are expanded and updated with the most recent research, including research conducted by the authors. New chapters on genetics and on medical disorders have been added to this edition. The final chapter has been expanded to include a theory of brain–behavior relationships that includes a three-dimensional understanding of brain networks and brain functioning. We are excited to provide this new edition with updated case studies that can illustrate how to evaluate children with usual and unusual disorders, so that practitioners are better able to serve the needs of all children, regardless of disability status.

1

The study of brain–behavior relationships is remarkably compelling and at the same time incredibly overwhelming. These relationships are difficult for professors to teach, students to learn, and practitioners to implement. Applying these neuropsychological principles in clinical practice seems impossible at first glance. Expertise in neuropsychological interpretation of test data requires diligent practice, a continued desire to better your interpretive skills, learning about theoretical and empirical advances in the field, and finding ways to apply this information in your daily practice of psychology. Hundreds of articles and books elucidating brain–behavior relationships are written each year. Although it is a daunting task to try to digest all the relevant neuropsychological literature, it is a noble goal, nonetheless. Moreover, applying these skills and the knowledge base to individual children requires clinical acumen—something that cannot be taught in any textbook or manual. Though the information contained in this book can help you utilize neuropsychological information in daily assessment and intervention practices, it is not a substitute for the training and supervised experience needed to become a board-certified neuropsychologist.

The goal of this book is to provide readers with a survey of the relevant brain–behavior literature and practices, but the material presented is not exhaustive. Many current training programs for school psychologists do not have substantial coursework in the biological bases of behavior. We provide a brief overview of brain structure, but it may be helpful for the reader to examine the resources listed in the chapter appendices. We also note that the knowledge base for our understanding of brain–behavior relationships is growing at a phenomenal rate. Implicit in this tremendous growth is that previously accepted ideas about the brain are now outdated. For instance, when most people think of the cognitive constructs subserved by the left and right hemispheres, they think of verbal and nonverbal skills, respectively. As we discuss in this book, this long-held dichotomous belief does not accurately reflect the true nature of hemispheric processing differences. Though not all scholars in neuropsychology would concur with our position, the theoretical and empirical advances made in recent years confirm the validity of the model we describe in the following chapters. The implications of these findings are dramatic and meaningful in daily practice, providing you with new insight into brain–behavior relationships. These novel insights form a conceptual framework for differential diagnosis and treatment of the learning and behavior disorders you encounter in your daily practice of psychology.

Making Neuropsychology User-Friendly

While most students and practitioners studying neuropsychology find the material fascinating or at the very least interesting, they typically complain that the material is inaccessible, too complex to master, or irrelevant in daily practice. We think there are four major reasons for these difficulties, and we offer possible remedies for each to overcome these criticisms.

The first reason has to do with neuropsychology nomenclature, or—simply put—the large number of big words that sound medical or biological in nature. School personnel recognize that medical issues have an impact on their children and often rely on medical doctors to provide information about diagnoses and treatment. However, medical doctors do not know school requirements and school personnel frequently do not understand the medical issues. Having worked in both settings, we can assert that the medical doctors rely on school personnel to understand the best treatment approach for the child in the school. The school neuropsychologist can serve as a liaison between the medical establishment as well as the school personnel. Such an interdisciplinary approach is superior to a typical multidisciplinary one. All team members need to keep in mind that children are their primary clients. As members of the team, school psychologists and neuropsychologists in the schools need to bridge the diagnosis–intervention gap and learning neuropsychological terminology and principles can make this happen.

Learning about neuropsychological terminology is a lot like learning a foreign language, with no one readily accessible to help you master the terms before they are used to describe concepts and techniques. Having taught neuropsychology to a variety of students at different levels of training, we understand this hinders their acquisition and application of the material. These words may be foreign to you just like when you try to communicate with someone who speaks a different language. You may experience a similar feeling when reading the material that follows. However, don't be discouraged if you come across a term you haven't heard of when reading this book. We suggest you be patient with yourself as this new learning will eventually become part of your lexicon and you will begin communicating using these new words! In our neuropsychological studies, we were always amazed at how many, many ways there were to convey comparable concepts or brain structures, so we attempt to use the same terminology throughout the book. We have also compiled a glossary of common neuropsychology terms (see Appendix 2.1) to assist readers with acquiring this vocabulary.

The second obstacle for those studying neuropsychology is related to depth of coverage. Many neuropsychology texts go into incredible detail regarding the anatomy and physiology associated with brain–behavior relationships. As is the case with statistics, the depth of coverage can become overwhelming, especially when it is conveyed in complex terminology. We could have expanded the material presented in this book into several volumes, but instead we have chosen to highlight major structures and functions without becoming overly detailed in presentation. For instance, this book does not include a discussion of the cellular basis of behavior (as many textbooks do), and the coverage of neurochemistry is limited. Although this information is certainly important for an understanding of the psychopharmacological treatment of psychological disorders, and further study is highly recommended, the cellular basis of behavior is of limited use in daily practice. Gender and racial issues are briefly addressed, but it is important for you to realize that the material presented is often cursory in nature. Although some additional information can be found in the In-Depth boxes in the chapters, further reading of the resources provided in the chapter appendices will help you become thoroughly knowledgeable in your areas of interest and practice.

The third difficulty learners experience has to do with the techniques used in neuropsychological research. Many think that neuropsychological principles have been derived from the study of adult patients and animal models with brain damage. This was true for most of the 20th century, but it is far from the case now. Noninvasive neuroimaging techniques, such as positron emission tomography (PET) and functional magnetic resonance imaging (fMRI), have provided us with great insight into brain–behavior relationships, in both typical and clinical populations. PET and fMRI have been used to study mental processes both in typical children and in those with disabilities. These are children very similar to those in your classrooms. We need to recognize that typical children and those with disabilities lie along a continuum, and that the brain processes described in this book apply to all children. The brain is directly responsible for learning and behavior. We all knew this, but now we can measure changes in brain functioning while children perform cognitive tasks and can visually depict these changes as they occur. However, it is important to realize that even these techniques require inferences about brain function, and that results may vary because of the tasks, methodology, and analyses used. We feel that when you are studying the neuropsychological literature, it is critical for you to review the participants, instruments, and procedures used in these studies. It is also important to realize that all studies have limitations, which are typically glossed over or minimized in some journal article discussions.

This is true for all research studies, not just neuropsychological ones. It is essential for you to become an "informed consumer" in reading about brain–behavior relationships. The most important part of any article is the "Method" section as it allows you to know how the study was conducted and who participated, and how researchers used inclusion and exclusion criteria that may have shaped the results found and conclusions drawn.

The fourth obstacle has to do with the real-world application of neuropsychological principles. Our experience suggests that many of those who study brain–behavior relationships take courses taught by experimental psychologists that have substantial interest in one particular area of the brain rather than the brain as a whole. Development is an important aspect of understanding the neuropsychology of children, but it is generally not addressed in many physiological psychology courses, where adult perspectives about brain functioning may be predominant. We feel that neuropsychological assessment and intervention principles should become integral parts of psychology training programs. In addition to neuro-anatomy and neurophysiology classes, we believe that courses in child neuropsychological assessment and intervention techniques, as well as neuropsychology practice and clerkships, should be developed.

We agree with others who call for the development of a psychology subspecialty called "school neuropsychology." The term *school neuropsychology* was originally coined by George Hynd and Jack Obzrut (Hynd & Obzrut, 1981). A school neuropsychologist is not only aware of brain–behavior relationships, but of their application in real-life settings, both for typical children and those with disabilities. The information presented in this book is but one step in a larger mission to bring neuropsychological principles to the forefront of educational and clinical practice. We realize that application of neuropsychological principles in school and clinical settings takes individual determination and system-level change. Many practitioners are already overwhelmed by their caseloads; adding additional measures and lengthening reports for the sake of diagnostic accuracy is laudable, but just not feasible for most. As we will argue, we believe that it is critical for practitioners to intervene so they may assess (more thoroughly). The only way you are going to free up your time to do thorough neuropsycho-logical assessments is to reduce the number of referrals for formal evaluation. To do this, you must rigorously adopt preventative intervention methods, pursue data-based multi-tiered interventions, and develop school-wide intervention assistance teams to help you (and of course, each other). To begin the change process, we provide you with a better understand-ing of brain–behavior relationships and of methods to apply this information when carrying out interventions for children with learning and emotional/behavior problems. You will be provided with real-life examples and Case Study boxes that highlight the application of neu-ropsychological principles in assessment and intervention practices.

The Relationship among Cognition, Brain Function, and the Real World

During a televised New York–Philadelphia baseball game, the complexity of brain–behavior relationships was revealed. The batter hit a line drive toward left center field. The quickly sinking line drive had just cleared the infield, and the left and center fielders converged on the ball simultaneously. As the ball veered slightly more toward center field, the left fielder stopped at the last second, and the center fielder dove to make an apparently spectacular catch. Although the dive was nearly perfect and the ball hit the webbing of his glove, it popped out. In the subsequent confusion, the left fielder finally picked up the ball and threw it to second base, but the runner slid safely beneath the tag.

What does this have to do with brain structure and function? Everything. One goal of this book is to help you, our readers, think about how brain–behavior relationships can be applied to real-life situations. By task-analyzing a ball player's actions, thinking about the various cognitive processes that led to the outcome, we can better understand the thinking skills necessary for completing the task. For example, when the ball left the bat, both the left and center fielders had to visually examine the direction, velocity, and trajectory of the ball to know that it was coming their way. They might have done nothing, thinking that the ball would be caught by an infielder, but they "knew" that the probability of this happening was small. So, visually tracking the ball, they "knew" that they must run toward where it was likely to land, and each other. They couldn't walk or jog to get to the ball; they had to sprint. The left fielder had to decide, at the last minute, to yield to the center fielder. This required combining knowledge of the ball's path and the actions of the center fielder. The left fielder had to have this knowledge, plus a way to stop his actions, realizing that it was in the best interest of the team's goal for the center fielder to catch the ball and make an out. Now the center fielder was also trying a similar strategy, but he may have been distracted by the left fielder coming toward him and then stopping abruptly, reflecting his skill at inhibition. Although the center fielder knew he had to dive and extend his mitt—coordinating eye, hand, and body to make a spectacular catch—the combined factors resulted in his failing to account for the impact of the ground on his mitt and how this impact would affect his closing the mitt to catch the ball. Since there was an apparent catch, neither the left nor the center fielder had planned well for the new situation—that the center fielder had dropped the ball. The delay in planning, organizing, and carrying out the throw to second base resulted in the runner's making it safely to second—a chance the runner might have not taken, had he not seen the play unfold as he rounded first base.

To summarize, there was a line drive to short left center field, the center fielder was charged with an error, and the player made it safely to second base. Why not just say it in those few words? We all watched the play unfold, and our summary adequately reflects what happened—or does it? Recall that the center fielder was charged with an error, meaning that the official scorer thought he should have caught the ball. Without evidence, the fans would have expressed their dismay, and the two opposing factions could have erupted in conflict over it. Something similar can happen in clinical practice when you are trying to decide whether a child's attention problems are due to an attention problem, or an auditory processing problem, or even oppositional behavior. To understand brain–behavior relationships, you must analyze the task demands of any given cognitive or neuropsychological measure. This task analysis explores the input demands, processing demands, and output demands of a given task. However, as we note later in the text, making a judgment just on the basis of input or output has often led psychologists astray in their attempts to understand brain–behavior relationships. Within the last dozen years, it has become increasingly clear that the processing demands of a task are essential for linking assessment to intervention, with input and output demands less relevant. With a thorough understanding of the neuropsychological basis of task processing demands, you will gain a better understanding of how children learn and behave in the classroom.

Returning to our example, let's task-analyze the missed catch. Catching a ball requires visual processes to identify where the ball is: the velocity, trajectory, and direction as it moves through space. A fielder must not only track the ball path, but also determine the speed of his own running and whether he needs to catch it on the run or engage a diving sequence to bring the mitt closer to where the ball will land. Prior knowledge of the size, shape, and density of the ball, and of his trusty glove, helps the fielder recognize the force the ball will exert on his mitt. The tactile sensation of the hand against the leather glove helps to identify the impact of the ball. The posterior part of the brain is involved in these processes. The anterior or frontal part of the brain is critical for eye–hand coordination to track the ball into the glove. After completing the running and then diving motor sequences, the fielder must reach out his arm and grasp the ball instantaneously as it hits his glove. Given that the center fielder in our example accomplished all these activities successfully, he should have caught the ball. However, within a split second, his anterior brain manager ("brain boss") should have helped the fielder monitor his performance (running/diving) in relation to the ball's position and exerted "executive" control, allowing the fielder to modify his behavior. The brain's executive could have provided the sensory system with direction to alter the glove's position and motor instructions to change the force of grasp to account for the glove's coming into contact with the ground before the ball arrived. And all of this might have happened if the brain boss had helped him to ignore the left fielder's actions, which would likely distract most of us attempting this feat.

This is, of course, a very difficult task to accomplish, but one that occurs regularly in professional sports and, of course, our daily lives. Think of a time you narrowly missed having an accident with another car, or bumped into someone on the street, or missed a step going down a flight of stairs. Many of the cognitive processes outlined above were required for you to avoid the accident.

Examining the input, processing, and output demands required in any activity will help you apply your knowledge of brain–behavior relationships in real-life situations, including the classroom or clinic. In this book we highlight the brain structures associated with the cognitive skills described above and help you to link cognitive and brain processes together so you may apply them in your life and psychological practice. While the following chapters and materials have been organized with this purpose in mind, deciphering how actions are related to brain functions takes regular practice and perseverance. As the old adage suggests, "Practice makes perfect." This is certainly the case when understanding brain–behavior relationships in the real world.

The Book's Purpose and Structure

The purpose of this book is to provide current information on brain–behavior relationships, as well as suggestions for applying this information in daily practice. Most chapters include both content and methods, with the former emphasized initially, and the latter becoming more prevalent in the last sections. The first chapter reviews practices in school psychology assessment of cognitive processes, and provides an overview of the promises and pitfalls of early attempts to link cognitive profiles to treatment (i.e., aptitude–treatment interactions). It explores early research into the cognitive and behavioral characteristics of children with learning disorders or disabilities. Chapter 1 sets the stage for an introduction of brain–behavior relationships in Chapter 2, and then this new understanding is adopted to further your assessment skills in Chapter 3. Chapter 4 provides a methodology to link assessment results to interventions and is designed to encourage the use of brain–behavior relationships within the context of a problem-solving consultation approach to service delivery, a model similar to one espoused in professional psychology. Chapters 5, 6, and 7 provide current brain–behavior research and intervention strategies for children with various types of learning problems, all within the paradigm offered in the earlier chapters. Chapter 8 provides a review of diagnostic and treatment for children with attention-deficit/hyperactivity disorder, autism spectrum disorder, and nonverbal learning disabilities. This chapter has been greatly expanded from the first edition of the book, including a comprehensive Case Study. Chapter 9 not only provides you with an understanding of how neuropsychological processes could be related to developmental psychopathology, but it also describes interventions designed to address behavioral strengths and needs. It also goes into detail as to the neuropsychology of commonly seen psychiatric disorders in children: depression, anxiety, and lesser seen disorders such as bipolar disorder. Chapter 10, a new chapter for the second edition, discusses chronic medical conditions that can negatively affect a child's performance in school, given this diverse population exists in your setting. It is designed to provide you with information on disorders that you will frequently encounter in your practice, including traumatic brain injury, cancer, and leukemia among others. Chapter 11, also new for this edition, provides a brief overview of genetic disorders as well as an explanation of appropriate assessment techniques and how to team with medical personnel. A Case Study is included to provide a guide for understanding the neuropsychological process involved in assessing a child with a significant genetic disorder. All the clinical chapters include comprehensive neuropsychological Case Studies and appendices provide additional information within each chapter.

The chapters in this book are both informational and applied. The application of brain–behavior relationships in clinical practice is difficult, and some diligence will be required on your part to ensure that the patterns and relationships discussed are relevant to your daily practice, which is the ultimate goal of this book. It is designed for practitioners—individuals who have experience administering and interpreting standardized and informal measures of cognitive, academic, and behavioral functioning. As such, it assumes a basic understanding of the areas of child development, learning, cognition, behavior, psychopathology, and brain–behavior relationships. It also assumes an understanding of individual, group, and system-level interventions, and of both direct and indirect service delivery models. Some of the information may be redundant with your training, but we have designed the book to meet the needs of practitioners who have varying levels of training and experience in the aforementioned areas. Given that the goal of this book is to help you develop a new way of thinking about how children learn and behave, the information and methods will help you analyze all types of data and interventions from this new brain–behavior perspective.

This book is not designed to provide you with the necessary information or skills to call yourself a neuropsychologist, which requires formal training and supervised experience. The Clinical Neuropsychology section (Division 40) of the American Psychological Association can provide you with additional information about neuropsychology training and credentialing. The American Academy of Pediatric Neuropsychology (AAPN) and National Academy of Neuropsychology (NAN) are additional resources, and the International Neuropsychological Society (INS) provides practitioners with a global perspective of neuropsychological research and practice. However, this book is designed to help you interpret test performance and behavior from a neuropsychological perspective—one we hope you will adopt in your assessment and intervention practices in the years to come. It is also about thinking and practicing psychology in a flexible and evolving manner. No book for practitioners has the answers to all your clinical questions; it merely provides new ideas and methodologies that you can incorporate into your own clinical worldview. This material should not be the end of your training in neuropsychological principles applied in school or clinical settings. Instead, we hope it will fuel your desire to further your neuropsychological knowledge base and interest in rigorously applying these principles in daily practice. We hope our work will open a new path for you—one that is fruitful for the children, parents, and teachers you serve in your educational or clinical setting.

Chapter 1

Assessment and Intervention Practices in Educational Settings

Foundations of Intellectual and Cognitive Assessment

The Relevance of History

For over a century, scholars, practitioners, and other stakeholders have debated the merits of using psychological assessment for educational purposes. Depending on the definition used, assessment (formal and informal) is a common practice in our work. We begin this chapter with an overview of the promises and pitfalls of assessment practices in the schools. A chronological review of assessment theory and practice, test interpretation, and identification of learning disabilities culminates in an overview of our recommendations for the practice of psychology in the schools. This overview serves as an important foundation for the remainder of this book, where we integrate apparently disparate fields within psychology, including cognitive theory, academic assessment, behavioral psychology, educational psychology, special education, and neuropsychology. The explosion of neuroscience has led to many great insights into learning and behavior, forming the foundation of the arguments presented herein.

Why examine the history of assessment practices in the schools in a book about neuropsychology? First, a historical context helps you understand how past, current, and probable future assessment practices are related and have changed over time. Examining these trends can provide you with a conceptual continuity of service delivery that advances your practice of psychology. Second, it is important to recognize that brain networks are responsible for intellectual, cognitive, neuropsychological, academic, and psychosocial functioning. Understanding the relationships among these domains will give you the necessary template to rethink long-held assumptions about the practice of psychology in the schools and will provide you with the necessary motivation to incorporate new ideas and skills into your existing practice of psychology.

Historical Views of Intelligence: The Debate Begins

Like so much else psychologists do, cognitive testing in particular has always existed in a sociopolitical context. Intelligence, especially the concept of g or general intelligence, has been associated with notions of a person's value. Because IQ measures have been used to deny immigration, support sterilization, segregate individuals into categories, and deny educational opportunities to entire groups of people, it is only fair to ask where the tests came from and what they are being used for today.

Three pertinent questions will form a framework for your examination of the following material:

1. What is the relationship between early conceptions of intelligence and current models of cognitive and neuropsychological functioning?
2. How have the content and process of cognitive assessment changed in relation to theory?
3. What are the benefits and costs of intellectual/neuropsychological assessment as a model of service delivery?

We hope that this historical perspective will help you gain a better appreciation for the strengths and limitations of the tests we use. That is, these measures are merely tools for use in a comprehensive, multifaceted model of service delivery. Tests are solely tools to help understand the child; it is how you interpret the tests to help children that is important in this discussion.

The assessment of individuals can be traced to early philosophers, but the first person who is typically associated with the systematic measurement of human abilities is Sir Francis Galton. Though his work in the late 1880s and 1890s at the University of London's Anthropometric Laboratory marked the beginning of scientific interest in testing mental ability, his notion that sensory discrimination and motor functioning form the basis of intelligence was overly reductionistic. Though Galton interpreted results solely on the basis of observable stimuli and responses, it is important to note that this was perhaps the last time that truly objective methods were used for assessing intelligence, because his items were least influenced by prior educational opportunity or experience.

Another assessment pioneer was Lightner Witmer, usually hailed as the first "school psychologist." He founded the Psychoeducational Clinic at the University of Pennsylvania in 1896. Witmer believed that experimental psychology ideas and findings needed to be applied in the real world. For that reason, he was concerned about the ecological and treatment validity of data gathered on individuals. He is credited with the first systematic attempts to link measurement of individual characteristics to specific interventions. These efforts at the end of the 19th century stimulated the ambitions of many who would follow; the pioneering work of Galton and Witmer served as a catalyst for many researchers and practitioners to examine the link between assessment and intervention.

Actual "intelligence test" development is usually credited as beginning with Alfred Binet (see Binet & Simon, 1905), who attempted to devise an instrument capable of determining the children who would benefit most from educational experiences. Binet developed his scale to measure higher-level reasoning and problem solving, but the actual items included prior knowledge and language-based questions that we would today recognize as "crystallized" items—those dependent on prior experience and educational opportunity. Although Binet designed his tool to be sensitive to individual differences and thought interpretation should be individualized for each child, his premise was dismissed when the concept of the intelligence quotient, or IQ, was introduced several years later.

Before you read further, what words do you think of when you think of IQ? Most people would think of the words "ability," "intelligence," "aptitude," or "potential," but how many would think of the word "achievement"? Ever since Binet introduced items that tapped crystallized and language skills, intelligence tests have been partly achievement tests. We *learn* things when we develop, and crystallized abilities—the abilities based on prior experience and education—are *learned* abilities. Unless all children have equal opportunities for learning, then differences on intelligence tests that include crystallized measures cannot be attributed solely to differences in ability. The scores on these measures are part ability, including neuropsychological processes, and part achievement, making their interpretation more challenging than solely considering them to be measures of "crystallized ability." We return to this point later in the chapter.

How did Binet's test become the first "intelligence test"? Binet's original scale was of hierarchically arranged items according to developmental age expectations. It was later adopted by Terman (1916), who added a scoring system that would change the nature of intellectual assessment. Terman's IQ, or "intelligence quotient," was originally computed by dividing the child's "mental age" (MA) by the child's chronological age (CA) and then multiplying by 100 to eliminate the decimal point. Since its inception, the IQ has been reified as the "true" measure of human intellect. Although some have questioned its utility, many have devoted their entire careers to attempting to validate the IQ as psychology's truly "objective" measure. Following Binet's lead, several decades later David Wechsler introduced another intelligence test, which was based on the works of Binet and the United States Army entrance exam tests. Though the Wechsler–Bellevue Scale (Wechsler, 1939) was designed to measure an individual's global capacity to act with purpose, Wechsler's Verbal and Performance subtests were thought to be clinical tools for examining individual differences in test performance (Kaufman, 1994).

Contemporary Views of Intelligence: The Debate Intensifies

It is important to realize that since the earliest days of mental testing, there have been disparate views about the structure of intelligence, and these differences continue today (see In-Depth 1.1 and Appendix 1.1). Spearman (1904) introduced us to the concept of *g*, or general intelligence, which assumes that intelligence is a single construct,[1] with IQ soon to become its de facto proxy. IQ was seen by early researchers as a meaningful measure of the brain's overall power, much like a motor's horsepower. Among modern researchers, Arthur Jensen (1998) is perhaps the most widely known of the *g* proponents. His body of work has explored the links between *g* and a variety of other measures, with fairly convincing evidence of its validity. Similarly, Linda Gottfredson (1997) contends that *g* is the best predictor of success in school, job training, and overall occupational attainment without attention paid to the experiences of the child, different cultural and ethnic influences, and most of all, the effect of poverty on later occupational success. Without these aspects factored into our understanding of ability, her arguments have been used to support conservative political agendas. In their book *The Bell Curve*, Herrnstein and Murray (1994) argue that *g* is predictive of various real-world outcomes, including educational attainment, income level, and likelihood of incarceration. However, it is important to note that this "seminal" work was flawed by the use of an *achievement* test to measure *g* (Roberts et al., 2000). Probably one of the most controversial *g* advocates is Rushton et al. (2010), who has examined race, gender, heritability, brain size, temperament, lifespan, family structure, personality, and criminality variables linked to intelligence.

Several writers, such as Paul McDermott, Joseph Glutting, and Marley Watkins, recommend interpretation of only the global IQ derived from cognitive testing; they note the importance of *g* in predicting school learning. Using hierarchical regression and based on their statistical tests, they stated that IQ was a strong predictor of achievement scores,

---

[1] Spearman also recognized there were some aspects of intelligence not subsumed under *g*, and identified them as *s* for special ability.

IN-DEPTH 1.1. Major Players in Intelligence, Test Theory, Research, and Practice

ADVOCATES OF GLOBAL INTELLIGENCE

Arthur Jensen saw general intelligence, or *g*, as the most important predictor of just about everything. In Jensen's view, selection of an appropriate test depends solely on its *g* loading, or how well it measures general intelligence.

Linda Gottfredson produces research that links general intelligence to success in a variety of learning environments, including later career and life success.

Paul McDermott, Joseph Glutting, Marley Watkins, and their colleagues have studied the use of profile and subtest analysis with a number of commonly used intelligence tests. Their conclusion, based on bifactor analyses, is that factors other than global IQ are not reliable enough for decision making.

THEORETICALLY/EMPIRICALLY ORIENTED ADVOCATES OF COGNITIVE STRENGTHS AND WEAKNESSES

John Carroll was a hierarchical theorist supporting *g*, but his true contribution to our understanding of the structure of intelligence beyond IQ has been unparalleled. His treatise synthesizes 512 databases of cognitive test data; this is great for researchers, but not for the faint of heart!

J. P. Das and **Jack Naglieri** adapted parts of Luria's neuropsychological model in their development of the Cognitive Assessment System (now in its second edition, CAS2), a measure of cognitive processes that minimizes assessment of crystallized abilities or prior knowledge, and has been used to demonstrate individualized aptitude–treatment interactions.

John Horn argued strongly against interpreting *g* and in favor of interpreting various cognitive processes and abilities. His extended *Gf-Gc* model (fluid and crystallized intelligences) is one of the components of modern Cattell–Horn–Carroll (CHC) theory.

Richard Woodcock is well known for both theory and test development. He recommended interpretation of the Woodcock–Johnson from a variety of perspectives, including the CHC clusters of abilities, specialized clinical clusters, and an integrated information-processing model (which includes consideration of the cognitive and noncognitive factors that affect performance).

PRACTICE-ORIENTED ADVOCATES OF COGNITIVE STRENGTHS AND WEAKNESSES

Colin Elliott argued for a model of both global and specific abilities, recommending interpretation of other cognitive abilities and inclusion of diagnostic subtests to analyze strengths and weaknesses.

Randy Kamphaus calls for a scientist-practitioner approach to stay abreast of the research findings and apply them to the interpretation of an individual child's performance.

Alan Kaufman and **Nadeen Kaufman** are the founders of the modern practice of research-based clinical interpretation of test performance. The methodology involves interpretation of a child's strengths and weaknesses, based on statistical information about the test and research information about what subtests actually measure.

(continued)

IN-DEPTH 1.1. *(continued)*

Kevin McGrew, Dawn Flanagan, Sam Ortiz, and their colleagues have combined Carroll's hierarchical model with Horn and Cattell's extended *Gf-Gc* model to form CHC theory. Their research-based cross-battery approach allows for comprehensive, individualized evaluations of multiple cognitive abilities.

Jerome Sattler is the author of the books "most likely to be owned" by psychologists everywhere. He compiles research and clinical information on assessment and test interpretation for comprehensive service provision.

ADVOCATES OF MULTIPLE INTELLIGENCES

Howard Gardner explores nontraditional areas such as musical and interpersonal "abilities"; although his humanistic theory is not grounded in empirical science, it compels others to value individual differences and is popular among educators.

Robert Sternberg developed the triarchic theory and measures of intelligence, with preliminary empirical support suggesting that all three aspects of intelligence (analytical, creative, and practical) are related to academic success.

ADVOCATES OF A "PARADIGM SHIFT"

Frank Gresham and **Joseph Witt** argue that intelligence testing is a waste of time, as the tests are not useful in developing interventions and are frequently disregarded during team eligibility determinations.

Dan Reschly and **James Ysseldyke** agree that intelligence tests are not useful for diagnosing mild disabilities or developing interventions; they called for a "paradigm shift" that eliminates standardized testing.

---

but subcomponent scores (e.g., factors, subtests) accounted for little "incremental validity" beyond that achieved by IQ (Glutting et al., 2006).[2] These findings are based on flawed methodology because the subtest scores are added to produce the IQ, and the *same subtests* are used to compute the factors. So if one enters factors first and then IQ, IQ shows no "incremental validity" (Hale et al., 2007).

More recently, Watkins and Canivez (2022) have used bifactor analysis to argue that after removing the effects of *g*, individual factor or index scores lack sufficient reliability to be used clinically. This argument overlooks the fact that clinicians do not interpret factor or index scores independent of *g*, but as the complex measures that they are. When factor or index scores are used to predict achievement or to develop interventions, they include the variance from general as well as specific cognitive functioning.

It is important to note that most *g* proponents do not deny the reality of other, more specific cognitive functions. They just question the utility of interpreting anything other than global IQ. The implications of these ideas are significant: No longer would practitioners need to waste time on clinical assessment or interpretation; they could simply give an intelligence

---

[2] Pedhazur (1997) used this very type of analysis (composite scores and subtest scores used to compute composites in the same regression equation) to show the problems with hierarchical regression of collinear data.

test and report the global IQ. However, this argument implies that IQ is an intransient measure of innate ability, and that no intervention, whether educational or sociopolitical (such as affirmative action), can alter the likelihood of individuals' success if they have a low global IQ.

Multiple versus Single Abilities

Beginning with the Thurstone (multiple abilities) versus Spearman (single ability) debate in the early 20th century, many researchers and clinicians have argued that clinically useful intelligence tests must measure a variety of functions rather than a unitary IQ (e.g., Guilford, 1967; Horn & Cattell, 1967; Thurstone, 1938). Multifactor theorists focus on cognitive functions derived from test data and basic cognitive science research, although neuropsychological research has recently come to the forefront in contributing knowledge of cognitive functions (Agate & Garcia-Barrera, 2020). Guilford's structure-of-intellect model explored the diversity of cognitive skills differing in content, operations, and product—concepts similar to the input demands, processing demands, and output demands in our cognitive hypothesis-testing (CHT) model discussed throughout this book. Another processing model—the planning, attention, simultaneous, and successive (PASS) model (Das et al., 1994)—has demonstrated relationships between cognitive processes and educational achievement, and this information can be used to guide intervention. Sternberg's (1997) triarchic theory adds creative and practical intelligences to the analytical abilities typically thought of as "intelligence." His ongoing body of research into the cognitive processes, experiences, and environmental context of intelligent behavior has demonstrated cognitive ability–treatment interactions at the school and university levels (Sternberg, 2018).

Many current theories of cognitive ability are hierarchical; that is, they assume the existence of both an overall g and a variety of important cognitive processes subsumed under g. McGrew (McGrew, 2009) has combined Carroll's (1993) hierarchical concept of intelligence with Horn and Cattell's (1967) multifactor model to yield what is known as Cattell–Horn–Carroll (CHC) theory. The first test developed specifically for this theory was the Woodcock–Johnson Tests of Cognitive Abilities (now in the fifth edition: WJ-V Cognitive; McGrew et al., 2025). Given the preponderance of evidence supporting CHC, it is not surprising that other measures (e.g., DAS-II NU, KABC-II NU, SB-5, WISC-V) also offer CHC-derived factors to summarize subtest performance (Elliott, 2023).

Taken together, the thorough analyses embodied in a cross-battery approach (Flanagan et al., 2013), and the extensive database used for linking CHC cognitive abilities to academic achievement domains (McGrew & Wendling, 2010), provides practitioners with irrefutable evidence that our understanding of cognitive processes has grown immensely, and the impetus to incorporate this knowledge into their daily assessment practices (Fiorello & Wycoff, 2018). Even more exciting is the convergence of neuropsychological and cognitive theory, providing the neuropsychological explanation for what researchers and practitioners have observed on modern cognitive and achievement measures (Fiorello et al., 2008), which provides an important bridge for bringing neuropsychological principles and practices into the schools (Miller, 2013).

Measuring Intellectual and Cognitive Functioning

Is Theory Quantifiable?

You probably believe in "intelligence" and "cognition" as constructs, but these questions remain: How do psychologists measure them, and do they do it well? Accepted by many contemporary theorists (Kaufman, 2009), the hierarchical model, with *g* at the top and several abilities underneath, is often adopted by intelligence test developers in part due to tradition, and in part due to practical considerations (e.g., determining intellectual disability, giftedness). Possibly because of the important role IQ has played in differential diagnosis and eligibility determinations, a test that does not provide a global IQ score is often deemed less useful. For example, in the *Diagnostic and Statistical Manual of Mental Disorders, Fifth Edition, Text Revision* (DSM-5-TR; American Psychiatric Association, 2022), the concept of intellectual disability depends on an overall measure of intellectual functioning in clinical settings. Similarly, educational decision making typically requires a global intellectual functioning score for identification of intellectual disability under the Individuals with Disabilities Education Act (IDEA; Etscheidt & Curran, 2010) in the schools.

As noted earlier, the earliest practical intelligence tests—the Stanford–Binet (Terman, 1916) and the Wechsler–Bellevue scales (Wechsler, 1939)—yielded IQ scores, but did not dismiss the relevance of underlying abilities and skills that could be clinically useful. Moving beyond the infamous Wechsler Verbal–Performance dichotomy, the Stanford–Binet Intelligence Scales, Fourth Edition (SB-IV; Thorndike et al., 1986) was designed to measure Verbal Reasoning (crystallized ability), Abstract/Visual Reasoning (fluid ability), Quantitative Reasoning, and Short-Term Memory, and was based on an early version of the CHC model. The SB-5 (Stanford–Binet Intelligence Scales, Fifth Edition; Roid, 2003) has moved even further toward assessing a variety of cognitive skills from CHC theory, measuring Fluid Reasoning, Knowledge (crystallized), Quantitative Reasoning, Visual–Spatial Reasoning, and Working Memory through both verbal and limited-language tests.

The Kaufman Assessment Battery for Children, second edition (KABC-II Normative Update; Kaufman, 2018) is designed to assess cognitive abilities according to CHC theory, with clusters measuring crystallized, fluid reasoning, visual processing, long-term storage and retrieval, and short-term memory. The KABC-II NU is based on neuropsychological theory which forms a different theoretical approach from the WISC-V and SB-5. Another test battery derived from CHC theory is the Differential Ability Scales, Second Edition (DAS-II NU; Elliott, 2023), which measures Verbal Ability (crystallized), Nonverbal Reasoning (fluid reasoning), and Spatial Ability in its core battery, and includes diagnostic subtests to test auditory and visual memory, phonological processing, working memory, and processing speed. The PASS model led to the development of the Cognitive Assessment System—Second Edition (CAS2; Naglieri, Das, & Goldstein, 2014), which yields a total score in addition to measures of Planning, Attention, and Simultaneous and Sequential processing.

The WJ-V Tests of Cognitive Ability (McGrew et al., 2025) are based on hierarchical CHC theory, and measure multiple abilities in addition to providing a variety of cluster scores, including an overall score. Even the Wechsler Intelligence Scale for Children—Fifth Edition (WISC-V; Wechsler, 2014) has embraced CHC theory, with five main factors (Verbal Comprehension, Fluid Reasoning, Visual–Spatial, Working Memory, Processing Speed), ancillary subtests that assess other CHC abilities (Naming Speed [Retrieval Fluency] and Symbol Translation [Learning Efficiency]), and a variety of interpretive and neuropsychological process scores in addition to the Full-Scale IQ (FSIQ). The WISC-V was developed to be administered either in the traditional paper-based fashion or using computer tablets, presaging the next stage of intelligence testing. All of these batteries provide an overall global measure of *g* in addition to their measures of specific cognitive functions. As can be seen, intelligence/cognitive tests have moved away from single constructs such as "intelligence" to encompass more diverse cognitive abilities, functions, and skills.

Another movement in current assessment practice is the increased use of a neuropsychological approach to assessment and interpretation strategies in school-based psychology practice (Decker et al., 2013; Schneider et al., 2013; Reddy, Weissman, et al., 2013). Some of the measures started as measures of ability and have now been either renormed or have been re-interpreted based on neuropsychological principles. The WISC-V Integrated (2014) extended the traditional "testing of the limits" into a formal neuropsychological assessment and is derived from a psychometric process approach, which selects measures to test various hypotheses regarding the child's strengths and weaknesses. The process approach, discussed in Chapter 3, is a valued hypothesis-testing practice among many psychologists and neuropsychologists.

The KABC-II NU can be analyzed from a CHC perspective (see Chapter 3) or a Lurian approach, allowing interpretation of learning, simultaneous, sequential, and planning processes, similar to the CAS2. Although the WJ-V was derived primarily from psychometric CHC theory (as previously noted), it drew on neuroscience research in its development and provides cluster scores based on neuropsychological concepts. This merging of cognitive and neuropsychological principles in the assessment of individual differences forms the foundation of this book. A growing body of evidence suggests that neuropsychology and cognitive assessment (particularly CHC theory) are intimately interrelated (Fiorello et al., 2008), and that knowing about both areas leads to better assessment practices and to interventions sensitive to individual needs.

Statistical Methodologies and Conceptions of *g*

How do research methodologies regarding intellectual testing and *g* affect you? Policy issues and legislation are based on these studies, often dictating practice guidelines that may or may not make clinical sense. One of the reasons why discussions of *g* are so contentious is that intelligence researchers use a wide array of statistical methods to extract different information from the test data. An understanding of the major methodologies used in the quest for, or dismissal of, *g* may shed some light on the conclusions drawn by competing constituencies. First, it is important to understand that any task (test or subtest) assessing cognitive functioning is measuring many different brain functions at the same time. Part of the variance in scores reflects psychometric *g*, the underlying factor most equated with general intelligence and IQ scores. Part of the variance is shared by other tests, and this variance can be represented by multiple factors, or it can be represented by *g*. Finally, "unique" variance—variance that is not related to other tasks—is considered specific to the subtest (its specificity). Subtests also have "error" variance, which is associated with any measure and can be related to things like test construction, administration time, or item difficulty. Different types of analyses often favor one portion of variance over another, giving you a different picture about the meaning of the subtest scores you obtain during testing. For instance, if all the subcomponent scores measure *g* and nothing else, then the test would have little use beyond IQ interpretation, but if they have different relationships with each other, and in some cases enough specificity, then they could be helpful in clinical interpretation.

Given the above discussion of psychometric *g* and IQ, it should not surprise you that the most common methodology for studying cognitive test scores is *factor analysis*. Exploratory factor analysis explores the data and is often used to examine the performance of many people on single or multiple measures. The intercorrelations of the derived scores are used to identify underlying factors that account for the common score variance, leaving the unique variance and error variance behind. When factor analysis is done on several cognitive tasks, a common factor *g*, common to all the tasks, is typically identified. This finding of a common underlying factor on all cognitive tasks is also referred to as the *positive manifold* effect (Brody, 1997). Many theorists have considered this one underlying factor to be *g*, an overall measure of cognitive ability or mental power, since some portion of it has been common to all complex cognitive tasks. Factor analysis is a process that is "atheoretical"; that is, it is based solely on data and not on theory. The danger of only using this type of analysis to understand measures of ability is that the interpretation may be based more on statistics than on reality. As many statisticians indicate, what the findings mean really depends on how the data are input and analyzed.

Spearman did *not* equate g and intelligence, arguing, "There is no such thing, only a general factor *in* intelligence" (Dreary et al., 2008, p. 72). Spearman made more explicit this disavowal: "When asked what g is, one has to distinguish between the meanings of terms and the facts about things. *g means* a particular quantity derived from statistical operations. This then is what the g term means, a score-factor and nothing more" (Dreary et al., 2008, p. 156). Spearman was reflecting here on the difficulties concerning the atheoretical basis for factor analysis.

Single-factor solutions, which many researchers label g, have been found for many different cognitive measures. This consistency provides convincing evidence of the construct's validity, right? Well, it is not so clear-cut as some would lead you to believe. First, it is important to note that you can take just about any measure—say, one that has anxiety and depression items—and achieve a single-factor solution. The various groups of cognitive tasks analyzed in this way each yield a single-factor solution, but is it the same factor being identified each time? The g measured by any particular battery is probably related to the person's potential, but also to many other factors as well. In addition, there are a number of different factor-analytic methods. Some of these emphasize identifying a common factor, and some use rotated factors to emphasize finding several meaningful factors that can either be treated as related (oblique) or separate (orthogonal). Since we know that cognitive skills are interrelated, it doesn't make much sense to do orthogonal rotations, and results using these rotations are inherently misleading. Factor analysis can also look for a hierarchical structure, with g at the top, specific factors underneath, and individual subtests at the bottom, or a bifactor structure, where g variance is all taken into one factor and the specific factors only contain the variance left after the removal of g. The choice of one model over the other is theoretical, not purely statistical. We posit that the hierarchical structure, with g arising from the underlying factors, reflects our conception of cognitive functioning. Interpretation of factor or index scores with g removed is not how cognitive functioning is assessed or interpreted.

Finally, choosing one or multiple factors during exploratory factor analyses often requires the researcher to use an eigenvalue cutoff of 1.00 to determine the number of factors, but there is no clear consensus on what eigenvalue should be used. If you set the eigenvalue cutoff high enough, you can almost always achieve a one-factor solution for a cognitive test, or if you drop it below one you can have many more factors. Interestingly, while older intelligence tests often led to single-factor solutions, modern ones now show that a multiple-factor solution often fits the data better (e.g., Keith et al., 2006). So while early tests were related more to *intellectual functioning*, modern tests are constructed to be more measures of *cognitive functioning which involves a broader understanding of what ability really entails.* We often hear clinicians speak to the fact that IQ is the most reliable score on a cognitive test, but it has to be. More diverse items and a more diverse set of answers mathematically ensures the IQ is the most reliable score *for large normative samples.* But is it the most reliable score for the student sitting in front of you? We argue here, and present evidence to support the argument, that IQ is not a reliable indication of overall ability for those whose subcomponent (e.g., factor, subtest) scores are disparate.

Another methodology used frequently in studying cognitive test scores is *regression analysis.* Regression analyses are used to examine the amount of variance in an outcome (or dependent) variable that is explained by the independent variables. There are many ways of constructing the regression equation, depending on how the independent variables are related. In a *hierarchical regression analysis,* whatever variable is entered into the regression equation first will keep all of its own variance, plus all of the variance it shares with variables entered later in the equation. Therefore, if the independent variables are related to each other, the order in which the variables are entered can significantly affect the results of the analysis. Cognitive subtest scores are used to calculate the IQ score and the factor scores, so both reflect the same underlying subtest variance. Therefore, a regression analysis that includes both IQ and Index scores is not justifiable as you are measuring the same thing twice.

What kind of analysis can you do with highly related scores (i.e., collinear data)? One option is *structural equation modeling*. This approach requires a priori theoretical model of how variables are related before you conduct the analysis. Measures are combined to define a factor, or *latent variable*. For instance, measures of working memory capacity and processing speed like the WJ-V Verbal Attention and Number-Pattern Matching might be combined to define the latent variable of Cognitive Efficiency. The relationships between latent and observed variables are defined via directional paths—visual representations of the causal links. For example, Cognitive Efficiency would be one cause of reading fluency, so there would be a path from the latent construct Cognitive Efficiency to an observed variable such as the WJ-V Reading Fluency cluster score. The analysis then calculates the strength of all the paths in a manner similar to regression analysis, and goodness-of-fit indices tell you whether your model fits the data well or needs to be modified. An interesting application is using the model to estimate the latent scores for individuals, breaking out the contributions of g and the CHC abilities (Schneider, 2013).

The Final Word: Is g Relevant for Psychological Practice?

Is global IQ relevant for psychological practice? In a special issue of the journal *Applied Neuropsychology*, we and several colleagues addressed this important issue (Fiorello et al., 2007). One of the most enduring constructs in psychometrics, global IQ *is* a good predictor of school and occupational success (Gottfredson, 2008). IQ is the *single* best predictor and is a strong indicator of how well a child will perform in an English-speaking U.S. school with no instructional accommodations, supports, or services. It is also an excellent predictor of a child's performance on standardized achievement tests, but evidence is emerging that using a variety of cognitive skills predicts achievement domains even better (Caemmerer et al., 2018). Although modern cognitive tests often contain strong predictors of outcomes, none measures all essential components of cognitive functioning (Bowman et al., 2001). This concern has led some observers to conclude that the movement away from g to explore the complexities of cognitive functioning will prevail in the future (Keith & Reynolds, 2018).

Even if global IQ is a valuable measure predictive of important outcomes, subtest performance will affect the overall score—a fact often ignored when clinicians focus solely on IQ. Consider a child with a hearing impairment. If you administer an intelligence test in spoken English, the results will predict the child's classroom success, because the inability to hear and comprehend language will strongly influence both the test score and classroom performance. While no self-respecting clinician would use this reasoning, the situation may not be as clear for children with visual–motor difficulties, language impairments, cultural differences, or emotional/behavioral deficits. If such differences are not addressed and accommodated during the assessment and interventions, the child will not succeed. The IQ will also predict this child's classroom performance well, but the error occurs when we assume that the child's limitations are due to a difference in intelligence. If a boy with limited English from Ukraine comes to the United States, will his low IQ score predict he'll do poorly in the local schools? Sure, but assuming he is intellectually disabled would be a significant mistake. Similarly, a child who is exposed to violent situations or who is underfed will also underperform on these measures and likely also underperform in school—but not because of a lack of intelligence.

Ethnic and cultural issues are also critical to consider. For example, a Black child typically grows up in a different culture from the dominant culture in U.S. schools. John Ogbu's (2002) research documents how "involuntary minorities," such as African Americans and Native Americans, perform poorly on IQ tests and in school not because of any inherent lack of intelligence, but because of cultural differences, prejudice, and resistance to being culturally assimilated. An IQ score accurately predicts school success because of a host of factors, only one of which is its measurement of cognitive functioning. Intelligence tests are *statistically* unbiased because they predict outcomes well, but as Ortiz and colleagues (2018) point out, what is at issue here is the concept of *fairness*. Even if a test predicts outcomes well, it is not fair if it leads to misconceptions about the innate ability or potential of certain groups of children. *A critical point here is that the fairness problem does not lie in the instrument or its construction; the problem is associated with clinicians who uniformly interpret low test scores as reflecting low global intelligence.* It is *unfair* to say that the low score of a child with linguistic, cultural, or ethnic difference reflects that child has lower intelligence, but it is fair to say those differences could potentially explain his or her lower score. As long as the seasoned clinician is aware of this reality and does not reify IQ as a measure of ability, there is no difficulty explaining why a low cognitive score could reflect sociocultural or linguistic differences.

As noted earlier, another major problem with intelligence tests as measures of "ability" is that most intelligence tests measure crystallized abilities—those skills acquired through formal and informal experiences and education. By definition, these skills are inseparable from prior learning or achievement, so they cannot be true measures of innate ability. Those who have enriched backgrounds and educational experiences typically score better on crystallized measures than those who come from impoverished or varied backgrounds. Does this mean that children from enriched backgrounds are necessarily smarter? We think not. Assessment of acquired knowledge—language development, general information, and other crystallized skills—is still extremely important to fully understand a child's current level of school functioning. However, considerable care is needed when inferences are made about a child's underlying cognitive ability or intelligence, unless it can be ascertained that the child has been exposed to mainstream U.S. language and culture to the same exact degree as the normative sample. Can you, as the clinician, make this judgment? Since it is impossible to separate out experience and directly assess the underlying brain function, we can never truly measure pure ability. Ever since Binet introduced the first "true" intelligence test, we have never truly measured intelligence—only a confusing blend of ability and achievement. In addition to ability and achievement variance, in many children there is likely variance related to neuropsychological processing strengths and weaknesses, which can also easily influence these scores, so, again, considerable care is needed when interpreting crystallized measures. This is an important point, because many clinicians continue to believe that there is a "true" IQ to be measured. It calls into question the validity of ability–achievement discrepancy as a method for determining specific learning disorders, given that these cognitive and achievement scores are interrelated by nature.

We feel that IQ overemphasis is one of the major problems in psychology practice. This overemphasis has led to inappropriate identification of impoverished and minority children as having intellectual disabilities (Coutinho & Oswald, 2000), to the flawed "discrepancy model" of learning disability identification (Siegal & Blades, 2003), and to testing practices that are irrelevant for individualized interventions (Stuebing et al., 2009). Obviously, this is a big problem, so what is the solution? We recommend extending interpretation beyond the IQ in assessing a student's cognitive functioning, but ensuring that the results reflect reality and are meaningful for intervention. In the chapters that follow, we outline a neuropsychologically based approach to cognitive testing that occurs within the context of a comprehensive evaluation—one that ensures both the ecological and treatment validity of the findings.

Principles of Effective Assessment in the Schools

Response to Intervention/Multi-Tiered Systems of Support

We begin this section by recommending that you practice intervention. Can psychologists practicing in today's administrative climate do the sort of comprehensive evaluation that we recommend in this book? The answer is no, not if every child experiencing academic or behavioral difficulties is referred for a comprehensive evaluation. Not only is this a serious drain on resources, it also takes time away from children who could best benefit from a comprehensive evaluation. We believe that you must *intervene to assess*. That is, providing interventions using a multi-tiered systems of support (MTSS) model and evaluating the student's response to those interventions must occur *first* to help a majority of children in need—not only in order to help children, but also to reduce the number of children referred for comprehensive evaluations. Including measures of the rate of learning to achievement testing can add to the accuracy of our diagnostic efforts and impressions (Speece & Ritchey, 2005).

Rather than completing a short evaluation that is not helpful, and making a diagnostic "leap of faith" based on limited test data on every child, we recommend that you get involved in the MTSS process at your school. Use assessment data on a regular basis to monitor student progress, encourage empirically based instruction, and provide interventions for struggling learners (Brown-Chidsey & Andren, 2012). School psychologists' knowledge of assessment, intervention, and consultation skills are applicable at every tier of an MTSS model (Flanagan et al., 2010; Hale et al., 2006).

Although there are several tiered approaches, the Hale et al. (2006) model uses a standard protocol approach in Tier 1 (high-quality general education instruction, universal screening, and progress monitoring), a problem-solving model in Tier 2 (e.g., differentiated whole group, small group, or individualized instruction), and for those who do not respond to intervention, a comprehensive evaluation using the methods described in this book is needed for special education identification and Tier 3 services (which can occur in inclusive or individualized settings). In this model, a comprehensive evaluation should only be conducted after we have evaluated response to intervention—one that provides a thorough integrated description of the child to help you develop individualized interventions (Hale, Fiorello, et al., 2010). In addition, early intervention in an MTSS model can prevent processing problems from becoming significant, because if we wait too long to accommodate learner differences, we can essentially make a problem more resistant to intervention (Koziol et al., 2013).

School psychologists have not traditionally been involved in early intervention for children with learning problems, so by the time we get the referral for evaluation, the problem is often significant enough that special education services are needed. As a result, too much of your time is probably spent administering standardized tests and writing reports, so our proposition that you conduct *more* comprehensive evaluations probably seems outlandish and impractical. We concur. We do not expect you to conduct comprehensive evaluations if your assessment caseload is too high. However, through implementation of an MTSS model you can effectively reduce the number of children who require comprehensive evaluations and special education services (Fuchs et al., 2012). Sharing your knowledge of brain–behavior relationships with educators and other professionals can foster differentiated instruction practices in classrooms and increase intervention efficacy in an MTSS model (Hale, Wycoff, et al., 2010; Sousa & Tomlinson, 2011).

After reading this book and learning the practices we advocate, you can help teachers recognize behavioral manifestations of certain disorders, and help them tailor interventions accordingly using appropriate cognitive, behavioral, or psychosocial strategies. Similarly, if a child does not show the neuropsychological characteristics discussed in this book, you can hypothesize that environmental contingencies are playing an important role in the problem behavior, and use functional behavior analysis in preparation of manipulating antecedent or consequent conditions to change problem behaviors (Tarbox et al., 2020). It does us little good to dichotomize childhood learning and behavior problems into a "internal" brain or "external" environmental problem, given the environment and brain develop in a reciprocal manner.

A thorough examination of screening data, response to instruction and intervention, and other school records can help you determine whether a formal evaluation is truly needed, because you can be more confident that the problem behavior is not just related to environmental determinants. Slow or delayed learners will benefit from response-to-intervention (RTI) approaches that will help them catch up with their peers; whereas children with disabilities need individualized instruction based on their processing strengths and needs (Hale, Wycoff, et al., 2010). Obviously, this is not an "either–or" phenomenon, but careful examination of available data can help shape referral questions and determine whether formal evaluation for disability determination is needed (see Application 1.1).

When a formal, comprehensive evaluation is required after a student fails to respond to systematic, research-based interventions, you will have collected some initial data to help formulate your diagnostic hypotheses, and these data can serve as a basis for developing the formal assessment protocol. You will also have developed important relationships with teachers and parents—relationships that will serve as a foundation during implementation of subsequent assessment and intervention activities. To reiterate, you must *intervene* with a majority of children who have academic and/or behavior problems before you can adequately *assess* the few children with complex neuropsychological problems and instructional needs that require more comprehensive evaluations.

Assessment Issues in RTI

Recommended models of RTI include a variety of assessment techniques, most based on forms of curriculum-based assessment (CBA) or curriculum-based measurement (CBM). We have come a long way from the early days of CBA when individual school psychologists developed their own materials from a school's curriculum. We can now choose from a variety of published assessment materials with adequate technical quality (see *www.rti4success.org*). We will provide some information here about the major measures that are available. They are listed in alphabetical order, not in order of preference or utility.

CBM measures are designed to be quick and repeatable and are used for three main purposes: Identifying an instructional level, screening to identify children at risk for poor achievement, and progress monitoring during an intervention. They are not intended to sample every skill, but to use a key indicator called a general outcome measure (GOM) to see if a student is making progress toward a long-term goal. Although the first (and still most common) measures focus on oral reading fluency, other measures have also been developed for reading comprehension; writing; and math computation, concepts, and application. As part of a comprehensive model of RTI, we recommend the use of validated benchmark measures and progress monitoring.

APPLICATION 1.1. Reducing Referrals through Data-Based Decision Making

Ensuring successful prereferral interventions requires adequate data collection. Some teachers may resist collecting formal data, so you must reinforce the necessity of data-based decision making, and decide collaboratively on the data collection methods that are feasible in each classroom. It does no good to have a data collection method that is so difficult that the teacher doesn't adhere to it. The data collection methods touted in training programs are great, provided you have a staff of graduate students or teacher's aides sitting around collecting data for you. The average teacher has a full classroom with students of various needs, and the last thing he or she needs is a complex data collection system. Keeping the data simple but meaningful will avoid the propensity of teachers to avoid data collection altogether or do a mediocre job at it. Some teachers refer students more often than others, and you must find these teachers and provide them with support to reduce referrals. I once consulted with a teacher who made many referrals for formal evaluation. When I asked her about her most recent referral, she said, "I wrote the three interventions on the sheet. They didn't work; he's still calling out in class. Why do you think I made the referral?" She believed she had tried "everything in the book" to overcome a problem behavior. But often the "problem" should not be seen as a deficit per se, but as a poor fit between the child and the environment (Bernstein, 2000). The three interventions attempted included moving the boy's seat (isolating and stigmatizing him), calling his mother (blaming Mom was not helpful), and sending him to the principal's office (the boy's preferred intervention—allowing him to escape classwork and get individual attention from the principal, whom he liked). Although the behavior had reportedly been going on "since the beginning of the year," the teacher had tried all of these "prereferral interventions" within a 2-week period, and no data were available to confirm or refute their efficacy. Although it was a lengthy consultation, we successfully intervened with this child, and he did not require a comprehensive evaluation. Whether you use observation methods, a scatterplot, permanent products, or some other data (see Chapter 4), collecting data is necessary to help reduce comprehensive evaluation referrals, and it is legally mandated. For many problems, a functional analysis will reveal that environmental determinants are primarily responsible for a child's poor academic performance or behavior problem. MTSS teams can help teachers solve problems and develop ecologically sound systematic interventions before formal referrals are made.

AIMSWeb

AIMSWeb is a system of benchmarking and progress monitoring tools. It includes measures of early literacy and numeracy, reading decoding and comprehension, spelling, written expression, and computation. The National Center on Response to Intervention (NCRTI; 2010) has rated its measures of early literacy and numeracy, oral reading, and math as having strong evidence of reliability and validity. However, most of the articles cited to support AIMSWeb are general articles on the usefulness of CBM, rather than direct evaluations of the AIMSWeb measures themselves. The AIMSWeb measures are part of a data management system that is subscribed to by a school or district, and cannot be purchased separately (see Shinn & Shinn, 2002; Shinn & Yoshikawa, 2008).

Dynamic Indicators of Basic Early Literacy Skills

The Dynamic Indicators of Basic Early Literacy Skills (DIBELS) was developed at the University of Oregon as a series of measures to assess the five major areas of reading: phonological awareness, the alphabetic principle, fluency, comprehension, and vocabulary (Kaminsky & Good, 1998). The NCRTI (2010) rates the measures as reliable and valid benchmark measures, without sufficient evidence of slope (rate of improvement) reliability and validity. The DIBELS measures are available free, although there is a fee for data management services. Several studies have supported the utility of DIBELS in progress monitoring and treatment response (see Cummings et al., 2011).

System to Enhance Educational Performance

The System to Enhance Educational Performance (STEEP) is a comprehensive approach for use in RTI, and includes a standard protocol intervention process and implementation fidelity measures in addition to the universal screening and progress monitoring measures. Implementing the model as a whole has been demonstrated to reduce referrals to special education and make those referrals more accurate—that is, the students that are referred for an evaluation are more likely to qualify for special education services than those referred by teachers—and to reduce disproportionality (VanDerHeyden, Witt, & Gilbertson, 2007). STEEP measures are available for early literacy, reading, reading comprehension, and math. The NCRTI (2010) has rated the STEEP progress monitoring measure of oral reading as having strong evidence of reliability and validity. The STEEP model is a system that a school or district pays for as a complete program that includes data management; the assessments are not available separately, but preliminary research efforts show they can be useful to help schools implement RTI with fidelity, and it is useful for monitoring academic progress (see Mercer & Howe, 2012; Witt & VanDerHeyden, 2007).

Using RTI to identify a student with a disability means that your identification process, not just the CBMs themselves, must meet standards of reliability and validity. Currently, there are multiple RTI methods being investigated for their utility in determining whether a child is a responder or a nonresponder, but none to date has shown reliable and valid results (Hale, Wycoff, et al., 2010). Using different models of RTI, such as low achievement, low growth, and dual discrepancy models, can lead to poor agreement and poor stability of identification over time (Barth et al., 2008; Beach, 2012).

RTI Alone Cannot Be Used to Make a Diagnosis

When IDEA (Etscheidt & Curran, 2010) was rolled out, advocates suggested that RTI could be used for determining whether a child had a specific learning disability (SLD) (e.g., Gresham, 2017). Although RTI is a necessary component in the evaluation of children for disabilities, as it helps rule out environmental reasons for underachievement, such as poor instructional practices (Harry & Klinger, 2007), it is not sufficient to determine the presence of a disability (Hale, Wycoff, et al., 2010; Reynolds & Shaywitz, 2009). There are many reasons why a child might fail to respond to interventions (Hale, Wycoff, et al., 2010), including problems with the intervention process such as selection of an appropriate intervention, the fidelity with which the intervention is implemented, the intensity of the intervention, and inconsistent criteria for judging response (Barth et al., 2008; Fuchs, 2003; Fuchs, 2012). Characteristics of the child other than a disability, such as English learner status (Rinaldi & Samson, 2008), lack of requisite background, chaos or trauma in the home, or targeting the wrong area (teaching reading when attention is the main difficulty, for example) may also lead to a lack of response. Perhaps that is why Balu et al. (2015) failed to find that RTI helped struggling learners, as there was little attention paid in their study other than providing more "intense" instruction for struggling readers. In this massive study of over 20,000 children in 13 states, Balu et al. found no effect for an RTI approach in improving academic outcomes. Authors of the study admit that decision rules regarding response/nonresponse and types of interventions attempted in the tiers were not controlled, so each school did whatever it deemed best practice. Hendricks and Fuchs (2020) reported that the determination of response/nonresponse in an RTI model was subjective at best, with different criteria and biases influencing classification. Continued concerns over the reliability and validity of using RTI as a model for SLD identification has led the National Joint Council on Learning Disabilities (NJCLD) to publish a position paper opposed to using nonresponse as a sole means for identifying SLD (Gartland & Strosnider, 2020).

The two RTI approaches advocated by Hale (2006), the standard protocol and the problem-solving approach (e.g., Fuchs & Fuchs, 2006), both need to be considered in practice. Standard protocol approaches are typically well-validated and have procedures for ensuring treatment fidelity, thus ensuring external validity in the decision-making process. However, they may not be well-matched to the individual child's difficulties, especially when there are multiple concerns. A problem-solving approach allows for an individualized approach and more targeted interventions, but may have less evidence of efficacy or generalizability beyond the child in question, so in problem solving it is important to ensure internal validity by carefully controlling antecedent and consequent events and ensuring treatment integrity (e.g., Batsch et al., 2007; Burns et al., 2008). We recommend using both approaches with a child before recommending a comprehensive evaluation—this way, the strengths of each approach compensate for the weaknesses of the other (Flanagan et al., 2010; Hale, 2006).

A fundamental problem with the use of RTI alone for diagnosis is that there is no *true positive* in learning disabilities identification using this approach; it is essentially circular (Fiorello et al., 2012; Hale, Wycoff, et al., 2010). Those who fail to respond have a learning disability; those who have a learning disability will fail to respond. Adding a comprehensive evaluation that includes assessment of cognitive and neuropsychological processing will allow for identification of the true positive child with an SLD—the child who fails to achieve due to a processing weakness. This integration of RTI with cognitive assessment is advocated by a wide variety of researchers and clinicians (Hale, Alfonso, et al., 2010; Wodrich et al., 2006). In addition, the legal IDEA (Etscheidt & Curran, 2010) Child Find and comprehensive evaluation requirements suggest a child must be evaluated in all areas of potential disability, which may necessitate identifying all areas of cognitive and neuropsychological processing that might be impaired (Wright et al., 2013).

The Importance of Comprehensive Cognitive Assessment

Only psychologists are trained to administer and interpret many of the cognitive and socioemotional measures discussed in this book. Other psychologist roles, such as developing and monitoring interventions, consultation with teachers and parents, counseling with individuals or groups, conducting skill-based groups, or even participating in individualized education plan (IEP) development, can be fulfilled by other professionals. It is up to you to help administrators recognize that cognitive and socioemotional assessments are essential to understanding many (but not all) children with unique needs. In addition, as the burden of mandated assessment practices has been lifted from psychologists' shoulders, the proverbial door has been opened for you to engage in innovative practices. No longer does a child need an intelligence test every 3 years—but this does not mean that cognitive, behavioral, or curriculum-based measures cannot be used to evaluate child changes over time (neurodevelopment coverage in subsequent chapters will highlight this point). You should use the changes in disability law wisely (e.g., Wright et al., 2013) to become involved in other roles and functions, so that you may provide individualized, comprehensive evaluations that have ecological and treatment validity.

You may wonder why we are adamant that cognitive and neuropsychological assessment must remain important components of psychology practice. Psychologists have a wide array of tools, and cognitive measures are some of the best made ones. They often have the highest technical quality (i.e., reliability and validity) of any assessment tools on the market (see Flanagan et al., 2012). We are convinced that cognitive assessment provides an abundance of valuable information about a student's functioning that cannot be obtained in any other way. A child's overt symptoms may have one or more underlying etiologies, and just treating the symptoms could have a negative effect if the wrong treatment is chosen. For instance, a child may have a reading comprehension problem but you can't tell if there are problems with rapid naming, attention, working memory, receptive, or expressive language based on the achievement score alone. A child with attention problems due to a thought disorder could be diagnosed with the inattentive type of attention-deficit/hyperactivity disorder (ADHD), and actually be harmed by treatment with stimulants, the most common treatment for ADHD. Case Study 1.1 highlights how essential neuropsychological assessment can be in recognizing and treating children with special needs.

The implications for Carlos in Case Study 1.1 are profound. Even if the majority of the cases we see with childhood problems do not have a clear biological etiology, missing one child with acute brain deterioration is unacceptable. Will a pediatrician pick this up during a routine well-child visit? Will a teacher or behavioral consultant recognize the changes? The answer is likely to be no, not until the condition progresses to a point when it becomes obvious that something is wrong (e.g., seizures, falling down, vomiting). Even a school psychologist who administers tests with no knowledge of brain functioning may disregard a student's drop in performance, thinking that the child was unmotivated during the assessment or that variability in scores is common. You are on the front line of children's cognitive, learning, and socioemotional needs—the first one able to recognize whether a child's attention problems are related to ADHD, absence seizures, or any other number of possible causes. Just pulling out a rating scale and finding clinically elevated attention problems will not tell you the type of problem a child actually has, and a child could actually be harmed if the wrong intervention is chosen (Hale et al., 2013). As the frontline cognitive assessment expert, you must remain vigilant to ensure the mental health of the children you serve. Even if you do not practice or have training in neuropsychology, it is crucial that you learn basic neuroanatomy and have access to information about it because you will see children with rare genetic diseases, traumatic brain injury, birth injury or difficulties, and those who survived cancer

---

Case Study 1.1. Saving Carlos's Life

Carlos was classified as having a learning disability and was receiving special education services when he came to the clinic for a second opinion. He had one "full" evaluation in second grade to determine eligibility. Subsequent team re-evaluations consisted of record review and some anecdotal data provided by his special education teacher. At each re-evaluation, the few team members required by law concluded that Carlos still had a learning disability and needed services. Frustrated by Carlos's poor progress and the team's refusal to reevaluate him more fully, his parents brought him to a private psychologist. When the cognitive results were compared to his previous results, it was revealed that Carlos had experienced a severe decline in overall functioning, and that his profile had changed dramatically. Follow-up evaluation and referral to a neurologist revealed the reason for the cognitive and achievement decline: Carlos had developed a brain tumor! If the team members had acceded to the parents' request for a full evaluation (as they legally should have), the cause of Carlos's continued school difficulty might have been identified and treated sooner.

and other formerly deadly diseases; this is likely more than you learned about in your training program (see, e.g., Semrud-Clikeman, Bledsoe, et al., 2013).

This frontline role certainly serves the needs of prevention and early intervention in the RTI approaches we advocate, but keeping vigilant for relationships between cognitive functioning and other sources of data can also yield new insight into a child's characteristics and needs. For instance, you may find cases when a child's history becomes critical in understanding their cognitive, academic, and socioemotional functioning. Some psychologists skip the history section or touch on it briefly, thinking that it is only important to talk about a child's current functioning. Others suggest addressing only the reason for referral. Limiting history and your evaluation questions, however, limits your opportunity to meet children's needs. Case Study 1.2 highlights the relevance of taking a more holistic perspective when you are trying to interpret cognitive assessment information.

Major Cognitive/Intellectual Assessment Instruments

If you have been careful in your use of standard protocol RTI and problem-solving RTI, and treatment integrity has been consistent, it is likely the child may have a disability requiring special education intervention, either in inclusive or pull-out settings. What becomes critical at this point is a comprehensive evaluation in all areas of suspected disability (Wright et al., 2013).

Cognitive assessment, using one or more of the major intelligence/cognitive assessment instruments, forms the basis of our cognitive hypothesis-testing (CHT) model. As will be discussed in Chapter 3, after the history, RTI, and observational data are reviewed, an

---

Case Study 1.2. Donald and His Orthopedic Disability

Due to begin high school in the fall, Donald was brought to our clinic by his mother for help with vocational planning. A review of the history revealed that Donald had experienced a birth trauma (right-hemisphere cerebral vascular accident or stroke) that led to left-arm/left-leg hemiparesis, some speech impairment, and a fairly serious visual impairment. He was receiving special education services with a diagnosis of orthopedic impairment. His IEP contained some physical adaptations and accommodations, but he was enrolled in regular academic classes. Donald had never received a comprehensive evaluation. Our assessment revealed significant cognitive impairment. Although he had adequate basic skills and language development, his fluid reasoning, visual–spatial skills, and higher-level comprehension skills were all well below average. Consistent with our findings, his academic performance had showed a steady decline over the years, because the use of right-hemisphere cognitive processes increases with age. Only his extraordinary level of motivation and effort had helped him survive the higher grades.

Think of what Donald could have accomplished if his school had done a full evaluation earlier. There would have been time for intensive interventions to remediate some of his difficulties—but, considering his age and years remaining in school, we were left with trying more compensatory strategies. In both this case and that of Carlos (see Case Study 1.1), the cognitive assessments revealed important information that drastically affected our interventions. In addition, both evaluations were conducted by psychologists from outside the school system and were paid for by parents. Both sets of parents sought outside help, but what if they didn't, what would have become of Carlos and Donald? As frontline advocates of children's needs, we need to recognize that cognitive assessment is a valuable component of what we do as psychologists. We cannot rely on others to make judgments about children's cognitive functioning when the stakes are so high.

initial cognitive assessment instrument is administered, and then the next step is to develop hypotheses about a child's cognitive strengths and needs based on these initial results. Most psychologists stop there. The CHT model takes the interpretive process further, in that additional cognitive, and/or neuropsychological measures are administered to examine the validity of the original hypotheses (Fiorello et al., 2012). This process continues until possible explanations for a child's classroom performance and behavior have been confirmed or refuted (Hale, Wycoff, et al., 2010). In CHT, an intelligence/cognitive test can be used as the main first-step instrument, or subtests from the measures can be used to develop and test hypotheses. It is essentially used as a screening tool for developing hypotheses that are later evaluated with additional measures (Hale et al., 2016).

In this section, we provide you with a brief overview of the major cognitive assessment instruments we feel are useful in formulating initial CHT hypotheses. They are listed in alphabetical order, not by order of preference or utility. Your choice of instrument should be based on the referral question, history, permanent product, RTI data, observation, and interview. We provide information about the constructs and processes tapped by individual subtests, in order to allow you to begin the process of analyzing a student's strengths and weaknesses. However, further in-depth analyses of these constructs should be individualized for each child, to avoid the tendency to take a "cookbook" approach. Resources such as those by Dehn (2013), Flanagan, Ortiz, and Alfonso (2013), Miller (2013), Naglieri and Goldstein (2009) and Sattler (2018) should be helpful in understanding the constructs tapped by these measures. In addition, we provide a number of forms helpful for the more fine-grained demands analysis of subtest performance in Chapter 4.

Differential Ability Scales—Second Edition

An adaptation of the British Ability Scales, the DAS-II (Elliott, 2007) is an increasingly popular cognitive assessment measure since its introduction in the United States. One important feature of the DAS-II is the separation of Verbal Ability, Nonverbal Reasoning Ability, and Spatial Ability tasks into cluster scores for meaningful interpretation. Since these clusters are composed of only two subtests, the core is fairly quick to administer. Another is the use of diagnostic subtests to assess short- and long-term memory, phonological processing, and processing speed. The DAS-II also has a preschool version available, although we focus on the school-age version as being most useful for CHT. Several DAS-II subtests are useful in looking at essential cognitive processes and memory. Table 1.1 presents the core and diagnostic DAS-II subtests and the constructs they purportedly tap, which are helpful in interpretation.

The DAS-II was most recently revised in 2023 and is now called DAS-II NU (Normative Update) School Age. We welcome this, as the DAS-II has many strengths for use in CHT. It was standardized on 3,480 children from ages 2 years, 6 months (2-6), to 17 years, 11 months (17-11), stratified on age, sex, race/ethnicity, region of the United States, and education level of the parents (as a measure of socioeconomic status [SES]). The sample matches the 2002 U.S. Census information very well. An oversample of African American and Hispanic children was also drawn, in order to allow for bias analyses. Reliability studies indicate that the GCA is reliable enough for individual decision making at the school-age level, with coefficients ranging from .95 to .97 across age levels. Individual subtests have average reliabilities ranging from .68 to .97. Some subtests at some ages do not have sufficient reliability for individual interpretation, most notably Recognition of Pictures for out-of-level testing above age 8, Picture Similarities above age 7, and out-of-level testing using Early Number Concepts and Matching Letter-Like Forms above age 6. The availability of out-of-level testing makes the

TABLE 1.1. Differential Ability Scales—Second Edition, Normative Update (DAS-II NU)

Subtest	Constructs purportedly tapped
Core subtests	
Verbal Ability	
Word Definitions	Vocabulary task; child defines words orally; task depends on lexical/ semantic knowledge and expressive language skills.
Verbal Similarities	Child expresses the similarities among three named objects of increasing abstractness; task requires verbal knowledge, concept formation, reasoning, categorical thinking, and oral expression.
Nonverbal Reasoning Ability	
Matrices	Multiple-choice matrix reasoning task; it requires fluid abilities/ deductive and inductive reasoning; multiple-choice response may foster trial-and-error approaches.
Sequential and Quantitative Reasoning	Fluid reasoning task requiring inductive reasoning; later items involve oral response to a pattern in a numerical series; task assesses both fluid reasoning and quantitative reasoning—may tap math skills if impaired.
Spatial Ability	
Recall of Designs	Child uses pencil and paper to reproduce visual designs presented for 5 seconds each; test of visual memory, visual–spatial orientation; visual–motor integration and motor skills also required.
Pattern Construction	Block Design-like task; it requires perceptual analysis and synthesis; it can be interpreted with or without time bonuses.
Diagnostic subtests	
Recall of Digits Forward	Test of rote short-term auditory–sequential memory; no working memory component; quick aural presentation of digits to discourage rehearsal.
Recall of Digits Backward	Test of auditory working memory, as elements must be reordered.
Recognition of Pictures	Visual memory; deliberately designed to make verbal labeling difficult.
Recall of Sequential Order	Working memory task using both verbal and pictorial material.
Phonological Processing	Auditory processing with analysis and synthesis of phonemic items presented auditorially.
Rapid Naming	Timed task requiring automaticity of naming symbols.
Recall of Objects—Immediate	Card is presented with numerous pictures, which are then named, and card is taken away; three trials to recall the objects with time limits; memory task with a learning component and both visual and verbal cues.
Recall of Objects—Delayed	The same objects are named after a delay; test of long-term memory, using both visual and verbal cues.
Speed of Information Processing	Speeded clerical task; child indicates by pencil the circle with the most boxes/highest number in a row; test of attention, visual scanning, and processing speed.

Note. Diagnostic subtests are optional.

DAS-II especially attractive for assessing children with disabilities. Also helpful are directions for administering the test in Spanish and American Sign Language and the availability of the Special Nonverbal Composite—though, as we have noted before, an assessment that avoids language and crystallized abilities has limited utility in neuropsychological assessment. The DAS-II provides extensive evidence of validity, including concurrent validity indices with the WISC-IV of .84, and predictive validity indices of .66 to .77 with the WIAT-II, .42 to .81 with the KTEA-II, and .69 to .82 with the WJ-III Ach. Factor analyses and the standard error of measurement (SEM) confirm the structure of the test, which shows increasing differentiation of abilities over time and a close match to CHC theory.

We especially like the way the DAS-II uses three main factors at the school-age level; it separates the Nonverbal Reasoning Ability cluster from the Spatial Ability cluster, thereby deemphasizing the traditional verbal–nonverbal dichotomy. We also like the addition of diagnostic subtests to explore strengths and weaknesses. The specificities of most DAS-II subtests are above .25 at all ages (with the exception of Verbal Similarities), sufficient to allow individual interpretation. The technical manual is extremely complete and helpful for designing an appropriate assessment for an individual child, and it also presents information about special-group studies and bias analysis. For studies regarding the DAS-II utility in identification of SLD, see Elliott et al. (2010) and Hale, Fiorello, et al. (2008).

The interpretation section is especially strong, providing a great deal of information about the cognitive processes required for subtest performance; this information makes the DAS-II very useful for CHT. Subtest performance should be used to generate hypotheses about functioning and subsequently examined within the context of all other information sources (Dumont, Willis, & Elliott, 2008). As with all the measures we discuss, the DAS-II has several drawbacks, necessitating the use of additional hypothesis-testing measures. First, it does not explore the complexity of language processes as well as some other cognitive measures do, and teasing out crystallized knowledge from language functioning is difficult. The assessment of memory is a good idea, but the DAS memory-related subtests alone are not sufficient for a comprehensive memory assessment. The Recall of Designs subtest is a measure of spatial skills, but interpretation is influenced by both visual memory and motor (praxis) processes. Finally, the DAS-II does not appear to have an adequate measure of executive function, although the Nonverbal Reasoning subtests are certainly affected by executive skills. We have conducted two studies examining the utility of the DAS-II in the prediction of reading and math achievement (Elliott et al., 2010; Hale, Fiorello, et al., 2008), which attests to the high amounts of achievement variance it accounts for, as well as some individual test and factor results that provide evidence of its diagnostic utility, which is further enhanced by Dumont and colleagues' (2008) *Essentials of DAS-II Assessment* book. See also McGrew and Wendling (2010) and Keith et al. (2010) as a further testament to the DAS-II construction, psychometric strengths, and diagnostic utility, and Flanagan et al. (2013) for using the DAS-II in cross-battery assessment.

Kaufman Assessment Battery for Children—Second Edition, Normative Update

The KABC-II NU (Kaufman, 2018) is a major revision of the original KABC that is designed to allow interpretation according to CHC theory or a neuropsychological (Lurian) model. A primary goal of the instrument is fairness in the assessment of children of diverse racial and ethnic backgrounds. An emphasis on process rather than knowledge in the subtests, together with the option to obtain a full-scale score (the Mental Processing Composite) without any crystallized subtests minimizes score differences between dominant culture and minoritized children. Options to obtain a nonverbal score, and to administer the test in Spanish, also add to its utility with minority children. Of course, for a thorough neuropsychological examination, crystallized abilities must be assessed as well. Table 1.2 presents the core and optional subtests of the KABC-II and the cognitive processes tapped by each one. The KABC-II normative update sample consisted of 700 English-speaking children ages 3–18, and the demographic characteristics of the sample closely matched the 2015 U.S. Census information. The normative sample was stratified on age, sex, race/ethnicity, parents' educational level, and geographic region. Children receiving special education services were included as they naturally occurred and were somewhat underrepresented in the sample. Children with an intellectual disability or identified as gifted were specifically recruited to ensure a broad range of ability was represented. Educational status at age 18 was examined to ensure that the proportion in high school and those who had dropped out reasonably corresponded with census information. Reliabilities for the overall scores (Mental Processing Index and Fluid-Crystallized Index) are strong across all age groups, ranging from .92 to .97, with all reliability exceeding .95 for ages 4 to 18. The Non-Verbal Index reliability ranged from .91 to .96 across all ages. Index scores are generally moderate to strong as well. Individual subtests are moderate to strong, with some exceptions. Gestalt Closure and Story Completion are weaker across numerous ages, and Number Recall and Hand Movements are weak at some ages. In addition, weak reliability was demonstrated for Word Order at age 3, Triangles at age 14, and Atlantis Delayed at age 6. Several subtests have alternate scoring available that eliminates time bonuses. The reliability of Pattern Reasoning remains strong without time bonuses, but Triangles and Story Completion show weaker reliability at numerous ages without time bonuses.

The KABC-II manual includes an interpretive guide that provides information about each of the scales from both a CHC theory and a neuropsychological/Lurian framework. Evidence of validity is relatively strong, with full-scale scores (FCI and MPI) correlated to the WISC-V at .65–.72 and correlated with KTEA-3 composite achievement scores at .49–.74. The manual also includes information about each subtest to aid in interpretation, including qualitative indicators that are particularly relevant to notice during the child's performance of that task. The qualitative indicators are listed on the test record form by each subtest, and a summary of those is available as well. Of course, you should not limit yourself to those particular observations, but this feature is especially helpful for novices to draw their attention to important features of a child's performance.

The KABC-II NU is linked with the KTEA-3, and some areas of processing, phonological processing and rapid automatized naming, are assessed on that instrument rather than the KABC-II NU. Research is beginning to show that the KABC-II is a powerful instrument, not only for identification of processing strengths and weaknesses, but also differential diagnosis, and planning intervention as well (see Kaufman et al., 2005; Reynolds et al., 2007; Kaufman, Kaufman et al., 2011). Finally, see Flanagan et al. (2013) for use of the KABC-II in cross-battery assessment.

Stanford–Binet Intelligence Scales, Fifth Edition

The SB-5 (Roid, 2003), the most recent revision of the venerable Stanford–Binet, returns to the tradition of measuring high-functioning and low-functioning individuals well, while updating the content to take advantage of modern cognitive/intellectual functioning theory. However, the SB-5 was last renormed in 2003, meaning that its norms are too old to recommend it for current use. SB-5 is designed to assess five basic constructs from CHC theory as described earlier (Fluid Reasoning, Knowledge, Quantitative Reasoning, Visual–Spatial Processing, and Working Memory), using both verbal and nonverbal formats. This was actually an important contribution often neglected by many test publishers. By developing factors that are cross-modal, a practitioner can actually be sure that the psychological process in

TABLE 1.2. Kaufman Assessment Battery for Children—Second Edition, Normative Update (KABC-II NU) and Selected Tests of Achievement (KTEA-III)

Test	Constructs purportedly tapped
Sequential/Gwm	
Number Recall	Rote auditory sequential memory for digits.
Word Order	Early items are rote sequential memory of spoken words, indicated by pointing to pictures. Later items have an interference task, rapid color naming, to make this a working memory task.
(Hand Movements)	Rote memory of visually presented sequences of hand movements; fine-motor skills and motor planning (praxis) is also required. Can informally assess handedness and mirroring.
Planning/Gf	
Story Completion	Child puts photos into a story sequence to make a meaningful story. Draws on inductive and deductive reasoning, visual skills and attention to detail, sequencing ability, and general knowledge.
Pattern Reasoning	A matrix reasoning task, designed to assess fluid reasoning, but may depend on visual–perceptual ability as well.
Learning/Gl	
Atlantis	Learning task where child must learn made-up names of fish, sea plants, and shells. Performance can be enhanced if syllabic clues are noticed and used.
(Atlantis Delayed)	Child is tested on the same material after a break.
Rebus	Learning task where child must learn symbols for words and "read" sentences using those symbols. Symbols have mnemonic properties, and the sentences draw on knowledge of English vocabulary and grammar.
(Rebus Delayed)	Child is asked to "read" sentences using the same symbols after a break.
Simultaneous/Gv	
Rover	Child must move a toy dog through the shortest path to his bone while following rules. Assesses executive functioning, planning, spatial scanning, counting ability, inhibition, and maintenance of rules.
Triangles	Child must reproduce abstract visual patterns with colored triangles. Draws on spatial visualization, spatial relations, praxis, and bimanual coordination.
Block Counting	Child must count the number of blocks present in a drawing of a three-dimensional construction. Requires spatial visualization and math ability.
(Gestalt Closure)	Child must identify objects from pictures presented in incomplete, "inkblot" style. Requires visual closure and general knowledge.
Knowledge/Gc	
Verbal Knowledge	Child must answer questions about vocabulary words to demonstrate their understanding. Draws on vocabulary and general knowledge.
Riddles	Child uses reasoning, vocabulary, and language development to guess what is being described by the examiner.
(Expressive Vocabulary)	Child names pictures of common objects.

(continued)

TABLE 1.2. *(continued)*

Auditory Processing (Ga) *(Achievement)*	
Phonological Processing	Child completes a variety of phonological awareness tasks—rhyming, matching sounds, blending, segmenting, and deleting sounds.

Rapid Automatized Naming (Gs/Gr) *(Achievement)*	
Object Naming Facility	Child must rapidly name objects.
Letter Naming Facility	Child must rapidly name letters.
Associational Fluency	Child must name as many words as possible falling within a semantic category or beginning with a specified sound.

Note. Subtests in parentheses are optional.

question is impaired if both subtests reveal a difficulty. For instance, when tapping working memory on the WISC-IV, it was only auditory–verbal working memory that was evaluated (fortunately this is not the case on WISC-V), so language processing impairments could explain the problem too. However, keep in mind, though, that many of the nonverbal tasks still have verbal directions. Table 1.3 outlines the tasks and processes involved in each subtest, summarized across age levels.

The SB-5 was standardized on 4,800 people ages from 2 to over 85 years, stratified on age, sex, race/ethnicity, region of the United States, and education level of the examinee or parents (as a measure of SES); it generally matches the demographic characteristics of the 2000 U.S. Census well. In addition, 6.8% of the sample were receiving special services (special education or clinical treatment), and 2% of the sample had been identified as intellectually gifted. Reliability studies indicate that the Full Scale score is highly reliable, with coefficients of .97 to .98 across all age groups. Individual subtests have average reliabilities ranging from .84 to .89, although some subtests have reliabilities below .75 at some ages. The SB-5 has good evidence of validity, including concurrent validity indices of .82 to .84 with the Wechsler scales, as well as predictive validity indices of .66 to .84 with the WJ-III Achievement and .53 to .80 with the Wechsler Individual Achievement Test—Second Edition. Factor analyses confirm that the structure of the test (verbal vs. nonverbal, and the five-factor model) is supported. Extensive studies of special groups are also presented in the comprehensive technical manual. The floor of most of the subtests is not adequate for low-functioning examinees until about ages 4-6, although Rasch-based "change-sensitive scores" are provided for the factor scores below the 2-0 age equivalent level. The ceiling appears adequate at all age levels. Full Scale scores can range from 40 to 160, and the interpretive manual allows for calculation of extended scores from 10 to 225 (Roid et al., 2003). This and the change-sensitive scores provide for interpretation below and above the typical 4 standard deviation range, making the SB-5 especially useful for low- and high-functioning individuals.

The expansion of the factors assessed by the SB-5 was a welcome addition, and it is more closely aligned than the SB-IV was with current cognitive and neuropsychological theory, making it useful as a cognitive screening tool or for hypothesis testing in CHT. As is true with all of these screening measures, a number of important cognitive skills are not adequately assessed on the SB-5, necessitating supplemental testing within our CHT model. The SB-5 yields factorially complex tasks, with interpretation complicated by the extended age range (2–85+). The actual process demands of a subtest vary depending on the level administered, which in turn depends on the student's age and performance on the verbal or nonverbal routing task; all this makes interpretation somewhat inconsistent from child to child, so

TABLE 1.3. Stanford–Binet Intelligence Scales—Fifth Edition (SB-5)

Subtest	Constructs purportedly tapped
Nonverbal	
Fluid Reasoning	Object series/matrix analogies; multiple-choice inductive reasoning, using objects/pictures.
Knowledge	Procedural knowledge at lower levels (child demonstrates named activity); child identifies or explains picture absurdities at higher levels.
Quantitative Reasoning	Variety of quantitative reasoning tasks, including block counting, manipulatives, multiple-choice visual quantitative series, and visual equations; spatial visualization or visual memory, in addition to reasoning ability, required on several items.
Visual–Spatial Processing	Formboard at lower level; form patterns (tangram-like activity) at higher level; task requires spatial visualization and visual–motor skills.
Working Memory	Object constancy, then block-tapping span, then a working memory version of block tapping; visual–sequential memory task, with working memory component at higher levels.
Verbal	
Fluid Reasoning	Lower levels require giving verbal descriptions of complex pictures, categorizing picture chips in different ways, and categorical labeling; higher levels involve verbal absurdities and analogies; reasoning ability and expressive language required.
Knowledge	Lower levels include body part naming and expressive labeling of nouns, then verbs; higher levels require defining words presented visually and aurally.
Quantitative Reasoning	Lower levels include oral counting and naming numerals; higher levels require solving word problems; pencil and paper are permitted, to minimize the impact of working memory.
Visual–Spatial Processing	Lower levels include use of spatial terms; higher levels include oral directions for map-like drawing and answering directional questions.
Working Memory	Lower levels require repetition of sentences; higher levels require answering a series of aurally presented questions, then repeating the last word, in order, of each question.

Note. Actual SB-5 tasks differ according to which levels are administered.

some instruction and practice is needed (see Roid & Barram, 2004). Much practice with many different types of children will be needed before you can acquire good "head norms" about this test. As a result, it is essential to task-analyze a particular subtest, and this task analysis may change for different children of different chronological ages. Riverside makes a technical note available (Roid, 2006) that provides information about linking assessment with the SB-5 to instruction and intervention, although we again caution you not to apply recommendations in a "cookbook" fashion. Please see additional citations about the use of the SB-5 in clinical practice in assessing processing strengths and weaknesses (Roid et al., 2009) and in the cross-battery approach (Flanagan et al., 2013).

Wechsler Intelligence Scale for Children—Fifth Edition

There have been five iterations of the WISC scales and subtests and indices have changed over the years. The WISC-V (Wechsler, 2014) has moved beyond the Verbal–Performance dichotomy and this revision utilizes recent theoretical advances and research findings on cognitive functions and processes to provide a five-factor model. The five factors are Verbal Comprehension, Visual Spatial, Fluid Reasoning, Working Memory, and Processing Speed. Niileksela and Reynolds (2019) compared all of the versions of the WISC and found that the constructs and indices tested by the WISC have generally remained fairly constant over the revisions. What variance was found was due to unique subtest variances and did not affect basic interpretation.

WISC-V also provides ancillary subtests that assess associative memory and naming speed. In addition to the FSIQ and the five Index scores, the WISC-V provides special index scores, including the General Ability Index, Cognitive Proficiency Index, Nonverbal Index, Verbal Working Memory Index, and Quantitative Reasoning Index. The scoring software allows for a pattern of strengths and weaknesses analysis that is compatible with our Concordance–Discordance Model (Hale & Fiorello, 2004). There is a Spanish-language version available (WISC-V Spanish; Wechsler, 2014).

The WISC-V has a normative linking sample with both the WIAT-III and the KTEA-3, adding to flexibility for the examiner. As with the WISC-IV, an integrated expansion adds 14 supplemental subtests to assess processing in more depth. Follow-up tests (such as multiple-choice versions of the Verbal Comprehension subtests) and supplemental tests (such as Spatial Span and Sentence Recall to explore working memory capacity and verbal–semantic memory) add tremendously to the interpretive power of the WISC-V. Table 1.4 provides information about the individual WISC-V subtests and their interpretation.

The WISC-V norming and clinical studies suggest it has strong evidence of reliability and validity. The standardization sample was stratified on age, gender, race/ethnicity, parental education level, and region of the United States. In addition to the update to more closely follow modern intelligence theory, the WISC-V was developed and normed to be administered in two distinct ways—either in the traditional paper-and-pencil format or using touch-screen tablets. Careful validation and equating studies make the versions comparable, although for individual students, you should evaluate the suitability of each version. The WISC-V thus appears to be a stronger instrument than its predecessors in that it too is aligned more closely with CHC-theory, and it remains a psychometrically sound instrument consistent with the Wechsler tradition.

While there are improvements in the stimuli and the addition of subtests that are useful, there is controversy surrounding the five factors of the WISC-V. The WISC-IV had four factors, and the Fluid Reasoning factor was added to the WISC-V. Studies have frequently found four factors for the WISC-V with the visual spatial and fluid reasoning factors sharing variance similar to the perceptual reasoning factor from the WISC-IV (Canivez et al., 2020; Canivez et al., 2017; Dombrowski et al., 2015). These studies have been conducted with typically developing children and with clinical samples with similar findings.

While this is an improved measure, there are still a number of important cognitive functions that are indirectly assessed or not measured at all by the WISC-V. For instance, there is no good measure of auditory processing or phonemic awareness, though this is assessed on the co-normed Wechsler Individual Achievement Test, Fourth Edition (WIAT-4). The WISC-V is very heavily culturally and linguistically loaded, making its use with minority children questionable. Moreover, two subtests (Picture Span and Figure Weights) were found to show differential findings in the African American sample and should be carefully interpreted when the scores differ from normative expectations (Graves et al., 2021). The normative

TABLE 1.4. Wechsler Intelligence Scale for Children—Fifth Edition (WISC-V)

Subtest	Constructs purportedly tapped
Verbal Comprehension	
Similarities	Expressive language needed to identify how two words or concepts are alike; task requires vocabulary/semantic knowledge, categorical thinking, and verbal reasoning ability.
Vocabulary	Early items require picture naming; later items require defining words presented aurally; requires vocabulary knowledge, crystallized abilities, and expressive language.
Comprehension	Child explains reasons for common social rules; task requires expressive language, implicit knowledge, and reasoning about social situations and conventions.
Information	Child answers factual questions from science, social studies, and the humanities; test of long-term memory retrieval and crystallized knowledge.
Visual Spatial	
Block Design	Child views a model or picture and reproduces it with red-and-white blocks; task includes time limits and time bonuses (untimed score available); measure of visual orientation, spatial processing, analysis and synthesis, and processing speed.
Visual Puzzles	Child views a picture of a complete shape and chooses which response options will combine to make the shape; each item has a time limit of 30 seconds; measure of spatial orientation, spatial processing, analysis and synthesis, and processing speed.
Fluid Reasoning	
Picture Concepts	Child chooses a picture from each of two or three rows to form a group with a common characteristic; measure of fluid reasoning and abstract categorical reasoning ability.
Matrix Reasoning	Pictorial analogies, including pattern completion, classification, analogical reasoning, and serial reasoning; multiple-choice responses; measure of fluid reasoning and nonverbal concept formation.
Figure Weights	Child views a picture of a scale with missing weights and chooses which response option will balance the scale; each item has a time limit of 20 or 30 seconds; measure of fluid reasoning and quantitative reasoning, processing speed.
Working Memory	
Digit Span	Consists of three tasks—repeating a series of digits presented aurally in forward, backward, and sequential order; total score is combined, but process scores are available for forward (rote auditory–sequential memory) and backward sequencing (attention, working memory, and executive function).
Letter–Number Sequencing	Aurally presented letter and number sequences, repetition of numbers in ascending order and letters in alphabetical order; test requires attention, auditory working memory, mental manipulation, sequencing, and simple verbal expression.
Arithmetic	Child solves orally presented arithmetic problems within a time limit; task requires increased working memory load and decreased mathematical ability, as compared to WISC IV arithmetic. *(continued)*

TABLE 1.4. (*continued*)

Processing Speed	
Coding	Child copies marks into symbols (younger) or symbols matched to numbers (older), according to a visually presented code; similar to Symbol Search, with more graphomotor and visual memory demands.
Symbol Search	Child visually scans and marks whether target symbols are in an array of abstract symbols; measure of visual perception of abstract symbols, scanning, processing speed, and graphomotor abilities (low).
Cancellation	Child visually scans an array of colored pictures, marking all of the animals; measure of visual perception, scanning, attention, processing speed, and graphomotor abilities (low).

Supplementary Subtests	
Picture Span	Child views one or more pictures, then selects them in order from a visual array; measures visual working memory.
Naming Speed	Child names pictures or letters and numbers as quickly as possible; child identifies quantity of squares in a box as quickly as possible. Measures rapid access of information from long-term memory, processing speed, fluency of symbol identification, fluency of quantity perception.
Visual–Verbal Association (Immediate and Delayed)	Child learns a series of rebuses in a controlled learning task and must recall them immediately and after a 20 to 30 minute delay; delayed task includes a recognition task; measures learning ability, long-term memory storage and retrieval, some reasoning ability involved in learning the associations based on visual cues, compare recall to recognition.

sample included only 13% of children who were African American, which is lower than the percentage of African American people in the general population (Council of Great City Schools, 2017).

Woodcock–Johnson V Tests of Cognitive Abilities and Tests of Achievement

The WJ-V series of tests (McGrew et al., 2015) differs in two ways from the other cognitive assessment tools presented here: it was designed specifically to assess the full range of cognitive abilities according to the CHC theory, and it attempts to minimize factorial complexity by assessing specific, narrow abilities. Subtests are designed to be cognitively complex while still remaining relatively clean measures of specific abilities, which often means that the executive function demands, such as working memory and focused attention, are increased. This means that the WJ-V is an excellent screening tool or a source of individual subtests for CHT, despite the fact that it was not designed primarily as a neuropsychological assessment instrument. The scoring software provides a wide variety of interpretive options, including a General Intellectual Ability, a Brief Intellectual Ability, and a *Gf-Gc* Composite score in addition to clinical clusters. Table 1.5 presents information about a variety of useful tests from the WJ-V battery.

The WJ-V standardization and norming indicates strong evidence of reliability and validity of the scores and excellent representation in the norms group and clinical study samples. Finally, although the WJ-V authors would probably not condone this, there is a tendency for practitioners to interpret these subtests with a "one construct, one subtest" mentality, which does not accurately reflect the cognitive skills required for the subtest (Hale & Fiorello, 2002).

TABLE 1.5. Woodcock–Johnson V Tests of Cognitive Abilities (WJ-V Cognitive) and Selected Tests of Achievement (WJ-V Achievement), and Virtual Test Library

Test	Constructs purportedly tapped
Comprehension–Knowledge (*Gc*)	
Oral Comprehension (Achievement)	Task measures knowledge of spoken vocabulary—naming, synonyms, antonyms, analogies; sensitive to word-finding problems, not complex language.
Oral Vocabulary	Child is asked to define words.
General Information	Task assesses knowledge of general information/vocabulary; child answers function questions about objects.
Picture Vocabulary (Achievement)	Task measures semantic knowledge of picture–word associations; sensitive to word-finding problems.
Learning Efficiency (*Gl*)	
Visual–Auditory Learning	Test of word–symbol analogy learning and associative memory; "reading" visual rebus sentences; ability to benefit from feedback.
Story Comprehension	Child is asked to retell a story read earlier.
Retrieval Fluency (*Gr*)	
Semantic Word Retrieval	Child names words starting with a specific sound, given time limit; measure of phonemic fluency and retrieval, speed of lexical access.
Rapid Picture Naming (Visual Test Library)	Confrontational naming of pictures under a time limit; test of rapid automatic naming skill, speed of lexical access.
Visual–Spatial Thinking (*Gv*)	
Spatial Relations	Task requires mental visualization. Block Rotation Task requires mental visualization and rotation.
Auditory Processing (*Ga*)	
Segmentation (Virtual Test Library)	Child is presented with words auditorially and must break them apart, first into component words, then syllables, then phonemes; an aspect of auditory processing that underlies spelling ability.
Sound Blending (Virtual Test Library)	Child combines phonemes presented aurally to form English words; test of auditory attention, phonetic coding, auditory sequencing, and assembly; underlies phonics ability.
Nonsense Word Repetition (Virtual Test Library)	Child listens to auditory presentation of a nonword and must repeat the utterance exactly; measures phonemic awareness and auditory working memory, memory for sound patterns; linked to language and reading disabilities.

(*continued*)

TABLE 1.5. (*continued*)

Fluid Reasoning (*Gf*)

Concept Formation	Child identifies rules underlying set formation, using simple geometrical figures; early items involve teaching and feedback; later items require use of "and" and "or" rules; inductive reasoning task with grammatical component.
Analysis–Synthesis	Child uses presented pictorial rules to solve color-combining problems; early items involve teaching and feedback; deductive/sequential reasoning task.
Number Series (Also measures *Gq*)	Child uses the mathematical principle underlying a number sequence to identify a missing number; quantitative reasoning task with no significant working memory load.
Verbal Analogies (Also measures *Gc*)	Child uses verbal reasoning to complete analogies given orally.

Processing Speed (*Gs*)

Letter-Pattern Matching	Child finds patterns of letters that match in a response booklet; the patterns to match are frequently used orthographic patterns in written English; measures visual scanning, perceptual speed, and orthographic processing.
Number-Pattern Matching	Child finds matching numbers from an array and circles them; measure of visual scanning and perceptual speed.

Working Memory Capacity (*Gwm*)

Verbal Attention	Child is presented auditorily with a list of mixed items and digits, then must answer a specific question requiring working memory, such as repeating just the colors, or naming the numbers in numerical order; measure of attention, auditory working memory, and executive function.
Numbers Reversed	Auditory working memory task; child repeats an aurally presented list of digits in reverse sequence; measure of attention, working memory, and executive function.
Animal–Number Sequencing (Virtual Test Library)	Child encodes and retrieves a list of mixed animals and digits presented aurally, repeating animals in order, then digits in order; increasing role of strategic planning; good measure of working memory and executive function.
Memory for Words (Virtual Test Library)	Child remembers a list of unrelated words presented aurally; measure of auditory–semantic memory without significant working memory component.
Understanding Directions (Virtual Test Library)	Child points to elements in a complex picture in sequential order, corresponding to an aurally presented direction; test of attention, working memory, language comprehension, and praxis.
Sentence Repetition (Virtual Test Library)	Child repeats sentences of increasing length; test of auditory–semantic memory and crystallized knowledge of syntax.

CHC is alluring because it helps practitioners look at processing patterns based on the most common finding for standardization samples. However, all cognitive assessment measures are factorially complex, so different patterns of performance can happen for different children. In addition, while CHC-based factor loadings using standardization samples can be a place to start, children with disabilities may have different factor structures or loadings consistent with neuroimaging evidence of differences (Decker et al., 2012; Elliott et al., 2010; Flanagan et al., 2011; Fiorello et al., 2009), so you need to consider the input, processing, and output demands (discussed in Chapters 2–4) of all measures you administer. With all that being said, the WJ-V provides numerous subtests covering a wide variety of cognitive skills, especially when you include the Achievement tests; it is thus a very useful CHT screening tool and source for supplemental tests for CHT evaluations. Some language tests are available in Spanish as well as English, and a Spanish-language version of the Third Edition Cognitive and Achievement measures is also available (Batería III Woodcock-Muñoz; Muñoz-Sandoval et al., 2005).

Intelligence Test Interpretation: Levels versus Patterns of Performance

Flanagan et al. (2013) provide a welcome format for comparing instruments and using additional measures in their cross-battery approach. Kaufman's (1994) "intelligent testing" approach moves from global (IQ) to specific (subtest profiles). He presents a detailed analysis of subtest constructs and recommends idiographic (individualized) analysis of common abilities. Sattler recommends a similar successive-level approach that culminates in a qualitative interpretation. Kamphaus et al. (1994) emphasize an integrative approach for combining qualitative and quantitative data about a child. He recommends a priori hypothesizing and hypothesis testing during the evaluation. O'Neill (1995) formalizes the process by providing an interpretative hierarchy, with Level 1 indicating scores and descriptors, Level 2 including conclusions based on statistical properties, and Level 3 individualizing the interpretation for high-level inferences. Finally, using more of a neuropsychological orientation, Poreh (2002) provides a quantitative approach to process assessment, similar to a cross-battery approach (Flanagan et al., 2013), and Decker et al. (2012) examine this approach to consider test base rates. This balance between cognitive approaches remains a challenge for even the seasoned cognitive assessment veteran, but clearly diagnostic clarity improves with careful attention to these interpretive issues (Decker et al., 2013).

As these scholars do, we argue that both nomothetic (normative) and idiographic (individualized) approaches have merit and are not antithetical. In Chapter 3, we present an applied neuropsychological perspective in our CHT model—one that allows for the integration of both product (levels of performance) and process (patterns of performance), and is sensitive to a child's background, environment, and behavior. Unfortunately, straight subtest profile or pattern analysis can be problematic for a number of reasons. Individual subtests are generally less reliable than cluster or global scores, which is in part a manifestation of the number of items that a summative score represents. In addition, these subtest measures are factorially complex (Flanagan et al., 2013), and using a "cookbook" approach of listing all possible skills and influences on a given score is not useful. Measurement errors, including administration errors, are also more likely to affect interpretation at the subtest level (McDermott et al., 2013), leading some opponents of subtest interpretation to admonish practitioners to "just say no" to subtest interpretation (McDermott et al., 1990). It is clear that the global IQ or a level of performance interpretation is appropriate for some children. When subtest variability is limited (e.g., flat profile), the global IQ seems to be the most parsimonious measure of a person's level of intellectual functioning. As we have noted earlier, IQ is a strong predictor of several important outcomes—generally those that are equated with success in our society (Gottfredson, 2010).

Although global IQ interpretation may be appropriate for some children, several have suggested that it should not be interpreted when factor or subtest differences are considerable (Hale et al., 2018; Prifitera et al., 2008). An examination of the pattern of performance in these cases is necessary because the IQ score is rendered uninterpretable by significant subtest or factor variability (Fiorello et., 2007). This belief is not merely a philosophical one. Our work (Elliott et al., 2010; Fiorello et al., 2007; Hale, Fiorello, Dumont, et al., 2008; Hale, Fiorello, Miller, et al., 2008; Hale et al., 2007) demonstrates that the WISC-IV IQ and the DAS-II GCA should not be interpreted for most children, especially children with disabilities. We have identified a variety of patterns of cognitive functioning that are related to different achievement areas (e.g., Hale, Fiorello, Miller, et al., 2008), and differences in patterns between typically developing children and those with disabilities (e.g., Elliott et al., 2010). Clearly, we now have extensive evidence that suggests the relevance of psychological processes in the prediction of meaningful academic (McGrew & Wendling, 2010) and psychosocial (Reddy, Weissman et al., 2013) outcomes.

This evidence leads us to tell you that *a Full-Scale IQ should never be interpreted when there is significant subtest or factor variability or scatter.* In addition, even if a child has a flat profile, it is important to recall that intelligence tests may be unfair for children with linguistic or cultural differences, and that IQ scores are intimately related to prior education and experience. In addition, even if a child shows little subtest variability, you must take into account what is actually assessed by the instrument, because no two intelligence tests use the same tasks or administrative format. The scores are not interchangeable but should instead be interpreted in light of the content processes and content knowledge required by each test. You must remember that IQ scores are probably *related* to ability, but they are not a direct measure of, nor should they be *equated* with, ability, as Spearman himself acknowledged in his discussion of *g* we reported earlier in the chapter. Because of subtest factorial complexity, the fact that each subtest taps multiple neuropsychological processes, and these vary as a function of individual differences (Lezak et al., 2012), the utility of collapsing these disparate scores into a single IQ is highly questionable (Hale et al., 2007; Hale et al., 2016).

Although this discussion should provide you with convincing evidence that IQ should not be interpreted when significant factor or subtest variability is present, our research findings have additional implications. You might conclude that interpretation of Index or factor scores is appropriate, but the situation is more complex than that. Children's Index or factor scores are partially related to ability, partially related to prior experience with the task, and partially related to neuropsychological processing strengths and weaknesses, so it is problematic to conclude they represent unitary measures of only one ability. As a result, further hypothesis testing is needed for each individual child. We do not want to suggest here that every child with significant subtest or factor variability has a disability, because profile variability is the norm, not the exception (Hale, Fiorello, Miller, et al., 2008). In fact, given that variability is the norm for a majority of children, including those with disabilities, we need to recognize that *cognitive* diversity is important to consider in society, in addition to more commonly considered aspects of linguistic, cultural, ethnic, racial, gender, and sexual identity diversity. This finding is consistent with the emerging literature (see, e.g., Rosqvist, Chown, & Stenning, 2020), where cognitive processes in and of themselves reflect meaningful differences in learning and behavior.

Since profile variability it so common (about 80 to 85% of all people), we are simply asserting here that significant variability warrants the interpretation of cognitive strengths and weaknesses, and that this interpretive strategy is both clinically justified and empirically supported. In addition, because these scores are so factorially complex and interrelated, a simple "cookbook" interpretation approach cannot be employed, as even cross-battery proponents recognize (Flanagan et al., 2013). Interpretation must take into account not only a child's performance on the test, but also other data from prior assessments (RTI, current testing, observations, background information, and the environment) (e.g., Functional Behavior Analysis results, see Steege et al., 2019).

Intelligence Test Interpretation: Idiographic Interpretation and Demands Analysis

Because a majority of the children we see in clinical practice show significant subtest and/or factor variability, we have no choice but to interpret cognitive processes. We must be careful, however, given that misinterpretation becomes likely, especially if processing hypotheses remain untested (e.g., if they lack concurrent and ecological validity).

Many clinicians in the field apparently agree with this conclusion, as almost 90% of school psychologists use factor scores, subtest profile analysis, or both in interpreting intelligence test results (Pfeiffer et al., 2000) and continue to consider processing characteristics in the identification of SLD (Machek & Nelson, 2007). If psychologists are analyzing intelligence test data beyond IQ, they need a methodology that is likely to lead to more reliable and valid conclusions—conclusions that have ecological and treatment validity. We have developed the CHT model's methodology with this need in mind. The CHT model allows you to form and test hypotheses about a child's performance on cognitive measures, and is designed to link those findings to intervention. Only in this way can we overcome the diagnostic "leaps of faith" that have plagued idiographic interpretation for so many years.

Another problem with traditional profile analysis that must be overcome for accurate idiographic interpretation is similar to the one found for IQ: focusing on the scores instead of on children. Our approach is to include all the normative scores in a report appendix and instead talk about the child in our reports. Few consumers of psychological assessment want to hear about standard scores, percentiles, and confidence intervals—they want to hear about the child of concern. The approach we present helps you recognize that different *children may achieve the same score on the same task, but for different reasons.* Just interpreting a score, without considering *how* the child approached the task, may obscure important differences. Consider the Wechsler Block Design subtest, which can be interpreted differently based on the errors displayed on the task. One child may glance at the design and put the blocks together correctly without looking at the model, clearly using the visual gestalt and visual–spatial memory to solve the problem. Another child may look at the design and then match one block at a time, in a methodical, step-by-step fashion. A third may use a trial-and-error approach, looking back and forth between the model and the blocks, and flipping the blocks over and over until they are in the correct position, using a match-to-sample strategy. Even if all three children obtain the same score, hypotheses about their cognitive functioning would be different, as will recommendations for intervention. This is a major reason why subtest and factor profile interpretation models can also lead to erroneous conclusions, and why any hypotheses derived be verified with additional measures and/or evidence from the classroom. Clinicians using scores for interpretation often assume that there are a finite number of ways to approach a task, instead of considering the process a child uses to solve the problem.

While acknowledging that factor or subtest analysis can lead to error if we are not careful, we even recommend looking at a child's performance on the subtasks within a single subtest. For example, we found the WISC-III Digits Forward and Digits Backward subtasks to be differentially related to attention problems: Digits Forward appeared to be a test of short-term rote auditory memory span, whereas Digits Backward seemed to be related to standardized attention, working memory, executive function measures (Hale et al., 2002). In addition, the Hale et al. study found that only Digits Backward performance was related to teacher ratings of attention problems. The WISC-V provides separate process scores for Digits Forward, Digits Backward, and Digit Sequencing, so while the former measures rote auditory sequential memory, the latter two are valid working memory measures. Our demands analysis provides a methodology for analyzing the input, processing, and output demands of individual cognitive tasks, so you can more easily describe a child's strengths and weaknesses in a way that will allow you to develop useful individualized interventions. By testing the hypotheses derived from the measures, and ensuring external validity, you can truly tailor an IEP to a child's needs. The CHT model and demands analysis are described further in Chapters 3 and 4, with forms and tables to assist you in the process.

Identifying SLD: The Concordance–Discordance Model

After IDEA (Etscheidt & Curran, 2010) initially only recognized ability–achievement discrepancy and nonresponse to intervention as methods of learning disabilities identification, researchers began to question the evidence and utility of these approaches (e.g., Hale et al., 2006). In part this was because they could not address the statutory definition—that children with SLD had to have a deficit in the basic psychological processes that led to poor achievement (e.g., Jang et al., 2011; Wright et al., 2013). The Learning Disabilities Association of America held a 2010 summit where major researchers in the cognitive and neuropsychological aspects of SLD argued for a processing strengths and weaknesses approach for SLD identification, which led to a 58-author white paper advocating the approach. In that paper, Hale, Alfonso, Berninger, et al. (2010) concluded:

- The SLD definition should be maintained and statutory requirements strengthened.
- Neither ability–achievement discrepancy nor failure to respond to intervention were sufficient for SLD identification.
- A third method approach was needed to identify the pattern of psychological processing strengths and weaknesses, with the weaknesses leading to the SLD.
- RTI was needed to prevent learning problems and provide more intensive interventions, but nonresponse should lead to a comprehensive evaluation in all areas of suspected disability and individualized interventions.
- Assessment of cognitive and neuropsychological processes should be used for both assessment and intervention.

   We recommend strategies where you look for patterns of performance on both cognitive and achievement measures using what we call the concordance–discordance model (C-DM). Essentially, you are looking for a pattern of strengths and weaknesses: strengths in cognitive functioning, processing weaknesses in cognitive functioning, and associated achievement weaknesses (see Figure 1.1). You are looking for concordance between the achievement deficit and the cognitive processing weakness because this is likely the processing deficit that is causing the SLD, and discordance between the achievement deficit and the cognitive strength (see In-Depth 1.2).
   The C-DM is a *processing strengths and weaknesses* model for identifying SLD consistent with the Hale, Alfonso, Berninger, et al. (2010) white paper on SLD identification. You will sometimes see this called a "third method" (Flanagan et al., 2010) because IDEA identifies three ways that SLD can be identified: the severe discrepancy method, the RTI method, or other research-based methods. An advantage of this method, especially if nonresponse in RTI is established prior to evaluation, is that it meets both statutory and regulatory IDEA

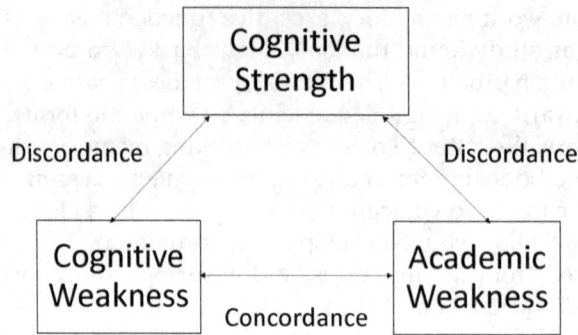

FIGURE 1.1. The concordance–discordance model.

requirements (Jang et al., 2011; Fiorello et al., 2012; Wright et al., 2013). Prominent SLD researchers Dawn Flanagan and Jack Naglieri also have similar models, with cognitive strengths, cognitive weaknesses, and associated achievement deficits at the core (Flanagan et al., 2010; Hale, Flanagan, et al., 2008), attesting to the value of this approach. With the deficit in the basic psychological processes established—something that neither discrepancy nor RTI can do and that is required by law (Wright et al., 2013)—you can be assured that a child who meets C-DM criteria meets SLD statutory and regulatory requirements, providing you with diagnostic confidence. Because of the way IDEA is written, your state or district may place limitations on the use of "third-method" approaches to SLD identification, so make sure the C-DM is acceptable before using it.

The empirical basis of this C-DM approach to SLD identification is now well-established at both the single subject and group levels of analyses, showing processing strengths and weaknesses associated with different learning and psychosocial deficits (Backenson et al., 2015; Fiorello et al., 2012; Hain & Hale, 2010; Hain et al., 2009; Hale, Alfonso, et al., 2010; Hale et al., 2013; Mascolo et al., 2009). These processing differences lead to several important SLD subtypes that show associated patterns of performance deficits on cognitive, achievement, and neuropsychological measures (Carmichael et al., 2014; Feifer et al., 2014; Kubas et al., 2014; Ortiz et al., 2014). A special issue of *Learning Disabilities–A Multidisciplinary Journal* shows empirical evidence regarding the utility of a processing strengths and weaknesses approach in identifying SLD subtypes and evaluation of ethnic minorities (see Fiorello et al., 2014; Mather & Tanner, 2014), but these studies suggest a multimethod approach instead of straight psychometric application of C-DM is required to accurately identify children with SLD.

There have been numerous attempts to discredit a pattern of strengths and weaknesses (PSW) and/or the C-DM model (e.g., Benson et al., 2020; Miciak et al., 2018), however, it should be noted that these research designs were undertaken with methodology designed to create a Type II error. For instance, Benson et al. (2020) used vignettes with school psychologists to see if they preferred a C-DM approach to nonresponse in an RTI model and ability–achievement discrepancy. The PSW vignette actually included multiple test results (e.g., more than one achievement measure), and it is unclear whether these are related to the same child, as if to show the respondent that there was no relationship between PSW and decision making regarding SLD identification. Miciak et al. (2018) also designed their study so only one processing weakness could be used to identify types of reading disorders, when our own research shows there are multiple causes. Perhaps this is why their studies failed to report published peer-reviewed evidence of the utility of PSW using C-DM; it would clue the reader into other lines of evidence that do not support their position.

IN-DEPTH 1.2. The Concordance–Discordance Model of Learning Disability Determination

Rather than using the much-maligned discrepancy model, we promote the use of a concordance–discordance model, which has three criteria that should be met for learning disability identification. Not only does this model represent a more accurate way to identify children with learning disabilities, but it could lead to more effective interventions, because it helps the team recognize each child's unique cognitive strengths and needs. When determining whether a child meets these criteria, we first look for a concordance between the deficient achievement area and the neuropsychological processes associated with that area and attempt to rule out other possible causes for the disorder. Second, we attempt to establish a discordance between the deficient achievement area and neuropsychological processes not related to the achievement area in question. Third, we look for a discordance between processing strengths and weaknesses. For example, as we discuss later in this chapter, a word-reading disorder can be due to deficits in phonemic awareness, orthographic coding skill, rapid automatic naming, processing speed, temporal sequencing of sensory input, or processing automaticity, or any combination of these (Miller & Tallal, 1995; Wolf, 2001). A comprehensive CHT evaluation may reveal deficits on measures of auditory processing and sequencing (the processing weakness cluster), and good performance on measures of nonverbal reasoning and visual–perceptual skills (the processing strength cluster). These subtest scores could be used to create composite weakness and strength cluster scores for the child. Based on these scores, the child should demonstrate a significant difference (in terms of standard error of the difference [SED]; see Chapter 3, Application 3.4) between the strength cluster and the weakness cluster, and a significant difference between the strength cluster and the achievement deficit score, but no significant difference between the weakness cluster and the achievement deficit score. Once you identify the deficit area in both processing and achievement, you need only to find a processing area unrelated to the achievement deficit (demonstrated by research), and you have both concordance and discordance—a process graphically represented in Figure 1.1.

In the CHT model, if *no* processing weaknesses associated with academic deficits are identified, this suggests that the difficulties may be primarily the results of other causes. Consistent with this line of reasoning, if processing areas thought to be *unrelated* to the deficient academic area are also deficient, then the child would be considered a low achiever, as all skills would be low. Although we generally adhere to the National Association of School Psychologists' position that children should be served without the need to label them, we believe that the concordance–discordance model can be used to identify children with learning disabilities more accurately.

We admonish practitioners not to become overly focused on statistical comparisons of data to determine eligibility for learning disability services. As noted throughout this book, you must use multiple assessment tools and collect data from multiple sources if you are to recognize a child's unique strengths and needs, and to ensure that your diagnostic and treatment decisions have ecological and treatment validity.

Not only is a PSW approach supported by the 58-expert white paper (Hale, Alfonso, Berninger, et al., 2010) and the law (Wright et al., 2013), it is also supported by empirical research. Although not exhaustive of all methods using a PSW approach, it is important to note that the C-DM/PSW approach has been used in multiple lines of research. It has been used to show the relevance for cognitive processes in reading (Elliott et al., 2010; Fiorello et al., 2006; Hale et al., 2001; Hale, Fiorello, et al., 2008), mathematics (Hale et al., 2001; Hale, Fiorello, et al., 2008), and written expression (Fenwick et al., 2016). It has also been shown to detect cognitive processing characteristics in children with SLD and emotional/behavior disability (Backenson et al., 2013; Hale et al., 2013).

Factors Influencing Intelligence Test Interpretation

Numerous additional factors can affect the conclusions you draw about a child's test performance, several of which we briefly review here, including test behavior, technical adequacy, linguistic/cultural sensitivity, and ecological validity.

In regard to test behavior, any interpretation must take into account the wide array of child behaviors displayed during testing. Although we all learn about this during graduate school, we tend not to notice the subtle variations in test performance that can affect interpretation (Hale & Fiorello, 2002). Sattler (2014) provides guidelines for observing specific behaviors that may indicate performance variability and psychological problems. These observations, combined with observations in the natural environment and input from parents and teachers, can provide important contextual information for interpreting the child's test performance. The reality is that some of the problems associated with idiographic subtest interpretation are related to child performance and examiner administration consistency (Hale et al., 2018; McDermott et al., 2013). In other words, some of the variance we are interested in is *trait* variance, while some of it is *state* variance, which will vacillate from between and within testing sessions; that is why repeated assessment, hypothesis testing, and establishing ecological validity are so critical in practice, as advocated in the CHT approach.

We will assume that you are already familiar with how to assess the technical adequacy of a test—an issue that has been covered extensively elsewhere and thus is not reviewed here. Good resources include Sattler's (2014) *Foundations of Behavioral, Social, and Clinical Assessment of Children,* Flanagan and McDonough's (2018) *Contemporary Intellectual Assessment, Fourth Edition,* and Bracken's (1988) classic article, "Ten Psychometric Reasons Why Similar Tests Produce Dissimilar Results." We would like to stress, though, that no test should be administered to a child unless its reliability, validity, floor, and ceiling are sufficient to permit you to draw conclusions about the child's performance. In addition, you should consider issues of content validity and sample space, to ensure that you are not drawing conclusions about a broad area of skills based on a very small sample of actual behavior. Also recall from our earlier discussion that construct validity, which is critical for interpretation, may vary among children with disabilities (Hale et al., 2013), so while the analyses provided in CHC factor analyses found in cross-battery texts (e.g., Flanagan et al., 2013), are a good place to start for interpretation given their converging relationship to neuropsychological processes (Fiorello et al., 2008), the findings are not uniform for all children.

We have previously discussed linguistic and cultural sensitivity in interpretation, arguing that crystallized abilities or skills are related to prior experience and education. Although crystallized skills are of critical importance in a psychological evaluation, it is essential to remember that they are significantly affected by a child's language, educational experience, and sociocultural background. We have argued that tests measure different things for different children, and this is certainly the case for many children with racial, ethnic, linguistic, cultural, and/or cognitive differences. The questions of test appropriateness raised here allow us to review "test bias," a statistical concept that determines whether the statistical properties of a test are the same for different groups. The following questions are often used to determine whether a test or task is biased:

- Is the item difficulty the same for all children?
- Is the reliability the same for all children?
- Is the test score prediction of school or occupational success the same for everyone?
- Is the underlying structure or model of the test the same across groups?

Since modern test developers examine these factors, no modern test of cognitive functioning is statistically biased. The absence of bias does not mean that a test is uniformly *fair* for all children, however. Fairness takes a child's linguistic and sociocultural background, and formal and informal educational opportunities, into account. An IQ score will not be biased as long as it equally predicts school success for all children, but it is not fair to conclude that children with linguistic, sociocultural, or experiential differences are unintelligent because they have a low IQ score.

The relationship between a child's environment and test performance is bidirectional if assessment and intervention are to have ecological validity. Comparing the conclusions about input, processing, and output demands that you draw from a child's performance to indicators of classroom performance and behavior will help establish the accuracy of your interpretations. For example, poor WISC-V Processing Speed performance may reflect a variety of problems, including limited attention to detail, visual acuity, visual scanning, processing speed, psychomotor speed, fine-motor coordination, graphomotor skills, and/or associative learning. Simply listing these in a report would be a meaningless "cookbook" approach, unrelated to the child's current functioning or to needed interventions. It is your responsibility as a clinician to evaluate these as hypotheses, comparing them to results from other tests and other evaluation information (see Case Study 1.3).

Although clinical judgment and teacher impressions are important for establishing ecological validity, you should, whenever possible, use direct observation and classroom behavior rating scales to obtain objective information about a child's behavior in the classroom. Systematic observations, whether you use time sampling, interval recording, latency/duration, or event recording, can provide important ecological validity information. Several formal coding systems have also been developed, such as the Achenbach System of Empirically Based Assessment (ASEBA) Direct Observation Form (McConaughy & Achenbach, 2009), or the Behavior Assessment System for Children, third edition—Student Observation System (BASC-3-SOS; Reynolds et al., 2015). We recommend starting with an anecdotal observation that codes a variety of child and teacher behaviors. After the informal observation, choose specific target behavior(s) and compare the child to a control peer. Sattler and Hoge (2005) provide a good overview of various observation systems. Another source of ecological validity information can come from behavior rating scales, which are easy to administer and score, and usually have good psychometric properties. As opposed to direct observation methods, ratings sample behaviors over an extended time, so they are useful for both diagnosis and treatment. It is important to keep in mind that parent and teacher ratings are subject to bias, due to differing expectations or tolerance for behaviors. Examples of broad classroom behavior rating scales that have good psychometric characteristics are the ASEBA Teacher Report Form (Achenbach & Rescorla, 2001) and the BASC-3 Teacher Rating Scale (BASC-3-TRS; Reynolds et al., 2015).

| Case Study 1.3. Jordan's Slow and Sloppy Work |

Imagine that you have a student, Jordan, who was referred for testing because she was slow to complete her written work. You found that her work samples showed messy writing, with some evidence of poor spacing and coordination. Her WISC-V results revealed poor Processing Speed performance and some difficulty with Working Memory. There are several hypotheses you would be likely to consider. Besides slow processing speed, which might also reflect attentional or affective problems, you might consider deficits in visual tracking, perception, visual–motor integration, fine-motor coordination, graphomotor abilities, or executive function. What further testing and observations might you use to test these hypotheses? You might do further testing with something like the Beery Developmental Test of Visual–Motor Integration to decide whether difficulties with visual–motor integration, visual discrimination, and/or fine-motor coordination were contributing to the problem. A computer-based test of attention (such as the Tests of Variables of Attention), or the CAS2 Attention or Planning scales, or the NEPSY-II Attention/Executive Functions subtests might help you decide whether attention or executive function problems were contributing. What behaviors might you see in the classroom that would help you evaluate these different hypotheses? Jordan might show signs of neglect of herself (e.g., appearing disheveled) or of the environment (e.g., missing information from the board). She might bump into other people or not catch baseballs well. Fine-motor problems might show up in difficulties with tying shoelaces or fastening her coat. Visual–motor integration problems might lead to a tendency to use "abstract" drawings in art class, as well as the messy handwriting and poor spacing already noted. Copying from the board could be difficult for Jordan, and she might fall behind during note taking or not write the correct information in her notes. Jordan's attention during activities not involving visual–motor skills, such as listening while the teacher reads a story, might indicate whether attention is a problem. And planning and other executive function deficits might reveal themselves in difficulties with transition times (such as getting ready to leave at the end of the day), playing age-appropriate games at recess, or completing complex multistep tasks (e.g., research papers). Finally, Jordan could be depressed, so you might look for signs of mood disturbance, such as flat affect, anhedonia, and withdrawal. It is your job as a clinician to consider all of this information in deciding on a probable cause for Jordan's difficulties, and to work with the teacher to design and monitor an appropriate intervention. This will ensure the ecological validity of your findings.

A Practitioner's Guide to Intelligent Cognitive Assessment

Before we leave our blueprint for the practice of psychological assessment in the schools, we think it is important to take a minute to review the major points presented in the preceding sections. This blueprint serves as a foundation for much of the material presented in later chapters. Table 1.6 provides a number of suggestions we originally presented in a journal article (Hale & Fiorello, 2001).

Are you a clumper or a splitter, or do you agree with us that you should be both? We think it is always better (more reliable and likely more valid) to interpret at the highest level possible. But if subcomponent scores measuring a factor do not hold together, you have to determine why, and that is where CHT becomes critical. So you clump whenever possible, split when you have to, and then clump again to add weight to your diagnostic impressions during case conceptualization. You may have other points you would add to this synthesis, and this is a good idea. However, probably the most important thing you can realize from this discussion is that intellectual/cognitive assessment is a part of what we do, but it is by no means the only thing we should do as psychologists. These measures are only *tools* for use in a more comprehensive service delivery model that includes assessment and intervention. In the chapters that follow, we will demonstrate the utility of CHT evaluations in helping children with their learning and behavior problems. This is the true test of any psychological measure or approach—the practitioner's skill at linking assessment to intervention.

Now that we have reviewed the basic issues related to intelligence/cognitive assessment, the factors involved in administration and interpretation of intelligence tests, and the commonly used measures of intellectual/cognitive functioning, let us turn our attention to several critical issues related to the practice of psychological assessment in the schools. These issues include identification of children with disabilities, complying with clinical and legal mandates, trends in service delivery, and linking assessment results to intervention.

Critical Issues in Assessment Service Delivery

Identifying Children with Disabilities

Unlike private practitioners, psychologists in the schools (or any other individual team members, for that matter) cannot identify a child with a disability. The multidisciplinary team determines eligibility, placement, and services under special education law. Therefore, you are not individually responsible for identifying the child's problem or proposing a solution. How does this affect your diagnostic practice? First, differential diagnosis is determined by examining whether a child meets diagnostic criteria specified by professional consensus. A neurologist has criteria for diagnosing epilepsy, a psychiatrist has criteria for diagnosing Tourette syndrome, and a speech–language pathologist has criteria for diagnosing developmental aphasia. A particular professional does an evaluation and diagnoses the child as having a particular disorder. What are the advantages and disadvantages of such diagnoses? Are they relevant for identification, eligibility, placement, or treatment?

Does having a disorder automatically make a child eligible for special education services? The short answer is *no*; the school's multidisciplinary team must review and gather

---

TABLE 1.6. A Practitioner's Guide to Intelligence Testing

- Intervene to assess. Reducing the number of referrals will result in better evaluations and ecological validity.
- Read recent theoretical, empirical, and practice-oriented literature on intelligence and its assessment.
- Explore neuropsychological literature for cognitive, achievement, and behavioral applications.
- Supplement core intellectual assessment tool with additional measures to ensure that all cognitive domains are assessed.
- Assess attention, memory, and executive functions as critical constructs related to school success.
- Interpret crystallized abilities in light of cultural, linguistic, and experiential background.
- Administer new measures of learning and memory to assess potential, rather than inferring it from crystallized measures.
- Interpret both level and/or pattern of performance based on individual child's profile.
- Interpret global intellectual scores only when there is no significant factor or subtest variability.
- Use demands analysis to examine input, processing, and output demands, but avoid "cookbooking," and test hypotheses to ensure ecological validity.
- Test assessment and intervention hypotheses over time, using single-subject experimental designs.
- Avoid confirmation bias; consider alternative hypotheses and interventions to meet child's unique needs.

Note. From Hale and Fiorello (2001). Copyright © 2001 the American Psychological Association. Adapted by permission.

additional information to decide whether the child is eligible. You don't have to be intimi-dated into providing special education for a child just because a physician wrote "Dyslexia—provide special education" on a prescription pad! In fact, the word "dyslexia" has little utility in and of itself, other than to suggest that the child has a reading disorder. Several times, I (Fiorello) have been asked by interns whether they can "diagnose" a child. I tell them that as licensed psychologists, they may be professionally qualified to diagnose a child as having a specific disorder. But does the diagnosis make the child automatically eligible for special education services? The answer is no. Even though you are a school professional and a mem-ber of the multidisciplinary team, you cannot unilaterally decide that a child is eligible. This can be frustrating when you know a child has a disorder and meets requirements for clini-cal diagnosis but does not meet the necessary IDEA criteria for services. It is important to remember that every referral must go through the team process to decide whether it meets all three eligibility questions:

- Does the child meet criteria for one or more of the existing disability categories?
- Does the child's disorder have an adverse impact on educational performance?
- Does the child need specially designed instruction to ensure a free, appropriate public education (FAPE)?

You probably have appropriate concerns about diagnosing and labeling children, but it is important to consider that many children suffer negative effects when their school prob-lems are obvious to teachers and peers, even without the label (e.g., see Riddick, 2000). A potentially more serious problem is the risk that a child's parents and teachers—and even the child—might have lower expectations because of the label or a self-fulfilling prophecy of failure (Rosenthal & Jacobson, 1968), although this tendency appears to decrease over time (Harris, 1991). Labels serve multiple purposes, but it is important to realize that they are only useful if they allow for accurate identification of child needs and help to identify appropriate services for the child. A label can tie together disparate problems, making them more under-standable and manageable for all involved in the child's care. Keep in mind that a label may also make it easier for students and families to find resources and access support groups.

Another consideration here is specificity of diagnosis and its relevance in schools. Given the broad categories (e.g., learning disorder, emotional disturbance), it does not seem rel-evant for entitlement purposes, but it is certainly relevant for intervention. Is a child's atten-tion problem due to ADHD, depression, learning disability, or a host of other possibilities? You cannot just have parents complete a checklist or respond to DSM-5-TR criteria and say, "Joey has ADHD, predominantly inattentive presentation." You must make every attempt to find out the exact nature of the attention problem, so that appropriate interventions can be attempted. For instance, Hale et al. (2011) showed that some carefully diagnosed children with ADHD did not have the disorder (e.g., "pseudo-ADHD"), or at least the type of ADHD that responds to medication, while those with "true" ADHD all responded to medication. We recommend the following principles for identifying or labeling children in order to maxi-mize the benefits and minimize the costs:

- Never avoid clinical labels because determining educational disability does not require them.
- Never use a label to "admire the problem"—ensure that it leads to appropriate inter-vention.
- Never label a child unless you believe that the label is accurate (e.g., to get services).
- Never use a label as an excuse for a child's continued difficulty or failures.

Complying with Legal Mandates

As you are well aware, the IDEA and Section 504 of the Rehabilitation Act (1973a, 1973b), and the Americans with Disabilities Act (ADA, 1990; ADA Amendments Act, 2008) are the major pieces of legislation governing the practice of psychology in the schools. Intended to serve the educational needs of children with disabilities, IDEA provides for identification of all district students with disabilities (i.e., "Child Find"); comprehensive evaluations of all areas of suspected disability; and specially designed instruction and related services to ensure that each child receives FAPE, which have been affirmed in the Supreme Court (Hess et al., 2010; Wright et al., 2013). Section 504 of the Rehabilitation Act and ADA are both civil rights laws that protect children and adults with disabilities from discrimination. Schools are required to provide reasonable modifications and accommodations to ensure that students have access to educational programs, but they are not required to develop an IDEA-specified IEP to serve the child. Instead, they should develop a 504/ADA plan that specifies the modifications and accommodations the student will receive.

What if a child has a significant disability (e.g., anorexia) but because their cognitive pattern (e.g., obsessive–compulsive disorder) leads to high achievement, they may not be showing significant academic deficits, but still need accommodations to overcome their psychosocial difficulties? Do remember that educational impact is not necessarily academic impact—a student may qualify under IDEA even with average achievement scores if there is adverse educational impact. But qualifying for protection under 504/ADA is different from that under the IDEA. The student must have a "physical or mental impairment that substantially limits at least one major life activity" (ADAAA, 2008), but there is little further definition of such terms as "substantial" or "limits." However, the amendments have clarified that "substantial" is not to be interpreted as significant or severe. As a result, qualifying as disabled under 504/ADA is typically less stringent than qualifying under the IDEA. As a result, team members may see 504/ADA qualification as a backup plan for any student who doesn't qualify for IDEA services. However, note that both require identification of a disability or impairment. If the student's disability does not fall into one of the IDEA categories (i.e., educational impairment required), or if the student requires accommodations but not specially designed instruction, the student can be served under 504/ADA. Your diagnosis, or that of an outside provider, may be one component of eligibility for a 504 plan. Many school districts use the same procedures for 504 as they do for IDEA, but they are not required to, so be sure you know and understand the procedures and regulations in your jurisdiction.

Sometimes the issue is not just serving children's needs; it also involves funding those services. Schools do not receive any federal money for providing 504/ADA accommodations, so from a strictly behavioral perspective, there is less incentive for serving children under these laws. This can be a real tragedy for some children, as needed services may be withheld until a struggling child falls far enough behind to qualify under the IDEA. Meeting children's needs should not be based on whether they fit categories or labels, but this is often the case. This is especially true in cases that are less clear-cut, when you may be pressured to identify a child as having a disability so that the child can receive services or not identify a child because the difficulties are not considered great enough. In such cases, legal and ethical expectations may come into conflict, leading you to a less than desirable outcome. As you are a child advocate, you must decide how to resolve the situation, and when in doubt, Child Find requires every school district to search for and identify children with disabilities residing in their jurisdiction (Wright et al., 2013).

You must remember that if children meet IDEA or 504/ADA criteria, they must be provided with services. However, it is important to remember that whether children are served under the IDEA or 504/ADA, they should be served in the least restrictive environment (LRE) to meet their needs. The fact that children are identified as having a disability doesn't mean that they cannot be fully served in a regular education or inclusive classroom, which is the preferred setting if it meets their academic and psychosocial needs. Being labeled with a disability doesn't automatically mean a need for segregation, as there is a long history of the detriments of special education segregation (Crockett & Kaufman, 2013).

Trends in Service Delivery

Since the original passage of Public Law 94-142, special education law has called for students to receive a FAPE in the LRE, while still receiving a continuum of services. The law requires that each child's needs must be individually assessed, eligibility must be determined, and *then* the team must decide where the instruction should take place. You should never decide to label a child because you have room in a classroom, or a team member has time to work with him or her. It is presumed that the primary placement should be in general education with supplementary aids and services, but if that is not possible, more restrictive placement options must be available. Three factors need to be taken into account when deciding what the LRE is: the academic benefits versus costs of each setting for the student; the socioemotional benefits versus costs of the settings; and the degree of class disruption that makes satisfactory education impossible. These factors lead to a very difficult ethical issue that schools must address. They are somewhat vague factors, but considerations worthy of examination nonetheless. They were also ever so important in the age of online learning during the pandemic. For instance, a student cannot qualify for special education if the achievement deficits are caused by a lack of quality, empirically based instruction.

Does this mean that the IDEA mandates inclusion? The answer is no. "Inclusion" and its predecessor, "the regular education initiative," are not part of the law; definitions in the research literature and schools vary, but inclusion is not synonymous with LRE. Inclusion is commonly defined as serving a student with a disability in a general education classroom with necessary supports and services (e.g., Lipsky & Gartner, 1995). The major difference is that the IDEA requires a continuum of placements to be available if education in the inclusive setting is *not* working. A child with an auditory processing disorder will struggle in a lecture class without a note taker, written notes/instructions, audio recording, or some other accommodation to meet his or her needs. As teachers become better trained in individual differences, they can provide differentiated instruction to meet the needs of many children with learning differences and disabilities (Gregory & Chapman, 2012; Hale et al., 2013). In addition, the IDEA considers resource room or pullout services to be part of the supplementary supports and accommodations provided in the LRE (Heumann & Hehir, 1994), whereas many inclusion advocates consider resource room placement as noninclusive (Vaughn et al., 2024). Full inclusion of a student with intellectual disability in an English literature class that studies Shakespeare is a clear example of a case when the LRE is not the general education classroom, because the student is unlikely to benefit from that instruction.

It is important to remember that the LRE is really the LRE *that meets the child's needs.* What does the research tell us about inclusion? When appropriate services and supports are provided, the outcomes of inclusion are generally positive both for the student with a disability and for his or her classmates (Alquraini & Gut, 2012; Boyle et al., 2011). But if a student with a disability is placed in a general education classroom without appropriate services, continued academic and peer difficulties can be expected (Fiorello et al., 1999). If general education teachers are provided with adequate training and staff resources, most are willing to serve children with disabilities in their classrooms (Mastropieri et al., 2013). However, the team members must ensure that the child's IEP services are provided in the LRE and must keep in mind that the LRE is not always the general education classroom. Thus, it is a team decision about how best to meet a student's instructional needs.

We have now examined your involvement in assessment and placement of children with disabilities, which have been the traditional concerns of psychologists practicing in the schools. However, these are not the only roles of school psychologists. Before we end this introductory chapter, it is important to consider one more area that has been largely neglected until relatively recently in the literature and in training programs. This role—one that is essential to serving the needs of children—may be the one that you feel least comfortable with: linking assessment results to intervention.

Linking Assessment Results to Intervention

Too many times, psychologists tend to see themselves solely as diagnosticians. As a psychologist conducting individual evaluations in the schools, you have *two* major objectives: identifying child strengths and difficulties (i.e., problem identification and analysis), and providing interventions to ameliorate the problems (i.e., instructional design, implementation, and evaluation). Linking assessment information to intervention is one of the main tasks of school assessment teams. Many years ago, before we had a good understanding of brain-behavior relationships, researchers examined aptitude–treatment interactions (ATIs) or the diagnostic–prescriptive model. The purpose of this work was to identify links between specific assessment results and interventions. Early ATI researchers focused on identifying modality or perceptual weaknesses in children (e.g., auditory or visual), implementing group interventions to strengthen children who apparently had the weak modality, and, finally, assessing whether the targeted ability or related achievement improved as a result of the intervention (see Ysseldyke & Sabatino, 1973; Hammill & Larsen, 1974). Reviews of that early research have consistently found limited support for either the modality or perceptual training model of instruction (e.g., Hessler & Sosnowsky, 1979; Kavale & Forness, 1999; Ysseldyke & Sabatino, 1973), or for matching academic instruction to students' strongest learning modality (auditory, visual, or kinesthetic) (Braden & Kratochwill, 1997; Kavale & Forness, 1999).

Because most ATI research occurred when investigators had poor assessment instruments and a limited understanding of brain functions, early ATI research failures have been attributed to a variety of reasons. Many cognitive constructs were poorly defined or poorly measured (Ysseldyke & Salvia, 1974). Often, heterogeneous groups were simply divided at the median to define "high" and "low" groups. Treatments were also poorly defined or implemented without integrity checks (Reynolds, 1988). Some studies have used the original Kaufman Assessment Battery for Children (Kaufman & Kaufman, 1983) simultaneous or sequential processing strengths to develop instructional interventions, but with limited success (Ayres & Cooley, 1986; Fisher et al., 1988; Good et al., 1993). However, as we will see in Chapter 3, this may be in part due to the assumption that the left hemisphere processes information sequentially and the right hemisphere processes simultaneous information—an assumption that does not fully reflect current beliefs about hemispheric functioning (Bryan & Hale, 2001).

Because of the failure to find ATIs, Ysseldyke and Sabatino (1973) recommended assessing and remediating academic skill deficits instead of searching for "aptitudes," a point echoed by Hammill and Larsen (1974) in his disavowal of ATI. It is interesting to note that the seeds of Ysseldyke's (2014) fervent "paradigm shift" position advocating elimination of intelligence/cognitive testing were probably sown after his own early ATI study was unsuccessful. As Braden and Kratochwill (1997) have noted, however, the fact that ATIs weren't established in the past doesn't mean that they can't be established in the future, especially at the single-subject level of analysis. Recall from your research training that we can reject or fail to reject the null hypothesis in research, we should never *accept* the null hypothesis. Changing the focus from the *content* of test items (e.g., auditory, visual) to the underlying psychological *processes* (Fiorello et al., 2007; Reynolds et al., 1997) may be the key to understanding the true nature of brain–behavior relationships for individual children.

Since these early studies, research on cognitive/neuropsychological processes and their relationship to intervention has developed, but no one calls them ATIs anymore, perhaps because we don't even know what an "aptitude" is. In fact, in modern research, speech–language pathologists, occupational therapists, and physical therapists frequently use single-subject designs to demonstrate these assessment-intervention associations. Psycholinguistic training, which identifies students' weaknesses and provides individualized, prescriptive instruction, has led to significant improvement in students' language skills (Kavale & Forness, 1999). Interventions focusing on vocabulary, verbal reasoning, and memory are more effective for students with SLD and language deficits than for typically achieving students (Hay, 2007); while phoneme/grapheme training is more effective than lexical/semantic instruction for students with word-level reading difficulties (Wise et al., 2007).

Another cognitive assessment-intervention study found that a mediated learning program was best for preschool special education students with language impairments, but that a direct instruction model was best for those with higher language skills. Performance on the CAS-2 (Naglieri et al., 2014) Planning, Attention, and Simultaneous and Successive Processing scales (PASS) has been linked to intervention with the PASS Remedial Program (PREP). Studies using the PREP have shown improvement not only in Simultaneous and Successive Processing scores, but also in reading and mathematics scores (Naglieri & Otero, 2017).

There have been numerous calls for cognitive assessment-intervention research studies that examine the multivariate nature of cognitive constructs, and that address the technical issues associated with treatment development and integrity (e.g., Braden & Kratochwill, 1997; Deno, 1990; Reynolds, 1988; Speece, 1990). In addition to improvements in the "cognitive" portion of the equation, the "treatment" portion needs attention as well. Two models, a deficit remediation model and a strength-based instructional model, are possible. When deficit remediation instruction is explicitly linked to academics, either during initial training or through a training transfer process, improvement in academic performance has been reported. Responsiveness to phonological and metacognitive instruction caused differential improvement in children with phonological, rapid automatized naming, and double-deficit groups (Lovett et al., 2000). Students with reading difficulties in a study by Helland (2006) showed different patterns of phonological, visual–spatial, and executive skills according to whether they demonstrated orthographic or phonological weaknesses, and they also responded differentially to interventions. As guest editors of the *Journal of Learning Disabilities,* Fuchs and colleagues (2011) ensured all studies in the special issue showed the relevance of cognitive assessment for intervention, but this work is seldom reported in pro-RTI studies.

The strength-based model has some theoretical support, but has been inadequately assessed (Reynolds, 1988). One study of students with orthographic and phonological deficits specifically addressed this, and found better response to interventions targeting their weaknesses than interventions using their strengths (Gustafson et al., 2007). However, a study of children with right hemisphere ("nonverbal") SLD showed that strength-based verbal mediation was effective in improving academic achievement and brain functioning (Tuller et al., 2007). Because group designs may obscure individual differences, single-case research using within-subject experimental methodology has been recommended as the preferred way to study cognitive assessment-intervention relationships (Braden & Kratochwill, 1997). In later chapters, we will argue that our CHT model (which is composed of neuropsychological interpretation of test data and verification of initial hypotheses), incorporates methods for ensuring ecological validity, and continual monitoring of intervention effectiveness until treatment efficacy is achieved. This research shows how to link assessment to intervention for individualized service delivery to children, leading to successful treatment outcomes for affected children (Hain & Hale, 2010; Mascolo et al., 2009). They make a convincing argument against strength-based instruction from a neurodevelopmental perspective, that we should be remediating, not compensating for, processing weaknesses.

Although we will address neuropsychological response-to-intervention later in this book, we would like to draw your attention to a special issue of the *Journal of Learning Disabilities* (see Fuchs et al., 2011) devoted to the relevance of cognitive processes related to intervention. In this issue, investigators showed the relationship between psychological and/or neuropsychological processes in serving children with reading difficulties and disabilities (Frijters et al., 2011; Fuchs et al., 2011; Helland et al., 2011; Larusso et al., 2011), math disabilities (Iseman & Naglieri, 2011), written language disabilities (Berninger & O'Malley-May, 2011), and ADHD (Hale et al., 2011). This special issue also reviewed many other studies that show these cognitive-intervention relationships. Probably the leader in establishing brain-behavior-intervention relationships is Virginia Berninger, who has dozens of studies for your consideration. Berninger and Dunn's (2012) book *Brain and Behavioral Response to Intervention for Specific Reading, Math, and Writing Disabilities; What Works for Whom?* is exactly the type of work we expect to see more of in the future.

As you can see, there is a great deal of information that can be derived from individual cognitive assessment, which is why we recommend that it always be a part of a comprehensive assessment. However, simply giving a test and reporting an IQ does very little to help children, whereas integrating RTI with cognitive and neuropsychological assessment into the CHT model will serve most children, including those with and without disabilities. Through teaching practitioners and educators about what has been termed "brain literacy," we can begin to provide instructional environments that are sensitive to individual needs (Walker et al., 2019). With this foundation in mind, let's turn to a model of brain functioning, one that will lead to a better understanding of psychological processes that will facilitate your ability to link assessment to intervention for children with and without disabilities.

SCHOOL NEUROPSYCHOLOGY

54

APPENDIX 1.1. FURTHER READINGS IN THE INTELLIGENCE DEBATE

Canivez, G. L., McGill, R. J., Dombrowski, S. C., Watkins, M. W., Pritchard, A. E., & Jacobson, L. A. (2020). Construct validity of the WISC-V in clinical cases: Exploratory and confirmatory factor analyses of the 10 primary subtests. *Assessment, 27*(2), 274–296.

Carroll, J. B. (1993). *Human cognitive abilities: A survey of factor-analytic studies.* Cambridge University Press.

Chen, J.-Q., & Gardner, H. (2018). Assessment from the perspective of Multiple-Intelligences Theory: Principles, practices, and values. In D. P. Flanagan & E. M. McDonough (Eds.), *Contemporary intellectual assessment: Theories, tests, and issues* (4th ed., pp. 164–173). Guilford Press.

Flanagan, D. P., Ortiz, S. O., & Alfonso, V. C. (2013). *Essentials of cross-battery assessment* (3rd ed.). Wiley.

Gottfredson, L. S. (1997). Why *g* matters: The complexity of everyday life. *Intelligence, 24*, 79–132.

Graves, S. L., Jr., & Nichols, K. (2016). Intellectual assessment of ethnic minority children. In S. L. Graves, Jr., & J. J. Blake (Eds.), *Psychoeducational assessment and intervention for ethnic minority children: Evidence-based approaches* (pp. 61–76). American Psychological Association.

Gresham, F. M., & Witt, J. C. (1997). Utility of intelligence tests for treatment planning, classification, and placement decisions: Recent empirical findings and future directions. *School Psychology Quarterly, 12*, 249–267.

Jensen, A. R. (1998). *The g factor: The science of mental ability.* Praeger.

Kaufman, A. S. (1994). *Intelligent testing with the WISC-III.* Wiley.

McDermott, P. A., Fantuzzo, J. W., & Glutting, J. J. (1990). Just say no to subtest analysis: A critique on Wechsler theory and practice. *Journal of Psychoeducational Assessment, 8*, 290–302.

Sattler, J. M. (2020). *Assessment of children: Cognitive foundations and applications* (6th ed.). Author.

Sternberg, R. J. (2018). The triarchic theory of successful intelligence. In D. P. Flanagan & E. M. McDonough (Eds.), *Contemporary intellectual assessment: Theories, tests, and issues* (4th ed., pp. 174–194). Guilford Press.

Watkins, M. W., & Canivez, G. L. (2022). Assessing the psychometric utility of IQ scores: A tutorial using the Wechsler Intelligence Scale for Children—Fifth edition. *School Psychology Review, 5*(5), 619–633.

Woodcock, R. W. (1993). An information processing view of *Gf–Gc* theory. *Journal of Psychoeducational Assessment (WJ-R Monograph)*, 80–102.

Ysseldyke, J. E., & Reschly, D. J. (2014). The evolution of school psychology: Origins, contemporary status, and future directions. In P. Harrison & A. Thomas (Eds.), *Best practices in school psychology: Vol. I. Data-based and collaborative decision making* (pp. 71–86). National Association of School Psychologists.

Chapter 2

A Model of Brain Functioning

A Developmental Perspective

Child Neuropsychology, or Neuropsychology Applied to Children?

A child is not a miniature adult. From the outset of our discussion on brain–behavior relationships, it is important to recognize that there are important brain differences between children and adults, which have implications for assessment and intervention (Yeates et al., 2009). Every child neuropsychology text will make this proclamation with great conviction, and then report literature on adult patients. There is much more adult neuropsychology literature than on child neuropsychology, so this limitation affects almost all neuropsychology texts, including ours. Our book is somewhat different, however, in that we focus on developmental issues and primarily report literature relevant to practice with children. Although there is less brain research on children than adults, this situation is changing at a phenomenal rate. With the advent of noninvasive neuroimaging techniques, there are more and more data both on typical children and on those with disabilities (e.g., Bednarz & Kana, 2019).

Although the brain changes throughout life, it is important to recognize that the most dramatic changes occur during childhood (Casey et al., 2005; Sowell et al., 2003). The broad conclusion that there are significant brain–behavior differences between adults and children is true, but recent findings continue to dispel myths about child brain function and dysfunction. Long-held beliefs that children with genetic or traumatic causes for their learning and behavior problems do not suffer the same deleterious effects as adults with these conditions are no longer considered accurate (Dennis, 2010). In fact, the opposite may be true; some studies have suggested more adverse outcomes for children, depending on the developmental level at which a disorder is first recognized and treated (Anderson et al., 2011).

In addition, it is important to realize that we are talking not just about neurodevelopmental issues applied to genetic conditions and brain trauma, but about the many types of learning and behavior disorders that have been linked to abnormal brain development (Arnsten & Rubia, 2012; Giedd & Rapoport, 2010). For example, there is now research that children of immigrants who move to the United States and who come from violent environments, have a higher incidence of autism (Dealberto, 2011). It is hypothesized that this incidence may be due to conditions in the country of origin as well as the stress of adapting to the new environment in the United States (Keen et al., 2010).

Development must be taken into account in any consideration of brain function and dysfunction. Brain development is inextricably related to the environment in a reciprocal manner, as Bandura (1978) posited many years ago. Although some clinicians diagnose attention deficits in 3-year-olds, this procedure is particularly challenging, even for seasoned practitioners. Based on what we know about the brain and executive functions at that age, we might *expect* a toddler to have attention deficits. Today's researchers are trying to do what was inconceivable many years ago—early diagnosis and intervention for children suspected of ADHD (e.g., Young et al., 2021). However, application of this research to individual children is difficult given the relationship between a child's brain development, his or her behavioral self-control, and what is expected from others in the child's world. One of us (Hale) usually says, "If children don't have attention deficits when they are 3 years old, I think something must be wrong." Discrimination of typical and atypical attention at any age is difficult, especially at this young age. This is why a dimensional perspective may be more advantageous than a categorical one. It is the relationship of the child's individual differences to their neurodevelopment that challenges even the seasoned veteran.

Surely, given that ADHD has deleterious effects on cognition, learning, and behavior, early identification of ADHD is a good thing; as we will see, however, the brain areas that help control attention are not well developed in preschoolers, and maturation of these areas is not complete until adulthood (Giedd & Rapoport, 2010). In fact, the last brain area to fully develop has to do with social and emotional behavior control (Lebel et al., 2008). This area is important for what we call "theory of mind"—the ability to take the perspective of others, a key ability for empathy. In fact, the uncinate fasciculus, a key white matter pathway that connects this emotional regulation brain area with subcortical emotional structures is not fully developed until after adolescence (Olson et al., 2015), which has direct implications for understanding emotional and behavioral disorders. This knowledge of neurodevelopment can inform our understanding of children's relationships with others. For instance, can we really expect rich intimate social attachment in a child or adolescent who has not yet fully developed the area of the brain important for perspective taking and empathy? How does this knowledge inform our judgments about children who have conduct problems and commit crimes against others?

It is important for all of us to recognize that neurodevelopmental changes occur in children, and at different rates for different children. Is the test performance we are seeing during an assessment due to these neurodevelopmental differences, to a genetic condition, to abnormal neural organization, to a "typical fall" head trauma, or to the psychometric characteristics of the test we're using? Only seasoned clinicians—investigators with a wealth of clinical acumen—can answer these questions. But rest assured, the answer is never easy to ascertain for a child; in fact, it isn't easy for *every* child we see if we do our job well. It is always a combination of factors that leads to the child's current status, to say otherwise is reductionistic and minimizes our potential in serving children and their needs. With these caveats in mind, let's begin our understanding with what we know about typical and atypical developmental changes and the brain.

Typical and Atypical Brain Development

Developmentally, many changes occur in the central nervous system (CNS) before birth, and they continue throughout life. There are four distinct phases of early brain development: the birth of neurons, cell migration, cell differentiation/maturation, and cell death/synaptic pruning (Kolb & Fantie, 1997). Once the neural tube develops, the process of cellular migration and neuronal differentiation can take place in earnest. As the brain is developing, neurons are differentiating and connecting with other neurons. The bumps (*gyri*) and crevices (*sulci*) are poorly defined during gestation, leaving the fetal brain looking somewhat like undifferentiated Jell-O until the last trimester, when gyri and sulci become better demarcated.

With sophisticated fetal magnetic resonance imaging (MRI), we can now see what structures develop at what times (Prayer et al., 2006), and this explains why newborns do what they do (e.g., basic bodily functions, some sensory and motor behaviors), and can't do other things (e.g., volitional behavior). At birth, the brain has the differentiated neurons in the correct place (for typical children), but the brain weighs only about one-quarter of its final weight. So the brain is almost all "there" at birth, but why is it such a fraction of its final weight? What continues to take place after birth, and at extraordinary rates, are the branching and connections of dendritic "trees" and the myelination of axons, which accounts for the majority of hemispheric growth after birth (Majovski, 1997; Giedd & Rapoport, 2010). *Myelin* is the substance that helps speed transmission of the nerve impulse, and modulates and synchronizes neuronal firing patterns, which is what "white matter" is all about. It grows steadily throughout neurodevelopment. Unlike white matter, gray matter shows a curvilinear U-shaped development. In other words, it increases and then declines (Gogtay et al., 2004). This conceptualization is important when we consider hemisphere function later in the chapter, because there is more gray matter relative to white in the left hemisphere, and the converse is true in the right.

As dendritic branching and myelination race forward at tremendous rates, a curious and seemingly opposite process is happening in the brain at the same time—the brain is actually *destroying* what it originally built! This process is called *pruning* (just like pruning a tree) and it is critical that this destruction occurs throughout the lifespan. The brain builds and destroys neuronal connections in an attempt to reach a "goodness of fit" between the child and the environment. In other words, the brain is trying to establish an equilibrium that optimizes beneficial pathways and minimizes dysfunctional ones. Essentially, the process is similar to Darwin's notion of natural selection. And one can see the direct devastating effects of lack of pruning in children with autism (Bauman & Kemper, 2005).

This presentation gives you the gist or "big picture" of the process of neurogenesis. This neurodevelopmental path reflects the development of complex cognitive processes through the process of cortical maturation (Waber et al., 2007). Although the process occurs throughout the lifespan, likely the most important changes occur during the first 5 years of life (Whitaker, Bub, & Leventer, 1981). The evolution of gray to white matter changes drastically with age (see also Giedd et al., 2004).

Cortical maturation begins with the primary zones (these regions "register" incoming or outgoing information). Maturation then progresses to the cortical areas that integrate information (association areas) and finally to the frontal lobe, which is the last and most important cortical area to fully develop (Giedd & Rapoport, 2010; Waber et al., 2007). As a result, different brain areas may be used to process information at different ages. This directly affects our interpretation of cognitive, neuropsychological, and/or achievement test results, with different conclusions drawn based on the child's developmental level.

It is important to recognize that neurodevelopment does not follow a strict linear trajectory—it shows periods of growth followed by a leveling off or a decrease in growth. In other words, it follows neurodevelopmental *stages*, much like Piaget and other developmental psychologists have posited (Epstein, 2001). The discontinuous nature of frontal lobe development is of particular importance, because changes in learning and behavior are associated with changes in the frontal lobe (Rubia et al., 2000). The frontal lobes, as discussed later, are the "brain boss" which governs all aspects of cognition and behavior—at least the volitional kind. Also as discussed later, many behaviors are unconscious or automatic (Gazzaniga, 2013), which attests to the importance of cerebellar function in governing daily actions, given its importance in automatic behavior (Koziol et al., 2013). This has dramatic relevance to understanding pathology, given that an automatic problem behavior may have been developed in response to environmental demands, and difficult to eliminate as a result. Not all behavior is volitional, even though Western psychology often places emphasis on cognitive control over behavior.

There has been much debate about the critical periods for brain growth and recovery of function following brain injury (Dennis, 2010), as related to the brain's plasticity (Meredith, 2015). It is obvious there is evidence that the young child's brain is malleable or plastic, and that sparing of a cognitive function following brain damage in children is often lost in adults (Hecaen, 1976). This finding became known as the Kennard principle. However, the notion that early rather than late damage is better is neither accurate nor a representation of Kennard's actual findings (Dennis, 2010). Early damage may result in limitations for both the function that is spared *and* the other functions as well, which may also be negatively affected (Fletcher et al., 1984). In the case of language recovery following left-hemisphere damage, the presumption is that the right hemisphere "takes over" for language functions, sometimes called "crossed lateralization" (Alexander & Annett, 1996). Unfortunately, some language functions, as well as some right-hemisphere functions such as spatial skills, may be lost. This is known as the "crowding hypothesis" (Teuber, 1975), because language is said to "crowd" out the spatial skills. However, as you will find out later, this "crossed lateralization" belief does not make good sense given current thinking about brain structure and function, because verbal and nonverbal skills are *bilateral*. In other words, the hemispheres are not specialized for verbal or visual *stimuli*; they are specialized for *psychological processes*, as suggested in Chapter 1.

Though it is now generally accepted that some cognitive and/or behavioral dysfunction will occur following brain injury to a child, the developmental stage clearly affects the manifestation of the cognitive and behavioral deficits observed (Dennis, 2010; Kolb & Fantie, 1997). The brain–environment interaction is by definition bidirectional, affecting how brain structures develop propensities for information processing, and placing constraints on brain plasticity (Meredith, 2015). Although we are only now beginning to sort through the relationship between genotype and phenotype from the field of epigenesis, it is clear that many psychological disorders have a genetic basis (see Goldstein & Reynolds, 2010). Many clinicians have heard the saying "The apple doesn't fall far from the tree," and this is something that must always be considered in our evaluations/history taking. As we develop a greater understanding of the genetic basis of childhood disorders, such as learning disorders and ADHD, we can begin to evaluate their unique developmental pathways, and possibly to determine different developmentally appropriate assessment techniques and intervention strategies for each condition. This has formed the basis of the revolution in research, where Research Domain Criteria (Insel, 2014) are used, rather than relying on behavioral criteria and categorical labels for neurodevelopmental disorders. See Chapter 11 for a discussion of childhood genetic disorders.

A Review of Major Brain Structures

A Semantic Road Map

In addition to the terms and definitions found in Appendix 2.1, the following terminology review will help you navigate the upcoming discussion of major brain structures. If this information is new to you, take a few minutes to study these terms and then quiz yourself. When one author (Hale) teaches brain structure and function in courses, one of the first tasks is to quiz students on their understanding of neuropsychology terms. If you are unfamiliar with these terms, much of what is written in this chapter will be very difficult to understand. Learning about brain–behavior relationships is a lot like learning a foreign language that must be mastered to understand the concepts presented and their application to clinical practice.

Recall that the central nervous system is primarily composed of *gray matter* (the nerve cells) and *white matter* (myelinated axons that speed transformation of information). You can think of gray matter as more like boxes, cabinets, closets, rooms, and buildings. White matter, by contrast, is more like hallways, paths, roads, and highways of the brain. Remember this metaphor later in the chapter, when we speak of the left hemisphere as having more boxes and rooms relative to the roads and highways of the right hemisphere.

Clusters of axons, or *tracts*, often connect different brain areas and are sometimes called *commissures.* The largest commissure is the *corpus callosum*, which serves to connect a majority of the left hemisphere with a majority of the right. In an intact brain, almost any information sent to one hemisphere is easily transmitted across this largest commissure. Many disorders affect white matter development, leading to dysfunction of the anterior and/or posterior portion of the corpus callosum, so the two halves of the brain don't work well or quickly together. A similar structure is the *cingulate*, which allows the front parts of the brain to communicate with the back parts, so it is not surprising that anterior functions are related to executive attention while posterior regions are related to evaluative and memory functions (Rolls, 2019).

Afferent is related to input, or projections entering into a structure; *efferent* is related to output, or projections leaving a structure. *Ipsilateral* means the same side of the body, and *contralateral* means the opposite side. Most information above the lower brainstem crosses over *(decussates)* from one side of the body to the other side of the brain. However, the increasingly important cerebellum subserves the ipsilateral and contralateral side of the body (Karavasilis et al., 2019). Structures are said to be *superior* or *dorsal* if they are on the top or in front, whereas *inferior* or *ventral* typically reflects bottom or posterior. Finally, *lateral* often refers to the side, away from the midline, and *medial* suggests the middle. There are many structures (especially subcortical ones) that are given different names or identified as belonging to different systems, depending on this directional template. The important details for you to remember are the general location of the structures and how they interact with each other.

Unless otherwise noted, the following eight excellent sources have served as the basis for much of the following neuroanatomical and neuropsychological material. These resources include a classic neuropsychology text (Kolb & Whishaw, 2023), two neuroanatomy and neuropathology texts (Mendoza & Foundas, 2007; Reitan & Wolfson, 1985), two child neuropsychology texts (Reynolds & Fletcher-Janzen, 2009; Semrud-Clikeman & Ellison, 2009), a pediatric neuropsychology text (Davis, 2010), a prominent neuroscience text (Gazzaniga et al., 2013), and a classic text on the left and right hemispheres (Springer & Deutsch, 1998). For those of you who prefer "active" learning or benefit from motoric input, I also recommend a neuroanatomy coloring book (Pinel & Edwards, 2007), which gets rave reviews from my students each term. All are highly recommended for further reading.

The Supporting Cast: Subcortical Structures Serving the Neocortex

Although the majority of this chapter focuses on neocortical brain structure and function (i.e., the occipital, temporal, parietal, and frontal lobes), it is important to review the major forebrain and brainstem structures involved in neuropsychological and cognitive processes. Table 2.1 presents the major forebrain structures (which also include the neocortex) and their purported functions. An excellent text written on subcortical structures is *Subcortical Structures and Cognition: Implications for Neuropsychological Assessment* (Koziol & Budding, 2009).

TABLE 2.1. Overview of Forebrain Structures

Brain area	Associated structures	Function	Associated activities
Basal ganglia/ striatum	Caudate, putamen, globus pallidus	Motor	Posture, tone, motor activity, response coordination, sequencing, attention, working memory, executive functions
Limbic	Hippocampus	Memory	Encoding/consolidation
	Amygdala	Emotion	Approach–avoidance, emotional valence
	Cingulate	Executive	Orientation, inhibition, monitoring

The basal ganglia have rich interconnections between cortical and subcortical structures, including the thalamus (sensory and motor relay structure) and the nucleus accumbens (reward center). Together these structures are part of the frontal–subcortical circuits (FSC) and are implicated in most neuropsychiatric disorders (Hale et al., 2009, 2018). Of the three basal ganglia structures, the caudate nucleus (excitatory-motivation for action), putamen (learning and appetitive behavior), and globus pallidus (inhibits action and inhibits inhibition), exert a subcortical executive regulatory role. According to Koziol and Budding (2009), the prefrontal cortex is responsible for determining what behavior to display, while the basal ganglia determine when this behavior is appropriate. Although these ganglia were originally relegated to a motor role only, our appreciation of their importance has grown in recent years; they are now known to be involved in executive, motor, and sensory functions (Middleton & Strick, 2000).

In addition, dysfunction of the basal ganglia structures and their frontal cortical–subcortical loops has been linked to several childhood disorders, including ADHD, obsessive–compulsive disorder, and the disorder that has symptoms of both, Tourette syndrome. For a practical example of how the basal ganglia affects behavior, let's consider the nucleus accumbens in ADHD (e.g., Goto & Grace, 2005). Because there is deficient dopamine function in ADHD, the nucleus accumbens is not stimulated enough, so pleasure is hard to come by for these children. That could explain why children with ADHD prefer highly stimulating and/ or dangerous activities–it gives them the pleasure they lack. It can also explain why these children often say they are "bored" and don't respond to typical behavioral interventions—they just don't find typical "reinforcers" reinforcing enough.

The amygdala is typically included as part of the limbic system, because it is involved in recognition and recall of emotional stimuli (Adolphs, Tranel, Damasio, & Damasio, 1995). Along with the orbital cortex, the amygdala has been implicated in autism, potentially explaining why affected individuals have poor social connectedness (Bachevalier & Loveland, 2006). The limbic system has been considered the "emotional brain" for many years, but the roles of the hippocampus (memory encoding, consolidation, and retrieval), and the cingulate gyrus (attention, motivation, error monitoring, and executive control) (Casey et al., 1997; Cohen, Botvinick, & Carter, 2000; Gehring & Knight, 2000), suggest that this conceptualization may not fully reflect the complexity of this system.

Although significant research efforts continue to provide understanding into the functions of these structures, findings often reinforce their complex rather than simplistic nature. For instance, given the importance of the hippocampus in memory encoding, consolidation (with the temporal lobe), and retrieval (e.g., Ritchey & Coker, 2013), careful attention must be paid to this structure if it is damaged or dysfunctional. For children who experience a great deal of stress or trauma, the hypothalamic–pituitary–adrenal (HPA) axis is dysfunctional, and it can interact with the hippocampus negatively impacting a child's memory (Bao et al., 2008) or their ability to learn and recall information in the classroom. Anterior cingulate dysfunction, common in many neuropsychiatric conditions, can lead to poor "online" monitoring of performance and slowed processing speed (Bush et al., 2000; Turken et al., 2008).

We now move to the brainstem (see Table 2.2). The diencephalon consists of four structures that regulate body functions. The thalamus is of particular importance because almost all sensory and motor systems are influenced, making it the "Grand Central Station" of the brain. With its close partners, the frontal lobes and the basal ganglia, the thalamus is now being implicated in several childhood disorders. The hypothalamus, with its involvement in the endocrine system and maintaining homeostasis, is considered the autonomic center of the brain. It affects drives related to eating, drinking, sexuality, and rest. It is near the optic chiasm, where the vision "crosses over" (see our upcoming discussion of the occipital lobe). Because it secretes melatonin, the pineal body of the epithalamus has been associated with circadian rhythms (e.g., sleep–wake cycles), which must be considered when assessing attention problems given the sleep deprivation literature (Arns & Vollebregt, 2019). Pineal tumors can occur during puberty, so dramatic changes in sleep patterns (outside the typical teenage experience!) should be evaluated further. The red nucleus and substantia nigra have rich interconnections with the basal ganglia structures, and, along with the cerebellum, are involved with regulation of motor functioning and learning.

Among the other brainstem structures, the cerebellum has gained a great deal of attention in recent years (Koziol & Budding, 2009). In fact, its involvement in many cognitive processes and its association with several psychological disorders suggest that it is almost a mini-brain unto itself. It is interesting that the cerebellum affects the ipsilateral and controlateral sides of the body, suggesting that it possibly serves the function of a cortical check-and-balance system, because the cortical areas all affect contralateral regions. In addition to motor functions, the cerebellum seems to be intimately involved in timing, learning, memory, and coordinating cognitive functions (Kolb et al., 2023)—the "how" of executive action (Koziol & Budding, 2009). Because of its interrelationship with the frontal–subcortical circuits, damage to the region called the cerebellar vermis can lead to a disorder called Cerebellar Cognitive Affective syndrome, which affects executive functions, spatial abilities, language, and emotion (Wolf et al., 2009). Finally, the net-like reticular formation, with its involvement in cortical tone, serves as an important mediator of attention as Luria's (1973) first functional unit—the unit for regulating tone, waking, and mental states. Although most think that cortical tone is outside the purview of neuropsychologists, it has become clearer that this tone influences processing, such as is the case with the cognitive–energetic model (Sergeant, 2005) of ADHD. As we will see, many of Luria's principles and much of his theory still dominate the field of neuropsychology today.

We have come to learn much more about these subcortical structures in recent years, and to appreciate the contributions they make during cognition. In fact, although humans can survive without the cortex (albeit their daily lives would be quite limited, as they would be entirely dependent on others for survival), they can't live without the subcortical structures. These subcortical structures are also implicated in many learning and other psychological disorders, so we must avoid a "corticocentric" view in assessing child learning and behavior problems (Koziol & Budding, 2009). However, many subcortical problems are likely to be recognized by physicians and neurologists, because their symptoms are often readily apparent and somewhat easier to assess than cortical dysfunctions. As a result, we place greater emphasis on the cortical brain areas in the following sections.

Cortical deficits are likely to be identified as "soft signs" that require further neuropsychological investigation. They are also more likely to present as learning and behavior problems in the classroom. However, we believe that practitioners should learn to identify the signs and symptoms of subcortical as well as cortical dysfunctions, as the processes

TABLE 2.2. Important Subcortical Structures

Brain area	Associated structures	Function	Associated activities
Diencephalon			
Epithalamus	Pineal body	Body rhythms	Sleep–waking and other activity cycles
Subthalamus	Links to midbrain and basal ganglia	Modulation	Movement
Thalamus	Lateral geniculate body	Relay station	Visual
	Medial geniculate body	Relay station	Auditory
	Pulvinar	Attention	Sensory filter
Hypothalamus	Pituitary gland	Homeostasis	Regulation of hunger–thirst, temperature, sleep, and hormones
Other subcortical structures			
Tectum	Superior colliculi	Vision	Visual modulation
	Inferior colliculi	Hearing	Auditory modulation
Tegmentum	Red nucleus	Motor	Voluntary movement
	Substantia nigra	—	(related to basal ganglia)
Cerebellum	Vestibulocerebellum	Body position	Balance, posture, eye movement
	Spinocerebellum	Gross motor	Sensory–motor integration for locomotion
	Neocerebellum	Fine motor	Movement initiation, maintenance, sequencing
	Pons/medulla	Sensorimotor	Ascending–descending tracts, cranial nerves
Reticular formation		Arousal	Level of consciousness

subserved by both types of functions are intimately related and often clinically inseparable. Essentially, we have typically been too "cortico-centric" in our approaches to neuropsychological understanding (Koziol & Budding, 2009). Instead, theoretical and empirical advances have made it clear that the cortex and subcortical systems interact in an interdependent way (Koziol et al., 2013), somewhat like a complex, interconnected, hydraulic system where dysfunction in one system can have a cascade effect on others, not only between cortical and subcortical systems, but within each as well.

The Three-Axis Model of Brain Functioning

Laws of Neuropsychological Functioning

To begin to understand how these cortical and subcortical structures interact with each ther to produce cognition and behavior, we have identified three important dimensions or "axes" to aid in interpreting cognitive processes from a neuropsychological perspective:

1. Posterior–anterior axis
2. Left hemisphere–right hemisphere axis
3. Superior–inferior axis

First, we describe each of the four lobes—the occipital, temporal, parietal, and frontal lobes. This section can serve as a guide for interpreting brain–behavior relationships on the posterior-to-anterior (input-to-output) axis.

Following this section, we discuss lateralization of function—the second important distinction necessary to explore the differential processing capabilities of the left hemisphere-to-right hemisphere axis. Simply put, the left hemisphere is specialized for processing detail-learned information and the right hemisphere is specialized for processing global-novel information.

Finally, we discuss the third superior–inferior axis. The posterior-to-anterior axis is affected by the anterior frontal regions, and their interactions with subcortical structures, including the frontal–subcortical circuits and cerebral–cerebellar circuits. This third superior–inferior axis is essentially our psychopathology axis, the one that can explain many of the emotional and behavioral disorders we see in children (Hale et al., 2018).

Before we explore the nature of these axes, it is critical to note what we term the two fundamental *laws of neuropsychological functioning* (Hale & Fiorello, 2004) in our exploration of brain–behavior relationships. It is these two laws or caveats that help us understand brain–behavior relationships, and in turn the results of our neuropsychological evaluations. The laws of neuropsychological functioning are:

1. No complex human behavior can be linked to one specific brain area; most brain–behavior relationships require an examination of interrelated and interdependent brain networks.
2. There is considerable individual variability in cortical organization and function; differences within individuals are often greater than differences between individuals.

The Posterior–Anterior Axis and Cerebral Cortex

Table 2.3 provides an overview of the four lobes of the cerebral cortex. The four lobes, as well as the limbic system and basal ganglia (described earlier), constitute the telencephalon. An oversimplified, but useful, distinction among the functions of the four lobes is as follows: The occipital lobe processes visual information; the temporal lobe processes auditory information; the parietal lobe processes touch or somatic senses; and the frontal lobe governs motor output (and all behavior, for that matter).

TABLE 2.3. Overview of Cortical Structures and Major Functions

Brain area	Associated structures	Function	Activities
Cortex	Frontal lobe	Motor	Praxis—drawing/writing
	Parietal lobe	Somatosensory	Gnosis—feeling/texture/pressure
	Temporal lobe	Auditory	Hearing—understanding/memory
	Occipital lobe	Vision	Seeing—objects/words/faces/color

To reiterate, the three posterior lobes are grossly associated with receiving afferent or input information, and the frontal lobe is responsible for efferent projections or output. However, all cortical structures have "superhighway" white matter tracts or commissures that allow information to be sent to or received from other brain areas. Thus, a frontal lobe problem can affect perception, whereas a posterior lobe problem can affect executive functions.

Before we begin to explore the function of each lobe in detail, it is important to review some important physical landmarks that will be referred to later. The two hemispheres are separated by the longitudinal sulcus or fissure, but commissures (connections) allow the hemispheres to communicate. The central sulcus separates the frontal motor area from the parietal somatosensory area. Simply put, anything posterior from the central sulcus is responsible for receiving afferent or sensory input; anything anterior is involved in efferent or motor output. However, as discussed previously, the anterior and posterior areas interact with each other, so that they are involved in almost every aspect of cognition.

The lateral sulcus (often called the sylvian fissure) separates the frontal (motor output) from temporal (auditory input) lobes, and one can see the central sulcus extends laterally to separate the frontal from parietal (somatosensory input) lobes. For the other demarcations, the boundaries are less clear. There is a reason for this: The occipital, parietal, and temporal lobes have intricate interconnections that are necessary for processing complex visual, somatosensory, and auditory information. So the parietal–occipital–temporal "junction" is not typically demarcated clearly, as this region processes all types of information, not just one sense. Given this caveat, the boundary between the parietal and occipital lobe is conveniently named the parietal–occipital sulcus, and the preoccipital notch is sometimes identified as separating the occipital lobe from the temporal lobe. Figure 2.1 illustrates the major gyri of the brain.

Luria's Working Brain and the Two Axes

Over 5 decades ago, the noted Russian neuropsychologist A. R. Luria provided us with a conceptual understanding of how the posterior–anterior and left–right axes work together

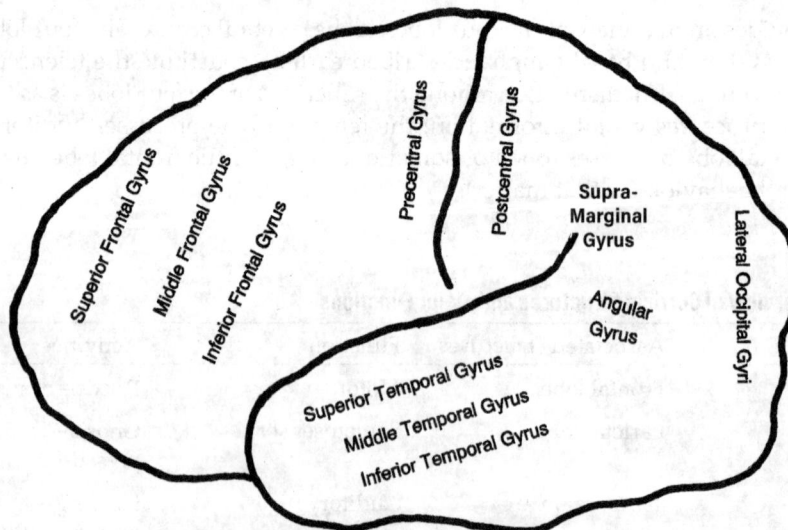

FIGURE 2.1. Lateral view of major gyri.

to produce complex behavior. Although parts of his theory have been questioned, and many of his initial findings about patients with brain damage have been elaborated and expanded upon, Luria's *The Working Brain* (1973b) still serves as a seminal work in neuropsychology. His ideas provide a conceptual understanding of the basics of brain–behavior relationships from both a structural and functional perspective, which will serve you well as you begin to explore the posterior–anterior axis represented by the four lobes of the neocortex.

According to Luria's (1973b) model (also see In-Depth 2.1), there are three *principle functional units* in the brain. As noted earlier, the reticular system and related structures are primarily responsible for Luria's first functional unit, which is the *unit for regulating tone or waking*. Luria noted that without the first functional unit, higher levels of cognition are unlikely. Quoting his colleague Pavlov, Luria noted that optimal cortical tone is critical for organized goal-directed activity.

You can easily envision this construct of cortical tone, especially when your morning coffee is wearing off! The posterior occipital, parietal, and temporal areas represent Luria's second functional unit—the *unit for receiving, analyzing, and storing information*. Although this suggests that the posterior regions are important for memory, research has supported that long-term memories for motor function are likely an anterior function (Kluen et al., 2019), important for production of written expression and spelling. The anterior (output) cortex is responsible for Luria's third functional unit—*the unit for programming, regulating, and verifying mental activity*. As the cortical area responsible for the third functional unit, Luria described the frontal lobes as the "superstructure" responsible for governing the entire brain. Although this claim about the frontal lobes may seem somewhat overzealous, current evidence suggests that Luria's contention is largely correct, especially for higher-level mental activities. The frontal lobes are the "brain manager" or "brain boss" (Hale & Fiorello, 2001), basically governing almost every aspect of volitional cortical functioning.

There are three basic tenets of Luria's process-oriented model: (1) The brain is hierarchically organized (from basic zones to complex zones); (2) the cortical areas diminish in specificity (from simple processing of stimuli to complex integration demands); and (3) the cortical areas increase in lateralization of function (from undifferentiated cells to unique hemispheric systems). To summarize, the three Lurian *laws of functional organization* (see In-Depth 2.1) are:

1. *Hierarchical organization*
   - Primary zones: clear brain–behavior relationships
   - Secondary zones: integrative association cortex
   - Tertiary zones: highest levels of cognition
2. *Diminishing specificity*
   - Primary zones: one function
   - Secondary zones: more than one function
   - Tertiary zones: many functions, not specific
3. *Progressive lateralization*
   - Primary zones: left hemisphere = right side of body; right hemisphere = left side of body
   - Secondary/tertiary: left hemisphere = detail–learned; right hemisphere = global–novel

Notice that the primary zones coincide with the somatosensory, visual, and auditory cortices for the second functional unit, and these get integrated in the secondary/tertiary of what Luria referred to as the *zones of overlapping*. The highest levels of *understanding* take place in the zones of overlapping. The frontal lobes are responsible for the third functional unit, with the secondary/tertiary zones being what Luria coined the brain *superstructure*. The

IN-DEPTH 2.1. Luria's Working Brain

Luria's first law of functional organization is his principle of *hierarchical organization* of individual cortical zones. This has to do with how information is processed and/or behaviors are produced. According to this model, the body sends afferent information to the subcortical structures and then to the *primary* cortical zones. There are three primary zones for the different senses—one each in the occipital (vision), temporal (auditory), and parietal (somatosensory) lobes. This information is then elaborated on in *secondary* zones or *association cortex*. Finally, there is the *tertiary cortex* or the "zone of overlapping," where all information is eventually processed, regardless of origin and type. It is in the tertiary cortex that the highest levels of comprehension and understanding take place.

According to Luria's model, input proceeds in a hierarchical fashion from primary to secondary zones and then to the zone of overlapping, the tertiary cortex. For motor functions, the opposite occurs: The tertiary cortex provides the idea and plan; next, the secondary motor cortex provides a motor program; and then the primary motor cortex dutifully carries out the act. Luria's notion *is* largely accurate in representing how the brain processes information and produces behavior, but current research suggests that there are multiple parallel pathways and processes, some of which bypass different zones.

However, Luria (1973b) correctly noted that these zones form an interdependent system, and that disruption in one zone is likely to affect another. It is well known that a focal brain lesion can cause initial loss, and then subsequent loss of function in the interconnected areas in the system—a process called *diaschisis*.

Luria's second law of functional organization suggests that there is *diminishing specificity* as one ascends the hierarchical zones (or *increasing* specificity as one descends the frontal motor route from tertiary to primary cortex). That is, the primary cortex is very specific in addressing only one sensory modality, whereas the tertiary cortex can address all of them. At the occipital–parietal–temporal "crossroads" described later, structural boundaries become blurred, and multiple complex cognitive processes take place within this "zone of overlapping."

Luria's third law of functional organization is related to the *progressive lateralization* of function. As information ascends the sensory hierarchy, and is processed by association cortex that is less modality-specific, it is more likely that subsequent processing will take place in one hemisphere or the other. Although some have interpreted Luria (1973a, 1980b) as suggesting that successive processes occur in the left hemisphere, and that the right hemisphere processes simultaneous information, this is an oversimplification of his theoretical and clinical presentation. According to Luria's model, it is not the type of information that distinguishes between the hemispheres; it is the manner in which they organize and represent information (Majovski, 1997). It is this third law—the one addressing lateralization of function—that has evolved dramatically since Luria's time. These changes are discussed in the section of this chapter on the left–right axis.

---

highest levels of *doing* occurs in the frontal lobes, in an area called the prefrontal cortex. These highest areas of understanding and doing are heavily connected with white matter tracts, so they influence each other in a bidirectional manner.

Concerning the development of new functions (e.g., learning new tasks), Luria (1973b) argued that there is a gradual development of cognitive skills from anterior to posterior: New skill acquisition requires more of the (anterior) third functional unit to operate and incorporate the new information, but once a skill is mastered or becomes routine, the (posterior) second functional unit becomes more important in performing the learned task (Goldberg et al., 1994), and then when it is completely automatic, it may in essence be largely a function of the cerebellum (Koziol & Budding, 2009; Poldrack et al., 2005). More importantly, as we describe later in the chapter, there appear to be hemispheric differences in processing novel and routinized information, so the anterior (new/novel)–posterior (old/learned) dichotomy is only part of the picture.

We now begin our discussion of the four lobes of the brain, but keep in mind that there is support for Luria's notion that the four lobes work together to perform most cognitive tasks, in a type of gradiential fashion (Goldberg, 2001). Again, keep in mind the hydraulic analogy, where each system is influencing the other, and function or dysfunction can escalate as multiple interdependent systems influence each other in a unidirectional or (often) a bidirectional manner.

As you will see, disruption or damage to one area is likely to affect the others. Is this pattern of performance due to primary dysfunction to a particular area, or is it due to another area that affects the performance you see? You will learn to ask yourself this question repeatedly in clinical practice. For instance, neglect of self and environment may look like ADHD–inattentive type, but it is caused by dysfunction of the parietal lobes, not the frontal–subcortical circuits that cause "true" ADHD (Hale, Reddy, Decker, et al., 2009). Why is this important for us to know? The frontal type of ADHD is more likely to respond to medication treatment (Hale et al., 2011; Carmichael et al., 2015; Kubas et al., 2012), whereas for the parietal lobe type (e.g., "pseudo-ADHD"), the influence of medication is likely equivocal or minimal at best. This is why differential diagnosis requires a thorough understanding of the complexity of neuropsychological processes before these processes can be related to achievement and/or behavior domains.

An Axis Divided: I. Visual Processes and the Occipital Lobe

Visual Pathways: From Eye to Occipital Lobe

Before visual information can be processed by the occipital lobe, the information must be processed by the eye and sent to it. Afferent information from the retina of the eye is sent to the occipital lobe mainly via the optic nerve, thalamus, and superior colliculus. The left visual field projects to the right hemisphere, and the right visual field goes to the left hemisphere in both eyes. Damage to the pathways can lead to loss of vision in one eye—or, if the damage is after the optic chiasm (where crossover occurs), then it is likely to cause loss of vision in half of each eye contralateral to the injury.

Several cranial nerves control horizontal or vertical eye movement, iris (pupil) size, and eyelid movement. When you are concerned about a child's visual functioning, it is important to check each of the visual fields (each eye has four quadrants) and look for differences in pupil size or reaction to light, as well as eyelid function. It takes only a penlight and a couple of minutes to check these things, and one of us (Hale) has found several children with cranial nerve damage, so it is worth the effort when "visual" processes are a concern.

After entering the lateral thalamus, two main types of pathways emerge from the lateral thalamus to the occipital lobe: the *M pathway*, which will eventually lead to processing of motion and contrast; and the *P pathway*, for eventual processing of contrast, color, location, and orientation. This visual division of labor continues and becomes more detailed in the occipital lobe, where the P pathway divides in two (one P pathway leads to perception of color and contrast, and the other to perception of location and orientation). Working in concert with the pulvinar, the superior colliculus affects these processes in the occipital lobe. It is responsible for detection and orientation to visual stimuli, and has been associated with visual attention (Poppel et al., 2020). However, as we will see later, the concept of attention is multifaceted and requires several interconnected brain regions.

Occipital Lobe Structure and Function

The occipital lobe has several distinct areas that process different aspects of visual stimuli and are depicted in Figure 2.2. Sometimes you will read descriptions of brain areas in terms of Brodmann's (1909) areas (e.g., 17, 18, 19), and sometimes you will read descriptions using a contemporary V nomenclature (V1, V2, dV3, VP, V4, V5). For the purposes of clinical assessment, it is important to note that different areas exist and do different things. The main occipital regions are functionally identified as the *striate*, or *primary visual cortex*, and the *extrastriate*, or *association visual cortex*. Simply put, the primary visual cortex receives or registers the information from the visual pathways just described, and then sends this information to the association cortex, where processing and interpretation begins. Interestingly, you can have scotomas (blind spots) from primary occipital lobe damage that are completely "filled in" by the association cortex, so that perception may be weak or slow, but the person's association cortex allows her to "see" everything (also called perceptual filling). What you might see in the classroom for a child like this is a compensatory nystagmus, as the child uses visual searching and scanning to help the association cortex "fill in the blanks."

Returning to the pathways, afferent information from the M and P pathways is received by the primary cortex. If a stimulus is located in the peripheral visual fields, it will be processed medially. If it is in the center of the visual field, it will be processed by the most posterior cortex. This suggests that damage to the most posterior part of the occipital lobe could lead to loss or partial loss of vision in the center of the visual field, but that such an injury is less likely to affect peripheral vision. The different aspects of processing are discussed in In-Depth 2.2, but for the remainder of this section, we refer to these areas as *primary cortex* and *association cortex*.

From the primary cortex to the secondary and other association areas, the pathways become quite complex and interrelated, but their distinction becomes important in our study of visual–perceptual brain–behavior relationships. These pathways extend *beyond* the occipital lobe to the parietal and temporal lobes, so differential diagnosis requires an independent understanding not only of the occipital, temporal, and parietal lobes, but of how they interact with each other. As stated earlier, the differentiation of the M and P pathways continues in the primary cortex and becomes elaborated in the association cortex. From there, the beginning of the *dorsal stream* (occipital lobe to parietal lobe) and *ventral stream* (occipital lobe to temporal lobe) becomes apparent in the association areas. The dorsal stream receives input that originated in the M pathway system, but the ventral stream receives input coming from both the M and the two P pathways.

To make the connection between the occipital and respective lobes, the dorsal stream requires the superior longitudinal fasciculus (frontal to parietal), and the ventral stream uses the inferior longitudinal fasciculus (occipital to temporal). Although an oversimplification, you may read literature that talks about the dorsal stream as the "where" pathway and the ventral stream as the "what" pathway (Ungerleider & Mishkin, 1982). Recognize that these two streams form the basis of many learning and possibly psychological disorders discussed later. In-Depth 2.3 provides you with a greater understanding of these important visual processes, but their functions are illustrated in Figure 2.2.

In our example of the baseball player diving for the ball in the Introduction to this book, he needed his dorsal stream—not only to track the trajectory of the ball, but also to be aware of his own body and glove position in relation to the ground and the other fielder's movements. Whereas egocentric (self) space is likely to be related to dorsal stream functions,

IN-DEPTH 2.2. The M and P Pathways

For the primary visual cortex, Gazzaniga and colleagues (1998) provide a nice summary of the three distinct processing areas related to the M and P pathways. As can be seen in the table below, the structures related to the two P pathways include some for color and contrast perception (called blobs) and some for form, location, and orientation (called interblobs). The M pathway is important for processing contrast and motion, and has been associated with reading disorders. This pattern is continued in the secondary association cortex, but here the structure of the cortex has led to a different distinction—one of "stripes" (thin, thick, and pale). As can be seen, the M pathway cells lead to perception of motion and contrast, whereas the two P pathways lead to perception of color, contrast, location, and orientation.

	M pathway		P pathway
		Occipital lobe structures	
V1	Layer 4b	Blobs	Interblobs
V2	Thick stripes	Thin stripes	Interstripes
		Cell stimulus response	
Contrast	High	High	Low
Location	Low	Low	High
Motion	High	Low	Middle
Color	Low	High	Middle
Orientation	Middle	Low	High

It is important to note that the pathways are responsive to other stimuli as well. This differential response is important, because damage to one occipital region but not another can lead to "blind spots" (scotomas) in the visual cortex, and to misperception of form, color, motion, or location. Individuals with these blind spots are usually not aware of them, because rapid eye movements (nystagmus) help compensate or "fill in" the missing information. Although this compensation is important, task performance may be impaired or slowed as a result.

---

allocentric (other) space is likely also to require the ventral stream. Because object perception and recognition are related to visual memory, the center fielder needed his ventral stream to recognize objects, people, faces, uniforms, the grass, the ball, and so on, consistent with evidence that visual association areas and the ventral stream are associated with long-term visual memories for faces and objects (Kosslyn et al., 1993). In addition, the ventral stream helped the center fielder realize that the left fielder's changing image suggested he was moving vigorously toward the center fielder and then stopping.

The ventral stream doesn't detect movement per se; it allows a viewer to recognize that regardless of his or her position, and the position of the object, it is still the same object. To attempt to catch the ball, the center fielder needed an understanding of his body in relation to other objects and their relative movement and shape, necessitating the interaction of the dorsal and ventral streams via the superior temporal sulcus stream. His dorsal stream helped the center fielder recognize the motion of the left fielder and his own actions in space, but this ventral stream helped him to recognize the different perspectives of the left fielder. The

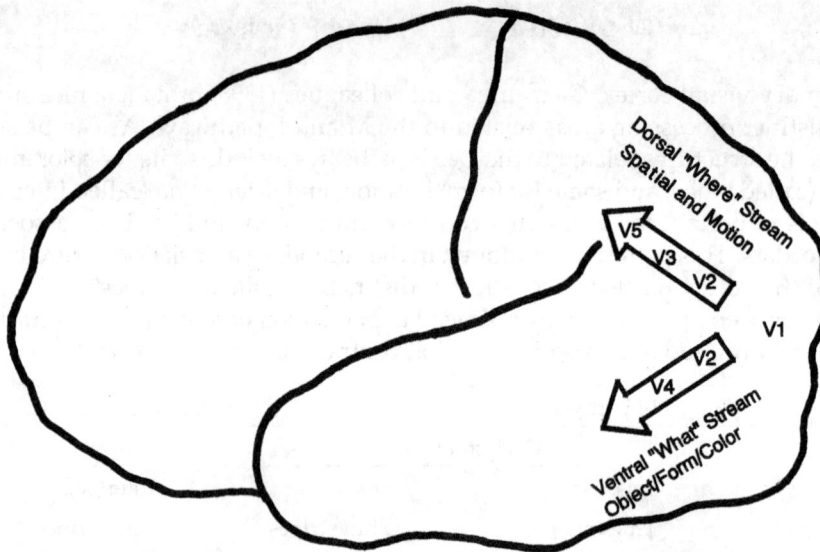

FIGURE 2.2. Structure and function of the occipital lobe.

fielder's actions, as well as such activities as driving or reaching for a door, require coordination of the two visual streams. However, because these streams project to different lobes, it is important to recognize their differential impairment and/or dysfunction. Further evidence for the relevance of the dorsal and ventral streams in psychological practice can be found in Application 2.1.

In addition to these two streams, the superior temporal sulcus stream, which is between the two others, appears to be important in *cross-modal matching*. I have seen several children who apparently had a problem with this stream. When a boy was asked to define words given orally, he was above average, because the input was auditory and the output was verbal. And although visual–spatial and visual–detail processing was adequate, he had a considerable problem pointing to pictures when given a vocabulary term, or naming pictures when shown a picture, so *cross-modal matching* was impaired. This can also influence reading words, where the sounds (superior temporal lobe) need to match up with the visual letters (extrastriate) cortex. These "streams" are more functional than structural, but they are likely influenced by the vertical occipital fasciculus, which connects association areas in the anterior occipital lobe, so the brain can compare/contrast how best to process incoming information.

Occipital Lobe Summary

To summarize the functions of the occipital lobe, it is the primary processor of visual information. It is thought to have the following attributes:

- Visual processes are both hierarchical and parallel. There is a check-and-balance system that allows some sparing of visual perception, even though there may be damage to small regions of the visual cortex. If this is the case, you will see a child display *nystagmus* (rapid eye movements) to compensate for the damage.

- The separate M and P pathways that project to the occipital lobe process different types of information. The M pathway is most closely related to contrast and motion. The P

IN-DEPTH 2.3. Further Examination of the "Where" and "What" Pathways

Milner and Goodale (1995) provide a more detailed examination of the "where" and "what" pathways that reflects their complexity. For the dorsal stream, V3A and VP are involved in recognition of spatial forms, and V5 is important for motion perception. As a result, the "where" stream may more accurately be considered the "how" stream. For the ventral stream, V3 is responsible for dynamic form recognition or object constancy, and V4 is important for color/form recognition. As discussed later, the dorsal stream is important for recognizing spatial relationships and motion, and the ventral stream is critical for perception and recognition of a variety of objects. They serve very different functions, but seldom work independently of each other in the real world. Differentiating the relative adequacy of the functions mediated by the dorsal and ventral streams can have implications for academic and behavioral intervention. For instance, a child with a writing problem may have difficulty with fine or gross-motor skills (probably a frontal lobe problem), but if the difficulty is related to spatial processing, and visual feedback to the motor system, the areas associated with the dorsal stream may be implicated, particularly in the right parietal lobe. If integration of the dorsal and motor systems is in question, the corpus callosum may be implicated, because spatial–holistic skills tend to require right parietal functions, and handwriting skills tend to require left frontal functions in right-handed people.

APPLICATION 2.1. Streams in the Classroom?

Take a minute to think about how the dorsal and ventral streams are relevant in the classroom. When are the dorsal and ventral streams needed in the classroom during a particular task? This task would require children to recognize objects, and then to guide their movements in response. Although there are many possibilities, one that comes to mind is copying notes from the board during a lecture—a common occurrence in the classroom, and one that gives children with some disorders considerable difficulty.

In this case, the ventral stream is specifically needed for recognizing the drawings and words on the board, and the teacher's shape and relative position (e.g., stretching an arm above the head and facing the board mean that the teacher is writing). The letters are symbols that represent words; they are objects, just as the teacher is an object. Children need the dorsal stream to guide their hands in forming and spacing the letters as they write. Of course, they must integrate this visual information with auditory information as well. All of this sensory information must be coordinated with the motor system, and managed by the "brain boss," the frontal lobe. When you think of all the complex systems that must be coordinated, it is no wonder that children with certain disorders have such a difficult time taking lecture notes in class.

pathway divides into two P pathways in the occipital lobe—one more related to contrast and color, and the other more related to location and orientation.

• After initial processing of information in the primary cortex, different pathways emerge in the association cortex: a dorsal stream that projects to the parietal association areas, and a ventral stream that projects to the temporal association areas. These are connected via the vertical occipital fasciculus, a white matter pathway that allows for the brain to "choose" the best pathway for processing incoming visual information.

• The ventral stream is important for recognizing objects and for integrating form and color, regardless of object orientation ("dynamic form").

• The dorsal stream is important for detecting motion and spatial relationships, and providing perceptual feedback to the motor system so that a person can respond to the environment.

• Both streams are needed for complex interactions between the individual and the environment; however, recognizing these functions can help you tease apart visual processes and determine whether they are differentially affected in learning and behavior disorders.

• The superior temporal sulcus stream is involved in cross-modal matching (auditory–verbal–visual) and integrating the dorsal and ventral streams. It is structurally supported by the vertical occipital fasciculus.

An Axis Divided: II. Auditory Processes and the Temporal Lobe

Auditory Pathways: From Ear to Temporal Lobe

The outer, middle, and inner ears have complex functions that translate sound information to electrical information in the auditory nerve via the cochlea. Because many children with reading problems have had frequent ear infections (otitis media), it is critical for referred children to be given audiological examinations to ensure adequate auditory acuity. However, as explained shortly, frequent ear infections can cause reading disorders even in the absence of frank hearing loss, because the association cortex learned the associations incorrectly.

The auditory nerve transmits information via the cochlear nucleus to the inferior colliculus, and two separate pathways emerge, with one going to the dorsal medial thalamus and the other to the ventral medial thalamus. The ventral pathway directly influences the primary auditory cortex, whereas the dorsal pathway influences the auditory association cortex. Unlike the visual system, where complete crossover takes place, auditory information is represented bilaterally. However, a majority of the afferent projections to the primary auditory cortex in the temporal lobe are contralateral. However, a sound made in the left ear is primarily sent to the contralateral auditory cortex of the right hemisphere (crossover), but it is also represented in the ipsilateral auditory left-hemisphere cortex.

Temporal Lobe Structure and Function

The lateral or sylvian fissure serves as an important landmark for separating the frontal lobe from the temporal lobe, and for locating the primary auditory cortex in Heschl's gyrus (see Figure 2.3). This superior temporal area, and the surrounding auditory association areas, is especially important for processing of language (Newman & Tweig, 2001). The tissue surrounding and within the superior temporal sulcus (STS), which separates the primary auditory cortex from the association and ventral stream areas, contains complex multimodal (i.e., pertaining to different senses) association cortex. The visual ventral stream described earlier is below this language region, in the lateral–ventral temporal cortex.

There are several important areas in the middle temporal lobe. This medial middle temporal cortex includes connections with the hippocampus (needed for forming new long-term memories, and also for retrieval) and limbic structures such as the amygdala (needed for affective tone or valence). However, as noted earlier, this is an oversimplified explanation of the medial areas, because they are part of an exceedingly complex interconnected circuit affecting attention, memory, and emotion.

There are multiple connections between the temporal lobe and other lobes—including the anterior commissure and the uncinate fasciculus (an important emotional–memory link between the frontal–temporal areas). The corpus callosum is involved as well to transfer information across hemispheres, the superior longitudinal fasciculus and cingulate are also involved in bringing posterior information to and from the frontal lobes. Clearly, the temporal lobe has several different important roles in cognitive processes. It participates in auditory processing and comprehension, memory consolidation and storage, emotional processing, and visual object recognition.

We now have an oversimplified understanding of the complexities of the temporal lobe. The superior and dorsal medial temporal areas are involved in processing sounds; the ventral–lateral area serves as the ventral visual stream; and the medial middle areas are involved in memory encoding and emotional valence, whereas the lateral middle areas are involved in long-term memory storage. Let's look at each of these independently.

First, the processing of sounds and language is of primary importance in the study of reading disorders. Even when they are detected as early as infancy (Molfese, 2000), auditory processing weaknesses can lead to poor phonemic awareness and reading disorders (Melby-Lervag et al., 2012). In addition to genetic studies, the Molfese infant study suggests that some causes of reading disorders are genetic or occur at some time prior to birth (see Chapter 5); however, others may be caused by auditory pathway or temporal lobe dysfunction/disruption, which can be caused by recurrent ear infections (i.e., otitis media), so an audiological examination should be undertaken whenever there is concern about reading. However, even when hearing is intact, a *history* of ear infections can result in reading impairment, but this may be related to the time when the ear infections occurred during development of the auditory association cortex.

Why would early hearing problems lead to reading difficulty if hearing is now intact? The answer takes us back to the difference between the primary and association cortices.

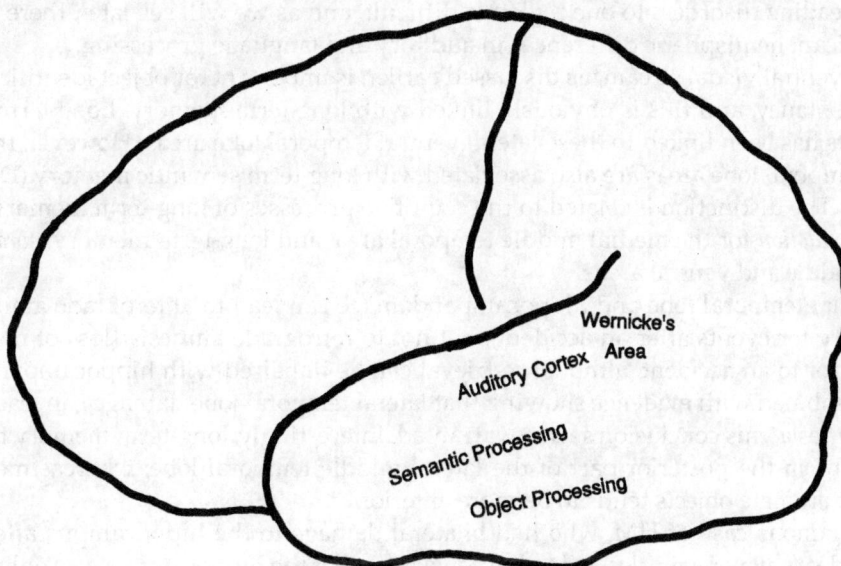

FIGURE 2.3. Structure and function of the temporal lobe.

When the young child was developing the association cortex during perception of speech, the sounds weren't correctly registered in the primary auditory cortex. As a result, the association cortex didn't perceive the sounds right in the first place, so it learned them wrong. The hearing was corrected, and now registration of the sounds in the primary auditory cortex is fine, but that adequate sound registration in the primary auditory cortex is misinterpreted by the association cortex, so the child still doesn't "hear" the sounds correctly. It is also possible that having many ear infections, which are incredibly painful, can lead to emotional and behavioral difficulties if not treated appropriately or sufficiently. During the time the young child is experiencing these ear infections, generally within the first 3 years of life, it is also the time the child develops basic trust. Think about how this could affect the child, the child's relation to the parent, and the child's view of the world. For these reasons a good history that details such difficulties is crucial for our understanding of the child.

As is the case with the visual cortex, auditory processing begins in the primary auditory area within Heschl's gyrus. High-frequency sounds are processed in the posterior–medial part of this area, and low-frequency sounds are processed in the anterior–lateral section. The sounds are elaborated and integrated in the association areas, where comprehension occurs in Wernicke's area, the multimodal superior temporal sulcus region (part of Luria's Zones of Overlapping), and the medial region (the insula). The primary cortex is involved in auditory attention and auditory sensory memory, which are short-lived. As noted earlier, it just "registers" the auditory input for further analysis by the association regions, as Luria predicted. Information is then integrated, organized, and categorized in the association cortex, allowing comprehension of auditory information to occur in the tertiary temporal region.

As noted in In-Depth 2.6, the tertiary areas of the planum temporale—including Wernicke's area—are involved in comprehension of language, regardless of the input modality (Michael et al., 2001). As mentioned earlier, this area has been found to be important in developing an association between sounds and symbols, with the closely associated supramarginal and angular gyri of the left parietal lobe, and it has been implicated in phonemic awareness, sound–symbol association (alphabetic principle), and reading skills. It is the temporal lobe boundary of the occipital–parietal–temporal multimodal "crossroads" area. However, linking reading disorders to one region is difficult, and as we will see later, there appear to be significant hemispheric differences in auditory and language processing.

The ventral visual stream, as discussed earlier, is important for object identification and object constancy, and this is obviously linked with long-term memory. Long-term memory for objects has been linked to these lateral ventral temporal lobe areas. However, the middle lateral temporal lobe areas are also associated with long-term semantic memory (Daselaar et al., 2002). The distinction is related to the cognitive processes of long-term memory *encoding* and *consolidation* for the medial middle temporal area, and long-term memory *storage* for the lateral middle and ventral areas.

Medial temporal lobe and hippocampal damage can lead to anterograde amnesia (loss of memory for events after an accident), but not to retrograde amnesia (loss of memory for events prior to an accident, although retrieval can be impaired with hippocampal damage). When combined with evidence showing that lateral temporal lobe damage can lead to retrograde amnesia, this conclusion seems warranted. Interestingly, long-term memory for objects tends to be in the posterior part of the lateral middle temporal lobe; whereas memory for people or animate objects tends to be more anterior.

The famous case of HM, who had bilateral damage to the hippocampus affecting his ability to learn new memories, led to the conjecture that the hippocampus was only involved in memory encoding and consolidation, however, this is not the case. There is evidence that the hippocampus also becomes active during long-term retrieval of episodic, semantic, and autobiographical memories (Burianova et al., 2010).

Why would a structure thought to be only related to forming new memories also influence our retrieval of old memories? It is possible that we *reconstruct* memories every time we try to retrieve a memory, thereby making it in essence a "new" memory. This could explain why memory retrieval is not entirely accurate, and calls into question the use of eyewitness testimony in court cases. If we are using current information to update memory and reconstruct it according to the current situation and processing demands, our memories would certainly be fallible and susceptible to influence. The search for *where* and *how* long-term memories are stored is further examined in In-Depth 2.4.

Interestingly, if the medial damage affects the amygdala as well, emotional memories may also be impaired, further making emotionally laden memories difficult to retrieve accurately. Studies of emotion and memory suggest they follow a curvilinear relationship—too little emotion and you won't learn something, but too much emotion causes memory problems as well. This has direct implications for our learning in classrooms. If a child is so bored and apathetic, or too emotionally distraught over some problem, then learning will likely be impaired. So teachers need to "pump up" their kids to learn, but at the same time not let them get too carried away. This also explains why active engagement is so important for learning. When you are bored, your cortical tone goes down, and so does your emotional status. Keeping children engaged and active during learning is an effective strategy during classroom instruction (Webb et al., 2014), and this finding has its basis in brain–behavior relationships.

Temporal Lobe Summary

To summarize the functions of the temporal lobe, it is the primary processor of auditory information. It is thought to have the following attributes:

IN-DEPTH 2.4. The Search for Memory

Although it is clear that memories and emotions are affected by medial temporal lobe damage, it is unlikely that long-term memories are "stored" in these structures. Instead, a growing body of evidence suggests that semantic long-term memory is stored in the left temporal lobe. For instance, whereas facial processing tends to be a right temporal lobe task, memories for familiar or famous faces is found in the left temporal lobe (Damasio et al., 1996). In fact, memories for living things (people, animals) tend to be associated with the left anterior temporal lobe, and memories for objects tend to be located in the left temporal–occipital region (Damasio et al., 1996). This is also supported by positron emission tomography (PET) studies that demonstrate temporal and frontal lobe activity during retrieval of past memories (Tulving & Markowitsch, 1997). Additional support comes from studies showing noun deficits following temporal lobe injury, but verb deficits following frontal injury (Daniele et al., 1994). These findings appear to show a lateralized effect, with long-term memories for semantic information likely to be found in the left temporal lobe (Gourovitch et al., 2000; Strauss et al., 2000; Wiggs et al., 1999). Left temporal lobe activation is common throughout learning trials, as part of the consolidation process for forming long-term memories (Kopelman et al., 1998).

These findings suggest that whereas long-term memory for learned information is likely to be associated with left temporal lobe functions, memories for hearing, vision, somatosensory, and motor functions are probably related to the same areas that perform those functions (Goldberg, 2001). *The implications are significant for both assessment and intervention.* If someone has a particular sensory or motor deficit, then the memories of those functions may also be impaired. This could account for the well-known finding that damage to the left-hemisphere motor regions can lead to apraxia.

● The superior–posterior temporal lobe is where auditory information is received from the ear and auditory nerve, with the main projections contralateral; however, there are also ipsilateral projections as well, which is unlike the other sensory systems.

● Comprehension of auditory information takes place in the auditory association areas, which include the insula, areas within the STS, and Wernicke's area (located within the planum temporale, an area often implicated in language comprehension and reading disorders).

● The ventral–lateral temporal lobe is where the ventral visual stream is received from the occipital lobe. It is important in object recognition and probably long-term memory storage for objects, but long-term memory is widely distributed, primarily to the areas that process or perform the information originally (i.e., visual memory in the occipital lobe, auditory memory in the temporal lobe).

● The medial middle temporal lobe serves as an important component of the cortical link with the limbic structures associated with attention, learning, memory, and emotion. The lateral middle temporal lobe is likely where memory for facts and details, especially in the left hemisphere, is stored. Long-term memory for inanimate objects tends to be more posterior, whereas memory for animate or living objects tends to be more anterior, in this region.

● Connections between the temporal lobes and other cortical areas probably serve different functions. The connections between the left and right temporal lobes are likely to be important for linking object recognition processes, and for linking temporal lobe functions with limbic functions. The temporal–parietal lobe connections are important for linking the dorsal and ventral streams. The connections with the frontal lobes may have to do with the medial temporal lobe functions and long-term memory storage and/or retrieval, as well as emotional memories. The temporal lobe connections with the occipital lobes are important for the ventral stream. In addition, the vertical occipital fasciculus in the anterior occipital region allows the brain to determine whether incoming visual information is best processed by the dorsal or ventral streams.

An Axis Divided: III. Somatosensory Processes and the Parietal Lobe

Somatosensory Pathways: From Skin to Parietal Lobe

The major pathways for the somatosensory cortex project from the brainstem to the parietal lobe via the thalamus. As is the case with vision and hearing, two pathways emerge. The dorsal pathway leaves the dorsal column of the spinal cord and projects to the thalamus, where it then goes to the primary somatosensory area. Consistent with this organization, the dorsal pathway is important for perception of touch, pressure, and proprioceptive movement. The other pathway leaves the lateral spinal column and projects to the lateral posterior thalamus and pulvinar, and then on to the somatosensory cortex. This lateral pathway is important for perception of pain and temperature. Consistent with what we have seen for the other sensory systems, the lateral pathway affects the secondary somatosensory areas, not the primary cortex.

Parietal Lobe Structure and Function

Figure 2.4 presents several pertinent parietal areas discussed in this section. As noted earlier, the primary somatosensory cortex processes touch, pressure, and movement for the body. Important distinctions can be made in regard to what parts of the body are represented

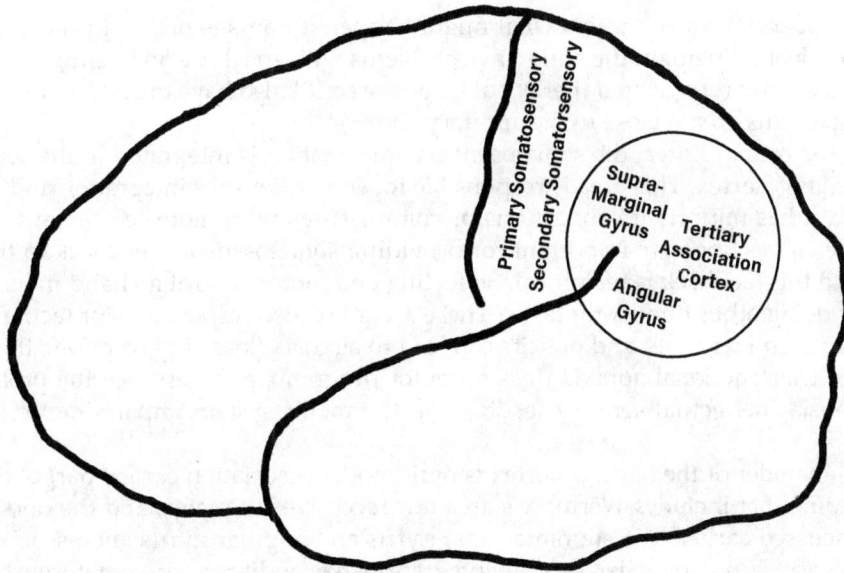

FIGURE 2.4. Structure and function of the parietal lobe.

in what parts of this primary cortex. Figure 2.5 presents the body area representations in the primary motor cortex (left side of figure) and somatosensory cortex (right side), called a *homunculus* ("little man" in Latin). As can be seen on the right, there are large amounts of somatosensory cortex for the hands and face, with smaller amounts for the limbs.

The disproportionate representation of somatosensory cortex allows for more sensitivity in important sensory areas (e.g., lips, fingertips), and less sensitivity in other areas. The organization of the cortex is important, because damage to the lateral somatosensory cortex can result in problems with facial feeling, whereas damage to the medial portion can result in loss of feeling in the feet. After medial area damage, a child is more likely to lose feeling in both feet, because of the close proximity of the medial somatosensory cortex in the left and

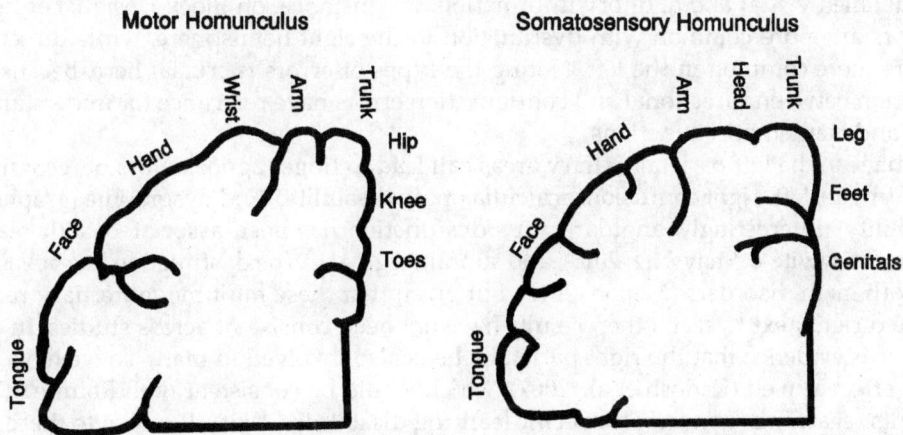

FIGURE 2.5. Motor homunculus and somatosensory homunculus.

right hemispheres. Can you guess what might happen if damage occurs in the lateral infe-rior section? Not only might the child have problems with speaking and eating (because the tongue and jaw are represented there), but he or she could also have problems with auditory processing (as this area is close to the auditory cortex).

From the primary area, the somatosensory information is integrated in the somatosen-sory association cortex. This area is responsible for somatosensory integration and interpre-tation, and it has important connections or commissures with motor cortex in the frontal lobe. These connections are important for providing somatosensory feedback to the motor system, and this feedback is reciprocal. So feeling and motor control go hand in hand when writing or doing other fine-motor tasks. These areas are also responsible for tactile recogni-tion of shapes and textures, and deficits can lead to agnosia (loss of perception); this in turn can lead to constructional apraxia (loss of motor program), so in essence the problem is a motor agnosia–ineffectual sensory feedback to the motor system impairs motor action or praxis.

The remainder of the parietal cortex is multimodal association cortex, part of the zones of overlapping that includes Wernicke's area (for receptive language), and the dorsal visual stream discussed earlier. The supramarginal gyrus and angular gyrus and associated tem-poral lobe areas, as noted earlier, serve to integrate visual, auditory, and somatosensory infor-mation. The superior temporal sulcus stream ends here too, so important for cross-modal matching. This is the parietal boundary of the occipital–parietal–temporal "crossroads," where the most complex forms of multimodal comprehension take place—Luria's tertiary area (see In-Depth 2.1).

These tertiary neurons are more likely to respond to many types of stimuli—not just auditory, visual, or somatosensory. Associated with the dorsal stream, this area is where important visual–spatial and motion information can be integrated with the other senses. Given the complexity of this region, it is not surprising that it has connections or commis-sures with the prefrontal cortex and frontal eye fields, discussed in the next section.

It is also crucial to recognize that this multimodal association cortex is the most lateral-ized tissue of any receptive cortical area, and that these differences have important ramifica-tions for understanding complex cognitive processes, including reading, math, and writing. The right parietal lobe is important for spatial processing and representations of objects in three-dimensional space, which fits well with our knowledge of the right hemisphere and understanding of global–holistic processes. Whereas the right parietal region is important for spatial relationships, the left parietal is important for directional orientation and integra-tion of detailed visual and auditory information. For instance, on Block Design, configura-tion errors are more common with dysfunction in the right hemisphere, while directional errors are more common in the left. Noting the types of errors is crucial here, because the dissociation between directional and configuration errors have relevance for understanding reading and mathematics functions.

Damage to the left parietal tertiary areas can lead to finger agnosia (loss of recognizing touch of finger), left–right confusion, acalculia (math disability), and dysgraphia (graphomo-tor disability). Interestingly, angular gyrus dysfunction has been associated with reading disorders (Shaywitz & Shaywitz, 2016), and supramarginal gyrus dysfunction has been asso-ciated with math disorders (Menon, 2016), but given that these multimodal tertiary regions are located right next to each other, results have not been consistent across studies. In addi-tion, there is evidence that the right parietal lobe is also involved in math, so we have a lat-eralized effect as well (Kadosh et al., 2007), which would be consistent with Rourke's (2000) arguments regarding "nonverbal" specific learning disabilities. We will return to these find-ings in Chapters 5 and 6.

Dysfunction or damage in these tertiary parietal regions can cause problems with sen-sory integration, self-awareness, environmental neglect (ignoring what is going around you), right–left orientation, and academic performance. Since self-awareness and environmental awareness are related to parietal lobe functioning, particularly the right parietal lobe, it is not surprising that damage to these regions can cause attention problems and poor self-aware-ness (Caggiano & Jehkonen, 2018). As noted earlier, these symptoms are quite similar to the symptoms seen in children with ADHD. However, a child who has attention problems due to parietal lobe dysfunction will probably not respond to stimulant medication or will respond only minimally, so differential diagnosis becomes crucial. A child with this type of attention problem cannot be detected by behavioral criteria alone, as highlighted in Case Study 2.1. The clinical question at hand is whether the attention problem is a bottom-up problem (e.g., a "primary" attention-deficit, due to right parietal dysfunction), or a top-down problem (e.g., executive attention problem caused by hypoactive frontal–subcortical circuits). Of course, it can also include the question of whether cortical tone or Luria's first functional unit (e.g., Sergeant's Cognitive Energetic Model, see Mahone & Denckla, 2017) could also explain the problem. In a case like this, only neuropsychological testing will reveal the true nature of the child's attention deficits, and thus allow for the appropriate intervention to be rendered. For instance, unlike ADHD that is related to executive control of attention, a child with parietal primary attention problems can use intact executive functions to self-monitor this tendency to ignore himself and his environment (e.g., Hale et al., 2006).

Parietal Lobe Summary

To summarize the functions of the parietal lobe, it is the primary processor of somatosensory information. It is thought to have the following attributes:

- The primary somatosensory cortex has different pathways. One projects to the pri-mary cortex and processes touch, pressure, and kinesthesis, while the other projects to the secondary cortex and processes pain and temperature.

- The primary somatosensory cortex is arranged like a homunculus ("little man"). Large portions of cortex are needed for sensitive areas, such as the fingertips and lips; less sensitive areas, like the limbs, have less somatosensory cortex. The lateral surface is more likely to be involved in facial areas, and the medial areas are related to the lower extremities.

- The secondary somatosensory association cortex has rich connections with both the primary areas and frontal lobes to control movements, and, with the dorsal stream, is respon-sible for spatial perception and guiding actions in response to the environment.

- The posterior–ventral parietal lobe, and associated temporal regions, are where the highest form of understanding takes place. The occipital–parietal–temporal "crossroads" serves as the important non-modality-specific higher-level processing zone. It has numerous interconnected and bidirectional connections with the frontal lobe, discussed in the next section.

- Parietal lobe dysfunction, especially on the left side, can result in difficulty with sound–symbol association for reading, perceptual–motor difficulties for writing, and arithmetic computation skills. Damage to the left parietal lobe is sometimes referred to as Gerstmann syndrome, characterized by finger agnosia, left–right confusion, acalculia, and dysgraphia. However, right parietal dysfunction also leads to math and writing difficulty, but seldom to reading problems.

- Parietal lobe dysfunction, especially on the right side, can cause neglect of oneself and the environment, leading to symptoms (poor attention and self-awareness) that appear to be

Case Study 2.1. The Untreatable Boy with ADHD

Michael had been diagnosed with ADHD, depression, and social skills deficits several years before coming to our clinic. Originally diagnosed via criteria of the fourth edition of the *Diagnostic and Statistical Manual of Mental Disorders* (DSM-IV) and behavior rating scales, Michael had been unsuccessfully treated with several types of stimulants and antidepressants for several years. In fact, his social and academic skills were reportedly deteriorating, despite years of special education support. His writing was also quite messy, and he was seeing an occupational therapist. Michael's parents, teacher, and physician were quite concerned at his poor treatment response.

   After the physician referred Michael to us, we met with the parents, who presented a clinical picture that just didn't quite fit with ADHD. Sure enough, Michael qualified as having ADHD according to DSM-IV criteria, but his neuropsychology was quite different. When he underwent our double-blind placebo medication trial of methylphenidate (Ritalin), he showed no differences in response on medication and on the placebo. We could see why others thought he had ADHD, as his behavior ratings confirmed problems with attention, self-awareness, and interpersonal relationships. However, further neuropsychological testing suggested that he had the classic signs of right parietal dysfunction, affecting the dorsal stream. His "motor" problems, originally thought to be consistent with his ADHD diagnosis, were actually related to poor visual feedback to the motor system. Both Michael and children with "true" ADHD have behavioral signs of ADHD, but the interventions we use will have very different effects on these two types of children. We ended up using social skills instruction to help Michael identify facial affect and prosody, and metacognitive ("thinking about thinking") strategies to help him monitor his performance and behavior—strategies that would be difficult for most unmedicated children with "true" ADHD.

ADHD. However, the differential diagnosis is critical, as this type of attention problem is unlikely to significantly benefit from stimulant treatment.

An Axis Integrated: Higher-Level Processes and the Frontal Lobe

Motor Pathways: From Frontal Lobe to Muscles

So far, we have examined the afferent system, with the occipital, temporal, and parietal lobes all related to sensory input. Whereas the posterior brain regions are important for understanding, the frontal lobe is responsible for regulation of *action*. Notice that the heading for this section starts with the brain (frontal lobe) and then extends to the periphery (muscles). Instead of the association cortex being the end of the path, as it is for the sensory systems, the motor system starts with the association cortex, where motives and plans for motor activity are developed. These areas are discussed in the next paragraph. After receiving the motor directions from the association areas, the primary motor cortex is charged with carrying out the action.

   The primary motor cortex has a similar body representation (homunculus) described in the parietal lobe section (see Figure 2.5). From this area, two separate pathways emerge: the ventral–medial and lateral motor systems. Simply put, the ventral–medial system is responsible for whole-body, or gross-motor, movement; the lateral system is responsible for skilled, or fine-motor, movements. A description of these systems, and of their interaction with subcortical and posterior cortical sensory structures, would be exceedingly complex and is beyond the scope of this text. However, recall that the basal ganglia, cerebellum, and cranial nerves all play important roles in motor as well as other cortical functions. As suggested earlier, the variety of sensory and motor connections with subcortical regions not only allows for complex behavior to emerge, but also serves a regulatory check-and-balance function. Think of these sensory and motor connections as a judicial system that keeps the congressional posterior lobes and the presidential frontal lobe in check.

Frontal Lobe Structure and Function

Depicted in Figure 2.6, the primary motor cortex is the cortical endpoint of motor programs, not the beginning, as is the case with the primary visual, auditory, and somatosensory cortices. Anterior to the primary motor area are the secondary motor areas—one related to body motor skills (e.g., writing) and one related to eye motor skills (e.g., visual tracking). The secondary motor area is divided into the lateral–inferior or *premotor* area, and the medial–superior or *supplementary motor* area. The premotor area affects motor functions indirectly through the primary motor cortex, and directly through cortical–spinal connections. Although there is some debate over the issue, the supplementary motor and premotor areas provide for different motor functions, depending on the type of activity and the amount of experience the individual has with a task.

The supplementary motor area is thought to regulate internally guided motor programs (e.g., getting dressed for the day, brushing your teeth); it is critical for developing and programming self-directed motor sequences. When you write letters during a spelling test or a written expression assignment, the supplementary motor area accomplishes this task (at least for someone who is proficient at it) in combination with expressive language regions in an area called Exner's area (see Chapter 7). The supplementary motor area is also important for bimanual coordination (using both hands together). Alternatively, the premotor area provides for movement in response to external stimuli (e.g., the center fielder's reaching out to catch that baseball, learning motor movements in a new video game). Consistent with these

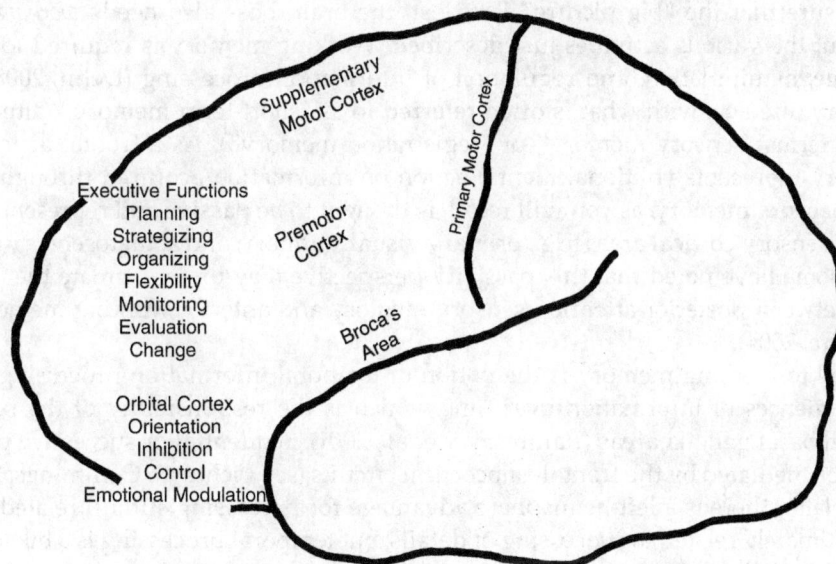

FIGURE 2.6. Structure and function of the frontal lobes.

propositions, the premotor cortex is active in learning novel motor sequences, but the supplementary motor cortex is more active during previously learned or routinized motor patterns (Nachev, Kennard, & Husain, 2008).

In our temporal lobe discussion earlier, we discussed its importance in storing long-term memories of facts, details, and words. However, this is long-term memory of *nouns*. Interestingly, the left motor association and prefrontal areas have been found to be related to memories for *verbs* (representing action) and imagined tool use (a motor skill) (Moll et al., 2000; Vigliocco et al., 2011). The other secondary motor area is the frontal eye field. It has numerous connections with cortical and subcortical structures to guide eye movements, which are important for visual search, scanning, and tracking (O'Driscoll et al., 2000). Consistent with the other secondary areas, one area is for self-directed movement, and the other is for responding to external stimuli. You will not be surprised to find that these areas have connections with the dorsal and ventral visual streams discussed earlier (e.g., M and P pathways), as well as subcortical areas involved in movement (see In-Depth 2.5).

To gain an understanding of the remainder of the frontal cortex, the prefrontal cortex, it is best to think of it as the "brain manager" or "boss" of the rest of the brain (Hale & Fiorello, 2001). It is Luria's (1973a) "superstructure"—the seat of all volitional goal-directed activity.

The dorsolateral prefrontal cortex serves as the highest cortical area responsible for motor planning, organization, and regulation. This area is often associated with "cognitive" executive functions. Before you continue reading, try to brainstorm all of the things a company executive or your boss does, and you will know the definition of *executive functions*. The boss does not do the work per se; he or she manages the workers, the work environment, and relations with the public. Similarly, the dorsolateral prefrontal cortex does not do the brain's work per se, but it is intimately involved in planning, organizing, strategizing, initiating, implementing, monitoring, evaluating, modifying, changing, and shifting (requiring flexibility) our behavior (Hale, Reddy, Wilcox, et al., 2009). These activities all require Luria's "superstructure" frontal lobes to govern all other brain areas, and with the basal ganglia and thalamus, serve as a gating or filtering mechanism for mental control of information (Shimamura, 2000), or at least conscious information (Koziol et al., 2013).

To ensure that the "big picture" isn't lost, the brain boss also needs *working memory* to carry out the various activities just described. Working memory is required for temporary storage, manipulation, and regulation of information processing (Dehn, 2008). Working memory interacts with what is often referred to as "short-term memory" (although we prefer the terms "sensory memory" or "registration memory"). As a frontal action, working memory represents volitional mental action on information acquired through sensory memory. Sensory memory, as you will recall, is thought to be passive and represented in the associated sensory cortical areas (e.g., primary visual, auditory, and somatosensory cortices); however, some have noted that this passivity perspective may underestimate the interrelationship between posterior attention/sensory memory and anterior working memory functions (Squire, 2004).

Related to working memory is the notion of temporal information processing, or processing sequences of information over time, which is the responsibility of the prefrontal and related basal ganglia areas (Rammsayer et al., 2001). Sequential or successive processes tended to be mediated by the frontal–subcortical circuits (see Lichter & Cummings, 2001). As discussed later, there is a left-hemisphere advantage for processing stimuli related in time, and it is intimately related to processing of details, but temporal processing is a bilateral phenomenon (Mauk & Buonomano, 2004). Many areas have been related to sequential processing, including the dorsolateral prefrontal, Broca's area, basal ganglia, and left parietal lobes,

IN-DEPTH 2.5. The Big Five Loops

There are at least five reciprocal frontal–subcortical circuits that are involved in the highest levels of self-management and emotion regulation. They are sometimes referred to as "loops," because information exchange is reciprocal. Lichter and Cummings (2001) provide us with the following understanding of how these interrelated circuits, born out of distinct physiological and functional systems, give rise to the complexity of human goal-directed behavior. All five circuits are related to the frontal lobe, basal ganglia, and thalamus. The dorsal system is responsible for executive control, and the ventral system is responsible for emotional tone, with both systems represented in dorsal and ventral areas of their related structures. The five circuits are as follows:

- Motor circuit—related to premotor, supplementary motor, and primary motor functions (ecological validity check: handwriting).
- Oculomotor circuit—related to frontal eye field, prefrontal, and parietal cortex functions (ecological validity check: reading words).
- Dorsolateral prefrontal circuit—related to anterior-lateral prefrontal executive functions (ecological validity check: turning words into equations during math word problems).
- Orbital prefrontal circuit—related to inferior-medial prefrontal functions (ecological validity check: raising hand and waiting turn during class discussion).
- Anterior cingulate circuit—related to anterior cingulate (ecological validity check: finishing work in a timely manner).

Deficits in the motor or oculomotor circuits can lead to problems with motor control and activity, or with visual attention and scanning, respectively. Dorsolateral prefrontal circuit dysfunction leads to the classic signs of attention deficits and executive dysfunction, such as problems with planning, strategizing, organizing, monitoring, evaluating, shifting, and changing behavior (Hale & Fiorello, 2001). Orbital prefrontal circuit dysfunction is often related to emotional lability and disinhibition or poor impulse control. Finally, anterior cingulate dysfunction can lead to problems with motivation, persistence, and on-line monitoring of performance. Hale, Bertin, et al. (2004) argue that children with ADHD probably experience dysfunction in one or more of these loops, especially the dorsolateral (inattentive type) and orbital (hyperactive–impulsive type) circuits.

---

so while sequential processing is likely a left hemisphere function, whether a sequencing problem is more anterior and/or posterior is worth clinical consideration.

Temporal relationships/timing also require multiple structures, including the dorsolateral prefrontal cortex (time relationships, such as "How long is going to take me to complete the task?"), basal ganglia (consistent application over time, such as "Am I doing this consistently over time?"), cingulate (keeping track of time, such as "Did I do this in the amount of time I thought it would take, or do I need to speed up?"), and cerebellum (motor timing when carrying out an act–no real thought here, just consistent motor performance). So the question "How soon do I need to leave to get downtown for the show?" is probably related more to cortical functions, whereas the timing of speech sounds or motor actions is probably more subcortical in nature.

As noted by Luria (1973), working memory is also important for both verbal fluency and nonverbal fluency (Baldo et al., 2001), which are related to locating and retrieving information from memory storage in the back of the brain. Damage to this prefrontal region leads to problems with organizing and segregating events in memory (Thompson-Schill et al., 2002) and posterior cingulate function also impairs memory retrieval (Pearson et al., 2011). Not only is working memory necessary for encoding of information into long-term memory storage, which is apparently the role of the left frontal areas; it is also needed for retrieval of semantic information from long-term memory storage, which seems to be the responsibility of the right frontal lobe (Babiloni et al., 2006; Stuss & Alexander, 2005). Although lateralization of encoding (new learning) and retrieval (accessing old memories) processes is currently a source of debate, there is convincing evidence that the frontal lobes provide the executive skills necessary for these functions (Wheeler et al., 1995). It is more likely that retrieval requires bilateral prefrontal cooperation (Stuss, 2011). However, if we must make a gross comparison, we use the hemispheric encoding/retrieval (HERA) model, where the left is specialized for encoding and the right for retrieval (Habib et al., 2003).

Executive functions are not just related to the individual's ability to interact with the *external* environment, they are also related to the *internal* state of the individual. Internal executive functions require the orbital region, part of the ventral prefrontal cortex. The orbital frontal cortex has intricate cortical connections with the temporal lobe (via the uncinate fasciculus) and subcortical connections (e.g., basal ganglia, thalamus, and amygdala) to help initiate and maintain performance, inhibit irrelevant responses or actions, and modulate emotional responsiveness. It also has a very important connection with a very small structure, the nucleus accumbens—the pleasure center of the brain.

In concert with the dorsolateral region, the orbital cortex mediates initiative and decision-making behavior, especially during complex probabilistic situations (Price & Devlin, 2011). Whereas cognitive impulsivity is probably mediated by the dorsolateral cortex, emotional impulsivity is likely a function of the orbital cortex. It is not surprising that the orbital cortex has an important role in both behavior and social control, and is often associated with the ability to take the perspective of others, or "theory of mind" (Stuss et al., 2001). The orbital cortex appears to be especially relevant for emotional as opposed to cognitive perspective taking (Hynes et al., 2006), making it critical for empathy.

As Koziol et al. (2013) have said, perception of emotion in the posterior regions is only one aspect of social competency; to have truly meaningful relationships with others, one must have empathy for the feelings of others. This makes the orbital cortex important for intimate attachment in friendship and love. In other words, if you have posterior regions intact, you may perceive someone is sad, but you need the orbital cortex to act on that perception before you say, "I feel your pain." Finally, if dysfunction can lead to too little or too much orbital activity, this could perhaps lead to indifference (e.g., psychopathy) or codependency (e.g., enmeshment) (Hale & Fitzer, 2015), but we are not aware of studies that have explored this possibility.

While the medial frontal cortex area (including the anterior cingulate and nucleus accumbens) is often identified during discussion of executive function, this area is sometimes also considered part of the limbic system. The anterior cingulate probably serves a crucial executive–attention function, ensuring efficient interactions between the multiple posterior and prefrontal areas (Shenhav et al., 2016). It is involved in responding to novelty, self-monitoring performance, inhibiting automatic responses, shifting cognitive set, motivation for action, and novel decision making (Bush et al., 2000; Kelly, 2009). Combined, these anterior areas serve as the executive attentional system, responsible for guiding and directing all other aspects of consciousness (Posner et al., 2016). (See In-Depth 2.5 for a further discussion.)

A discussion of the frontal lobes also has to include another motor area of interest to school psychologists and speech–language pathologists: the well-known Broca's area. Broca's area is an important site for expressive language, but it is also involved in syntax (the rules of language) and possibly other motor functions (Friederici, 2018). It is connected to Wernicke's area by the arcuate fasciculus—an important commissure that will be discussed further in Chapter 5. Interestingly, an area adjacent to Broca's area that includes the supplementary motor cortex, is known as Exner's area. Discussed earlier and in more detail in Chapter 7, Exner's area appears to be important for written expressive language (Nakamura et al., 2012). It represents the motor script or movements associated with spelling, which could explain why some children decode words well when reading, but have difficulties with written spelling.

As we can see, Luria's (1973) description of the frontal lobes as the "superstructure" above all other brain areas seems appropriate. It is interesting to note that few early researchers focused on the structure and function of the "silent" frontal lobe (for a discussion, see Goldberg, 2001), because several studies had shown that frontal damage did not result in decrements in "intelligence" as measured by IQ tests. Like many of the findings reported in this book and in the field, this conclusion may have more to do with the measures and methods used than with brain–behavior relationships. Early intelligence tests depended a lot on crystallized knowledge, and so would be less impaired after frontal damage.

If you assume that intelligence tests measure innate intelligence, and that intelligence is not harmed by frontal lobe damage, then you might conclude that studying frontal lobe functioning is not very important. On the contrary, as we have seen, the frontal lobes are the source of higher-level cognition; they serve as manager of the anterior–posterior axis, as well as of the left–right axis, and as discussed later, interrelated with subcortical structures in the superior–inferior axis. Unfortunately, few intelligence tests tap these higher executive processes well, and even neuropsychological measures may not fully tap the true nature of these functions. While dramatic decrements in intellectual functioning may not occur with frontal injury or dysfunction, subtle and additive negative effects can be seen on intellectual measures (Hale et al., 2012), which might lead others to inaccurately suggest those with frontal dysfunction are less "intelligent." We will return to this issue in the next chapter.

Finally, it is important to note at this point that the prefrontal cortex is not the seat of all executive functions, since additional cortical and subcortical circuits are needed to ensure efficient executive control, as discussed in the superior–inferior axis section. These cortical–cortical and cortical–subcortical circuits are required for all complex mental activity.

Frontal Lobe Summary

To summarize the functions of the frontal lobe, it is primarily involved in motor activity. It is thought to have the following attributes:

• The primary motor cortex has a "little man" structure similar, but not identical, to that of the primary somatosensory cortex. The head's motor activities are associated with the lateral portions, and those of the lower body are linked with more medial sections.

• The primary motor cortex is linked to two separate areas of association cortex: the premotor and supplementary motor cortices. The premotor cortex is more responsible for directing movements in response to the environment and is involved during learning of motor scripts. The supplementary motor area is more involved with self-directed movement and is active during previously learned or routinized motor skills. Motor skill learning has also been linked to the motor frontal-basal ganglia-thalamic circuits, and cerebrum–cerebellum circuitry, and the influence is bidirectional.

• The oculomotor circuit is important for visual tracking and saccade, which not only relates to visual scanning of the environment and determining relationships among visual stimuli, it also plays a role in visual sequencing of letters during reading decoding, so the M pathway detects motion during decoding activities.

- The prefrontal area consists of the dorsolateral prefrontal cortex, the orbital frontal cortex, and the medial section (including the anterior cingulate). These regions have rich interconnections with almost every area in the cortex, and either directly or indirectly with almost every subcortical area, especially the basal ganglia and limbic system.

- The dorsolateral and orbital cortices can be differentiated from each other. The dorsolateral region is in charge of executive function and working memory activities or *external* executive function; whereas the orbital frontal region is responsible for behavioral and emotional regulation, or *internal* executive function.

- The anterior cingulate also plays an important role in this executive "superstructure," including responding to novelty, self-monitoring of performance, inhibiting automatic responses, shifting cognitive set, motivation for action, and complex decision making.

- Part of the lateral frontal association cortex includes Broca's area, long identified as the source of expressive aphasia. It is located between the executive area and the facial motor areas; it is involved in symbolic expression, including language, and has been associated with language rules and other motor activities. It is connected to the posterior speech zones via the arcuate fasciculus. The adjacent Exner's area likely plays a similar role for written expression and spelling.

The Left–Right Axis and the Cerebral Hemispheres

Early Findings: The Dominant and Nondominant Hemispheres

Before the late 20th century, there were basically two brain–behavior camps: the "localizationists," who argued that separate brain areas are responsible for unique mental processes, and the "antilocalizationists," who argued that the brain is an "equal-opportunity" organ and that all parts are involved during all cognitive processes. Gall's phrenology was an early and unsuccessful attempt at supporting the localizationist position, whereas Lashley argued in favor of a mass action and equipotentiality for all cognitive processes (Das & Varnhagen, 1986). The seminal works by Paul Broca and Carl Wernicke in the late 1800s furthered the localizationist cause, as they identified damage to the left-hemisphere association areas in several patients with expressive and receptive aphasia. Since language was thought to be a left-hemisphere process, researchers concluded that visual–spatial skills must be a right-hemisphere process—a finding they then confirmed in numerous studies. These verbal–nonverbal results, often based on studies of patients and animals with brain damage, predominated during most of the 20th century.

The relationship between left-hemisphere language functioning and right-hand preference (handedness) provided further evidence for the localizationists. The localizationist camp gained greater recognition as this concept of "cerebral dominance" permeated the early neuropsychological research efforts. Studies demonstrating anatomical hemispheric differences confirmed the left hemisphere's propensity to control language and handedness (Galaburda et al., 1978). These arguments, especially when combined with findings suggesting that language problems (aphasia) and many types of motor problems (apraxia) are more likely to occur following left-hemisphere damage (Liepmann, 1908), led to the reification of the left hemisphere's role as the "dominant" hemisphere and the right hemisphere's role as the "minor" hemisphere (Goldberg, 2001). Because children with learning disorders were found to have a greater incidence of left-handedness, several concluded that incomplete hemispheric dominance can result in learning disorders (Geschwind, 1983); this led some to try to "correct" left-handedness in children. What followed was a plethora of "dichoto-mania"—theories and measures that claimed to reflect processing differences between the hemispheres (see Table 2.4).

Despite the overwhelming belief in the dominant-verbal and nondominant-nonverbal dichotomy, there were vocal opponents to these localizationist views. Noting the ability of young children to acquire language following left-hemisphere damage, Lenneberg (1967) took up the antilocalizationist cause by arguing that the hemispheres are equally capable of developing language, but equivocated by arguing that lateralization is gradually realized through adolescence. Supported by the finding that brain damage occurring early in life is less debilitating than damage occurring in adults—a concept discussed earlier known as the "Kennard principle" (Kennard, 1938)—many suggested that the brain may be equally capable of performing all tasks.

Although the Kennard principle has taken on a life of its own that did not actually reflect Dr. Kennard's work (Dennis, 2010), those supporting the "earlier brain damage is better" per-spective led to the popular belief that humans only use a small portion of their brains, and that much "brain power" is untapped, left in reserve should something go awry. These findings and beliefs led many to view localization of function as a worthless endeavor and to regard functionalist views as more pragmatic, especially in work with children. This gave clinicians treating brain damage in children a sense of optimism that the children could recover, regard-less of the insult; however, subsequent research suggests that such optimism may not be war-ranted (Anderson et al., 2011; Cioni et al., 2011; Dennis, 2010), as noted in Application 2.2.

As is the case for many debates in psychology, the "truth" about damage and recov-ery lies somewhere between the localizationist and antilocalizationist perspectives. When it comes to lateralization, controversy over whether the hemispheres act independently, inter-actively, or in domain-specific ways is likely to continue, as arguments can be made for both invariant and progressive lateralization (Kinsbourne, 1997). As we have seen, brain areas have many different structures and functions, but the brain also has an amazing ability to recover following an insult, and the same insult does not always produce the same behav-ioral outcome in all children (Dennis, 2010). That is why we need to be on our clinical toes! We must recognize that each child is unique and malleable, and that intervention has much to do with the success of a child's outcome, regardless of the nature or cause of the deficits or strengths.

TABLE 2.4. Theories of Differences in Left- and Right-Hemisphere Processing

Left hemisphere	Right hemisphere	Source
Leading	Automatic	Jackson (1868/1958)
Verbal	Nonverbal	Weisenberg & McBride (1935)
Analytic	Holistic	Levy (1974)
Routinized	Novel	Goldberg & Costa (1981)
Sequential	Simultaneous	Kaufman & Kaufman (1983)
Local	Global	Delis et al. (1986)
Microstructural	Macrostructural	Glosser (1993)
Fine	Coarse	Beeman (1993)
Successive	Simultaneous	Das et al. (1994)
Concordant/convergent	Discordant/divergent	Bryan & Hale (2001)

APPLICATION 2.2. The "Benign" Head Injury

It seems as if we are hearing a good deal from parents or teachers about kids hitting their heads and suffering no long-term consequences. About half of the children we see in the clinic have scars on their heads—evidence of past injuries (especially now that shaved or very short hair is back in vogue). Discussing the incidents with the parents during an interview, we usually get similar responses: "She fell from the high chair and hit her head on the table," or "They were throwing rocks, and one of the other boys mistakenly hit him," or "He fell off his bike and hit his head, but he only got a headache." The next sentence is usually "You know, these things happen to children; they fall and hit their heads all the time." True, children fall and children hit their heads, and many children apparently suffer no long-term effects. However, the children we see are often said to have learning and attention problems of unknown origin, but a careful examination often reveals a possible genetic, physical, or environmental determinant in a majority of these cases.

One of us (Hale) remembers one child who was in a car accident and hit his head. When he asked the parent about possible indications of brain trauma (headache, nausea, vomiting, dizziness, etc.), she replied, "Oh, no, he was fine, but he did get the flu that night." She never returned to the hospital to get this "flu" evaluated, and the boy could have died. We are especially bothered by emergency/rescue television dramas that discuss children who "miraculously" survive brain trauma. Yes, a child's brain is remarkable in its ability to recover function after even a serious cerebral insult, but such a child is likely to experience considerable attention and learning problems, with the length of coma directly related to the degree of impairment. This is not to say that we should automatically assume that every little bump and scrape leads to significant head injury, but we should be ever vigilant for the possibility that a reportedly "minor" incident has indeed affected a child's brain and his or her current functioning.

Similar to early conceptualizations of posterior–anterior brain functions, much of the initial work in hemispheric differences was based on measures and methods that limited accurate interpretation of left–right differences. Early conceptualizations were often based on adults with brain lesions or animal models. Just as many researchers and practitioners neglected the frontal lobes in early research, since frontal damage did not apparently affect "intelligence," early lateralization researchers were overly focused on measures of language and prior learning, which are more likely to be impaired following left-hemisphere damage. In other words, the methods and measures shaped the questions, and the results easily confirmed those early predictions.

Contemporary Interpretation of the Left–Right Axis

As much of our discussion has indicated, it is not surprising that these early beliefs have been modified or dismissed as we gain a greater understanding of hemispheric function. Although it is not completely inaccurate, the suggestion that the left hemisphere is "verbal" and the right is "nonverbal" is an oversimplification of hemispheric differences. Do you ever wonder why the auditory–verbal and visual–spatial intelligence subtests do not always hold together, even though you've been taught that they reflect left- and right-hemisphere processes, respectively? What about the Cognitive Assessment System successive and simultaneous model, or the Kaufman Assessment Battery for Children sequential and simultaneous model?

Though subtest scatter can certainly be related to the differential cognitive processes described in the previous sections, it is also related to left–right differences. However, as noted earlier, the original conceptualization of the left- and right-hemisphere processes was often based on the performance of adults with brain damage on verbal and nonverbal tasks. The findings of these early lateralization studies probably told us more about the tasks used than about true differences in hemispheric functioning (Poppel et al., 2020). It is now clear that hemispheric asymmetries are *process-specific*, not stimulus-specific (Kolb & Whishaw, 2021).

The advent of functional neuroimaging techniques helped to dispel early misconceptions about hemisphere differences. We now can study typical adults and children engaged in mental activities. Results from these and other studies confirm that verbal *and* nonverbal cognitive processes occur in *both* hemispheres. As we will discover, *the hemispheric division of labor is determined by the neuropsychological processes required, not the stimulus (input) or response (output).*

This essential tenet of hemispheric function is an important distinction—one that will advance psychological assessment and intervention practices in the years to come. When we could not correlate brain activity with mental processes, we were left with interpreting input and output we saw during testing, much like a behaviorist must rely on observation of overt antecedents, behaviors, and consequences to make judgments about children. Although stimulus input and motor output remain important, we must now examine neuropsychological processes as well. This has important implications for understanding all child disorders, especially children with specific learning disabilities, as discussed in Chapter 1.

As one would expect, given this premise, current neuroimaging research suggests that *both* hemispheres are likely to be engaged during most tasks, with most coordination occurring through the corpus callosum (although anterior and posterior commissures also play a role on some tasks), and executive circuits ensuring the hemispheric division of labor occurs on a gradient (Goldberg, 2001). It is the hemispheric division of labor that differs from one task to another, depending on the processes required, and individual differences in response to task demands. When discovered during their research, this fact baffled many researchers, as they found right-hemisphere involvement during language processing and left-hemisphere involvement during visual processing. However, within the neuropsychological paradigm shift we will discuss, this fact makes perfect sense. After reviewing the literature on hemispheric differences in In-Depth 2.6, we provide a greater understanding of why the old conceptualizations must give way to a new understanding of hemispheric processing differences.

The new synthesis evolved from the seminal work of Goldberg and Costa (1981), updated in Goldberg's (2001) highly readable and highly recommended treatise on frontal lobe functioning, *The Executive Brain*. Their work, in combination with the other findings presented below, provides us with the impetus to pursue this neuropsychological paradigm shift—a dramatic shift from focusing solely on input and output demands, to interpreting them in relation to neuropsychological processing demands.

A Monumental Step in the Right–Left Direction

Based on physiological differences and other clinical evidence, Goldberg and Costa (1981) concluded that the right hemisphere has a greater capacity to deal with informational complexity and multimodal representations, while the left hemisphere is specialized for tasks requiring single-modal representations that are well known and automatic. Therefore, the right hemisphere specializes in processing disparate information, whereas the left hemisphere is specialized for processing routinized codes. This is not to suggest that that the hemispheres work independently.

It is not surprising that Goldberg, as a student of Luria, sees the hemispheres as interconnected and mutually dependent. The hemispheres necessarily work concertedly on most

IN-DEPTH 2.6. The Asymmetrical Brain Divided

Although at one level the left and right hemispheres are symmetrical, there are numerous structural differences between them—not only in terms of their general anatomy, but at the cellular level as well. Of the physiological differences, several are related to auditory and other temporal lobe processes. The left planum temporale and insula are often larger than their right-side counterparts, and this asymmetry has important implications for language representation. The sylvian fissure is longer and the occipital lobe is wider on the left side. The postcentral gyrus and other secondary somatosensory areas have been reported to be larger on the left; this is similar to the pattern found in the frontal motor areas, including Broca's area. Interestingly, Broca's area is buried deeper on the left and has more surface area on the right. Asymmetries favoring the right side include a larger Heschl's gyrus, because there are two of them in the right hemisphere; a larger occipital–parietal–temporal association area; and a wider frontal lobe, especially the prefrontal cortex. Most importantly, the right hemisphere is heavier and contains more white matter than the left, but gray matter is disproportionately represented on the left. As a result, the left hemisphere has more primary cortex and does more within-region processing, whereas the right hemisphere has more association cortex and does more between-region processing.

---

tasks, with the major difference being related to how much they are involved in any given activity. According to Goldberg's (2001) gradiental theory, the interconnected nature of brain systems makes it difficult to determine whether symptoms are related to one structure or another, and damage to one system will necessarily affect another. Our left/right axis interpretation approach fits this basic premise: dysfunction is not seen as an either/or phenomenon (i.e., a left hemisphere or a right hemisphere problem); instead it is a *how much* one. Accordingly, when it comes to left–right hemisphere differences, a skilled clinician has to ask *how much* is the left hemisphere involved and *how much* is the right hemisphere involved in processing a particular task, producing the behavior we see, or making the inferences we make about the source of dysfunction or disability.

One research group has shown bilateral hemisphere activation during many different types of cognitive tasks, but their conclusions are somewhat different from ours. Historically, Belger and Banich (1998) conclude that information complexity determines the amount of hemisphere involvement, which is somewhat consistent with the position just stated. However, they conclude that as information complexity increases, an individual is likely to "recruit" the right hemisphere to help out the left hemisphere. This fits well with earlier notions about the "dominant" left hemisphere, but it also fits nicely with our model. In this old model, the left hemisphere was always considered to be the dominant and most primary hemisphere. More current theories suggest that the hemispheres are important for different reasons based on the activity or cognitive process that is involved (Gazzaniga et al., 2013). If an activity requires novel (or more complex) processing, then the right hemisphere will predominate. If a routinized, automatic code exists to aid in processing the incoming information, the left hemisphere will predominate.

Explicit language is a well-routinized code. It is symbolic (letters, words, and concepts) and highly structured (syntax and grammar), so it is not surprising that conventional explicit language use is better represented by left-hemisphere processes. This model does not supplant the left/verbal–right/nonverbal dichotomy per se; instead, it recognizes that the hemispheres are specialized for different processes, not different stimuli. Most verbal processes, especially those tapped by standardized measures that require a "correct" answer, require the left hemisphere's specialization for routinized codes. Conversely, the right hemisphere is specialized for global, holistic, novel processes. As a result, it is responsible for solving complex nonverbal performance tasks—tasks that require integration of multiple sensory, motor, and executive skills. The "hemisphere load" argument does not truly encompass this apparent difference between the two hemispheres, as suggested by the evidence presented in the following sections.

Empirical Examination of Left–Right Processes

Let us explore the empirical evidence supporting this new model of hemispheric interaction. As noted earlier, previous studies that had adults with brain damage perform dichotic listening or visual field tasks predominated during the early study of hemispheric differences. Given these early methods, which focused on stimulus inputs and motor (either speech or fine motor) outputs, clear and convincing evidence for the left hemisphere as "verbal" and the right hemisphere as "nonverbal" emerged (Springer & Deutsch, 1998). The concept of cerebral dominance was probably invoked to explain how a nonverbal behavior (carrying out motor acts or praxis) could also be carried out by the left hemisphere.

Despite this early convincing evidence, the advent of neuroimaging techniques and other technologies led researchers and clinicians to revise their thinking about hemispheric processes. The convergence of these findings within the theoretical framework described earlier is both enlightening and exhilarating. These technologies have allowed us to move beyond this stimulus–response mentality to one of understanding neuropsychological processes—a perspective that is congruent with Goldberg and Costa's (1981) propositions about novel/right–routine/left processes more than four decades ago.

If you ask many people, they will tell you that music is a right-hemisphere process. One area of research supporting these novel–automatic distinctions involves the processing and playing of music. With its distinctively nonverbal quality but auditory demands, the early findings that music was processed in the right hemisphere seemed to confirm that this hemisphere is specialized for nonverbal processes. Early research confirmed that deficits in processing of melody and other nonverbal sounds were associated with damage to the right, but not left, hemisphere—a finding confirmed from stroke data in adults (Sihvonen et al., 2019).

Like many of our early beliefs about brain function, the right hemisphere-music connection is not so straightforward. Left-hemisphere damage is likely to cause disruptions in temporal or rhythmic musical interpretation, but right-hemisphere damage limits understanding of pitch and melodic contour (see Peretz & Zatorre, 2005). Experience with music likely plays a role along an expert/left hemisphere-novice/right hemisphere gradient, as adults are more likely than children to use left hemisphere processes when processing music (Koelsch et al., 2005).

In support of this assumption, music processing for novices reveals a right-hemisphere advantage, while concert musicians use the left hemisphere for music skills (Beeman & Chiarello, 2013), and left-hemisphere damage can lead to aphasia for words and music in musicians, especially for familiar musical pieces (Sihvonen et al., 2019). This finding is consistent with a positron emission tomography (PET) study of concert musicians that showed bilateral activity during listening, reading, and playing of classical music, but the activity was greater in the left hemisphere, especially in occipital–parietal and frontal association areas (Sergent et al., 1992). As is the case with language, the left Broca's area appears to be important for processing oral, written, and musical syntax (Sammler et al., 2011). It is also important to recognize that for advanced musicians, music is a language. Similar to when you learned your language, the right hemisphere was dominant but after you mastered (automatized) the language, the left hemisphere became dominant. When would an expert musician use right hemisphere skills more? Probably when they are learning or creating a new musical piece, or improvising during a solo on stage, both of which would require a novel approach (right hemisphere) to the routinized musical knowledge (left hemisphere) they already possess.

Therefore, auditory processing of music is consistent with a right/novel–left/routine perspective. Could this theory also apply to language? One line of research has focused on the acquisition of linguistic processing skills in children. Using an electrophysiological technique called *event-related potentials*, Dennis Molfese and his colleagues have measured the brain activity of children in response to auditory-phonemic stimuli for over 40 years. They have even followed these children longitudinally, and found that *bilateral* auditory processing skills 36 hours after birth predicted whether children would have reading disorders (Molfese, 2000). Molfese et al. (1990) have consistently demonstrated this bilateral activity during phonemic processing in young infants, but as language skills develop, the left hemisphere is responsible for most auditory–verbal skills.

Could it be that early language acquisition requires right-hemisphere processes? The findings by the Molfese research group certainly confirm that bilateral processes are important, and that auditory-verbal processing undergoes a significant reorganization in the first years of life. These right–left differences seem to be related to the amount of familiarity or experience infants have with stimuli, regardless of the modality (e.g., verbal–nonverbal), and to initial versus later processing demands (Molfese et al., 1990). Cerebral blood flow studies confirm that the right hemisphere is dominant for cognitive processing during the first 3 years of life (Chiron et al., 1997), and with findings that right-hemisphere damage early in life leads to language deficits later (Lidzba et al., 2017). Pragmatic language has also been affected by right hemispheric damage (Parola et al., 2016). *Pragmatic language* is the ability to communicate verbally and nonverbally in a situation as well as the use of rhythm and prosody. This type of disruption to language understanding can significantly affect social and emotional bonds with caregivers and peers.

For many years, people thought that people who are deaf use their right hemispheres to process American Sign Language (ASL), because it is *nonverbal* (Poizner & Battison, 2017). After all, ASL does not require auditory–verbal skills; it requires visual recognition of hand movements to understand language, and motor skills to express oneself. If it is visual–motor, it must be a right-hemisphere task, right? The answer is no. Studies have consistently shown that the left hemisphere is used for processing ASL (Poizner & Battison, 2017), and that left-hemisphere damage leads to aphasia-like symptoms in deaf signers (Hickok et al., 2009). This finding may be because the left hemisphere preferentially processes grammatical structures, or it could be due to the fact that language is an automatized skill, as we have suggested here. However, hemispheric findings should be tempered by the type of sign, with lexical signs being produced by the left hemisphere, while classifier signs are related more to right hemisphere functioning (Hickock et al., 2009). Finally, while praxis is a visual–tactile–motor phenomenon, it is well known that apraxia and aphasia are more likely to occur following damage to the left—not right—hemisphere (Utianski et al., 2020).

Though there is overwhelming clinical evidence that language deficits (for both verbal language and ASL) occur following left-hemisphere damage, they also occur following damage to the "nonverbal" right hemisphere. When cases of "crossed aphasia" following right-hemisphere damage were discussed in the clinical literature, it was generally concluded that these individuals must have had language lateralized to the right hemisphere. Clinicians and researchers originally accounted for these differences by suggesting that language is not always lateralized to the left hemisphere. However, studies in the late 20th century began to shed light on this apparent paradox.

Indeed, language processes are represented bilaterally in all individuals; the different *neuropsychological processes* are what determine the participation of each hemisphere. Our traditional aphasia instruments readily tapped typical language processes, and adequately assessed individuals who were afflicted with traditional left-hemisphere aphasias. The left hemisphere appears to be specialized for closely related words, single interpretations, and semantic integration, but the right hemisphere is important for exploring multiple word meanings and distant semantic relationships (Beeman & Chiarello, 2013). The findings that people with right-hemisphere damage are more likely to have difficulty with comprehending voice intonation or prosody, drawing inferences, understanding metaphors, recognizing humor, analyzing multiple word connotations, and interpreting implicit or figurative speech (see Bryan & Hale, 2001) suggest that these individuals miss the "gist" of social discourse (Semrud-Clikeman & Glass, 2010). Although they are not typically deficient in understanding grammar because it is largely rule-governed, they have difficulty with complex syntactic structures (Balaban et al. 2015). Because they are overly focused on routinized literal interpretations and expressions during discourse, children with right-hemisphere dysfunction fail to adapt to the subtleties of social exchange and linguistic complexity (Beeman & Chiarello, 2013).

Individuals with right-hemisphere dysfunction have no difficulty with typical language tasks, but they may have difficulty retrieving verbal information from long-term memory. They also experience significant difficulty with inferential thinking and abstraction. Recall that activation in the left frontal areas occurs during encoding, and that retrieval requires right frontal activation (Stuss & Alexander, 2005), but that both frontal areas are involved in more complex memory tasks. At first glance, this seems to run counter to our right/novel–left/routinized distinction. But it makes perfect sense if we consider that encoding requires convergent processes to categorize and place information in long-term memory, and that retrieval requires a divergent search for information. The left frontal processes during retrieval are involved in prototypic semantic connections (e.g., "cool" = low temperature), whereas the right hemisphere represents diversity beyond immediate associations, examining indirect or implicit associations (e.g., "cool" = good) (Schwartz & Baldo, 2001).

This explains why children with depression (more likely to be related to left frontal dysfunction), have difficulty with encoding (Jorge et al., 2004), whereas children with ADHD are more likely to have a problem with retrieval (Hale et al., 2013). However, as we will see in Chapter 9, the relationship between psychopathology and hemispheric function is just now emerging (e.g., Hale et al., 2018).

In addition to the linguistic and memory-related aspects of right-hemisphere deficits, children with such deficits are likely to have difficulty adapting their language and behavior during social exchange, largely because they can't recognize subtle differences in behavior and flexibly explore multiple word/phrase connotations during discourse. For instance, imagine saying, "Don't put all your eggs in one basket," to Mary, a person with right-hemisphere dysfunction. She might respond, "Well, I put my eggs in the refrigerator," or "I don't have any eggs, and I don't even have a basket to put them in." Her literal interpretation is that you were giving advice about what she should do with her eggs, and that she should put some of them in the basket, but keep some of them outside the basket. As discussed further in Chapter 8, right-hemisphere disorders result in both verbal and nonverbal deficits.

We may not readily recognize these right-hemisphere problems at first, or may not detect them with standardized intellectual and achievement measures. However, these are some of the atypical children we see—those who show good routinized skills, and get decent IQ and achievement scores (at least during the early school years), but appear to have significant psychosocial problems and behavior disorders. Preferring to use left-hemisphere *convergent* processes that are *concordant* with their existing thoughts, children with right-hemisphere dysfunction are unlikely to integrate new *discordant* social information flexibly as the conversation proceeds, or to engage in the *divergent* thinking necessary to adapt reliably to the social situation (Bryan & Hale, 2001).

The left-hemisphere detail—fine and right-hemisphere global—coarse distinction has been validated as well. In visual field studies, the right hemisphere appears to be specialized for global perceptions, such as gender and novel faces, and the left hemisphere can visually identify known or famous persons (Ishai et al., 2005) and even famous landmark buildings (Gorno-Tempini & Price, 2001). This may be because the left hemisphere is specialized for high spatial frequencies, whereas low spatial frequencies are processed by the right hemisphere. In an ingenious experiment, Delis et al. (1986) asked patients with left- and right-hemisphere damage to draw the figures they saw. The patients with left-hemisphere damage typically drew the shape intact (i.e., if the letter was an M, they drew the M). In contrast patients with right hemispheric damage drew letters that were disorganized and did not show the full figure. (if the letter was an M, they twisted it around so that it was not recognizable)

These left/local–right/global processes are consistently found in empirical studies, but their relation to spatial frequency is still debated (Evans et al., 2000; Stiles, 2008; Hubner & Volberg, 2005; Weissman & Woldorff, 2005). However, this fits well with our understanding of hemispheric function. The left parietal lobe is sensitive to local stimulus characteristics like direction, orientation, and patterns of stimuli, whereas the right parietal lobe is sensitive to global, holistic, spatial configurations (Suchan et al., 2002)—a distinction that is useful in understanding performance differences on traditionally "nonverbal" tasks, such as WISC visual processing and fluid reasoning tasks. This global–local distinction also fits nicely with our novel–routine perspective, as the right hemisphere looks for multiple pieces of information to obtain the "big picture," and the left hemisphere is focused on specific details and predictable stimuli.

Finally, the right/novel–left/routinized distinction is accumulating supportive evidence on a regular basis, mostly from patient and neuroimaging studies. These studies are perplexing for those with a verbal–nonverbal orientation, but are quite consistent with the novel–learned position we present. For instance, there has been some debate over convincing evidence that visual imagery (e.g., visualizing your favorite lake in the woods) is a left temporal–occipital (ventral stream) phenomenon. This doesn't make much sense from a verbal–nonverbal perspective, because it is visual. However, because visual imagery requires memory, it is likely to be related to previous learning, so it is a left-hemisphere task. As a result, dreams that are meaningful or vivid tend to elicit left-hemisphere function, whereas vague, abstract imagery in dreams is associated with the right hemisphere (Gazzaniga & Miller, 2009). It is interesting to note that recommendations for children with left-hemisphere dysfunction often include use of visual imagery, because it has been presumed to be a right-hemisphere function!

In keeping with our novel-automatic hemispheric perspective, Henson et al. (2000) found that right occipital activation was common during initial exposure to visual stimuli, in keeping with the traditional role of the right hemisphere; once the participants were familiar with the stimuli, however, the homologous left-hemisphere region was active. Bilateral frontal activity, especially on the right side, has been found during initial learning of motor sequences, but this activity declines with learning (Muller et al., 2002; Staines, Padilla, & Knight, 2002).

Because of its role in working memory, frontal lobe activation is highest during initial learning stages, and there is a gradual shift from right to left frontal lobe activation when learning takes place (Lebel et al., 2019). This activation does not appear to be due to the verbal–spatial dichotomy; rather, the type and complexity of processing are what determine prefrontal activation for working memory tasks. Kiyonaga and colleagues (2017) found the ventral region to be responsible for active maintenance of information in working memory, and the dorsal region to be responsible for manipulation and monitoring of ventral processes, with right-sided activation greater during the complex working memory task.

Implications of the New Left–Right Axis

If the verbal–nonverbal dichotomy no longer accurately represents the left and right hemispheres, we must understand how verbal and nonverbal information differs in terms of the neuropsychological processes of each hemisphere. The right hemisphere gets the "big picture"; it processes novel, holistic, global, and discordant information. It likes new ideas and perspectives. The left hemisphere is more concerned with rote, detailed, local, and concordant information. It likes what it already knows. An interesting application of this pattern would be related to personality, with left hemisphere dominant people favoring details, history, and getting things right, whereas right hemisphere dominant people are more likely to be free thinkers, who are always forgetting minutia but are tolerant about it, and toward those who try to judge them.

Hemispheric specialization is certainly critical for learning new things and response to novel versus well-known situations. As a new task begins, right frontal executive and working memory demands are high, and then as a task becomes well-learned this shifts to the left posterior region, a sign that the task has been mastered. This perspective for the familiar Stages of Learning, makes sense with the research data. As suggested, during initial learning or processing of novel stimuli requires a great amount of right hemisphere and frontal activity, with a gradual shift to it being stored in the left hemisphere as it becomes automatic. However, to generalize and extend the known skill, right hemisphere activation is necessary to apply the knowledge or skill to a new circumstance or setting, or think of a creative use that builds upon this stored knowledge set. So as can be seen, what teachers do in classrooms is help children learn content by shifting it from the right frontal to left posterior regions.

Although it is interesting to note that the novel–learned perspective fits nicely with data supporting the *Gf*–right hemisphere to *Gc*–left hemisphere approach to understanding intelligence (Fiorello et al., 2007; Pallier et al., 2000), it is important to be aware that most of our classroom instruction and even our tests require veridical or correct decision making, so even on our most "right hemisphere" visual–spatial tests both hemispheres are required on virtually all measures requiring "correct" answers. Obviously, response format makes a difference: A multiple-choice format taps the left hemisphere to a greater extent, and a free-recall format taps the right. Not many tests ask for multiple answers (a right-hemisphere function), but instead directs respondents toward a single definitive response (a left-hemisphere function).

So our left brain likes details—our right brain says don't bother with them! That is because our right hemisphere processes information in a coarse fashion to explore multiple associations; the left hemisphere is specialized for making finely detailed distinctions (Beeman, 1993). The following two sentences highlight these differences:

"He stopped at the bank because he had to make a deposit."
"He stopped at the bank because he had to stay dry."

You probably needed less time to comprehend the first sentence than the second sentence, because "bank–deposit" is a common association and was easily processed by your left hemisphere, whereas the less common "bank–dry" association required additional processing time. To make this second association, you needed more right-hemisphere activity to explore multiple meanings of "bank" in reference to "dry." The association between "bank" and "money" is such a strong one that you may have thought after reading the second sentence, "Is he going to buy a raincoat or an umbrella, so he has to get money at the bank?", but then you probably thought to yourself, "OK, 'bank' refers to 'river bank.' " Had we included the word "river" in the second sentence, both sentences would have required familiar associations of course, so the left hemisphere would have been equally responsible for comprehending both sentences.

It is no wonder that traditional aphasia tests, as well as most academic skills, tap left-hemisphere cognitive processes, because these tests and skills require correct, explicit answers. How are right-hemisphere processes important for learning? The answer is that right-hemisphere processes are *essential* for learning, but we typically don't assess these processes well with our standardized measures. Without the right hemisphere, learning new information becomes difficult if not impossible—a finding consistent with neuropsychological studies of children with "nonverbal" learning disorders, who often acquire language later than other children (Rourke, 2000). Not only do these children have difficulty acquiring new skills; they are unlikely to generalize known skills beyond highly structured tasks and situations. They may perform reasonably well on veridical tasks that require correct answers, but they can't provide adaptive responses, which is the real key to success in society (Goldberg, 2001). All the facts and details in the world can't help a person overcome considerable problem-solving deficits and an inability to adapt to novel situations.

Learning is about acquiring new information, and children with right-hemisphere dysfunction are likely to prefer relying on previously learned information rather than adjusting to the novel demands of a new learning situation. This may not be a problem during early learning experiences, as these children use their good rote learning skills to acquire basic academic skills. They enjoy rote drill and instruction, so in many ways they are perfectly adapted for early educational experiences. However, as the demands of learning become more self-directed, and as information becomes more complex, implicit, and ambiguous, these children are likely to have significant difficulty. This pattern has implications for psychosocial functioning as well.

If children cannot adapt to new learning and social situations, they are likely to be perceived as unmotivated, oppositional, or preoccupied. Combined with limited self-awareness and difficulty recognizing the feelings and situations of others (i.e., poor "theory of the mind"), these children are at considerable risk for interpersonal problems (Surian & Siegal, 2001). The resulting alienation, as Cicchetti and Rourke (2004) have noted, can have devastating effects on psychosocial adjustment. However, because these children typically have positive academic experiences, we are often left to wonder: Do these children end up in classrooms for behaviorally disordered or seriously emotionally disturbed students because no one recognizes their neuropsychological deficits? To close our discussion of the second axis, let's look at some examples that highlight how the left and right hemispheres work together when presented with a problem (see Application 2.3).

The Superior–Inferior Axis and Frontal–Subcortical Function

The final axis of interpretation is the superior–inferior axis. You have already learned quite a bit about it because it essentially reflects the subcortical (e.g., basal ganglia, thalamus, cerebellum) and cortical (dorsolateral, orbital, cingulate, oculomotor motor circuits) structures previously discussed. The reason why this axis is important to consider in relation to the two

APPLICATION 2.3. The Civil War: Whose Side Are You On?

When you are asked a factual question such as "Was Illinois part of the Confederacy or the Union during the Civil War?," you must use language comprehension, long-term memory to access facts about geography and the U.S. Civil War, and expressive language to give the answer. But there are three types of people out there. There is a group who will know where Illinois is, and will know enough about the Civil War to know that it was in the Union. All of these people will probably require left-hemisphere, routinized processes. However, if you don't know where the Mason–Dixon line was located, or much about geography in the United States, right-hemisphere processes will have to come into play. You'll need to think about what you know about Illinois, or Google the state, and to make some associations: "Illinois—Chicago, it's cold in the winter, it's the Windy City, it was a cattle town and industrial town at the time of the Civil War," and so on. Also, you'll have to try to think of the Mason–Dixon line separating the Confederacy from the Union during the Civil War, and try to recall where major battles took place. You may try to visualize the various regions of the country, and to locate the Midwest.

All of these processes require left-hemisphere functioning, but the right hemisphere is active as well, because it has to help you explore and connect the proverbial dots. But the right hemisphere is also involved in the people who know *too much* about Illinois during the Civil War. How can that be? Certainly, industrial Chicago and northern Illinois wanted to stay in the Union, but many in southern Illinois supported their Confederate neighbors in the struggle to secede from the Union. The right hemisphere is required to give this answer: "Illinois was in the Union, officially, but the issues were hotly contested by Illinois politicians." This example also highlights how individual differences in prior knowledge, or crystallized abilities, can influence cognitive and academic performance. (By the way, the nickname "Windy City" came from the talkative politicians in City Hall, not the weather!)

---

posterior–anterior and left–right axes is that the superior–inferior axis is likely to be impaired in children with emotional and/or behavior disorders. In other words, the superior–inferior axis is the psychopathology axis. This relationship will be further discussed in Chapter 9.

Koziol and colleagues (2013) provide us with a conceptual foundation for understanding the frontal–subcortical and cerebral–cerebellar circuits and how they influence behavior and emotion. They suggest a two-tiered approach to how the superior–inferior axis allows for successful adaptive behavior based on environmental demands and prior learning. As noted earlier the frontal–subcortical circuits work to transfer knowledge and skill so that they can be performed in an expedited manner (Heilman & Rothi, 2003).

In other words, we want to be able to call up a predictable behavior script for a given task demand—the right behavior for the right situation (e.g., Saling & Phillips, 2007). A large portion of our behavior—as much as 95% (Radel et al., 2017)—is automatic; in other words, the learning has become second nature and doesn't require conscious attention to the task. This frees up our mind to "multitask" and think of other things. So the relationship of the "what" prefrontal region, the "when" basal ganglia, and the "how" cerebellum work together to determine if we need to process information actively, or engage a script we already have in place.

The frontal–subcortical circuits and cortical–cerebellar circuits are both involved in this third axis because they serve to determine whether a behavior already exists to respond to environmental demands, or whether an adjustable, novel behavior is required. They work as loops or circuits because the structures receive afferent and send efferent information back and forth to determine if modifications in behavior are needed to adjust to environmental demands.

As noted earlier, the frontal–striatal–thalamic circuits originate in the cortical regions, where they stimulate the excitatory striatum, which is then modulated by the globus pallidus. The circuit then influences thalamic sensory and/or motor functions, which in turn influences the frontal regions that generated the initial intention, thereby modifying the "what" function of the prefrontal cortex. Although there are some differences, the dorsolateral, orbital, cingulate, oculomotor, and motor circuits generally work in this circular fashion to influence volitional behavior. To add to the complexity of the cortical–subcortical influences on behavior, it would appear that these circuits work to balance each other when dysfunctional (Hale, Reddy, Wilcox, et al., 2009), which could account for the "comorbidity" of disorders (e.g., depression and anxiety, ADHD and conduct problems).

Although volitional behavior begins with the prefrontal regions, the basal ganglia have a more important influence on cortical function and behavior than was previously realized. According to Heilman, Valenstein, Rothi, and Watson (2004), the prefrontal-basal ganglia connections help us determine when to start or not start a behavior in response to environmental demands, and when to persist or inhibit behavior in relation to this decision. So the basal ganglia are not really movement structures, but regulation of intention ones. In addition to motor action, they also influence cognition, emotion, and motivation. Since basal ganglia projections send efferent information to the thalamus, the sensory and motor systems are influenced, which in turn allows the cortex to adapt flexibility to environmental circumstances.

Although the cerebellum–cortical circuit is less volitional in nature, it is important in governing action. Originally thought to fine tune and amplify motor functions, it has become clear that the cerebellum is involved in cognitive, affective, and appetitive behavior (Ackerman, 2008; Ito, 2008). Not surprisingly we have sensory–motor, cognitive, affective, executive, learning/memory, and automaticity regions of the cerebellum (Stoodley & Schmahmann, 2010). Through these interacting elements, the cerebellum works to influence a behavior's rate, rhythm, and force, or the "how" of a behavior. As noted earlier, it serves an important timing and automaticity function for procedural learning and quick efficient performance of known behaviors (Horowitz-Kraus, Vannest, Gozdas, et al., 2014).

Although automaticity is important for adaptive behavior and freeing of consciousness (Bruya, 2010), it can also play a debilitating role if problematic behaviors are automatized. Take, for instance, cerebellar cognitive affective syndrome, which can lead to internalizing or externalizing behaviors depending on the type of dysfunction. The condition results from cerebellar dysfunction, particularly in the area of the vermis, and leads to attention, executive, working memory, cognitive flexibility, language, and fluency deficits. If this syndrome is suspected because other signs of cerebellar dysfunction are found, it would be important to consult with a neurologist for further evaluation.

These two systems, the volitional frontal–basal ganglia–thalamus circuit and the automatic cerebral–cerebellar circuit, are called into play depending on whether a situation requires flexible problem solving or can be automatically responded to with an automatic script. Automatic cerebellar behaviors are preferred because they free up cognitive and higher-order cortical functions for things like planning and organizing future goal-directed behavior. When problem solving, the comparing and contrasting of known and novel aspects of a situation is what essential executive control is all about (Ardila, 2008; Miller, 2019). As with any other brain system, too much automaticity can cause significant problems where behavior is avolitional and reactive, while too little automaticity makes doing things slow and laborious, with new learning required each time. In the latter case, working memory is always overwhelmed, so higher level and new learning become quite difficult. These issues will be further addressed in Chapter 8.

The Integrated Brain: The Three Axes Summarized

You may wish to review Figure 2.2, which highlights the three axes combined, and how the posterior–anterior axis is interrelated to the superior–inferior axis in that they are both influenced by the frontal–subcortical circuits.

Simply put, the posterior–anterior axis governs input and output respectively. While the highest levels of understanding are in the tertiary zones of overlapping in the back of the brain (i.e., occipital–temporal–parietal lobes), the highest levels of doing (including executive control) are in the tertiary superstructure in the front of the brain (prefrontal cortex of the frontal lobe). The left and right hemisphere participate in verbal and nonverbal functions, so the belief that each hemisphere has sole responsibility for verbal or nonverbal skills is outdated. Instead, the left hemispheric functions are automatic, explicit, and detailed, while the right hemispheric function is novel, implicit, and global–holistic in orientation. Finally, the frontal–subcortical circuits include two circuits actually, the volitional frontal-basal ganglia–thalamic circuit and the automatic cerebral–cerebellar circuit.

Although this chapter gives you a good idea of how the brain works, it is only a start. The ideas presented here are complex and difficult to digest. For many readers they are quite novel. It is, after all, mostly "frontal" at this point, placing high demands on the executive system. To make it automatic will take a great deal of practice and additional reading. Brain–behavior relationships are not easily mastered, but with experience and application, they become quite useful in practice. In our graduate classes, we have students use brain coloring books, which are inexpensive and useful in consolidating our understanding of brain structure and function. The coloring is useful because students use Exner's area to get active in their own learning!

APPENDIX 2.1. GLOSSARY OF NEUROPSYCHOLOGICAL TERMS

a-   Prefix that means "without," but often can reflect "difficulty with" as well (see **dys**).

Absence seizure   Disorder characterized by brief lapses of attention; may be mistaken for ADHD.

Acalculia/dyscalculia   Inability to perform/difficulty in performing mathematical operations.

Afferent   Signal that is going toward the central nervous system (CNS) and from lower to higher levels of processing.

Agenesis/dysgenesis of corpus callosum   No development or (more typically) partial development of the corpus callosum—a disorder that interferes with efficient transfer of information between hemispheres.

Agnosia   Complete or partial failure to recognize stimuli, even though senses are intact; associated with problems in sensory association cortex.

Agonist   A drug that facilitates the effects of a neurotransmitter.

Agraphia/dysgraphia   Inability to write/difficulty in writing.

Anarthria/dysarthria   Inability to speak/difficulty with speech, caused by motor cortex or cranial nerve damage.

Anomia/dysnomia   Total or partial inability to name things or find words, common in Broca's or nonfluent aphasia.

Anosodiaphoria   Indifference, typically caused by right parietal lobe dysfunction.

Anosognosia   Failure to recognize deficits, typically caused by right parietal lobe dysfunction.

Antagonist   A drug that inhibits the effects of a neurotransmitter.

Anterior   Toward the front.

Anterograde amnesia   Inability to recall events/learn new information after a brain insult.

Aphasia   Loss of or difficulty with receptive and/or expressive language.

Apperceptive agnosia   Difficulty in recognizing objects, though senses are intact.

Apraxia   Inability to understand/difficulty with voluntary movement, due to sensory and/or motor deficits.

Aprosodia   Inability to understand/difficulty with understanding speech prosody, primarily due to right temporal lobe damage.

Asomatognosia   Loss of or difficulty with body awareness, primarily due to right parietal lobe damage.

Association cortex   Higher-level cortex that integrates across sensory and/or motor functions.

Astereognosis   Inability to recognize/difficulty with recognizing objects by touch, typically due to parietal lobe dysfunction contralateral to the affected hand.

Ataxia   Muscle coordination problem leading to irregular motor performance.

Autotopagnosia   Inability to name/difficulty with naming body parts, such as finger agnosia.

Bilateral   Pertaining to both sides of the body.

Broca's aphasia   Nonfluent aphasia resulting in halting/absent speech, low verbal fluency, and word-finding problems.

Coarse processing   Right-hemisphere processing that explores multiple aspects of stimuli simultaneously.

Commissure   White matter that connects the two hemispheres.

Concordant/convergent thinking   Left-hemisphere process of looking for similarities among stimuli and arriving at a single answer; contrasted with **discordant/divergent thinking**.

Concussion   Injury to the brain resulting in a temporary loss of consciousness; likely to lead to subtle impairments often undetected by standard assessments.

Conduction aphasia   Type of fluent aphasia characterized by poor word repetition but adequate comprehension of language.

Constructional apraxia   Inability to perform/difficulty in performing complex graphomotor or visual–motor constructional movements, despite adequate elementary vision and motor functions. Problems with writing and puzzles/blocks could be due to this disorder.

Contralateral   Pertaining to the opposite side of the body.

Contralateral neglect   Tendency to ignore stimuli on the side of the body opposite the injury; probably due to parietal disorders, more often right parietal (affecting left side of the body).

Coup injury   An injury to the brain in which the head is hit by a moving object (e.g., a baseball).

Coup–contrecoup injury   Common deceleration injury in which the moving head hits an object (e.g., a wall), causing a contusion to the brain (coup), and then the brain moves back and forth, causing another contusion to the opposite side of the brain (contrecoup).

Crossed aphasia   Term invoked to explain language deficits after right-hemisphere damage, based on the assumption that the individual must have right-hemisphere language localization; now probably explained by known right-hemisphere language processes.

Cross-modal   Integrated across senses and/or motor systems; assumed to be related to the integrity of white matter transmission of information.

Crowding hypothesis   The belief that undamaged brain areas can "take over" for damaged brain areas, resulting in some **sparing of function**, but that both the spared and original functions subserved by the undamaged brain area are subsequently depressed.

Declarative memory   Prior knowledge or crystallized abilities; probably related to the integrity of the medial and lateral temporal lobes.

Decussation   Crossed sensory and motor pathways, which allow the right brain to control the left side of the body and the left brain to control the right side of the body.

Deep dyslexia   Use of a sight-word approach to compensate for poor phoneme–grapheme correspondence; thought to be right-hemisphere reading.

Developmental deficit hypothesis   The assumption that brain-based learning and behavioral problems are due to developmental deficits suggesting brain dysfunction; largely accepted as a result of research refuting the **maturational lag hypothesis**.

Diplegia   Damage to the midline motor cortex, which causes muscle weakness/paralysis of the legs more than the upper body.

Diploplia   Double vision, or seeing multiple objects as one.

Discordant/divergent thinking   Right-hemisphere process of looking for multiple possibilities among stimuli and brainstorming multiple answers; contrasted with **concordant/convergent thinking**.

Distal   Going away from the point of reference.

Dorsal   The anterior/superior part of the brain.

Dorsal stream   The "where" occipital–parietal stream, necessary for perceiving spatial relationships and self-perception in relation to the environment.

Double dissociation   Controversial method of establishing localization of function in patients with brain damage; involves demonstrating that damage to one area leads to a neuropsychological deficit, but damage to another area does not.

Dys-   Prefix that means "difficulty with."

Dysarthria   See **anarthria**.

Dyscalculia   See **acalculia**.

Dysdiadochokinesis   Shifting from one motor response to another; related to prefrontal and premotor functioning.

Dysgenesis of corpus callosum   See **agenesis of corpus callosum**.

Dysgraphia   See **agraphia**.

Dysnomia   See **anomia**.

Efferent   Signal that is going from the CNS and from higher to lower levels of processing.

Executive functions   "Brain manager" functions for planning, organizing, strategizing, implementing, monitoring, evaluating, changing, and modifying behavior; thought to be functions of the prefrontal cortex and basal ganglia.

Explicit memory   See **declarative memory**.

Fine processing   Left-hemisphere processing that examines details and specificity of stimuli.

Finger agnosia   Inability to recognize or difficulty with recognizing fingers by touch.

Fluent aphasia   See **Wernicke's aphasia**.

Gerstmann syndrome   Finger agnosia, right–left confusion, acalculia, and agraphia resulting from left parietal damage.

Global processing   Right-hemisphere processing of multiple aspects of stimuli for a holistic "big picture" ("whole" of part–whole relationships).

Grapheme   Smallest group of letters that conveys meaning.

Gray matter   Neuron cell bodies, more common in the left hemisphere; contrasted with **white matter**, which is more common in the right hemisphere.

Gyri   The "hills" or "bumps" in the brain that have valleys (**sulci**) between them.

Hemianopia   Loss of vision in one visual field in both eyes, resulting from damage posterior to the optic chiasma in the hemisphere contralateral to the visual field loss.

Hemiparesis/hemiplegia   Muscular weakness or paralysis of one side of the body.

Hierarchical organization   Principle suggesting that processing is least complex in primary areas and most complex in tertiary areas; works in concert with **parallel processing**.

Homunculus   Literally, "little man" in Latin; the arrangement of known body area representations in the somatosensory and motor cortex. The legs are represented in the medial areas, and the face is represented in the lateral areas.

Hyperlexia   Well-above-average word reading without adequate comprehension, possibly related to **Wernicke's aphasia** or right-hemisphere dysfunction.

Ideational apraxia   Difficulty with the concept of a motor activity, even though the individual motor acts can be carried out; probably due to frontal–basal ganglia or temporal lobe damage.

Ideomotor apraxia   Difficulty with carrying out the individual motor acts, even though the individual maintains the concept of the motor activity; probably due to problems with supplementary motor cortex.

Implicit memory   Automatic performance of a routinized skill; likely to be related to cerebellar/basal ganglia and frontal circuits.

Inferior   Toward the bottom of the brain.

Ipsilateral   Same side of the body; the cerebellum affects motor functioning on the same or ipsilateral side of the body.

Kennard principle   The belief that early CNS damage is less likely to result in long-term deficits than later damage; unlikely to be uniformly true.

Kindling   Initially contested finding that repeated seizures result in further brain damage.

Kinesthesis   Movement perception or position of body parts, related to parietal lobe functioning; important for providing feedback to the motor system.

Lateral   Toward the side of the brain or body.

Lesion   Any damage to the CNS.

Local processing   Left-hemisphere processing of single aspects or minutiae of stimuli, for a detailed "part" analysis.

Maturational lag hypothesis   The assumption that brain-based learning and behavioral deficits are due to developmental delays; largely replaced by research supporting the **developmental deficit hypothesis**.

Medial   Toward the midline of the brain or body.

Morpheme   The smallest meaningful part of a word (e.g., "mean-ing-ful" has three morphemes).

Multimodal   Association cortex that processes more than one type of information; see **tertiary cortex**.

Nonfluent aphasia   See **Broca's aphasia**.

Nystagmus   Rapid eye movements that can result from cranial nerve damage or can serve as a compensatory mechanism to "fill in the gaps" when there is damage to the occipital lobe.

Object constancy   Identification of objects as the same objects, regardless of the viewpoint; a ventral stream function.

Papilledema "Bulging eyes," signaling cerebral spinal fluid increase due to brain damage.

Paragraphia Writing the wrong word; see **paraphasia**.

Parallel processing Simultaneously processing information in multiple ways; works in concert with **hierarchical organization** principle.

Paraphasia Saying the wrong word (semantic paraphasia) or letter (phonemic paraphasia).

Pathognomonic signs Symptoms that are clearly diagnostic of a known disorder; also known as "hard signs."

Perseveration Saying or doing the same thing over and over again; suggestive of frontal–basal ganglia dysfunction.

Phoneme Smallest unit of sound in words.

Plasticity The ability of the brain to change structure and function to compensate for damage to other areas. See **crowding hypothesis** and **Kennard principle**.

Posterior Toward the back.

Pragmatics The functions of language in relation to the environment; probably governed by the right hemisphere.

Praxis Movement governed by the premotor cortex (in response to the environment) or supplementary motor cortex (self-directed).

Primary cortex The first cortical zones to process information (superior temporal, posterior occipital, anterior somatosensory), or the last cortical zone to carry out a motor activity (posterior frontal).

Procedural memory See **implicit memory**.

Prosody Rate, rhythm, and intensity of speech; related to right-hemisphere functioning.

Prosopagnosia Inability or difficulty in recognizing faces; probably due to right (unfamiliar) or left (familiar) ventral stream, depending on familiarity with the face; also occurs with right parietal dysfunction.

Proximal Close to the point of reference.

Ptosis Drooping eyelid, indicating cranial nerve (oculomotor) damage.

Retrograde amnesia Loss of preinjury memory following brain damage, suggesting more global cortical destruction. See **anterograde amnesia**.

Right–left confusion Poor orientation to self or other (including object); symptom of left parietal lobe dysfunction.

Scotoma Small blind spot due to occipital damage, compensated for by nystagmus.

Secondary cortex Intermediary cortex between **primary cortex** and **tertiary cortex** that perceives input (sensory) or prepares for output (motor).

Semantics Prior knowledge of the meaning of language; probably related to left temporal lobe functioning.

Short-term memory Short-lived rote memory for stimulus input; requires **working memory** for higher level processing.

Sleep apnea Difficulty with breathing; can cause sleep disruption and subsequent attention problems.

Sparing of function See **crowding hypothesis**.

Stereognosis Recognition of objects by touch; probably requires both parietal lobe somatosensory and temporal lobe long-term memory store.

Sulcus The "valleys" between one gyrus and another in the brain (see **gyri**).

Superior Toward the top of the brain.

Surface dyslexia Phonological letter-by-letter approach to reading, with extreme difficulty with sight words or morphemes; probably impairs reading fluency and comprehension.

Syntax Language rules for putting words together; likely to be a left frontal function.

Tertiary cortex Luria's sensory "zone of overlapping" (occipital–temporal–parietal junction) and motor "superstructure" (prefrontal cortex), which govern the highest levels of cognition.

Ventral The posterior/inferior part of the brain, contrasted with **dorsal**.

Ventral stream The "what" visual stream between the occipital and temporal lobes, providing object recognition.

Visual agnosia   Inability to recognize/difficulty in recognizing objects; likely to be a ventral stream problem.

Visual neglect   Inattention to stimuli in the contralateral hemispace; probably due to parietal lobe damage, especially in the right hemisphere.

Wernicke's aphasia   Fluent aphasia characterized by clear speaking without meaning ("word salad"); also difficulty with language comprehension; due to damage to Wernicke's area.

White matter   "Superhighway" pathways allowing for intermodal connections and complex behavior; more prevalent in the right hemisphere, and contrasted with **gray matter**, which is more prevalent in the left hemisphere.

Working memory   Executive function memory that "works" on information in short- and long-term memory; important for encoding to and retrieval from long-term memory.

Note. **Bolded** terms within definitions are defined elsewhere in this glossary.

Chapter 3

Neuropsychological Approaches to Assessment Interpretation

Developmental Neuropsychological Assessment

Developmental Differences in Practice

The developmental differences among children can be significant and can have tremendous implications for neuropsychological interpretation of assessment data (Semrud-Clikeman et al., 2012). Moreover, as noted in Chapter 2, children are not merely small adults; their test performance is both quantitatively and qualitatively different from that of adults (Lee et al., 2005; Yeates et al., 2009). As a result, applying neuropsychological principles in school settings requires substantial training, skills, and clinical acumen, plus an awareness of the broader developmental context. This is what makes child neuropsychology different from adult neuropsychology.

In working with each child, developmental criteria should shape the nature of the assessment, interpretation of results, and recommendations for intervention. Therefore, different assessment practices should be used for different children (e.g., flexible battery approach; Baron, 2016; Lezak et al., 2004). Interpretation should vary depending on the child's unique patterns of performance within the context of his or her current developmental level.

One cannot simply use a template report, and substitute the words "above average," "average," or "below average" for a test and the psychological process or construct it purportedly measures. It may measure different things for different ages or different types of children. For instance, the excellent empirically based cross-battery approach documented by Flanagan et al. (2013), and supported in some neuropsychological models (Miller, 2013), is based on large-scale sample factor analyses that have not explored clinical samples. In our studies we have examined clinical samples, and in many cases found differences in cognitive test predictors of academic performance (e.g., Elliott et al., 2010; Fiorello et al., 2006, 2007; Hale et al., 2008). This is entirely consistent with neuroimaging research that shows children with disabilities use different brain areas to process information than typical children (Simos et al., 2007).

A child's age, developmental level, and brain-based strengths and weaknesses dictate how the child approaches a task, the responses displayed, the scores obtained, and how we interpret the results. If we ignore this reality, we will be inclined to make the cardinal mistake in psychological test interpretation—using a "cookbook" approach. This ignores what makes us different from adult-oriented psychologists and psychologists not trained in neuropsychology. We work with children who are growing and changing right in front of our eyes. This leads to an important distinction regarding interpretation of scores from the same child upon retesting, a point we will return to later.

Standardized test administration is a part of the picture here, because there is risk in qualitative interpretation without knowledge of psychometric issues associated with our tests (Reynolds & Mason, 2009). Our position about flexible test interpretation does not mean that you should deviate from standardized test administration practices or ignore factor analytic studies that show the most likely psychological process tapped by a measure (e.g., McGrew, 2009). Instead, it suggests our rapport building and maintenance activities will vary from child to child; response styles and subtest/factor patterns will vary substantially, and summative scores (e.g., global IQ) provide little insight into the developmental nature of the child's psychological processing strengths and weaknesses (Clements et al., 2011; Decker et al., 2012).

For instance, it would be inappropriate to conclude that a 7-year-old girl who gives only 1-point responses on the Wechsler Intelligence Scale for Children Similarities subtest has good "abstract verbal concept formation," just because her summative score is above average. That pattern of performance suggests good knowledge of words and concrete categorization of similarities among words, not good abstract verbal concept formation. The point is that standardized tests must be administered in standardized fashion, but flexibility in *interpretation* is required. This is not to say we don't want to test the limits when children don't understand tasks or processing demands interfere with optimal performance. In cases where test performance improves following testing of the limits, we may report two scores: One for standardized administration and the other for testing the limits performance, using only the standardized administration scores for deriving index or global scores. Thus, testing the limits can provide insight into clinical profile interpretation that is unrecognized when only the normative data administration and interpretive approach is used.

In some cases, we will interpret standard scores in our report differently if we observe that there was cognitive or behavioral interference with performance. For instance, a child with ADHD may have subtle decrements in performance due to variable attention and responding, poor impulse control, limited persistence, language formulation or retrieval difficulties, and limited frustration tolerance (Hale et al., 2012). All of these things might bring down the score one or two points, but the global scores could drop quite a bit if this performance interference is uniform.

What becomes critical for the best practice of school neuropsychological evaluation is good neuropsychological observation of the child during testing (Hebben & Milberg, 2009). Clinical observations and idiographic interpretation must be developmentally sensitive, with practitioners recognizing each assessment session is different, even with the same child. This flexibility in observation and interpretation is important, but some people think that it is contrary to a neuropsychological approach to interpretation. Indeed (and unfortunately), many view a neuropsychological orientation as one that focuses on static, intractable brain lesions with all strengths and weaknesses viewed as alike, regardless of developmental level (Semrud-Clikeman & Ellison, 2009). This view of neuropsychological assessment interpretation is quickly becoming passé with the advent of modern neuroimaging results, which show a picture much more consistent with a Lurian (1973) process-oriented model of interpretation (Fiorello et al., 2009; Schneider et al., 2013). The brain is a dynamic, changing, malleable organ, one that does not stay the same, and it shouldn't. It varies for different individuals and within individuals, making our jobs much more difficult. That's why we *need* people to do psychological assessment; otherwise machines could do the job!

Consistent with these arguments, the medical model, static lesion orientation is seldom supported by the current neuroscience literature or by those who practice neuropsychology today. What we know now is that some of the variance in a test score is due to *trait* variance, or what is stable in the child's processing profile, but some of it is also *state* variance, the dynamic interplay of child, examiner, prior experience, the test materials, and the environment for that day. Why do we know this? Because test scores are highly reliable *within* any given test administration (i.e., internal consistency), but they are less stable *between* test administrations (i.e., test–retest reliability).

What changes during assessments is *state* variance, and it can influence our understanding of the traits we are after. Children have different cognitive and emotional states when they take tests. They like to do the things they are good at, but don't like the things they struggle with. This basic fact of human nature is sometimes ignored in psychological assessment. Clearly, this effort pattern is likely to increase profile variability, particularly for children with executive dysfunction. Children also learn as they take the tests, so no two test administrations *should* be the same with the same child. Finally, tests vary in terms of how comfortable each child will be with any particular task. A hyperlexic child loves to read single words, but may become upset if you ask a nonliteral comprehension question.

In fact, Luria (1973a) would argue it would be a problem if a child did get the exact same score on the same test with each subsequent administration, which would suggest the child didn't learn from his or her previous experience. This is why *repeated assessment* is necessary for confirming or refuting hypotheses derived from any single test administration. While curriculum-based measurement corrects for state variance in monitoring achievement, most psychologists do not repeatedly assess children over multiple sessions before they write their reports. Most psychologists conducting comprehensive evaluations schedule one day of testing and try to take this snapshot as if it were a definitive assessment of all the trait variance they seek, neglecting the points just noted. The reality is that no single score on a given day can accurately reflect a child's functioning in any particular area, so we must test children over multiple days (at least two). This fact is the primary reason why we cannot sit a child down on any single day and make high-stakes decisions about their psychological processes, because state variance needs to be accounted for when drawing any diagnostic or treatment conclusions.

Most practitioners recognize the dynamic interplay between brain development and experience, which shapes and modifies a child's development course in a bidirectional manner (Riccio et al., 2010). As a result, most neuropsychologists today place greater emphasis on understanding children's processing deficits than on determining whether they have localized brain damage. The "pin the tail on the lesion" mentality is a great risk for many beginning neuropsychologists. Many readers will be surprised to know we don't put brain structures in our reports (unless medical history specifies a brain area affected); instead, we use our knowledge of brain structures and functions to talk about psychological *processes*. It is the processes that matter for assessment and intervention, not the structures. So while we report slow processing speed, lethargy and apathy, poor motivation and persistence, difficulty with decision making, and limited error monitoring, we're thinking the problem is likely due to cingulate dysfunction.

Although children tend to obtain developmental milestones at certain ages, each child is unique in his or her acquisition and manifestation of skills (Reddy, Weissman, et al., 2013). Assessment practices must examine both the vertical (i.e., nomothetic) and horizontal (i.e., idiographic) developmental variations at each level, because each child shows skill differences in progressing from one developmental level to the next, and the manifestation of psychological processes during test administration and everyday life will vary accordingly (Semrud-Clikeman & Ellison, 2009). For instance, a child may have brain dysfunction that is not readily manifested until later in development, or when needed for competent perfor-mance. In other words, the dysfunction might only become manifest when children "grow into" their deficit as a result of brain development processes (Dennis, 2010).

Continuum of Typical and Atypical Development

Important to these developmental processes and psychological test interpretation is how the brain develops under typical and atypical conditions. Typical brain development fosters more specialized brain regions and functional interconnectivity, and this development provides insight into how atypical development results in neurodevelopmental disorders (Uddin et al., 2010).

What do "typical" and "atypical" mean? It is important for you to recognize that there is no clear dichotomy; the brain's various structures and pathways develop along a continuum of typical and atypical development *for each individual child* who is struggling academically or behaviorally. This continuum is also evident in cognitive functioning, a point we made in Chapter 1, where we indicated that a vast majority of children display profile variability. A few systems function in relatively autonomous fashion, but most are highly related to each other and influence each other in reciprocal fashion. When one system is dysfunctional or impaired, it influences the others. As a result, understanding a child's idiographic *pattern* of psychological test performance in relation to normative strengths and weaknesses becomes critical in neuropsychological assessment and interpretation (Decker et al., 2012).

A child's chronological age can serve as a starting point for expected physical, cognitive, and brain development (Dennis, 2000), but developmental strengths and weaknesses must be examined in relation to each other, in what has been termed *empirical profile analysis* (Flanagan et al., 2011; Hale, Wycoff, et al., 2010). Some subtest score deviations are to be expected, but developmental benchmarks can be used to guide appropriate interpretation of test data, because what is appropriate at one developmental level may be problematic at another (Semrud-Clikeman & Ellison, 2009).

Brain development is dramatic during infancy and childhood, and corresponding changes in performance can be expected at each developmental level (Molfese et al., 2010). Interestingly, more brain functioning is not better brain functioning! We know that as white matter connectivity increases throughout child development, gray matter is also being pruned to allow for the most efficient brain functioning possible (Giedd et al., 2007; Waber et al., 2012). These typical brain development studies suggest more brain function is actually not better; instead, more *efficient* brain functioning is better. For a practical example, think of the construct of processing speed. Is slowed processing speed a sign of difficulty with white matter development or actual dysfunction, as is the case with traumatic brain injury (e.g., Backenson et al., 2015; Spitz et al., 2013)? In your practice, you must decide whether a child's presenting problem is due to a delay in brain development, a brain deficit, the environment, or (as is most likely) some combination of the three.

This neurodevelopmental context has specific relevance for psychological test interpretation. For instance, most children should master most of the calculation skills required for the Wechsler Arithmetic subtest by the early school-age years. For very young children, poor mathematics knowledge can account for poor WISC-V Arithmetic performance, a task thought to tap auditory working memory and fluid reasoning. For older children, however, other plausible explanations for poor responding should be entertained, including limited auditory attention, receptive language, working memory, fluid reasoning, and/or executive function (Flanagan et al., 2010). Uniformly interpreting Arithmetic as a measure of quantitative skills is both inaccurate and misleading (Breaux et al., 2017). Even just saying that it is tapping working memory could be misleading because it actually may be a better measure of fluid reasoning (Keith et al., 2006).

In addition, while summative test results can convey normative differences for a child, the practitioner must relate these findings to the developmental demands a child faces in the environment. For example, a child who is not expected to clean his or her room will be unlikely to meet this developmental criterion on an adaptive behavior inventory. If a skill has not been attempted or expected by parents, in our opinion, the child should not be considered to have a problem if they have not developed the skill. This finding applies to cognitive functions as well; a child who plays with blocks or Legos will likely do better on visual–spatial tasks than a child who reads novels for fun. As a result, you must always consider and ultimately determine how moderator (i.e., environmental) variables influence the child's basic neuropsychological processes, and the behavior displayed in the classroom. While this book presents brain distinctions that are meaningful, the intersection of brain and environment is something that must be considered in every evaluation we conduct.

Conducting Developmentally Sensitive Evaluations

Good assessment with children requires a balancing act. Rapport is important, as is small talk during breaks. However, you are more formal when conducting assessments than you would be during a therapeutic relationship. (Of course, you shouldn't test children with whom you have this type of relationship.) You have to be business-like with good boundaries during the evaluation, but also be pleasant and friendly at the same time. As young children are quite variable in their response to assessment demands, you must try to be quite enthusiastic and engaging during an evaluation. One of us (Hale) prefers to act like the tests and the testing materials are the most interesting thing in the world! Multiple sessions may be required for younger children. It does no good to test a child for 6 hours and then determine that the results are invalid because of fatigue or motivation problems, which will often occur toward the end of a long testing session.

During testing, it is important to maintain rapport while moving quickly through the measures, keeping the child engaged and interested in the test materials. We show interest in test materials by saying things like "Wow, let's see what we are doing next!" and "Now we're going to work on something really awesome!" It's important that you have an enthusiastic voice and hand gestures, facial expressions, changes in prosody to communicate your interest in testing. The focus of the session is the test and test performance, however, so while you should be affable and pleasant, it is important to remain more formal, even if the child tries to engage you in off-task conversation. If this happens between tasks, provide minimal responses and then turn again to your best friend in the room—the test materials.

As noted earlier, children (like all people) prefer success over failure, and will put forth more effort on tasks that come easy to them. Alternatively, they may need more encouragement and even redirection on tasks that tap their weaknesses. Recognizing this state variance source can be critical in interpreting the meaning of profile variability. It is not appropriate to reinforce accuracy with your words, but regular reinforcement of effort is good practice. You must keep your finger on the pulse of the child's performance and comfort with the task demands, within and between subtests, to provide the child with the necessary support to maximize his or her performance.

Supplemental instructions (if allowed) are frequently needed for young children and should be provided as necessary. These instructions, of course, depend on the nature of the task. For instance, a memory test item cannot be practiced prior to administration. Young children also speak, read, and write differently than older children. Whereas errors of articulation, grammar, and letter sequencing or reversals are common in young children, these could be signs of dysfunction in older children.

As young children explore their vocabularies and language formulation skills, they commonly use words inappropriately. Similarly, young children have poorly developed graphomotor (paper-and-pencil) skills, but this is not to say they have a constructional apraxia. Obviously, sorting out what is developmentally appropriate performance, and what is impaired performance, requires the use of normative data. If impairment is suggested, it may be useful to look at the performance of a younger child in the manual (sometimes available for graphomotor tasks) to see how the child you are evaluating compares to younger children.

Our understanding of cortical development (Giedd et al., 2007; Waber et al., 2012) and Luria's (1973a) model can provide us with insight into the developmental issues affecting neuropsychological performance in children. According to Luria, the developmental progression begins with the first functional unit and the primary sensory and motor areas; it then proceeds to the secondary areas; and it finally moves to the occipital–parietal–temporal "zone of overlapping" and frontal "superstructure," which are the last areas to reach full maturity, often late in early adulthood (Gonzalez-Escamilla et al., 2018).

The brain essentially develops from subcortical to cortical areas, posterior to anterior areas, and primary to tertiary regions (Chu-Shore et al., 2012). This neurodevelopmental trajectory is why infants focus on sensory and motor experiences, school-age children are concrete thinkers, and higher-level "abstract" thinking occurs in adolescence. Not surprisingly, neurodevelopment just so happens to roughly coincide with Piagetian stage theory (Bolton & Hattie, 2017). Although the developmental periods Piaget noted have been questioned and further elucidated since Piaget's initial writings, there is a neurodevelopmental explanation for why we go from sensorimotor behaviors to formal operations in thought. It also explains why well-learned or routinized behaviors are preferred using assimilation to novel ones that require reconceptualization (accommodation) of constructs (schemas). Additionally, socioeconomic, cultural, and ethnic issues, as well as response style (e.g., reluctant to respond when uncertain) may influence higher-level thought.

It is important to note that the developmental timeline is both dynamic and relative, so there is a great deal of intraindividual differences in cortical maturation. It would be inappropriate to conclude that children have no prefrontal activity before they reach school. In fact, different executive functions are likely to develop at different ages (Stuss & Knight, 2013). For instance, sustained and selective attention are typically developed by school age; inhibition and problem-solving skills are developed by middle childhood; and planning and foresight are accomplished by adolescence (Pennington et al., 2019), which is why different executive functions have different effects on academic achievement at different ages (Best et al., 2011).

Although there has been some variation in findings, this general developmental perspective is worth noting and adopting in practice. For instance, most infants are engaged in simple sensory and motor acts, and reflexive behavior predominates. As secondary cortical areas become functional, reflexive behavior diminishes, and symbolic behavior emerges in childhood. Finally, the development of tertiary areas allows for complex understanding and volitional behavior to predominate in adolescent and adulthood.

Similarly, hemispheric differences continue to emerge throughout development. It is also important to recognize that young children engage in more effortful processing and that they become increasingly automatic in the execution of complex behaviors with age (Koziol et al., 2013), suggesting a gradual developmental shift from right- to left-hemisphere processes during task performance (Giedd & Rapoport, 2010). What may be a novel task for one child may be routinized for another, even at the same chronological age. As can be deduced from Chapter 2, the distinction between routinized skills (automatic) and effortful skills may dramatically affect both a child's performance and the interpretation of the results (Fiorello et al., 2009).

This finding is especially relevant for children with disabilities, as they are likely to display effortful processing because they have not automatized skills that other children in the classroom may have already mastered. For instance, children with adequate decoding skills but poor visual memory may have difficulty with sight-word reading. Because all of their energy is spent on the word attack process, their working memory is overtaxed to remember what sentences mean, which in turn leads to poor reading comprehension, even if word recognition errors are minimal. This is also why children with disabilities often feel exhausted after academic learning, because they have not routinized what others in the classroom have and require more—not less—brain functioning when attempting academic tasks. This is one reason we should focus our efforts on remediating deficits, not compensating for them (Hale et al., 2018).

Developmentally appropriate assessment techniques are meaningless unless we can link them to developmentally appropriate interventions. As alluded to in Chapter 1, linking assessment to intervention requires an understanding of developmental neuropsychological processes and of differences in pedagogy from one age level to the next (Fischer & Daley, 2007). For instance, a child with right-hemisphere dysfunction may not need reading comprehension instruction in the early grades because comprehension is often about explicit facts from the passage or knowledge of vocabulary. However, the same child may require extensive help as he or she enters middle school (Fuchs et al., 2017), because the child is likely to have difficulty with implicit and inferential questions—questions that are seldom asked in the early grades.

Whereas remediation may be important for young children, compensatory strategies become essential for older children, depending on the nature and severity of the deficits. At all levels, some compensation and some remediation will likely take place; it is the amount of each that varies according to developmental level and level of severity. Developmentally sensitive interventions take into account the chronological age of the child, and the child's relative strengths and needs, as highlighted in Case Study 3.1.

Most schools have curriculum scope and sequence charts that can help you determine developmentally appropriate teaching sequences. Through task analysis of the goals and

---

Case Study 3.1. Terrance's Dislike of the Resource Room

One of us (Hale) once conducted a clinical interview with Terrance, a boy who had received special education resource room services for several years. The author asked Terrance what he thought about his teacher and the services he received. Terrance said that he liked the help and the teacher was nice, but that he didn't like being in the class and being a "sped." He hated being pulled out of his regular class, and he wished he was like the other boys in class—not "stupid" like the rest of the "speds."

What led Terrance to these feelings? Some of this could be related to the appropriateness of his placement, or to his segregation from peers. In asking about it, the author's early behavioral training became important in understanding Terrance's perspective. From Terrance's perspective, the resource room was a punisher, because the teacher always focused on the one subject he had a difficult time with and liked the least! He seldom experienced success in this class, and the focus was always on what he couldn't do.

Helping children like Terrance experience high rates of success by teaching at the instructional rather than the frustration level requires an understanding of developmentally appropriate curricula and teaching techniques. In addition, interspersing remedial activities (resolving weaknesses) with compensatory ones (teaching to strengths) allows you to use the Premack principle (use compensation to reinforce remediation) effectively to foster motivation and perseverance.

objectives, teaching successive steps, using scaffolding to bridge new and old content, and shaping success through differential reinforcement, we can help many children make developmental gains. If we have unrealistic objectives or overwhelming tasks (i.e., instruction occurring at the frustration level; less than 70% accuracy), our help will become a punisher for a child. After years of experiencing failure, older children can become disillusioned and oppositional toward those trying to help them. They may skip classes or become defiantly disruptive in the classroom in an attempt to avoid showing their weaknesses to their peers. Their social awareness tells them that it's better to look "bad" than to look "dumb." We don't do a very good job of helping older children and teens understand their disabilities or normalize their experiences for them. During evaluations, one author (Hale) always asks children who have prior diagnoses what their difficulty with learning is, and unfortunately, they often respond by saying "I'm dumb." This sense of inadequacy can lead to secondary depression—a sense of learned helplessness that nothing they can do will help them overcome their perceived inadequacy. That misattribution needs to be overcome with success if we are to have a meaningful impact on a child's learning and behavior.

Part of the problem is related to the labeling and self-fulfilling prophecy; the child described in Case Study 3.1 has come to believe there is something wrong with him, and after repeated failure he becomes a "disabled" youth (Blum & Bakken, 2010). Helping children understand their disability does not convey a message that they must fit some label or there is something wrong with them. Instead, we normalize individual differences for them, noting they are the norm, not the exception. It is no wonder that many of our children with differences dislike special education and school in general; it is an aversive experience for them, one that focuses on their weaknesses.

One of the keys to successful feedback and educating children and parents about disability is helping them to see that it is a cognitively diverse world we live in. With over 80% of *typical* children having at least one cognitive strength and weakness, as do most children with disabilities (Hale et al., 2007), cognitive diversity is a fact of life. Normalizing their experience by suggesting that all of us have developmental differences in cognition and behavior can help alleviate this problem. In addition, older or more impaired children may benefit from recognizing their strengths rather than focusing solely on their weaknesses (DeMatteo, 2021). Operating from a developmental and historical perspective, you can truly understand the dynamic and ever-changing relationship between brain and behavior—a key to successful assessment practices and intervention strategies for children of all characteristics and needs.

The Scientific Method in Neuropsychological Assessment

Examining Response-to-Intervention Data, Referral Questions, and Previous History

As discussed in Chapter 1, the systematic early intervention efforts (e.g., RTI) you have attempted will provide you with a good starting place for formulating hypotheses about each child's strengths and needs, and for developing your assessment battery. RTI data can also establish an important requirement under IDEA. IDEA requires that there is adverse educational impact for disability determination and service delivery, and repeated CBM results documenting below standard performance can aid in this matter. After you examine the RTI data, the referral question(s) can further define the nature of the child's difficulties and help shape the battery. Unfortunately, many referral questions are written from a global perspective, with summative rather than objective terminology. For example, a referral might read, "Johnny is out of control, he's mean, he can't stay seated, and he refuses to follow classroom expectations." You could conclude that Johnny has some problem with following teacher directions or completing work, and that he probably displays some negative behaviors (e.g., name calling, hitting, destroying property) toward his peers and/or the teacher. These assumptions can get you in diagnostic hot water, so after you receive the teacher referral, it is critical to clarify any vague or ambiguous information.

Even if the teacher or parent can pinpoint the overt symptom of the problem in a child (e.g., inattention, poor sustained attention, difficulty completing work, blurting out answers), it is still up to you to determine if the problem is due to inappropriate expectations, developmental delay, a learning disorder, another psychiatric problem, or whether it is truly ADHD (Hale, Reddy, Decker, et al., 2009). Although we focus primarily on high-incidence disorders such as SLD and ADHD in this book, as they are the most common referral problems (Pennington et al., 2019), it is important to be aware of other disorders and environmentally determined problems that can look like SLD or ADHD. In fact, it is best to think of attention problems as being a symptom like congestion in a cold—it exists in many disorders, only one of which is ADHD.

Referral information can provide an important link between the environment and subsequent assessment data, but it is important to realize that the teacher could be partially or completely wrong about the problem behavior. Because the referral question tends to represent the teacher's opinion and is influenced by the teacher's perceptions and interpretations (Sattler, 2024), you must keep an open mind when addressing the referral question. In our opinion, this common phenomenon is one of the biggest problems associated with problem-solving consultation that relies on teacher impressions to define the problem and develop interventions: What if the teacher is *wrong*? When a teacher says that a child has a "learning problem," you should consider multiple possible reasons—both neuropsychological and environmental—for the learning problem, only one of which could be SLD (Hale, Wycoff, et al., 2010), a point made clear in Chapter 1.

In addition, teachers rarely say that their teaching techniques are at fault, even though we know that environmental determinants are the cause of some problematic classroom behaviors. In fact, one of the reasons why MTSS has been seen as useful alternative to traditional school psychology practices is that it helps so many children who would be labeled under traditional "test and place" models. These children are served in an MTSS model because they do not have disabilities, but are instead "instructional casualties" or the result of ineffectual teaching or of teaching poorly differentiated to meet their academic needs (Fuchs & Fuchs, 2006).

In fact, it has been argued that disability is in essence a poor "goodness of fit" between the child and the environment, so it is important to help teachers realize that differentiated instruction tailored to individual differences can be the key to helping children overcome problem behaviors and poor achievement (Bender, 2012). Even if the teacher is found to be a source of the problem in the end, it is critical to use your consultation skills to help the teacher reframe his or her impressions so that they are congruent with the objective data, as suggested in Case Study 3.2. Otherwise, you've eliminated an important opportunity to work collaboratively with the teacher following your comprehensive evaluation. In other words, we have to avoid the "blame game" of saying this is a child problem, a teacher problem, or a parent problem—as all three people are part of the solution. In fact, we argue that the more teachers are "brain literate," the more they are able to recognize that differences in student learning and behavior are interrelated to their instructional methods (Walker et al., 2019).

Case Study 3.2. Reframing Juan's Referral Question

One of us (Hale) consulted with a kindergarten teacher who was frustrated with Juan's "disruptive" behavior, and complained that he was always in time-out. She said he needed special education for his "outrageous and uncontrollable behavior," which is hardly behavioral terminology. A functional analysis revealed that he only called out, talked to his peers, and played with objects during teacher lectures to the whole class. The teacher never engaged Juan during these times; moreover, she always conducted the lectures from the front of the room, and Juan sat in the back row. Finally, the time-out chair was in a play area in the back of the room, with a walled partition separating the child from the rest of the class. The time-out, which should last only the length of the child's age, was for over 20 minutes. Peering over the partition, Hale noticed Juan quietly playing with the boxes of toys during time out. Needless to say, Hale did not think that an evaluation was necessary.

In meeting with the teacher, Hale showed her the results of his observation, and brainstormed possible things she could do to help Juan. They eventually agreed to change Juan's seat to the front, to increase his participation by calling on him, improving teacher proximity, and to make time-out less appealing by removing all interesting objects from the time-out area. These interventions resulted in a decrease in Juan's disruptive behavior. Had these strategies not worked, then a formal evaluation might be necessary, with our major concern being a problem with auditory attention, auditory processing, or language comprehension.

Reviewing historical information gained from teachers and parents is also critical in the initial stages of comprehensive school neuropsychological evaluation. Too often we come across school psychology evaluations that have limited or even no history. At times this may be due to time constraints, but important information can be obtained through questionnaires and self-made developmental surveys. However, whenever possible, conducting a thorough medical, developmental, family, social, academic, and school history can shed substantial light into the nature, severity, and chronicity of the problem, as well as determine other mediating factors contributing to it (McConaughy et al., 2013).

We often say to our students, "If you can't find at least one plausible reason for a child's disability during an interview, then the interview has not been effective." Many school psychologists may say "the history is none of my business" or "I'm more interested in what the child can do now, not what happened in the past." But it is important to remember that *pediatricians, neurologists,* and *psychiatrists* often make their diagnoses on the basis of reported history alone. In fact, a thorough history that attends to all relevant information, and considers neuropsychological issues when asking questions, may be one of the most important data sources for both assessment and intervention purposes.

As a result, be thorough when conducting clinical interviews of children, parents, teachers, and other allied providers (e.g., occupational therapists, counselors) if possible. Parent and teacher informants can give you a foundation of understanding to develop your assessment battery. They will also help you recognize how the environment plays a role in the child's current level and pattern of psychological functioning. This information is analyzed to consider what type of evaluation is needed. If the child appears to have a cognitive/neuropsychological problem, then the theory of the child's strengths and needs is developed. This is the first step in CHT (Hale & Fiorello, 2004). The theory must be tested however, using multiple data sources. This leads to the next steps in CHT—hypothesis, data collection/analysis, and interpretation, which in turn lead to a more advanced theory about the child's functioning, as depicted in Figure 3.1. This sequence continues until the theory is sound and is used to develop, implement, monitor, and evaluate interventions, all within this scientific method.

THEORY → HYPOTHESIS → DATA COLLECTION → INTERPRETATION

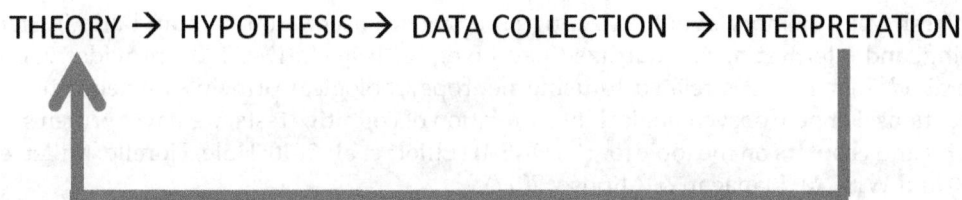

FIGURE 3.1. Sequence for cognitive hypothesis testing.

Conducting a Screening Battery Assessment

Sometimes psychologists have standard batteries they administer to all children. This "fixed-battery" approach has some advantages which we will discuss, but instead we think it is important to choose a flexible-battery approach. This involves choosing instruments based on multiple factors and it is similar to what is advocated in the cross-battery approach to cognitive assessment (see Chapter 1; Flanagan et al., 2013). We think choosing the best instruments for the child should be child dependent, in other words, in the child's best interest, not solely based on examiner preference for one tool over another.

Your choice of assessment tools should occur in stages, beginning with what we call the screening battery evaluation (this is different from what most people consider a screening, being much more comprehensive). Choosing the screening instruments depends on the MTSS data previously collected and the initial teacher, parent, and/or child interviews regarding the referral question(s). At this initial assessment stage, you should address environmental, historical, and prior intervention issues thoroughly, as factors such as educational, cultural, linguistic, medical, emotional, behavioral, psychosocial stressors, and expectations because they can all influence current functioning and test performance.

At this screening stage, include behavior ratings and interviews (with a teacher, a parent, and [if applicable] the child); a systematic classroom observation; assessment observations; a standardized measure of intellectual/cognitive functioning; and a standardized achievement measure that at least covers multiple areas such as reading, math, and writing. Even if a teacher or other educational evaluator conducts the team achievement evaluation for multidisciplinary team decision making, we believe that you should still collect some achievement data, as this will help you formulate your diagnostic impressions and intervention recommendations. Understanding the relationship between cognitive processes and academic processes is the key. Although this basic "screening battery" should be administered to all children, the specific measures used should be chosen based on the child's history, language, and culture, and there are circumstances in which you may wish to use additional measures (or eliminate others). To be clear, we see the standardized intellectual/cognitive measure (e.g., DAS-II-NU, KABC-II NU, SB-5, WISC-V, WJ-V) as a *screening tool* of psychological processes, not a stand-alone measure of them.

The initial screening evaluation should take place during one session, if possible (with adequate breaks offered, depending on the child's developmental level). However, teachers can be reluctant to have children tested over an extended period. At one extreme, a teacher may tell you to test a child only during one class period, which is typically less than an hour. This should be avoided, as repeated test sessions can disrupt rapport and violate standardized test administration requirements. Because your evaluation will subsequently follow this child throughout his or her academic career, you must make every attempt to get valid data.

For administering and scoring the tests, excellent sources such as Flanagan et al. (2012, 2013), Groth-Marnat (2009), Reynolds and Kamphaus (2003), and Sattler (2024) are available to refresh your memory about collecting assessment observation data and administering, scoring, and interpreting standardized psychological tests. In-Depth 3.1 provides you with several additional issues related to using neuropsychological principles when conducting evaluations. For neuropsychological interpretation of cognitive tests, we have written several articles and chapters on the topic for the DAS-II (Elliott et al., 2010; Hale, Fiorello, Millet, et al., 2008) and WISC-V (Flanagan & Alfonso, 2017).

After completing this initial evaluation, most psychologists score and interpret their data and write their reports. What we see as a *screener* of psychological processes, the average psychologist sees as a *comprehensive evaluation* of them. The average psychologist bases diagnostic and treatment recommendations on the observations, interviews, rating scales, assessment impressions, test results, and interpretation of data. This is certainly appropriate if the data obtained are all within normal limits. We should not continue to test children with numerous measures in an attempt to find a deficit that may not exist (Lezak et al., 2012), because as the number of measures increases, the likelihood that one will be deficient becomes likely (Casaletto & Heaton, 2017). This is the Type I error that we are told to avoid in statistics—saying that there is a problem when there is indeed none. The null hypothesis is that there is "no problem," and we should reject the null hypothesis only when there is convincing evidence of deficient performance that is impacting the child's academic and/or socioemotional life experience.

As a result of the limitations of profile analysis (Watkins et al., 2005), for most cases, you cannot stop after administering our single intellectual/cognitive test, even if there is an apparent problem based on the intellectual/cognitive test data. It is imperative that you validate apparent findings with additional tests that have better sensitivity and specificity for the disorders you are expected to identify (Hale et al., 2016). Typical school psychology practice does not afford an opportunity to confirm your clinical impressions. Many of us test too many children and as a result we are seldom thorough enough due to time demands and/ or a lack of training. We are instead asked to make diagnostic "leaps of faith," which serve to limit our effectiveness in understanding children and helping them learn and behave in the classroom.

After presenting the cognitive hypothesis testing (Hale & Fiorello, 2004) approach to psychological test interpretation during workshops, many psychologists proclaim they don't have the time, training, or experience for the sophisticated approach recommended. We, the authors, argue here three points to help you reconsider this commonly-held position:

1. With fewer formal evaluations (due to an effective MTSS system), you can be more thorough in your comprehensive evaluation efforts for the children who are nonresponders to intervention (Hale, Wycoff, et al., 2010).
2. You cannot interpret global scores when there is significant subtest variability within factors (Hale et al., 2007); you must instead go beyond these global scores to interpret within and between subtests, or conduct empirical profile analysis (Hale, Flanagan, et al., 2008).
3. Since profile analysis is prone to interpretive or administrative error (McDermott et al., 2013; Watkins et al., 2005), you must validate initial clinical impressions of your screening battery assessment to confirm or refute hypotheses derived from the profiles with other data sources.

As a result, the screening stage of assessment is designed to help you generate hypotheses about a child's strengths and needs, and then you must test these hypotheses with additional data sources until you have the concurrent validity to support your interpretation of a child's processing strengths and needs. You then need one final validation step–you

IN-DEPTH 3.1. Administration and Interpretation Issues

The following issues can affect the validity of your interpretation and the utility of your assessment results:

● *Maintaining rapport requires talking to the child at his or her developmental level, but not violating standardized administration and scoring of the measure.* Too often children's global test scores change because of administration differences—a source of error that can be avoided. The bottom line is that you must adhere to the manual's directions and score the behavior you obtain from the child.

● *If you think that the results do not reflect the child's current functioning, you should test the limits (TTL) to obtain maximal performance.* When you are using TTL results, report a score according to standardized administration, then calculate another using the raw score obtained during TTL, and report both scores. Only use the standardized administration score in calculating any index or global scores, though! Don't assume that a child can do something if he or she doesn't; objectivity in administration and scoring is paramount.

● *Rigid adherence to the test manual and directions is likely to interfere with rapport, so supplement standardized instructions with rapport-maintaining activities.* Maintaining rapport requires minimal "casual conversation" between subtests and "checking in" with children to ensure they are motivated and understand what is expected of them. It does no good to report extremely low scores or numerous "spoiled" subtests, which render the overall evaluation invalid (although this does happen from time to time).

● *If doing so is not contraindicated, you should supplement or paraphrase instructions or ask the child what he or she is supposed to do, to ensure that the child understands the task.* After using standardized instructions, you may need other techniques to ensure that the child understands the task demands, unless such techniques are explicitly contraindicated in the manual. As this is *not* possible for memory, fluid reasoning, and executive function tasks, you must administer such tests as specified, and then report any deviations that occurred during your TTL. You can't decide to change the wording of instructions because they are poorly written (even though some are), because the children in the norming sample also had those poorly written instructions. However, you may have to modify your administration and interpretation after the child performs very poorly with the standardized procedure.

● *You must describe any deviations from standardized administration, indicating that the results may not be valid and that interpretation should be made with caution.* Psychologists are often reluctant to say that their results are invalid, as if this suggests they did something wrong. However, scores that you judge as invalid should not be reported. Although reporting that the results are invalid limits your findings, this option is better than, for example, having a child fly through a timed task and receive a low score because he or she didn't attend to or understand the directions.

● *Because a child will have higher motivation for preferred tasks than for difficult ones, you must record all responses and behavior during testing.* We all have a tendency to like the things we are good at, and to dislike things that are difficult for us. During testing, it is important for you to be energized and motivated, so the child will work hard during the evaluation. In your observations, note whether motivation waxes and wanes, or whether affect changes, within or between subtests. A good dose of empathy can encourage and support children when they have difficulty on test items, as will be the case on any subtest where they miss multiple items on their way to a discontinue rule. Avoid the tendency to discount low scores because of "low motivation"; the low motivation is quite likely *because* of the difficulty the child has with the task.

(continued)

● *Scribble observation notes all over your protocol, and write down all responses, regardless of whether they are correct or not.* Sometimes "seasoned" psychologists barely write anything on protocols, just the scores. This tells us little about a child's performance and behavior. Also, noting only error responses provides clues to the child about his or her performance.

● *Subtest demands and a child's neuropsychological profile can influence test-taking motivation and behavior.* What hemisphere is more likely to be involved during the beginning of a subtest? You may think of the right hemisphere, because the task is novel when it is first introduced. However, the correct answer depends on the type of task and the individual's proficiency on the measure. For instance, on most achievement measures, the earlier the item, the more the left hemisphere will be engaged because the answer is automatic; the right hemisphere will be more involved during later, more complex items. The beginning of novel cognitive tasks requires right-hemisphere processes until the child becomes accustomed to the task demands and chooses a problem-solving strategy. Input, processing, and output demands can even change during a subtest. For instance, initial Block Design performance can deteriorate when the block lines are removed from the stimulus design. This unexpected task change happens in the middle of the task, so the early–late principle varies according to the nature of the task demands.

must ensure that a processing deficit found during assessment actually impacts the child in the real world. In other words, your results must have ecological validity. If you don't find evidence of ecological validity, it doesn't mean that the problem doesn't exist. Instead, it could be compensated for or is not necessary for the current classroom environment. In cases like these, we like to say in the recommendations section that this is an area of concern that should be monitored, rather than it is a guaranteed problem that should be directly addressed at the present time.

Cognitive Hypothesis Testing and Successive Levels of Interpretation

Whether you are conducting a problem-solving consultation with or without standardized cognitive and neuropsychological data, you should use the scientific method (i.e., theory, hypothesis, data collection, analysis, interpretation) when conducting evaluations and/ or interventions. A plausible theory calls for an empirical test of its validity. The scientific method is not just about research, it is also sound psychological practice. This is what it means to be a *scientist-practitioner*.

Since the screening battery assessment only gives you a theory of processing strengths and weaknesses, you must develop hypotheses to test your theory before arriving at firm conclusions regarding the theory's validity. In conducting this hypothesis-testing approach over the years, many of our theories regarding individual children have been supported during subsequent testing, but others have not. For instance, one of us (Hale) had a child who had a very low score on a listening comprehension subtest, but no other data suggested a listening or comprehension problem, and it was ruled out during the hypothesis testing stage. This finding during hypothesis testing is fairly common in our experience, which is a good reminder why using a single cognitive test profile analysis is likely to lead to interpretive error. Sometimes a low score is meaningful, but hypothesis testing confirms or refutes the relevance of this score for differential diagnosis and intervention/treatment recommendations.

The RTI approach has incorporated this important approach to assessment. By using repeated curriculum-based measurement, we can get a better understanding of a child's academic achievement, and how that changes with repeated measurement and over time. Similarly, with repeated measurement of psychological processes, we can get a better idea of how the child's brain processes information. The "one-time-snapshot" approach of most psychologists doing their entire battery in a sitting ignores this clinical reality. As stated before, if we want to draw conclusions about a child's current functioning, we need to know how that functioning varies from day to day, test administration to test administration. Only then can we have a good diagnostic picture of the child, a picture that can also lead to effective interventions.

To overcome this problem, a minimum of one additional testing session is needed on another day. Based on the intellectual/cognitive and other data gathered before this second test session, you will have developed a testable theory of a child's processing strengths and weaknesses. You then choose additional measures to test the various hypotheses, collect and interpret the data, and evaluate the validity of your initial theory, once again, using the scientific method in practice. This is what our CHT model is all about.

CHT is not unlike approaches that have been advocated by other neuropsychologists (see D'Amato & Hartlage, 2008; Fletcher-Janzen, 2005; Lezak et al., 2004; Miller, 2013). However, unlike other empirical methods that focus on overt behavior, CHT calls for you to go one step further. CHT requires examination of the *input, processing,* and *output demands* of the tests you administer, and relating the findings to all other obtained data. Of course, the input and output demands are easy to see, but *processing* demands are more difficult to ascertain. All we really have are observable and measurable behaviors from which to draw inferences about neuropsychological processes. This actually provides job security for us! We need well-trained psychologists to administer and interpret psychological tests; otherwise, we'd only need bachelor's level psychometricians or even just computers to generate scores and generic reports. This is also why we admonish practitioners to avoid "cookbook" approaches to interpretation.

As noted previously, just looking at observable input and output demands led to over a century of misconception about how the hemispheres process information, and many misguided attempts at establishing aptitude–treatment interactions (ATIs) as a result. There are no "visual" or "auditory" learners. As you learned in the previous chapter, you have to be more specific than that and refer to the psychological processes involved (e.g., auditory sequential, visual–spatial). Consistent with fMRI research, our research suggests *processing* demands are more important than input or output demands when it comes to psychological test interpretation (see Fiorello et al., 2009; Hale, Alfonso, Berninger, et al., 2010).

Each hypothesis derived during the initial screening evaluation should be subsequently evaluated for its validity. There are numerous measures available to test hypotheses, and most are easy to administer and score (see Chapter 4). It is important to critically examine these measures carefully before use—not only to ensure their technical quality—but also to examine their characteristics in relation to the child's functioning. Although your instrument choice will depend on the initial results, it is often important to use measures of attention/ concentration, learning, memory, and executive function during hypothesis testing, as these are the most common processing demands in many disorders (Hale, Reddy, Decker, et al., 2009; Reynolds & Voress, 2009).

You must be selective in choosing measures, as excessive testing will lead to fatigue and poor test performance (Strauss et al., 2006). It does no good to test a young child for 6 or 8 hours in a single day just to complete the testing and have them "impaired" on the last measures because they are exhausted. So choose the right measures for the hypotheses generated—the ones that will give you the most bang for your buck. Exactly which measures you administer will depend on the data previously acquired, the technical characteristics of the measures, the constructs tapped by the tests, and the number and types of hypotheses you have developed. However, you must be flexible in understanding the results of individual subtests, and not remain tied to one interpretation conclusion for each subtest, as highlighted in Case Study 3.3.

When you are choosing additional measures for hypothesis testing, it is important to make sure that the tests vary according to simple–complex, rote–novel, and single-modality–multiple-modality demands, and to look for similarities and differences on the measures that tap similar constructs (Sattler, 2024). It is also important to consider what test publishers or CHC theory (Flanagan & Alfonso, 2017) says a test purportedly measures, but you can't be rigidly tied to that research for interpretation. For instance, we tested a child who appeared to have receptive and expressive language problems on the WIAT-4 but no other indications of a problem with language on any other measures or during conversation, including above average WISC-V Verbal Comprehension Index scores. In testing out hypotheses, the child's language was fine—it was the cross-modal (visual–verbal) demands on the WIAT-4 that resulted in her low score. This cross-modal matching problem, which is related to the superior temporal sulcus stream/vertical occipital fasciculus discussed in Chapter 2, fit well with the other assessment data, whereas the receptive and expressive language problem did not.

From the previous chapters, it should be clear that even the simplest of tasks requires cooperation among almost every brain area. Therefore, you need to examine the various instruments available to you and choose several measures within the context of what you

---

Case Study 3.3. Benjamin's Auditory Processing Problem

Benjamin, aged 10 years, 3 months, apparently had an auditory processing problem. He had difficulty following class directions and frequently asked for repetition. Examination of his permanent products, and of his Wechsler Individual Achievement Test—Second Edition subtest data, revealed he was well below average in reading and spelling—apparently due to sound–symbol association deficits (presumed dysfunction in the superior temporal gyrus, angular gyrus, or secondary visual areas). However, on the Woodcock–Johnson (WJ-IV), Benjamin's *Ga* Sound Blending subtest score was significantly below average (supporting the hypothesis), but his Incomplete Words subtest score was in the average range (refuting the hypothesis). Interpreting the WJ-IV *Ga* cluster was obviously inappropriate (a significant subtest difference), so an examination of the subtests was in order. Was this subtest difference due to motivation, subtest construction, or differences in test demands? Benjamin seemed to try hard on both tasks, but an examination of the subtest sample space revealed very little at the upper age ranges, so a couple of errors could account for a fairly large SS difference.

Although this could possibly explain the difference, an examination of the task demands revealed an important distinction between the subtests: The Incomplete Words subtest requires auditory closure, whereas Sound Blending requires sequencing and phonological assembly skills. Further analysis of phonemic processing (left hemisphere), global processing (right hemisphere), and sequential processing (frontal lobes) helped delineate the exact nature of the problem. Benjamin did have phonological processing problems due to difficulties related to the superior temporal lobe, but he compensated for these by using good auditory closure skills on the Incomplete Words subtest. Several children with this deficit do well on this subtest; they hear part of the word (even if they miss some phonemes), and are still able to provide a plausible response. Concluding that they have adequate auditory processing skills on the basis of the *Ga* cluster score would be inappropriate and misleading, which is a risk with interpreting global or factor scores when significant variability exists (Fiorello et al., 2001).

know about the child's history, the existing data, and brain–behavior relationships. You may have a good idea of why the child is failing his math tests or getting in arguments with his peers, but further data analysis is required to confirm your diagnostic impressions. However, an equally important and critical component of the CHT model is trying to *refute* your hypotheses too; that is, you must try to maintain the null hypothesis or run the risk of confirmation bias. When teaching CHT, we often focus on the probable, likely, and unlikely causes for performance to avoid this bias.

You should reject the null hypothesis only when you have considerable evidence to support your conclusions. Don't fall into a pattern in which you look for confirming evidence and avoid other data that do not fit with your hypothesis. Instead, keep an open mind, and explore multiple possible explanations for the child's behavior. Table 3.1 highlights important questions to ask yourself when interpreting test results, especially when the subtest data don't fit well with your other findings. As suggested in the previous chapter, we all tend to be more comfortable drawing conclusions about assessment data and arriving at single explanations (e.g. preferring left hemisphere "correctness") than considering multiple plausible explanations.

Which measures should you use for CHT? In Chapter 1, we described several intellectual/cognitive assessment tools, and subtests that can be used for hypothesis testing. In Chapter 4, we describe a number of neuropsychological assessment tools we find useful in CHT. We primarily report measures that have good psychometric characteristics, but we realize that many clinical tools have a long history of use in clinical neuropsychology and can be helpful for establishing concurrent validity of findings. After all, Luria (1973a) could do a neuropsychological evaluation with what he had in his pocket!

Although there will always be a place for clinical tools in neuropsychological practice, it is important to realize that CHT and the application of neuropsychological principles in daily practice are difficult enough. As a result, we do not want to support continued use of "clinical" tools that have not been standardized or received enough empirical support if well-standardized tools are available. Clinical acumen and idiographic interpretation are enhanced when we use measures with adequate technical quality, which is especially important given we argue that deviation from straight score interpretation is often a necessity.

We also recognize that some neuropsychological measures, especially process-oriented ones, will not be constructed with traditional psychometric principles in mind. Take for instance the Halstead–Reitan Trail Making Test, Part B. The traditional outcome variable for this test is time to completion, and so this is the variable examined in both research and clinical practice. However, in our ADHD research we found that the *errors* made on this test were important diagnostically for children with ADHD and were sensitive to medication treatment response (Hale et al., 2009; Kubas et al., 2012). Even though this very popular test discusses errors and the need to correct them, no one thought they were worth considering over the years because the error base rate was too low in the standardization population. But we test clinical populations, and what may be true for standardization samples may not be

TABLE 3.1. Seven Questions for Effective Interpretation of Performance Variability

- Are subtest input, processing, and output demands reflective of the construct of interest?
- Could a particular input, processing, or output demand change the subtest score?
- Does the subtest measure something different for a child because a particular strategy was used?
- Is the subtest sensitive to and specific for the construct of interest?
- Does the subtest have adequate technical characteristics?
- Could the child's behavior before, during, or after the subtest help explain performance?
- Did a change in my interaction style or test administration affect the results?

true for clinical ones. This is what makes nomothetic interpretation on the basis of normative samples so problematic.

Recall that your assessment tools and your administration, scoring, and interpretation should meet the criteria described in the *Standards for Educational and Psychological Testing* (American Educational Research Association, American Psychological Association, & National Council on Measurement in Education, 2014). You need to examine test coverage, content validity, and comprehensiveness (Groth-Marnat, 2009; Sattler, 2024). Many tests may be sensitive to deficits or dysfunction (e.g., attention problems), but have little specificity (ADHD-only attention problems), so no instrument can be used alone to make a clinical judgment about diagnoses or psychological processes. That is why a multiple-source, multiple-measure, repeated assessment approach is so critical in CHT. As discussed in In-Depth 3.2, the use of clinical tools must be limited to supporting empirical judgments, not the other way around.

After you have carefully collected additional data during the hypothesis-testing stage, you should reexamine all of the data to determine whether your original theory was accurate. Some data will be consistent, while other data may not be. Determine why the data may not fit and try to explain why. It is important to look at all data, not just supporting evidence that confirms your hypotheses (Fiorello et al., 2009). Confirmation bias is unfortunately too common a problem in psychological assessment and intervention (Nickerson, 1998).

There are many reasons why the data may not fit, one of which is that your original theory was not quite right. Too often we hear psychologists suggest an inconsistent score was due to the measure or the child's poor motivation when it actually reflects an important psychological process missed by the evaluator. Again, this is another unfortunate result of poor training and/or confirmation bias. However, another example of this phenomenon occurs when we feel obligated to find a smoking gun showing that a child has a disability when, in actuality, he or she does not. After several weeks of instruction and case study work in one author (Hale's) neuropsychological assessment class, he often brings a case with no verifiable disorder. The child's performance variability was largely due to interest and motivation. His students often say it must be one problem or another, even though they can't find the evidence in the protocol to verify these hypotheses. At the end of the day, we must rely on the multiple sources of data we have to make judgments, and keeping an open mind to address all data is critical in CHT.

Despite these concerns, careful nomothetic and idiographic interpretation of data, combined with historical, observational, and prior intervention data, will lead to a well-supported theory of the child's processing strengths and weaknesses. If your theory appears to be accurate, and confirmed during hypothesis testing, then a crucial search for ecological validity can be undertaken. Only after ecological and treatment validities are established can you be entirely sure that your theory regarding a child's processing strengths and weaknesses appears to be a good one.

The Missing Link: Ecological and Treatment Validity

Ecological validity is one of our biggest concerns about practitioners' adopting and using CHT and the *demands analysis* strategies. Many educators complain that neuropsychology has everything to do with diagnosis, but nothing to do with intervention. This is likely the biggest problem with neuropsychologists—they may be great at differential diagnosis and identification of deficits, but how these relate to real-world outcomes is often missing in neuropsychological reports. Without this critical validity dimension, the report will be filed away in the child's record, and not used to benefit them beyond determining a disability and need for services.

IN-DEPTH 3.2. The Value of Clinical Judgment

Is there a place for clinical judgment in CHT? In addition to examination of normative data, "clinical norms" (sometimes referred to as "head norms") may have to be used when you are interpreting neuropsychological data (Reynolds, 1997). Although a qualitative clinical approach provides you with tremendous insight, it is difficult to learn; it does not allow for verification of results; and it does not readily allow for determination of treatment efficacy (Rourke, 1994). However, we don't want you to assume that qualitative, clinical approaches are meaningless. Instead, we stress that diagnoses should not be made in the absence of adequate norm-referenced measures (Reynolds, 1997). Test scores are only useful insofar as they allow for clinical interpretation (Lezak, 1995), and understanding the processes a child displays during testing can have intervention implications (D'Amato et al., 1997). You should not get stuck on psychometrics, i.e., fixating on numbers that may or may not accurately represent the child's true level and pattern of performance.

Every child is a single-case study, in which you must decipher the relationships among overt behavior, psychological processes, and neuropsychological systems (Bernstein, 2000). Ultimately, while the numbers remain important, and their consistency helps determine the confidence you have in your conclusions, it is up to you to make appropriate clinical judgments. There is often an inherent trade-off between sensitivity (detecting a problem) and specificity (discriminating among problems), so we must strive for a balance between the two (Reynolds, 1997). It is important to remember that the costs associated with diagnostic error are constant; a Type I error (identifying a problem when none exists) is as bad as a Type II error (identifying no problem when one exists). Good diagnostic decisions are based on both actuarial and clinical factors (Willis, 1986).

Although finding objective data to support inferences can be difficult, understanding how these inferences relate to the child's daily functioning is critical. There is growing empirical interest in the ecological validity of neuropsychological assessment results in relation to typical populations (Spooner & Pachana, 2006) and whether results suggest impairment or deficiency (Silverberg & Millis, 2009).

In addition, there has been increased interest in how assessment results are related to intervention, such as enhancing practical everyday skills (Hale, Alfonso, et al., 2010; Marcotte & Grant, 2010). Your job is to bridge the gap between neuropsychological knowledge, assessment results, and a child's everyday life. For each child, you will need to find evidence in the classroom, the home, or some other setting that relates your test findings to the natural environment. Without confirming evidence of ecological validity, no matter how convinced you are, your findings should at best be considered a working hypothesis.

Ecological validity data are acquired through examination of all existing data; follow-up direct observations; and consultation with parents, teachers, and/or the child. Finding ecological validity data are not as difficult as you think, as described in Application 3.1. Try to develop lists of ecological validity signs on your own to store in a "ecological validity dictionary." You can compare the behaviors described with the test results for each child, and then use that in a bank of test results—real-world example connections for use in subsequent cases. Some helpful ecological validity examples tied to various brain areas can be found in Appendix 3.1.

There are several sources that can provide you with the ecological validity evidence you need. Parent and teacher reports should be analyzed for concurrent validity, and children should be encouraged to discuss their own perspective as well (DeMatteo, 2021). However, it is important to note that children who have disabilities, especially those affecting executive function, may not be good informants. Parents could have the same disability the child has, limiting the relevance of their input. Finally, it is well known that interrater reliability is poor on most rating scales (Frick et al., 2010), so it is important to ascertain how much ratings reflect reality. As is the case with cognitive and neuropsychological assessment, it is important to determine how much of the rating scale variance is due to child in question, the environment the ratings come from, and the informant.

Many people think informant reports are "real-world" indicators of a child's functioning, and that neuropsychological tests are "laboratory" measures that may not relate to everyday life. It's important to recall that informant rating scales measure someone's *opinion* about the child in their environment, which is affected by that person's perspective. To truly determine if ratings have ecological validity, it would be important to observe the child in the natural environment to establish *criterion-related validity*. Unfortunately, this is rarely accomplished in psychological research and behavior rating scale construction.

As a result, no one data source is the gold standard for differential diagnosis of any childhood disorder. You should compare and contrast your assessment results with other data sources and determine what could account for any discrepancies obtained. It is amazing to find how parent or teacher perspectives can shed light on clinical data. For instance, during an initial interview, a mother described her son as inattentive, unkempt, and socially inept. He showed poor visual–spatial skills, inattention and poor self- and body awareness during testing, so she was asked to talk about his language understanding and prosody. She said that he had a hard time understanding jokes, and that he couldn't tell whether she was angry or happy when she talked to him. However, the teacher did not recognize this pattern at school. This is not an uncommon occurrence, given the difference in setting demands or differential tolerance of problem behaviors and the observer's perspective. Discrepancies may suggest different behavior in the home and school, but may suggest different expectations as well (Sattler, 2024).

In addition to a parent report, a teacher report, and a child self-report, it is important to establish ecological validity by determining how the assessment results affect classroom

---

APPLICATION 3.1. **Auditory Processing Problems in the Classroom**

Think of some things you might see during an observation that might suggest an auditory processing problem in a child. During interviews and observations, we have seen the following signs of ecological validity for auditory processing problems:

- Asks to have questions repeated.
- Does not understand oral directions or displays perplexed look during such directions.
- When repeating words or sentences, substitutes words that sound similar.
- Does not recall some or most of a phrase just heard.
- Does not pronounce words clearly.
- Fails to take notes, or looks at other children's notes, during lecture.
- Relies on context clues and discussion before answering questions.
- Performs better on written than on oral exercises.
- Uses sight-word approach when reading, and avoids decoding unknown words.
- Has spelling errors that do not make phonemic sense.
- Reports being confused in classroom, especially when it is "too loud."
- Has limited verbal interactions during noisy, unstructured activities.
- Asks for frequent help during oral activities.
- Uses both hand and facial gestures or props to further communication efforts.
- Has receptive language problems, despite a normal audiological examination.

behaviors (through direct observation), classroom performance (through examination of permanent products, such as classroom assignments and tests), as well as behavior in other environments. Direct observation in different settings and time periods not only helps you establish ecological validity, but also lays the foundation for intervention development, implementation, and evaluation.

In this interpretive quest based on careful analysis of data, sometimes you might get a gut feeling about a child you can't pinpoint. What about those pesky clinical hunches you have regarding a child, and what should you do with them? You may have clinical beliefs about your child's performance and underlying characteristics, but they should be considered tentative working hypotheses until you have established ecological validity.

There is a place for these hunches in reports, but they are only found in the recommendations sections. The word choice is delicate in these circumstances. For example, the examiner may suspect that a child has experienced a traumatic event but all informants deny it. It is appropriate to include in the report the following comments:

"Although not explicitly discussed during the evaluation, the data suggested Sarah might have experienced an event or situation in the past that causes her distress, concern, and worry today. Although the exact source or cause of these feelings remains unknown at this time, it would be helpful to explore this possibility further with Sarah within the context of a supportive, therapeutic relationship."

As a neuropsychologist, you must weave a tapestry that reflects the clinical picture of the child. As stated earlier, quantitative and qualitative data are interrelated and essential to substantiate clinical conclusions (Lezak, 2009), and both types can be used during consultative sessions to establish ecological validity and develop intervention plans. However, you must remember that even qualitative clinical judgments need objective support. At the same time that you search for support for your clinical judgments, work just as diligently at ruling out other possible causes for your findings (Hale & Fiorello, 2004).

If these attempts are thorough and ecological validity is established, you will hear from parents and teachers what we have heard on numerous occasions—the rewarding phrase, "How did you get to know him so well?" This accuracy in comprehensive evaluation serves two important purposes. Not only do you get the child's clinical picture and diagnosis right, but it also helps open the door for you to be involved in subsequent intervention efforts, because you have gained considerable credibility in the eyes of others on the team.

Discussing Evaluation Results and Planning Interventions

In CHT, the school neuropsychological evaluation is not the end product; it is the *beginning* for linking assessment to intervention. Once you have established ecological validity, and your data support your conclusions, you now have a theory as to why the child is having a particular difficulty. This theory is then discussed with the parent and teacher as part of a problem-solving process, where you and the teacher agree about the nature of the problem and possible remedies. This leads us to an essential aspect of the CHT model—developing individualized interventions that lead to child success. Once you have developed, implemented, and evaluated a successful intervention, you've accomplished the last important validity dimension—treatment validity.

Your knowledge of neuropsychological theory and principles puts you in a unique position of helping other team members recognize the underlying processes that contribute to what they have seen in the "real world" (Fiorello et al., 2009). However, it is important for you to avoid the temptation to "label" the problem during this discussion. In other words, don't "admire" the problem. We left-hemisphere types want a definitive answer—the cause of a problem—and then we might "glorify" it by talking about how bad it is. In reality, no matter how accurate your assessment results, it is never that clear-cut, and the problems associated with labeling are too numerous to list here.

It is best to talk about the child's current functioning in order to avoid the expectancy effects that are likely to result if the child is labeled (Sattler, 2024). This conversation should build upon previous discussions and should focus on understanding the nature of the child's strengths and needs, not on bringing finality to the process by assigning a label to the child. Your credibility with the teacher will be enhanced if you use examples of what you've seen in the classroom and during testing, as well as what the teacher reported during the interview. If these intersecting data points are illuminated during your evaluation presentation, you are more likely to have buy-in from stakeholders when it comes to intervention recommendations.

Allen and Graden (2002) provide us with several important problem-solving tips to remember when we enter the problem-solving phase with teachers, parents, and children:

- All children have the potential to learn.
- Learning is an interaction between the child and the environment.
- Assessment and intervention require multidimensional approaches.
- Problem solving is about solutions, not "problem admiration."
- Service delivery is about meeting children's needs, not solely determining eligibility.
- Assessment and intervention are necessarily idiosyncratic to the child and situation.

Evaluation and intervention are two sides of the same coin. What you did at the beginning of CHT, you continue during the intervention phase—you use the scientific method for intervention. The problem-solving model takes over within this paradigm. What is different from other problem-solving paradigms (e.g., Albritton & Truscott, 2014) is that you use neuropsychological data with other data sources for problem identification, problem analysis, plan development, implementation, plan evaluation, and recycling. Using this information, you and the teacher, parent, and possibly the student brainstorm possible intervention strategies, develop an intervention plan, and agree on the methodology for carrying out and evaluating the intervention. Data collection begins, and you modify and recycle your hypothesis as necessary.

The fact that you have a good understanding of the problem doesn't mean that the intervention you choose will automatically work. As we noted earlier, the CHT model begins with the collection of intervention and evaluation data; it does not end with it. Just as a hypothesis needs recycling after you refute it, the same is true when it comes to interventions. It would be great if the neuropsychological data led to the "cure" or the exact intervention needed to help the child overcome his or her deficits, but this is seldom the case. Even if there is a clear link between the evaluation results and proposed empirical intervention, that intervention must be tailored for the individual carrying it out within a given environment.

Sometimes you have to change—or add to—the intervention; sometimes you have to change the time or materials or setting. Sometimes the measurement system needs to be changed. Sometimes efforts are needed to improve treatment integrity. In working with teachers during this process, the first attempts may be overreaching and not feasible to continue over time. In a relationship of equal footing, it is important to come to an agreement as to how the intervention will continue and the amount of effort required to be successful. Such conjoint consultation has been found to be very successful in working with teachers and children where there is not a power differential—in other words, both professionals are experts (Sheridan et al., 2013). If the collaborative problem-solving model is used effectively and the consultee owns the intervention, we can almost always achieve success for each child.

Neuropsychological assessment data do not clearly point to a specific intervention. The CHT results only give you a better understanding of the problem and a greater likelihood of choosing an appropriate intervention that will be sensitive to the child's individual needs. Assessment of intervention efficacy, or establishing treatment validity, is still required. If your original intervention theory does not appear to be entirely accurate, a new theory should be developed and tested. The hypothesis testing is repeated until you have convincing evidence regarding your theory's validity and the child shows documented gains in the problematic areas. The comprehensive evaluation is not the endpoint; you need to monitor the child's learning and/or behavior over time. This is possible, given that a majority of referrals are now handled by MTSS services.

Good interventions are adaptive, flexible, and ecologically valid (Fiorello et al., 2009). In our opinion it does no good to have children learn to draw in the sand when they need to learn to write with a pencil on a piece of paper. One of the biggest drawbacks of specific interventions that are designed to improve brain functioning, but that do not include naturalistic task demands, is that they are seldom generalized to the classroom setting (Rossignoli-Palomeque et al., 2018). Use interventions that focus on the skills required in the classroom or other naturalistic setting.

Listed in later chapters are a number of excellent sources to help you develop a good understanding of interventions in academic and behavioral areas; however, they must be realistic, adapted to the individual situation and the resources available (Brown-Chidsey & Andren, 2012). The teacher is an excellent resource for developing interventions. You may also wish to consult with the special education teacher on curricula and teaching methods that have worked for them in the past. You cannot be a jack-of-all-trades and you do not want to be a master of none. What you do want is to know what your limitations are and then find supportive colleagues to help you in those areas.

We disagree with problem-solving advocates who suggest that the teacher should know all the intervention strategies, and that your job as consultant is merely to facilitate the teacher's decision making. True, that is one of your objectives. However, if you can demonstrate a knowledge of, and interest in, the teaching process, this will give you much more credibility (Hale, Fiorello, et al., 2010). The field has not done a good job of individualizing interventions in the past (Reynolds, 2010), so it is up to you to establish individual assessment-intervention relationships at the single-subject level (Hale & Fiorello, 2004; White & Kratochwill, 2005). In your efforts to help individual children, you should build a "theory of pedagogy" to truly link neuropsychological assessment findings to effective interventions.

Interpreting Test Results from a Neuropsychological Perspective

Specifying the Interpretive Sequence

One of the most common ways to interpret neuropsychological test data is to follow the procedure for interpreting the Halstead–Reitan Neuropsychological Test Battery outlined by Reitan (1974). Reitan specified four steps in the interpretive process:

1. Levels of performance.
2. Patterns of performance.

3. Left–right differences.
   - 3a. Left–right differences.
   - 3b. Posterior–anterior differences.
   - 3c. Superior–inferior differences.
4. Pathognomonic signs.

As you can see, we elaborated on Step 3 to reflect our three-axis interpretive model, so Step 3 includes interpretation of the left–right axis, the posterior–anterior axis, and the superior–inferior axis. Let us now turn to issues associated with each level of interpretation.

The levels-of-performance interpretation compares the individual's performance to that of the normative group for the measure in question. By its very nature, it is a developmental examination of how the child compares to his or her same-age peers. This is the normative developmental or vertical interpretation described by Bernstein (2000). As it is the nomothetic approach to interpretation, it serves to help us define the nature of the problem at a gross level. This level of performance approach has dominated Western neuropsychology since its inception (Luria & Majovski, 1977), but it is not without its limitations, especially when score variability precludes global or factor score interpretation (Hale et al., 2007).

The level of performance or nomothetic perspective is contrasted with the examination of Reitan's (1974) patterns of performance—the systematic analysis of intraindividual strengths and needs. This level of analysis is essential for developing hypotheses about cognitive characteristics and individualized interventions. The interpretation of left–right differences, as the term implies, requires examination of the hemispheric functions. We further this level of analysis by adding a posterior–anterior and superior–inferior component. Pathognomonic signs are considered frank signs of brain damage, although there is some concern that not all pathognomonic signs are purely the result of brain damage. Instead, they may be better seen as gross signs of atypical brain development, organization, or function. Let's explore each of these steps in further detail.

Levels of Performance

Although a levels-of-performance or nomothetic approach to interpretation is essential for understanding a child's developmental level, there are advantages and disadvantages associated with this type of interpretation. In the Reitan approach, the intelligence test serves as a nomothetic foundation from which all neuropsychological test data can be compared. It is therefore the global "baseline" from which deviations (either above or below) in neuropsychological test data can be compared (Reitan & Wolfson, 1985).

One advantage of nomothetic interpretation is that it is generally a simpler approach to understanding child performance; one score is easier to interpret than many. The law of parsimony is an alluring law to follow. As a result, nomothetic scores are more familiar to both professionals and laypeople, and results are easier to communicate to others. This approach is easier to interpret (or as we suggest, does not require interpretation). It is also less prone to error because it is easy to write up in a report—for example: "On the WISC-V, a measure of intellectual and cognitive functioning, Logan obtained a Full Scale Standard Score (SS; mean = 100, SD = 15, higher scores = better performance) of 110, with 95% confidence of his true score falling between. . . . " This type of report writing is common in traditional psychology practice. We do start our interpretation of intellectual/cognitive tests with some statement of overall performance, so the reader can get a nomothetic picture of the child's level of performance.

Nomothetic approaches allow concrete conclusions to be drawn. No one can question the sentence in the previous paragraph because it just states the facts. However, as discussed previously, there are certain problems associated with interpreting intellectual and other measures solely from a levels-of-performance perspective, especially when individual variability in performance is evident, which is the case for most children we test (Elliott et al., 2010). For children with significant factor or subtest variability, global scores are essentially abstractions that represent a conglomerate of many different skills, making it virtually impossible to determine what cognitive or behavioral characteristic they actually represent (Lezak et al., 2012). A nomothetic approach to psychological test interpretation is also based on the assumption that the same relationships (e.g., positive correlations) and patterns (e.g., low, average, high) among subcomponent scores are found in typical and atypical populations, which is not the case (Hale, Fiorello, Miller, et al., 2008).

Rather than conclude that the nomothetic/normative approach is irrelevant, we need to see the scores for what they are worth. These normative scores provide a developmental benchmark to help determine how the child's performance is related to that of peers and can be used to determine how gross performance changes over time (Bornstein, Putnick, & Esposito, 2017). In addition, normative scores are readily provided and interpreted by other professionals, so they provide others with an opportunity to see how the child's performance differs on various measures or with different examiners.

For clarity of communication, we suggest you use standardized measures that provide an SS that reflects performance in relation to the appropriate normative sample. Regardless of the derived score reported in the manuals, we prefer to put *all* scores in the same metric, because it is easier for others to interpret and provides for associated percentile ranks. Any normative score (e.g., *T*-score, *z*-score) can be converted to an SS via the equations listed in Application 3.2. We also suggest converting measures so that higher scores reflect better performance. For instance, if the Time score on the Trail Making Test (Trails Time) for a child is lower than the mean (i.e., faster performance), the child would have an SS below 100; however, using simple addition, the amount below 100 is how much the "real" SS would be above 100 (e.g., a calculated SS of 88 on Trails Time would equal an SS of 112). On the bottom of your data summary page, it would be important to acknowledge this change in reporting so all scores are comparable on a common metric.

In addition to putting scores in common metrics, we prefer to use relative descriptors based on these norms rather than putting actual scores in the body of the reports. Similarly, we talk about the child and their processing strengths and weaknesses, not the tests and scores. As discussed later, this information can be put at the end of the report in an appendix table or figure. It is distracting to have numbers and statistical concepts in the middle of your clinical impressions and is meaningless for many people who read the report. We typically start our intellectual/cognitive test interpretation section, and the academic achievement section, with a nomothetic paragraph before getting into clinical interpretation for each (which, by the way, often dismisses the global scores because of within-scale variability). In addition to scores, we prefer to use common performance descriptors for all norm-referenced tests. Table 3.2 presents the labels recommended by the neuropsychology profession. We also advocate the use of confidence intervals, which provide readers with an understanding of the imperfect nature of measurement of human performance.

You may be wondering about the use of age equivalents (AEs) or grade equivalents (GEs). We feel that these scores are some of the most dangerous scores available to us, because they are often used by laypeople for levels-of-performance interpretation, but they are psychometrically unsound (Sattler, 2024). Try to avoid reporting AE and GE scores, or if you must report them, make sure you add a note indicating that they are not valid for diagnostic purposes, comparison of children to each other, or monitoring treatment response.

Even the reporting of SSs and percentiles should be undertaken with extreme caution. As discussed in Chapter 1, the results of our large-sample studies on the validity of IQ scores

APPLICATION 3.2. **Converting to Standard Scores**

Use the following equations to compute first a z-score, and then a standard score (SS).
1. z-score = (raw score − population mean)/population standard deviation
2. SS = 100 + (z-score ′ 15)

Example: Let's say Sam is a 10-year-old boy who obtained 25/30 correct on a cancellation task. The mean number correct (*M*) for Sam's age is 25.68, with an associated standard deviation (*SD*) of 3.11. The following steps will give you the SS for Sam's performance:
1. z = (raw score − M)/SD
    z = (25 − 25.68)/3.11
    z = −.68/3.11
    z = −.219
2. SS = 100 + (z-score ′ 15)
    SS = 100 + (−.219 ′ 15)
    SS = 100 + (− 3.29)
    SS = 97

Then you look up the percentile rank associated with an SS of 97 (found in most test manuals or statistics texts), and you see that this rank is 42, or the 42nd percentile. This metric also helps put things in perspective when *SD*s are high. For instance, let's say Sam earned a total of 14 right out of a possible 40 on the "List-Learning Test." The *M* for his age is 32.39, which at first glance suggests that Sam performed quite poorly on this measure. However, his SS is also based on the *SD*, and in this case, the *SD* for his age is 17.80. Although Sam got fewer than half the items on the test, his SS is an 85, which is just low average.

---

suggests that significant subtest or factor differences precludes the use of a Full Scale SS for any purpose other than a coarse estimate of overall functioning (Elliott et al., 2010; Fiorello et al., 2007). These large-scale studies suggest that you should *never* report an IQ score whenever there is significant subtest or factor variability. Otherwise, you are reporting a score that is really composed of several different underlying abilities or skills (Lezak et al., 2004), and any interpretation of that IQ score would be considered inappropriate, especially for clinical populations (Hale, Alfonso, et al., 2010). The one exception would be for identifying an intellectual disability, where a measure of overall performance is necessary to make a diagnosis (Schalock, Luckasson, & Tassé, 2021). Individuals with an intellectual disability will often still show variability in their performance, which may be helpful in developing interventions, but which should not be used to rule out the diagnosis (Fiorello & Jenkins, 2018).

How do you determine whether the factor or subtest scores underlying the IQ score are significantly different from one another? We do not recommend ipsative analysis, which involves collapsing the disparate subtest scores into a mean subtest score and then determining whether any one subtest differs from that mean. As is the case with the global IQ, collapsing these subtest scores into any underlying mean score obscures important diagnostic information, because the very tests that are discrepant from one another are part of the mean score. Instead, we prefer to conduct pairwise comparisons of subtests or factors, in what is framed "empirical profile analysis" (Hale et al., 2008). The examiner must be aware that as the number of pairwise comparisons increases, the likelihood of a false positive or Type I error increases, and this fact has been used (appropriately) to criticize profile analysis (Kaufman et al., 2015). Therefore, planned comparisons such as within-factor and subscale comparisons make the most sense, as noted in Application 3.3.

Most test manuals have charts in the appendices to help you determine whether

TABLE 3.2. Levels-of-Performance Descriptors

SS	Performance descriptor
130+	Exceptionally high
120–129	Above average
110–119	High average
90–109	Average
80–89	Low average
70–79	Below average
69 or below	Exceptionally low

Adapted with permission from Guilmette et al. (2020). Copyright © 2020 Routledge.

APPLICATION 3.3. **Interpretation of Variable Profiles**

Examine the following Differential Ability Scales (DAS) profile. It highlights the statistical concepts suggesting that we need to interpret scores beyond the global General Cognitive Ability (GCA) score.

GCA = 106

Verbal Ability = 103	Nonverbal Reasoning Ability = 99	Spatial Ability = 109
Word Definitions = 55	Matrices = 40	Recall of Designs = 54
Similarities = 50	Sequential and Quantitative Reasoning = 59	Pattern Construction = 58

Using what we call a "top-down/bottom-up" examination of this DAS protocol, we can determine whether a levels-of-performance interpretation is valid. Going "top down," we see that the GCA is composed of the three global Verbal Ability (SS = 103), Nonverbal Reasoning (SS = 99), and Spatial Ability (SS = 109) composite scores. When we examine the appendix in the test manual, we see that none of these scores are significantly different from each other at the .05 level, so at this point the GCA is still valid. Next, we look within each of these factors to determine whether the subtests are different. There is no significant difference between the Word Definitions (T = 55) and Similarities (T = 50) subtests, so we go "bottom-up" and find that the Verbal Ability factor SS of 103 is valid. Similarly, there is no difference between the Recall of Designs (T = 54) and Pattern Construction (T = 58) scores, so we find the Spatial Ability SS of 109 to be valid. At this point, nothing we have found suggests that we should interpret anything but the GCA. However, the 19-point difference between Matrices (T = 40) and Sequential and Quantitative Reasoning (T = 59) is highly significant; from a "bottom-up" perspective, therefore, the Nonverbal Reasoning SS of 99 does not truly reflect a unitary construct, and thus invalidates the GCA.

---

subtest–subtest or factor–factor differences are significant. If the critical values in the table are in decimals, always *round up* for every critical value. For instance, if the critical difference between Subtest A and Subtest B is 4.01 in the table, then you must have a 5-point scaled score difference for it to be significant. Make sure you use a $p < .01$ table (or, if necessary, a $p < .05$ table). If there are significant differences between the subtests that make up a global factor or IQ score, we believe that the global score should not be interpreted—or even reported, for that matter. If you feel compelled (e.g., you have been told) to put invalid global scores in your report, indicate that they are invalid because of significant factor or subtest variability. Case Study 3.4 can help you address this issue.

What about tests or measures that do not have significance tables for determining score differences? What about comparisons across measures? Issues related to standardization of the instrument, such as type of normative sample, gender differences, cross-cultural representation, disability representation, and the time when the norms were generated, do influence your interpretation of performance on different measures (Pennington et al., 2019). While taking these factors into account, you must develop a method for comparison of generated SSs on different measures.

There are several different methods for determining significant score differences, the best of which is probably a regression approach (see Flanagan & Alfonso, 2017); however, this may not be feasible for you as a school practitioner, because few cross-instrument regression equations have been calculated and reported in the manuals. This is especially true if you have significant subtest/factor differences and you are asked to use the invalid global score. One approach that we find particularly useful and less cumbersome is the standard error of the difference (*SED*), described in Application 3.4; this provides you with a method for comparing SSs across measures.

Where should you conclude your interpretation? The answer is relatively straightforward for us: If there are no significant subtest or factor score differences, then go ahead and interpret the global IQ score, as it appears to be a reliable and valid indicator of the child's current level of performance. This is, of course, an ideal situation—one where the child's assessment behavior and results suggest that he or she consistently exhibited at a certain level of performance on the measure. In a report for this type of child, you would merely report the global score and then provide general descriptions of the various subtests administered. You would not report differences among subtests because you did not obtain any meaningful differences.

Unfortunately, our results discussed earlier suggest that this "flat" profile is fairly uncommon among the children we see in the field (only approximately 20% of children show flat profiles), and it is even rarer in children with disabilities. One exception is children with intellectual disabilities, who show less variability on cognitive measures (Blum & Holling, 2017), but this may be due to subtest floor effects. Our research also confirms that there are high "base rates" for significant discrepancies (i.e., most children show factor differences), but our results suggest that even for typical children with variable profiles, the global IQ should not be interpreted (Elliott et al., 2010; Fiorello et al., 2007). While base rates are important to consider when determining how significant a score difference is relative to the standardization

---

Case Study 3.4. Written Report on Mobina

The following text from the report on Mobina will help you meet the need to report global scores that are not valid for interpretive purposes:

On the Woodcock–Johnson IV (WJ-IV), a measure of intellectual and cognitive functioning, Mobina obtained a General Intellectual Ability (GIA) score of 105, with 95% confidence of her true score falling between 99 and 111. This score is a standard score (SS), where the average score is 100 and the standard deviation is 15. This means that 68% of all children Mobina's age score between 85 and 115. This score places her in the average range and at the 63rd percentile compared to her same-age peers. This global score suggests that she is performing at a level similar to, or greater than, 63% of her same-age peers. However, this score should be interpreted with caution, because there were significant differences among the subtests that are used to calculate this global score.

APPLICATION 3.4. The Standard Error of the Difference and Residual

The standard error of the difference (*SED*) takes into account the reliability of the measures being compared, and requires the same *SD* for each score. It does not take into account the correlation of the measures. It is defined as follows:

$$SED = SD\sqrt{2 - r_{xx} - r_{yy}}$$

The *SD* will be 15 for your analyses (all scores are converted to SSs). The r_{xx} is the reliability of the first subtest for the given age level, and the r_{yy} is the reliability of the second subtest at the same age level. Let's see whether a 20-point difference between an intelligence test and an achievement measure is significant. Twenty points seems significant, but let's see. On the "Ability Test," Fred earned an SS of 105 (r_{xx} = .89); on the "Reading Passages" test, he earned an SS of 85 (r_{yy} = .72). We plug these SSs into the equation:

$$SED = 15\sqrt{2 - .89 - .72}$$
$$SED = 15\sqrt{.39}$$
$$SED = 15\ (.624)$$
$$SED = 9.37$$

This is the critical value for *SED*, and the SS difference (105 – 85) must exceed this for it to be significant at the 68% confidence level. We prefer to use the 99% or 95% confidence level. To do so, the *SED* must be multiplied by 2.58 (p = .01) or 1.96 (p = .05) to obtain the critical value. If we do this, 2.58 × 9.37, we get a critical value of 24.16, and we would need a 25-point difference (we must always round up) between the Ability Test SS and Reading Passages SS for there to be a significant difference. Notice if we use the less stringent p = .05 level, our 20-point difference is significant because the *SED* is 19 (1.96 × 9.37 = 18.37). Again, we must always round up, so that a critical value of 17.0001 would require at least an 18-point difference for significance.

Although this method can be used to compare SSs on the same metric, the more appropriate (and complex) method takes into account the correlation between the two scores being compared. This is obviously the preferred method for comparison, but you must have the correlation coefficients between the two measures. Often you can find these coefficients for commonly used measures in test manuals (in the standardization section), but often you must use the simple difference approach described above if the correlations are not available. Again, the following regression-based approach (the standard error of the residual, or *SER*) is the preferred method for calculating whether two scores are different, but it requires the correlation between the two measures.

Let's say that there is a correlation of .55 between the Ability Test and Reading Passages. The first thing we need to do is to find the predicted Ability Test score. It is calculated by first computing a *z* score, which is easy enough; then multiplying this by the correlation to get the predicted score; and then changing back to a predicted SS from which the achievement score will be subtracted.

1. z_{AT} = (raw score – *M*)/*SD*
   z_{AT} = (105 – 100)/15 = .33

2. $z_{(AT\ predicted)} = r_{xy}\ z_{AT}$
   $z_{(AT\ predicted)}$ = .55(.33) = .1815

(*continued*)

3. $SS_{(AT\ predicted)} = 100 + (z_{(predicted)} \times 15)$

$SS_{(AT\ predicted)} = 100 + (.1815)(15) = 102.72 = 103$

4. Discrepancy difference $= SS_{(AT\ predicted)} - SS_{(RP)}$

$= 103 - 85 = 18$ points

So, if the *SER* we calculate is less than 18, we will reject the null hypothesis of no difference between the tests, and there will be a discrepancy. To calculate the *SER*, we first need to calculate the residual score reliability, which is defined by the following formula:

1. $r_{residual} = r_{yy} + (r_{xx})(r^2_{xy}) - 2r^2_{xy}/1 - r^2_{xy}$
2. $r_{residual} = r_{yy} + (r_{xx})(r^2_{xy}) - 2r^2_{xy}/1 - r^2_{xy}$

$= .72 + (.89)(.55^2) - 2(.55^2)/1 - (.55^2)$

$= .72 + (.89)(.3025) - 2(.3025)/1 - .3025$

$= .72 + (.269225) - (.605)/.6975$

$= .55086$

Now we can calculate the *SER*, which is defined by the following formula:

$$SER = SD\sqrt{1 - r^2_{xy}}\ \sqrt{1 - r_{residual}}$$
$$= 15\sqrt{1 - .3025}\ \sqrt{1 - .55086}$$
$$= 15(.83516)(.67018)$$
$$= 8.39560$$

We need to multiply this value by 1.96 for $p < .05$ ($1.96 \times 8.39560 = 16.455$) and round up to 17, which suggests that we need a 17-point difference for these scores to be significant. Our critical score was 18, so the scores are different. However, if we take the more rigorous route ($p < .01$), we obtain a value of 22 ($2.58 \times 8.39560 = 21.661$); this exceeds our 18-point difference between ability and achievement, so there is no significant difference at the .01 level.

Notice how these *SER* values are *lower* than the values we obtained using the simple *SED* formula described earlier. Therefore, you are more likely to reject the null hypothesis (i.e., there is a difference) with the *SER* than you are with the simple *SED* formula. Given that the *SED* is a much simpler formula, we'd suggest using the *SED* first and stopping there if you have significance, because you will also have significance if you use the *SER*. Similarly, if the difference between your test scores is much lower than the *SED* critical value, you could take a chance and suggest that there is no difference. However, keep in mind that the *SER* is related to the correlation between the two test scores, so "eyeballing" it may lead to error. If the difference between test scores is close to your *SED* critical value, but does not exceed it, you should calculate the *SER*. Keep in mind that you're more likely to make a Type II error (failing to reject the null hypothesis when it is indeed false) with the *SED*. In other words, when you use the *SED* formula, you are more likely to conclude that there is no difference between the scores when there actually *is* a difference, so in many ways it is the more conservative approach for determining whether two scores are different from one another. Using *SED*, you are more likely to have a false-negative result (no score difference when there actually is one) than a false-positive one (score difference when there isn't any).

sample, just because a child falls into a "typical" base rate range does not mean he or she doesn't have a disability. For children with variable profiles (i.e., significant subtest or factor differences), it is important to consider combining subtests into new factors, but when the data are not consistent, we feel that interpretation must go beyond nomothetic approaches to the idiographic level of analysis. We must interpret patterns of performance—the difficult, controversial, and often maligned practice we previously discussed in Chapter 1.

Patterns of Performance

As stated earlier, idiographic analysis should be avoided if possible, because interpretation of global factors is preferable to analysis of subtest scores (Flanagan & Alfonso, 2017). We were all taught that the IQ was the most reliable score and so you could place the most credence in interpreting this score, with subtest scores being the least reliable. Just because global scores are more reliable for large-scale populations does not equate to them being reliable for individual children, especially children with disabilities (Hale et al., 2010). However, it is critical to ensure you don't confuse normative reliability (large-scale typical populations) with intraindividual reliability (individual child).

The above point is key. If you have significant factor or subtest differences for a child you are testing, you do not have a reliable global score. You must go down from the global IQ score to the factor scores. You may have a reliable factor score (i.e., the subtests that compose it are consistent), and so you can interpret it. However, if the subtests that compose the factors are also variable, you have no choice but to go to a true pattern of performance or idiographic analysis, especially if you wish to understand the true nature of brain-related dysfunction (Clements et al., 2011; Lezak et al., 2012).

Interpreting patterns of performance requires considerable clinical acumen—something that can only be acquired through extensive training, careful observation, and supervised experience. This book will help you build upon the ideas already presented, but analyzing a child's patterns of performance requires discordant/divergent right-hemisphere processes to think of multiple possible explanations for profile variability, in addition to concordant and convergent left-hemisphere skills (both of which have been discussed in Chapter 2). Problem solving requires exploring multiple possibilities before formulating a plan (Shinn et al., 2013). If you are to be a good problem solver during assessment, your frontal and right-hemisphere skills will be critical in interpreting the profiles. When examining individual children, you must look at all aspects of their behavior and environment, and establish the concurrent, ecological, and treatment validity if our CHT model is to be helpful to you in practice.

An individual's test performance cannot occur in a vacuum (Lezak et al., 2012). Individuals are not scores, so we admonish you to avoid using a "cookbook" approach to subtest interpretation. Subtle qualitative differences in a child's performance across and within measures may be reflective of meaningful brain–behavior relationships, and these differences will be obscured if the focus is on test results only (Fiorello et al., 2009; Golden, Espe-Pfeifer, et al., 2000; Hale, Alfonso, et al., 2010). Instead of focusing solely on scores, we advocate a process approach—one that emphasizes Luria's (1973a) individualized assessment methodology and provides a strategy for maximizing the richness of clinical data.

The Boston process approach, developed by Kaplan and colleagues (see Milberg et al., 2009), objectifies qualitative differences in child subtest data. Kaplan (1990) has argued that the problem with both fixed and flexible neuropsychological test batteries is that interpretation is based on correct or incorrect item performance, whereas the problem-solving process approach can provide insights into neuropsychological processes that have direct implications for intervention. To accomplish this, it is not enough just to examine the outcome of performance (i.e., right or wrong); rather, it is necessary to determine how the child arrived at a particular answer. This approach is very similar to the tactics used in what has been referred to as *dynamic assessment* (e.g., Haywood & Lidz, 2006).

The process approach is inherently child-centered, sensitive to the unique characteristics of children and their environment. As stated earlier, we must recognize that the brain functions as a set of interdependent systems, doing the best it can to process and respond to task demands in a gradiental fashion (Mikadze et al., 2019). Individual functional brain areas attempt to accomplish tasks that might typically be performed by a dysfunctional area, albeit not as successfully. This has been called the "complementary-contribution principle" (Bernstein, 2000). In the absence or dysfunction of one system, another system does the best it can to accomplish the task, which is consistent with neuroimaging data. Neuroimaging data often show that when a test is used to assess a child's deficit area, the child shows a deficit, *and* a compensatory overactivity in other areas, perhaps to make up for the weakness (Hale et al., 2013). How do these systems interconnect, cooperate, or inhibit one another? It is your job to determine how the pattern fits together—a task that not only requires idiographic analysis of performance, but also allows for verification of results by means of the CHT model.

When conducting CHT, you clinically examine a child's pattern of performance both within and between measures, because you cannot determine what one score suggests without analyzing other scores and data (Fiorello et al., 2009; Hale et al., 2013). You go beyond the typical input and output observations made by most psychologists, and focus on neuropsychological processes, which can shed light on important child strengths and weaknesses. Identification of strengths not only helps you avoid pathologizing the child; it also lays a foundation for subsequent intervention development (Hughes et al., 2017). As argued earlier, focusing on input and output demands leads to misconceptions about hemispheric functions, and failed aptitude-treatment interactions. The multifactorial nature of subtests requires fine-grained analysis of input, processing, and output demands, as well as systematic testing of the limits, if we are to realize the full potential of our clinical tools for evaluation of hypothesized strengths and needs.

Whereas the normative approach provides little insight into individual differences in academic performance and behavioral functioning, this idiographic orientation allows us to establish important linkages to cognitive, academic, and behavioral functioning. It can serve as an integrative framework for interpreting apparently disparate behaviors. However, we must be extremely cautious, because our own heuristics and biases can influence our interpretation (Bernstein, 2000). We must realize that subtest variability could be due to many factors, so interpretation should proceed only with the greatest of caution. We need to recognize that children with the same disorder may have different symptoms, and that similar symptoms can be caused by different disorders (Hale et al., 2013; Sattler, 2024). Variability among "cognitive phenotypes" is common, and even when these may look superficially alike, they may involve fundamentally different cognitive processes. It is your responsibility to determine the nature of the expressed characteristics, and careful clinical analyses can clarify an otherwise confusing array of data (Lezak et al., 2012).

The key to successful CHT is recognizing the multifactorial nature of subtests, identifying the consistency among cognitive constructs tapped by the measures, and attempting to link them to brain functions. Many resources are available to aid in this process. A good place to start is the CHC literature (Flanagan et al., 2013; McGrew & Wendling, 2010), but other works for the DAS-II (Elliott et al., 2010; Hale et al., 2008) and WISC-V (Flanagan & Alfonso, 2017) may be helpful.

Demands analysis, as introduced in Chapter 1 and elaborated on in Chapter 4, provides you with the tool to recognize the similarities and differences among the subtests. We also provide two appendices in this chapter (Appendices 3.2 and 3.3) that you can reproduce for interpretive purposes. These forms allow you to take notes and generate hypotheses about a child's performance, based on the four-quadrant demands analysis approach described in the next section. It is important to realize that demands analysis does not allow you to ignore the nomothetic or quantitative aspects of subtest performance. It requires you to recognize the limitations of qualitative analysis, and to consider the technical characteristics of subtests (e.g., sample space, unique and shared variance, and standard error of measurement), when drawing conclusions about child performance.

Although poor technical quality has been a problem with neuropsychological assessment tools in the past, this is changing, and a majority of the instruments we list in Chapter 4 have excellent technical quality. Clinical and qualitative information is important, but neuropsychological assessment requires an examination of how test reliability and validity affect performance and interpretation (Franzen, 2013). We agree that demands analysis is inherently more difficult and more prone to error if not undertaken with the greatest of care and empirical rigor. However, it can shed new light on seemingly random variations in subtest performance, especially if you consider the posterior–anterior, left–right, and superior–inferior axes discussed in Chapter 2.

Left–Right, Posterior–Anterior, and Superior–Inferior Differences

In addition to the left–right differences noted by Reitan (1974), we add the posterior–anterior axis as a concurrent level of analysis. Simply put, the posterior region is for understanding *input*, and the anterior region is for accomplishing *output*. The left and right hemispheres work side by side, with the right hemisphere responsible for discordant/divergent processes, and the left hemisphere carrying out concordant/convergent processing demands (Semrud-Clikeman & Ellison, 2009).

Recall that Luria's (1973a) second functional unit is the one responsible for the interpretation of incoming sensory information, and the third functional unit is the one responsible for motor output and higher-order executive functions. These functions become increasingly lateralized as one ascends the hierarchy; however, as we have discussed, the left–right axis does not represent a verbal–nonverbal distinction, but rather a rote/crystallized–novel/fluid distinction. We can think of stimuli—regardless of whether they are auditory, visual, or somatosensory—as being processed by both hemispheres, with the division of labor directly related to whether there is a "descriptive system" available to process it (Goldberg & Costa, 1981).

This "descriptive system" idea can be related to Piaget's notion of a schema. If there is a schema or descriptive system to process the information, the left hemisphere is likely to carry out the task. The more rote, automatic, well-learned, or local a task is, the more likely the left hemisphere is to process it with an existing schema (i.e., assimilation). The more novel, ambiguous, or global a task is, the more likely the right hemisphere is to process it and attempt to create a new schema in the left (i.e., accommodation). Most tasks will have some novel aspects, but novel problem solving requires the use of existing knowledge and skills, so bilateral performance is expected on just about any task that taps multiple psychological processes. This rote–novel distinction does not suggest that findings supporting left- and right-hemisphere differences on the WISC Verbal–Performance scales are invalid (Mellet et al., 2014). Instead, the model should help you recognize that interpretation must go beyond the typical verbal–nonverbal dichotomy, and that bilateral activity is the rule rather than the exception, especially when processing most complex tasks.

Our new dichotomy can also be used to describe the posterior–anterior axis as well. The more a task requires fluid reasoning or novel problem-solving skills, the more the frontal executive system will be involved (Decker et al., 2007). Given our understanding of hemispheric differences, it is the *right* frontal lobe that will be responsible for fluid reasoning and executive tasks, but recall that bilateral activity is likely. What about the left/storage–right/ retrieval dichotomy? Recall that putting new information into memory requires consolidation with existing knowledge (a left-hemisphere function), but retrieval requires considering multiple memories for words and concepts, as well as several possible responses (a right-hemisphere function). As the task becomes more automatic and crystallized, the posterior areas are more likely to respond to the task—especially in the left hemisphere, an area specialized for crystallized knowledge (knowledge gained through experience and education). Again, it is important to realize that all areas are likely to be involved in most tasks; only different degrees of involvement are required, a point highlighted in Application 3.5.

Because most brain areas are involved in many tasks we administer, we must exercise extreme caution in drawing inferences about particular brain areas being affected or damaged (Baron, 2018). For instance, a child may have difficulty with executive functions that could be related to the cingulate; limited motor skills because of poor dorsal stream feedback to the motor system; or problems with implicit language comprehension due to right temporal dysfunction that results in expressive language problems similar to "jargon aphasia." We must avoid the "pin-the-tail-on-the-lesion" mentality that will neglect the interconnectedness of the brain systems that govern complex behavior (Koziol et al., 2013). Such a mentality also neglects the finding in many brain-based disorders that other neural systems may be recruited to solve the problem and that everyone's brain is as unique as a fingerprint. It is possible to have the same area damaged in traumatic brain injury, and yet show different deficits.

Keeping this important gradiental orientation in mind, we can begin to break down the

APPLICATION 3.5. Brain Functions and Stages of Learning

For a better understanding of brain–behavior relationships in the classroom, it is important to relate brain functions to the stages of learning described by Smith (1981). During the initial *acquisition stage* of learning new information, regardless of the modality (e.g., auditory, visual), right-hemisphere resources are required. The more novel or unique the new information, the more the right hemisphere will be required, and the activity will be more frontal, because executive demands will be high. The left hemisphere is working simultaneously with the right to develop a descriptive system or schema to process the information for the future. There's then a gradual shift from right- to left-hemisphere processes as tasks become learned (Goldberg, 2001).

Left-hemisphere processes are necessary for both the *proficiency* and *maintenance* stages of learning. This is because the proficiency stage's objective is quick and efficient (fluent) performance, and the maintenance stage's objective is retention over time. Not only do both of these stages rely heavily on left-hemisphere processes, but posterior systems become more involved. *Proficiency* is the process of consolidating the skill into long-term memory and developing automaticity so that the task can be performed both accurately and quickly. Once proficiency is achieved, the skill must be stored in long-term memory for later use, so *maintenance* requires the left-hemisphere areas (mainly posterior) associated with long-term memory storage. This right-to-left shift in learning and retention of skills then changes again in the *generalization* and *adaptation* stages. To generalize skills, a child must use right-hemisphere skills to modify his or her behavior to cope with the novel application of the skill in new settings or situations. Finally, to capitalize on this knowledge in the *adaptation* stage and to recognize its use in novel problem-solving situations, substantial right-hemisphere involvement is required, and again executive demands are high. It is important to recognize that hemispheric activity in learning is not an either–or proposition. Instead, there is a gradual shift from right (especially right frontal) to left (especially left posterior), and back again as the child progresses through the learning stages.

posterior–anterior and left–right axes into four quadrants, as depicted in Figure 3.2. Simply put, the right posterior hemisphere is specialized for global, coarse, or novel processing of stimuli, and the left posterior region is specialized for local, detailed processing of automatic or routinized information. Similarly, the right frontal region is important for brainstorming multiple ideas and carrying out complex motor programs requiring adaptation and change to environmental demands. Alternatively, the left frontal region would appear to be the area that brings closure, categorization, and compartmentalization of ideas, as well as the region that organizes concepts and develops motor programs to carry out complex actions (including familiar aspects of expressive language). Let's explore each of these quadrants in further detail.

Right- and Left-Posterior Quadrants

At an input or primary cortex level, the right posterior region will be primarily responsible for left-side hearing, visual field, and somatosensory feeling, and the left posterior region will be responsible for these functions on the right side of the body. Finger agnosia (inability to recognize touch of fingers) and astereognosis (difficulty with recognizing objects by touch) may occur following damage to either the left or right parietal area. Damage to the left primary somatosensory area affects the right hand, and damage to the right area affects the left hand. However, this left–right dichotomy is not as simple as it seems (see In-Depth 3.3), because complex tasks require more right-hemisphere involvement, and simple, routine tasks require more left-hemisphere involvement. So feeling a three-dimensional object with the left hand will be processed almost entirely by the right parietal lobe. Put it in the right hand and now you need both hemispheres, the left parietal to feel the object and the right parietal to recognize the global spatial elements of it. Similarly, this would make it easier to recognize numbers or letters drawn on the right hand than the left, since the left hemisphere is likely to be the place these symbolic representations are stored.

   At a processing level, the right posterior region is especially good at recognizing unfamiliar or global relationships among stimuli parts, especially when multiple sensory modalities

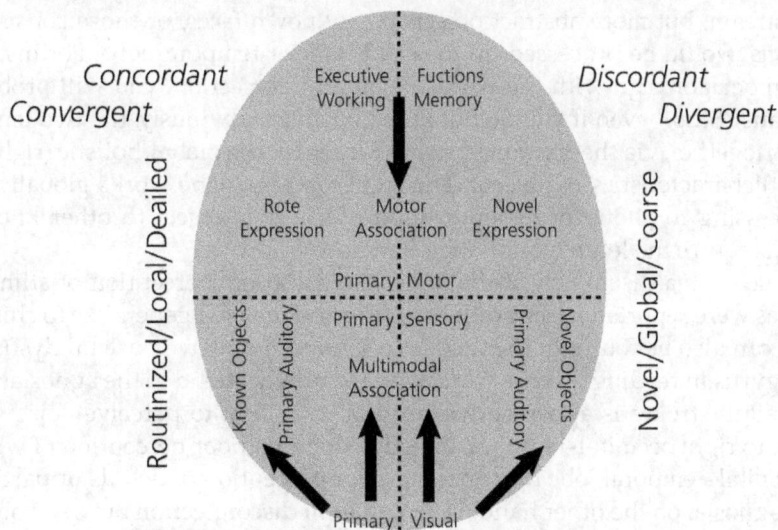

FIGURE 3.2. Four-quadrant analysis of brain function.

IN-DEPTH 3.3. Simple versus Complex Sensory–Motor Tasks

Consistent with our reconceptualization of the two hemispheres, it may be the complexity of the task that determines the nature of a sensory–motor deficit: Right-hemisphere dysfunction may interfere with complex, novel tactile–motor skills, whereas simple, routinized tactile–motor skills may be more likely to occur with left-hemisphere dysfunction (Francis et al., 1988). These findings provide another clear example of how more complex or multimodal integration skills require right-hemisphere involvement. Because there is much more primary than association cortex in the left hemisphere, single-modality or simple, routinized somatosensory processing is likely to be attempted by the left posterior hemisphere.

In this lateralization quest, we must recall that integrity of the corpus callosum and motor areas (i.e., frontal lobes–basal ganglia–cerebellum) plays a role in Francis and colleagues' (1988) conclusions as well. Surely damage to the left frontal cortex can cause right hemiparesis, but the motor tasks we use are likely to require contralateral activity as well; it is the amount that varies, based on the simple–complex dimension. As we can see, the dichotomy is not a simple one between the left hemisphere/right body and the right hemisphere/left body. Instead, you must examine the task performance in relation to other tasks, and determine whether performance deficits are due to input, processing, and/or output problems.

---

are involved. It is specialized for coarse processing rather than detail processing. It is also important for recognition of objects, especially when the objects are presented in a unique or novel perspective (ventral stream). As we have seen, processing novel faces and changes in facial expression requires the right ventral stream—hence the importance of this stream in social perception. Developmental prosopagnosia, or inability to recognize faces, is likely to be caused by dysfunction or damage to either temporal lobe ventral stream (Wilson et al., 2010); again, however, the details of facial recognition would be lost with left-hemisphere dysfunction, whereas right-hemisphere dysfunction would lead to global face recognition deficits.

Common objects and faces may be more likely to be processed by the left ventral (temporal lobe) stream, but more abstract objects or unknown faces, or those consisting of new configurations, would be processed by the right inferior temporal lobe. For instance, if you encounter an octagon sign with the word *Alto* at an intersection, you will probably realize that this means "Stop," even if you do not know Spanish. Obviously, the two temporal lobes need to work together, via the commissures, to recognize the global/holistic (right) and local/detailed (left) characteristics of objects. The right temporal lobe works globally at a coarse level of processing to allow for generalization of the new object to other known objects, which would require the left temporal lobe functions.

What follows is a discussion of the agnosias that affect perception of stimuli. Historically, agnosias were reported in the adult literature and may not generalize to children. Child case reports can also be found in the literature. Children do have parietal dysfunction (e.g., the angular gyrus in reading), so it is worthwhile to briefly attend to the agnosias. A disorder common to adult strokes is apperceptive agnosia, or failure to perceive objects visually; it could be due to right occipital–temporal lobe dysfunction (poor perception of whole objects) or to left occipital–temporal lobe dysfunction (poor perception of details or parts of objects). Associative agnosia, on the other hand, is an apparent disconnection between object perception (which is intact) and its semantic label. A child who cannot do cross-modal (e.g., verbal–visual) matching, even though visual and verbal skills are both adequate, will show this pattern. The need to crossover was a problem for a child with associative agnosia. Whereas apperceptive agnosia may result from dysfunction occurring earlier in the ventral stream (i.e., the occipital lobe), associative agnosia may occur at a later point (i.e., the temporal lobe), with the superior temporal sulcus region being particularly important for this cross-modal matching. Spatial relationships, movement perception, and body awareness are primarily processed in the dorsal stream of the occipital–parietal areas. Although these agnosias are often seen in adult patients with brain damage, the zones of overlapping may be delayed or dysfunctional in children, so nonetheless it is important to think of these perception problems.

Dysfunction in the parietal lobe (especially the right) can lead to several additional types of agnosia, including limited awareness of self (asomatognosia) and the environment (neglect), usually in the contralateral hemispace. In addition, because this region is responsible for providing visual–spatial feedback to the motor system, constructional apraxia is often the result of right parietal lobe dysfunction and may be more appropriately termed *constructional agnosia*. The right posterior ventral region is the area most likely to maintain ongoing perception of both facial affect and verbal prosody during social discourse. If the dysfunction is more superior, a prosodic agnosia could result; if it is more inferior, prosopagnosia and object agnosia could result. An easier way to think of these conditions is that affected children tend to ignore themselves and what is going on around them, which is similar to ADHD–inattentive presentation.

This right posterior area is also responsible for examining verbal incongruities, such as metaphor, idiom, sarcasm, and humor, as well as other types of implicit communication (both verbal and nonverbal). For these tertiary-level deficits, the occipital–parietal–temporal "crossroads" in the right hemisphere is likely to be affected. However, it is important to recognize that these novel higher-level interpretive processes are much more likely to require frontal involvement. Because these complex interpretive skills may not be needed at a young age, they may not be clinically manifested until the age at which they are required (Horton et al., 2010).

The homologous left-hemisphere regions play comparable roles, but they focus on different aspects of the stimuli. The left posterior quadrant is involved in local processing of detailed stimuli (making fine distinctions between one stimulus and another). It is also important for orientation and directionality of stimuli and is responsible for processing of well-known routinized information. So much of long-term memory is probably localized to this quadrant in the areas that process that information (Gazzaniga et al., 2013). Prior knowledge of places, objects, facts, details, and relationships will all be localized to this region, particularly to the temporal lobe. However, as nouns are likely stored in the left posterior region, verbs are likely to be stored in frontal regions. Interestingly, and related to this, memories of people tend to be more anterior in the middle temporal regions, whereas memories for objects tend to be more posterior.

Gerstmann syndrome, characterized by finger agnosia, dysgraphia (problems with writing), dyscalculia (problems with math calculation), and right–left confusion (due to body awareness and direction), can occur following left parietal lobe damage. Early reports based on adult cases have been challenged, with some wondering if the syndrome actually exists. However, left parietal functions have been associated with finger agnosia, somatosensory problems in handwriting, math calculation impairment, and left/right confusion (Roux et al., 2003), so it is worth discussing briefly here. It is interesting that left/right confusion (e.g., letter reversals) often co-occurs with reading deficits caused by left parietal dysfunction. It is not surprising that some types of apraxia (difficulty with carrying out motor activities) can be related to parietal lobe damage, because of limited body awareness or representation of posture (Pisella et al., 2019). Because phonemes are the basic sound units of language, the left posterior temporal lobe is probably responsible for phonemic awareness, analysis, and segmentation. Posterior and medial to this region, problems with receptive language, known as Wernicke's or fluent aphasia, are likely following damage to the parietal–temporal tertiary areas.

The posterior ventral parietal (i.e., angular gyrus, supramarginal gyrus) and associated occipital regions are more likely to be involved in the written aspects of language (Seghier & Price, 2013). Obviously, any of these areas can be associated with comprehension deficits; however, because of the left hemisphere's propensity for fine, routine, and automatic processes, oral and written language comprehension are likely to be impaired. However, the rote–novel hemispheric distinction plays a role here, with left-hemisphere language areas responsible for explicit comprehension, and the right-hemisphere language areas responsible for implicit comprehension (Male & Gouldthorp, 2020). We will return to these topics in later chapters.

Right- and Left-Anterior Quadrants

For the primary cortical areas, recall that the right frontal lobe is involved in motor control of the left side of the body, and that the left frontal lobe is responsible for right-side motor control. Recall that the secondary areas are differentiated by whether the motor skill is self- or other-oriented. The secondary area (the supplementary motor cortex) is responsible for self-directed movements, and the lateral secondary area (the premotor cortex) is responsible for movement in response to external stimuli. Because the supplementary motor area is responsible for internal motor scripts, it is not surprising that this area is connected to the prefrontal cortex and basal ganglia. The premotor area has connections with the parietal cortex and cerebellum, because it is important in responding to environmental stimuli.

Recall that during new skill learning, the premotor area is more active, but as skills become automatic or routinized, the supplementary motor area (in conjunction with temporal lobe, limbic structures, and cerebellum) is best suited to perform the learned task (Ruan et al., 2018). However, this distinction has been debated in recent times; the nature of the stimuli may be what determines the extent of premotor and supplementary motor area involvement, with both areas likely involved to some degree.

Because the left hemisphere is involved in fine, detailed, and routinized activities, it is not surprising that the apraxias, even though they are "visual–motor" difficulties, are more commonly associated with left-hemisphere dysfunction. They often go hand in hand (pun intended!) with aphasia. Damage to the supplementary motor area of the left frontal lobe can result in difficulty with developing a motor plan, and/or with carrying out a complex or routinized motor task.

Although posterior left-hemisphere dysfunction can also cause ideational apraxia (in which the child cannot think of the concept/idea of what to do) or ideomotor apraxia (in which the child has the concept, but cannot carry out the steps) (Chang & Yu, 2016), these problems can also occur following left frontal quadrant dysfunction. However, since these apraxias are the result of prior learning and knowledge, they are more common with left-hemisphere dysfunction and are less likely following right-hemisphere damage.

As noted earlier, constructional apraxia is more difficult to evaluate and requires considerable clinical attention. Like the other apraxias, it could be due to problems with motor control (left secondary motor cortex). However, it can also be caused by parietal dysfunction in either hemisphere. In the right hemisphere, dysfunction can lead to problems with spatial and motor movement feedback to the anterior motor system and left parietal somatosensory problems (sensory feedback to the right hand) can lead to problems with somatosensory–motor feedback. Left posterior parietal dysfunction can also lead to orientation problems, resulting in reversal errors. Because these functions tend to be differentially processed by the two hemispheres (right, spatial/holistic feedback; left, motor and somatosensory control), hemispheric integration is required, and agenesis of the corpus callosum can also lead to constructional difficulties (Berlucchi, 2012).

You must try to determine whether a child's problem is with somatosensory functioning/orientation/movement (left parietal), global spatial feedback (right parietal), motor functioning (left frontal motor area), or integration (corpus callosum), because you would attempt different remediation strategies for each type of deficit. Obviously, a child who has handwriting problems due to constructional apraxia should develop these skills by practicing handwriting, but different complementary intervention techniques for both handwriting and associated deficits are worth exploring. In addition, differential diagnosis is needed to determine whether occupational therapy services are required. We will return to interventions for handwriting in a later chapter.

Differentiating between the higher functions of the right and left frontal lobes has been difficult, possibly because most "frontal" tasks require *correct* rather than *adaptive* responding (Burgess & Stuss, 2017). The limited empirical evidence for lateralized frontal lobe functions is less difficult to accept if we recall that both hemispheres are likely to be involved in most cognitive tasks; it is just the amount of involvement that varies. It would appear that the right frontal region is likely to be involved in many aspects of brain functioning, especially those that require novel problem-solving or fluid abilities.

The right frontal region works with posterior regions to examine incongruities among stimuli, using divergent processes to examine discordant information. This area works to produce behavior that is flexibly consistent with the current situation, maximizing the likelihood of success. The use of novel problem-solving skills/fluid abilities seems to follow a U pattern during child development. Novel problem-solving skills are greatly needed in infancy to learn sound–symbol associations and the nuances of functioning in the world. These skills are not needed as much during the early school years, when rote memorization and recall of facts and details predominate.

As we will discuss in a subsequent chapter, children with right frontal dysfunction are more likely to be recognized for their unusual behavior and social alienation during these years than for their academic deficits. Academic, occupational, and social pursuits are more likely to be impaired during initial learning in very young children, and then again in adolescence and adulthood, which can be frustrating for these children, because they were such good students in the early school years. As these children leave middle childhood, they have developed a very left-hemisphere, concrete understanding of the world; however, with the onset of adolescence and formal operational thought, the need for novel problem-solving/ fluid abilities increases, as adolescents begin to question the validity of their earlier concrete beliefs.

Most research does not differentiate between right and left frontal areas which may be due in part to the limited attention the frontal lobes have received until very recently. Executive functions are all about self-regulation and task management. They are likely to be bilaterally represented, but their dynamic nature suggests that the right hemisphere is probably more involved than the left. The right hemisphere is likely to be involved in executive strategizing, inhibiting, monitoring, evaluating, shifting, and changing performance—all important tasks in solving novel problems (Hale et al., 2013; Stuss, 2011). Planning and organization skills, also considered executive tasks, are also likely to require right frontal functions, but because the left frontal region is associated with temporal relationships and categorization, these executive tasks may be more bilateral in nature.

Consistent with Luria's (1973a) notions about the frontal lobes and memory, retrieval of information from long-term memory appears to be somewhat more closely related to the right frontal lobe than to the left. This is not because long-term memories are located there, but rather because retrieval requires a comprehensive (discordant/divergent) search pattern through the vast catalogs of information that are probably located in the left posterior regions. Working memory demands are high for long-term memory retrieval (Barbey et al., 2013), because a person must keep the retrieval question in mind, find the appropriate long-term memories, and determine whether the ones located are the ones needed. Likewise, during novel problem-solving tasks, working memory requires retaining and acting upon novel information that has not yet been coded into long-term memory.

Expressive language skills (namely, in the area of affective prosody) and the implicit messages discussed are likely to be influenced by right frontal areas (Patel et al., 2018). If you see someone with a monotone, or someone who has difficulty modulating his or her voice (i.e., it is always too loud or too quiet), right frontal dysfunction could be the cause. Implicit expressive language appears to be a right inferior frontal lobe task. Because visual attention requires a search strategy, the right frontal area, especially the frontal eye fields, may be more involved in visual selective attention and scanning.

The left frontal lobe is responsible for looking for concordant information and integrating information in a convergent, ordered fashion, so it is not surprising that this lobe is involved in understanding of temporal relationships and consolidating information into long-term memory. As a result, working memory plays an important role in memory consolidation in the left hemisphere (Barbey et al., 2013). For this reason, categorical and convergent thinking and behavior (e.g., determining how two words belong to a category) are likely to be left frontal tasks. Certainly, the left frontal region is responsible for explicit expressive language, and Broca's or nonfluent aphasia is more likely following damage to this region. Broca's aphasia is known for halting speech and poor adherence to grammar. Why does Broca's aphasia lead to poor grammar? Because grammar is all about rules, and rule-governed behavior is what the left hemisphere thrives on.

Not only is the left frontal lobe the source of rules; it is also responsible for temporal (i.e., time-related) information processing. It helps the posterior regions organize information in a step-by-step, sequential, or successive fashion. Of course, all of these skills are necessary for language processes, but the left hemisphere's propensity for fine, detailed, and routinized processing is what makes symbolic communication lateralize to that hemisphere (Romeo et al., 2018). Considering the left-hemisphere processes to be sequential or successive in nature is not wrong per se; it just fails to recognize the true nature of the left hemisphere, because it focuses on input and output demands. The left hemisphere likes rules, details, prior knowledge, and order, making it an ideal candidate to respond to most aphasia tests, and most achievement tests as well. In fact, it can be argued that *any* test requiring a "correct" response is really tapping left-hemisphere concordant/convergent functions.

The Superior–Inferior Axis

We've already talked quite a bit about this axis. The "superior" part of this axis is the same as the "anterior" part of the posterior–anterior axis of interpretation. So how does the superior part differ? In the past decade or so, we have learned such a great deal about our frontal–basal ganglia thalamic circuits (frontal–subcortical circuits) and our cerebral–cerebellar circuits. We have given these critical interactions "axis" status because of how these circuits govern both automatic and volitional behavior, and are the source of most emotional and behavior disorders or psychopathology (Koziol et al., 2013).

When emotional and/or behavioral disorders (i.e., psychopathology) are being hypothesized, one should consider this superior–inferior axis as being the likely source of the problem. It is difficult to assess, because we don't have any real "subcortical" neuropsychological tests. Nonetheless, we can start to see relationships and patterns in the data that could suggest this psychopathology axis is the likely cause. While there are more "frontal" or "cerebellar" types of tasks, these are not localizing tests because whether the problem is more one or the other, it is likely that both will be affected. In fact, we can expect subtle decrements on many tasks, including cognitive ones (Hale et al., 2013), if a child has executive dysfunction. As a result, understanding the pattern of performance is essential for recognizing a superior–inferior axis problem like ADHD, OCD, depression, or other neuropsychiatric conditions.

What does one look for when examining this superior–inferior axis? Surely, our tests that tap "executive function" are a good start. Unfortunately, while many have good sensitivity to executive function deficits, most of these measures do not have adequate specificity for *different* types of executive dysfunction. Since these tests are not specific for brain areas, results are often influenced by other factors and psychological processes, so a process approach may be necessary for understanding patterns within and between executive measures. For instance, a low score on the Wisconsin Card Sorting Test could be due to a lot of things. A child with OCD may be unable to shift gears to think of other possibilities. A child with ADHD may have difficulty maintaining focus and thus lose the solution that had been established. It's also likely that a child with ADHD may not profit from the feedback that is provided during the test telling the child his/her answer is right or wrong. These are all examples of difficulty with the ability of the frontal lobes to monitor success and failure. So while executive dysfunction may or may not be apparent given a total nomothetic score, a pattern may emerge that highlights the type of executive dysfunction displayed. With your knowledge of the circuits and their influence on emotions and behavior, and a careful examination of behavior ratings and other behavior/personality measures, you can piece together whether a child's attention problem is due to ADHD, depression, anxiety, or some other disorder affecting the superior–inferior axis.

Although discussed more in the subsequent chapters, one of the most prominent and consistent findings for children with executive dysfunction is *inconsistent* performance (Stuss, 2011)! As noted in the last chapter, executive dysfunction leads to problems with the what (prefrontal), when (basal ganglia), and how (cerebellum) of a child interacting with the world (Koziol & Budding, 2011). According to this model, what to do is decided by the frontal lobes, whereas the basal ganglia knows when to carry out the executive act, and the cerebellum provides the amplitude or how the behavior is carried out.

This circuitry doesn't just affect emotions or behavior, it also affects how a child learns in the classroom and approaches tasks, including our test materials during evaluation. If a child doesn't plan before responding to a test item, she may respond impulsively and make a careless error. On the other hand, someone who reflects too long on a task before responding may have difficulty responding quickly and efficiently. This behavior can vary during testing as well, with what is often known as the speed–accuracy trade-off pattern (Standage et al., 2014). If a child has an anxiety disorder that makes him not respond (because of difficulty with decision making), the child instead might respond quickly and without deliberation, because if he doesn't respond quickly, he may not respond at all. Someone who is anxious and can't decide might have slow processing speed, as can someone with depression who is lethargic or apathetic, or someone with ADHD who is distracted off-task and loses track of what he's doing. Once again, it is understanding idiographic patterns of performance that can help illuminate important performance distinctions deemed irrelevant from a nomothetic perspective.

The key in interpreting superior–inferior axis function is, in part, related to how well you observe behavior, and to gathering as much intra-individual data as possible on executive function performance on our measures. Part of the difficulty with relying on nomothetic data (instead of idiographic process data) for executive measures is that these measures are frequently insensitive or nonspecific for the disorder, or how the child copes with the disorder. As noted earlier, we found Trails B errors to be sensitive to ADHD (Hale, Reddy, et al., 2009) and medication response (Kubas et al., 2012), but we were the first to produce normative data on errors because most people have just analyzed time to completion on this task.

Understanding the pattern and how it relates to volitional (e.g., dorsolateral prefrontal–dorsal cingulate circuits), emotional/behavioral (e.g., orbital prefrontal–ventral cingulate circuits) or automatic (e.g., cerebral–cerebellar circuit) is important for us to consider both for learning and adaptive behavior (Reddy et al., 2013). Through examination of these circuits, and understanding circuit dysfunction in different disorders, we can piece together the complex pattern of the child, understand his or her disorder(s), and make targeted recommendations for intervention. Accurate interpretation of the third superior–inferior axis is critical given that we will likely need cognitive, behavioral, and/or medication treatment for affected children.

"Red Flags" or Pathognomonic Signs

The last area to consider after level of performance, pattern of performance, and left/right differences (including posterior–anterior/superior–inferior axes) is what has been termed pathognomonic signs, which are taken to represent clear signs of brain damage. Although "soft signs" are common in neurodevelopmental disorders, "hard signs" of brain damage are less common outside medical or rehabilitation settings. However, it is worth familiarizing yourself with them because they may be evident in a child who has a severe disability. In addition, because schools are often not well versed in symptoms and outcomes associated with brain damage, you can be an important team member who can share your insight with others regarding brain injury, recovery, and transition to schools following a traumatic incident (Hale, Metro, et al., 2010).

Pathognomonic signs are what we like to call "red flags," because they tell us that a child's processing is different from that of typical children the same age. There are some clear signs of brain damage that we should look for in our evaluations. For instance, a marked unilateral sensory or motor deficit, abnormal reflexes, changes in pupil size or eyelid function, visual field loss, and hearing loss can be considered clear signs of brain damage.

As can be seen in Table 3.3, Lezak et al. (2012) specifies several symptoms of brain damage, some of which you may have seen in your practice. It is important to recognize that discrimination of these signs is often difficult, so you must exercise caution when making inferences about these symptoms and brain damage. Some practitioners consider some of these symptoms "soft signs"—that are less predictive of brain damage and are quite common in children with disabilities. Soft signs such as motor overflow (different limb or finger movements from those the child is attempting to produce), motor incoordination, left–right confusion, motor weakness on one side, distractibility, hypo- or hyperactivity, and emotional lability are better interpreted as signs of dysfunction than of damage.

Alamiri et al. (2018) differentiate between "developmental soft signs" (DSSs) and "neurological soft signs" (NSSs). DSSs are considered abnormal only if they persist or fail to develop within a developmentally appropriate time period. One DSS you regularly assess is a delay (compared to typical same-age children) in meeting developmental milestones. Several other DSSs we have seen include motor overflow, poor left–right orientation toward self or other, immature pencil grasp, poor fine or gross-motor coordination, motor impersistence, poor gait/posture/stance, tactile extinction during simultaneous stimulation, and speech articulation problems.

Soft signs are considered abnormal (SSAs) if noted at any developmental level and include many of the symptoms presented in Table 3.3. Since neither DSSs nor SSAs are frank pathognomonic signs, they should be seen more as signs of neuropsychological dysfunction than as signs of brain damage; indeed, some consider them nonfocal neurological signs. We must not forget that presenting problems such as developmental delay, learning difficulties, or immaturity, though commonplace, may be among the first signs of a true neurological problem (Baron et al., 2018).

TABLE 3.3. Possible Signs of Pathological Brain Function

Category	Signs and symptoms	Behaviors
Executive	Perseveration	Repetitive speech or other motoric behavior
	Impersistence	Inability to initiate/maintain behavior
	Confabulation	Distorted thoughts/incongruent associations
Motor	Lateralized differences	Motor speed and coordination/strength difficulties
	Gait/balance	Walking/standing difficulties
	Activity level	Hyperactivity or hypoactivity
Somatosensory	Lateralized differences	Touch sensitivity/symbol recognition difficulties
	Somatic complaints	Abnormal somatosensory experiences
Language	Dysarthria	Slurred speech
	Dysfluency	Articulation problems
	Verbal output	Rambling speech or poverty of speech
	Paraphasias	Letter/word substitutions
	Retrieval difficulties	Word-finding problems
Visual–spatial	Visual field problems	Loss of one or more visual quadrants
	Constructional apraxia	Problems with copying designs (both blocks and drawing)
	Spatial disorientation	Location problems/poor spatial judgment
	Right–left disorientation	Self/body part indentification wrong
	Neglect	Self or environment: Left > right side

Common Interpretation Problems and Solutions

Before we leave our discussion of the neuropsychological approach to test interpretation, it is useful to explore where you might go wrong when implementing the CHT model. Despite your best intentions and efforts, you may make a mistake in your administration, scoring, or interpretation of neuropsychological and cognitive tests. Recognizing this possibility, you must be vigilant to reduce the chances of diagnostic error. One of the important characteristics of the CHT model is that the findings are incorporated within a larger problem-solving model, so that built-in corrections for error can take place during the intervention phase, when data-based decisions regarding efficacy are made. We must always remember that our hypotheses are just hypotheses until treatment validity is established. Nonetheless, we must still attempt to increase our self-awareness as clinicians and be on guard for common interpretation problems, as highlighted in In-Depth 3.4.

The CHT Approach to Report Writing

Terminology Issues and Audience

As stated in the Introduction to this text, using neuropsychological principles in practice does not provide you with the training and experience necessary to become a neuropsychologist. Therefore, it is critical that you ultimately discuss a child's *behavior*, not his or her

IN-DEPTH 3.4. Common Interpretation Errors and Possible Solutions

Lezak (1995) suggests that the following are the most common interpretation errors. We provide you with a brief discussion and our recommended solution for each one.

Problem 1: Overgeneralization of results
Discussion: Overgeneralization can happen within a child or across children. Some examiners have a tendency to draw broad-reaching conclusions from limited amounts of data, or to determine that the same conclusion should be drawn if the performance profile for one child is similar to that of another.
Solution: Avoid "cookbook" interpretations and the use of report templates.

Problem 2: Failure to find the problem
Discussion: Clinicians tend to miss problems when they rely on summary data that obscures diagnostically important differences, such as when they conclude from the summary score that there is or is not a problem.
Solution: Explore performance within and across subtests, and focus on neuropsychological processes, not subtest stimulus and response differences.

Problem 3: Confirmation bias
Discussion: In CHT, we develop and test neuropsychological hypotheses—but what if a child performs adequately on a measure we hypothesize the child will perform poorly on? Could this mean that we picked the wrong measure, or that it doesn't measure what we think it does, or that maybe we just have the wrong hypothesis?
Solution: When we have contradictory evidence, we may need to go back to the proverbial "drawing board" to develop a new hypothesis. We can't ignore contrary evidence, but must incorporate it within our diagnostic conclusions.

Problem 4: Misuse of data
Discussion: Sometimes we have a tendency to be overly cautious and underinterpret data, and at other times we draw dramatic conclusions with very little support.
Solution: Use the incremental validity of the objective results, and the outcome of your ecological validity investigation, to temper your interpretations.

Problem 5: Failure to consider base rates
Discussion: Significant performance differences are fairly common, both between and within measures. They are not in themselves diagnostic. Although our research findings suggest that significant differences must be analyzed at the subtest or factor level (Fiorello et al., 2001), it is critical that you determine why the differences occurred, and not automatically conclude that they represent underlying pathology.
Solution: To avoid false positives, you must ensure that the performance differences reflect a consistent problem (in both your testing results and your ecological validity sources) that interferes with academic achievement and/or psychosocial functioning.

---

brain, in your reports and conversations with parents and other professionals. Although we have come a long way in our understanding of brain–behavior relationships, we still know much more about developmental neuro*psychology* than about developmental *neuro*psychology (Rourke, 1994). Given our knowledge of the interrelationships among cortical systems, and the interplay among cortical and subcortical functions (Koziol & Budding, 2010), we must always recognize that children's problems are influenced by complex interactions of neuropsychological, behavioral, and environmental factors.

There are many different approaches and orientations in report writing. Mather and Jaffe (2016) provide many different reports from well-known clinicians in the field that highlight similarities and differences in report writing style. Schneider and colleagues (2018) have written a useful book on report writing that includes many samples as well. Flanagan (2024) has an edited text on clinical report writing that focuses on integration of clinical information. Some clinicians prefer writing narratives about children, with few tests or scores presented in the report body. Others focus more on objective results, and include a great deal of psychometric information, with little interpretation beyond reporting factual results. In our experience the former is more useful and user friendly for consumers, but clinical inference is often high. While "number reports" are easy to write, the focus on nomothetic scores is antithetical to our process approach.

The idea behind these number reports is that you know what the child did, but you don't know why she or he did it.

When you are writing reports and communicating results, use examples of the child's behavior you saw during testing, and comments that others have made, in an attempt to establish consensus among team members and parents, and use the all-important requirement of ecological validity. Engaging others in your feedback keeps them interested and invested in the findings. This type of interactive communication style during feedback helps maintain rapport and shared understanding—critical components of establishing a cooperative and collaborative parent relationship (Postal & Armstrong, 2013). Try to focus on the child's positive attributes, as well as his or her deficits and needs. Too often we focus on what is wrong with a child (Baron, 2000), instead of recognizing that the child can do something, even if it is below expected levels. The power of "positive reframes" in report writing can have a profound impact on how you write reports and communicate results, as noted in Case Study 3.5.

Most trainers suggest that you should avoid using psychological jargon and use standard terminology in reports, presenting the findings in a clear, succinct way, so that both professionals and nonprofessionals can understand them (Miller & Wang, 2019). Although you will hear similar beliefs echoed in almost every trainer's lecture on report writing and follow-up consultation, we believe that accomplishing this is not that simple. Yes, it is a good idea for your reports to be understood, but we think it is difficult to write a brief report that truly conveys the complexity of a child in simple terminology.

Many practitioners think they write reports that others can understand, but in reality,

---

Case Study 3.5. Violet's Feedback Session

When we sat down to discuss the team's results and recommendations for Violet, a child with a moderate intellectual disability who had spent years in special education, no one expected the meeting to be very long. This was because Violet was a pleasant, compliant, and hardworking girl with significant intellectual and adaptive deficits. She always seemed to have a smile on her face, even when she was struggling. During the feedback session, one of us (Hale) primarily focused on what Violet *could* do and what was the next developmental step for her.

  Approximately halfway through the presentation, the mother began to sob uncontrollably. Hale stopped the feedback to ask why and to provide support. Violet's mother reported that she had listened to these team meetings for years, and never once had anyone said anything good about her child. Although her global perception was probably skewed (Hale was sure someone had said something positive about this nice child), it was a strong sentiment nonetheless. The positive approach obviously went a long way toward helping the mother understand her child, and gave her hope for her child's advancing beyond her current level of performance.

most reports are not written so that an average adult can understand them. If the average adult doesn't know what you're talking about, think of what it must be like for a parent with an eighth-grade education or a disability. Either you can write a 20- or 25-page CHT report that conveys the child's performance in simple terms or defines all complex terms (but is too long for anyone to read), or you can write a brief report for professional use. We prefer the latter approach. After you write the brief professional report, we suggest you take the summary paragraph and recommendations, and write a parent letter that describes the results in lay terminology. One author (Hale) has found this to be highly successful and take very little time once the professional report is completed. You are probably gasping, "What, more work, after all this hypothesis-testing stuff?" We'd like you to consider a few things before you dismiss this strategy outright:

- Writing 7-page reports takes a lot less time than writing 17-page reports.
- Once a summary is written, modifying it does not take a lot of additional time. (Try this on your current reports; "step back" from complex presentation. It is easy!)
- We have found parents to be highly appreciative of the letter approach. (They also receive the actual report for further information which you can explain.)
- You will have additional time to write the parent letters because referrals are reduced by MTSS.

In the feedback session, it is important to present results at a level that is understood by both the teacher and parents; you should note that the detailed professional report and parent letter will provide additional information. Resist the temptation to provide a diagnostic label or make predictions about possible outcomes. During this time, it is important to use examples parents and teachers have provided, and to encourage descriptive statements from them in order to foster consensus. Parents may have difficulty accepting the results and may experience a variety of emotions during the feedback session, so you must be attentive to their reactions (Postal & Armstrong, 2013). To foster comprehension for all, use examples or lay descriptions of function if you choose to use a more complex term (e.g., "Lisa has graphomotor reproduction deficits, which means she has a problem with connecting what she sees and what she writes or draws with a pencil").

By providing insight into the child's current functioning, and showing how this is related to the environment, you may be effectively disrupting a system of homeostasis (DeMatteo, 2021)—one that has been in place for some time and can be seen as adaptive, albeit dysfunctional. Also, recall that some parents you are talking with may have the same disorder as their child, which could affect their understanding and acknowledgment of the child's problem. The feedback session not only informs parents and teachers of the results, but it begins the intervention process as well. You may find the concept of therapeutic assessment helpful as you consider the feedback session as the beginning of intervention (see Finn, Fischer, & Handler, 2012).

Distinguishing between Certainty and Inference in Reports

One of the most daunting tasks for psychologists is turning observed behavior and test scores into an accurate interpretation that leads to effective interventions (Baron, 2000). Faced with an overwhelming amount of data, you may find yourself struggling to conceptualize how the results are related to brain functions, and how your interpretation is related to academics and behavior. It is important to recognize that test scores are not necessarily related to brain pathology, and also that a typical score does not necessarily mean there is no dysfunction (Lezak et al., 2012), because children perform tasks in different ways.

Recall the complementary-contribution principle and the gradiental approach to interpretation: Children can use various intact brain structures in an attempt to adapt to different task demands. That is why your observations are so essential to CHT interpretation. As noted previously, you should be extremely cautious when test results are inconsistent, and avoid discussion of cause–effect relationships (Sattler, 2024). It is important to use qualifying terms when you write about behavior (*may, could, appears, seems, apparently, reportedly, likely, probably,* etc.). Unless you have neuroimaging or other neurological evidence (e.g., from a medical or imaging report), you cannot say with certainty that a single brain area is damaged or even dysfunctional. You can, however, use your knowledge of neuropsychological principles and functions to understand which systems are functional or dysfunctional, and how these systems are likely to influence academic achievement and psychosocial functioning. Even when there is direct evidence of brain damage, and it is consistent with your obtained data, you may want to minimize your discussion of the brain, because it only serves to increase the likelihood of "problem admiration." Instead, focusing on strengths and needs saves you from the uncomfortable position of responding to the question "Is this what causes my child's problem?"

Report Sections

This section of the chapter will remind you of some important report-writing considerations within the context of the CHT model. We all get into writing ruts that make our reports less informative and more boilerplate, so that they do not reflect the truly unique nature of a child's functioning. In addition to the following material, Flanagan's (2024) book and Sattler's (2024) chapter on report writing are fine sources for refreshing your skills. In our opinion, the best reports require three things: revision, revision, and more revision. Although reports are objective, concise documents, there is an "art" to writing them well. Well-written reports convey information about children in interesting and compelling ways. Good report writers vary their sentence structure and word choice. They provide evidence to support conclusions, as well as examples that highlight ecological validity. Word choice is particularly important, because it conveys the strength of your diagnostic convictions. The stronger your data, the stronger your interpretive conviction, and so you use stronger terms to convey the information. The ramifications of using the words *could, should,* or *must* in recommendations are considerable. Although we advise use of qualifying terms when writing about behavior, do not qualify your *findings* with words such as *appears, might be,* etc. These terms make it seem like you are unsure of what you found—either it is there in the data or it isn't. Don't temporize.

If your report is written well, it will become an important document that may follow a child for the rest of his or her academic career. Although report styles differ and will vary according to site needs and administrator demands, we recommend following these basic CHT sections, described below: the reason for referral; relevant background information (medical/developmental, family/social, academic/school); classroom observations and functional analysis (as necessary); assessment observations; cognitive/intellectual assessment (sometimes referred to as a screening); cognitive hypothesis testing; academic functioning; psychosocial and behavioral functioning; summary; and recommendations.

Reason for Referral

As noted earlier, the reason for referral should address the concerns presented by those making the referral, but it should also consider other possible referral issues (such as the findings of MTSS interventions and progress monitoring). It is important to be descriptive if possible, and to avoid overly general summative statements such as "behavior problems." The reason for referral is preferably brief—a short paragraph at most.

Relevant Background Information

Background information can provide you with both the foundation for establishing possible disorder causes, and data for establishing ecological validity. Good clinical interviews with the teacher, parent, and child will provide you with opportunities not only to develop hypotheses about a child's functioning, but to obtain concurrent validity evidence as well (Semrud-Clikeman & Ellison, 2009). The clinical interview is not only about gathering information; it helps establish important relationships with those who will eventually carry out the interventions and monitor their efficacy. We prefer to include three paragraphs in the history:

1. *Medical/developmental history.* This section includes the gestation and birth history; any medical illnesses or accidents; vision and hearing status; and acquisition/delay of developmental milestones. If you do not recognize a medical condition, or are told of an accident involving possible head trauma, explore these thoroughly. Keep in mind that parents may not remember correct terminology—one of us (Fiorello) had a parent report that her son had had a stroke, but after a lot of information gathering, she discovered that her son had suffered heat stroke, a very different event. Even if doing so delays your report, you must obtain the necessary permissions and releases of information to fully understand a medical incident. If you do not understand terminology from the report, look it up in a medical dictionary. Don't just repeat what was in the medical report, but instead identify the possible implications for current psychological functioning. Apparently innocuous conditions or accidents can provide you with the evidence you need to understand the child's test performance and behavior in the environment.

2. *Family/social history.* Interpretation always occurs within a context; it varies depending on individuals, their life circumstances, and current environment (Lezak et al., 2012). Many school practitioners think that the home environment is not relevant for school diagnostic or intervention decisions. This is a serious omission. Not only can home circumstances affect current psychological functioning, but they can also provide insight into the contingencies that shape a child's experience. In addition, many conditions discussed in Chapters 5–8 have a genetic basis. Understanding that a child may have a genetically based disorder not only aids in diagnosis; it also helps you tailor your feedback to family members and your recommendations for the child. This subsection can also include a list of the child's preferred free-time activities and social relationships, which can be seen as possible reinforcers and thus can serve to guide intervention efforts. You might also list any psychosocial stressors a child experiences outside the school setting. Always conclude this paragraph with an indication of whether there is an immediate or extended family history of psychological or learning disorders. In addition, I find it helpful to add a sentence or two about what the child likes to do and what he or she is successful at. Moreover, it is also helpful to include, if you have the information, how the family views the child's temperament.

3. *School/occupational history.* From the first educational experiences to the child's current placement, the school history provides the reader with information regarding the child's adaptation to the instructional environment. It should include a summary of both positive and poor academic performance, as well as peer and teacher relationships. Finally, this subsection should include information regarding the MTSS strategies previously attempted and

the outcome of each and any CBM/whole group test results, as well as the child's current functioning in academic areas, and peer and adult relationships.

Classroom Observations and Functional Analysis

As noted earlier, careful observation is critical not only for differential diagnosis, but for intervention development as well. The functional observational data collected will help you generate hypotheses about the child's interactions and coping strategies in the classroom that directly lead to intervention (Sattler, 2024; Steege, Pratt, et al., 2009). At a minimum, classroom observations should include an anecdotal or narrative recording; a systematic observation using event, latency, duration, time sampling, or interval recording (with a comparison peer); and a functional analysis, where the determinants of the target behavior are explored. The comparison peer can be chosen by the teacher, but this could lead to picking someone who is not representative of the class, and so we like to choose a child at random. A comparison with the referred child can be very useful. For example, if acceptable behavior in that classroom is to be out of the seat a great deal, recording out of the seat incidents would be misleading. Contrasting the target child's behavior to another peer can be very helpful in providing a yardstick as to what behaviors are of concern and what are accepted in that particular setting. Depending on the child, this section can be one to three paragraphs long. One author (Hale) typically concludes this section with a table and discussion of the systematic observation (often using momentary time sampling), highlighting both the child and peer results for the reader.

Assessment Observations

Assessment observations should provide a synopsis of the entire evaluation; they are like a behavioral summary of the results, without extensive interpretation. If interpretation is offered during observations, observable and measurable behaviors that support the interpretation must precede or follow it. These observations should include the child's reliability as an informant, personal appearance, rapport with you, approach to both novel and routine tasks, cooperativeness and motivation, reaction to failure, frustration tolerance, need for encouragement, comprehension of instructions, oral expression characteristics, and general level of affect (Semrud-Clikeman & Ellison, 2009). It is important to describe the following in your assessment observation section:

- The child's adaptation to testing and response to rapport building.
- Whether the child understood and complied with assessment demands.
- The child's responses to visual, auditory, and motor demands.
- The child's receptive and expressive language characteristics.
- The child's attention, impulse control, motor activity, and executive behaviors.
- The child's range of affect and frustration tolerance.
- Need for testing accommodations, such as structure and redirection.
- Whether current assessment results are reliable and valid indicators of the child's functioning.

In these descriptions, it is best to focus on the child's behaviors, not on their absence (Sattler, 2024). In addition to reporting testing behaviors, be sure to indicate how the child responded to the testing situation, and whether performance was consistent between and within measures. Different behaviors may emerge during intellectual/cognitive, academic, and psychosocial assessment, and these should be noted. Finish this paragraph with a statement that reflects your thoughts as to whether the results are reliable and valid. Many assessors tend to say that results are valid regardless of testing behavior, but do not be afraid to report that a child's behaviors interfered with maximal performance, at least on some of your measures. If effort or performance validity measures are used to assess compliance, it is useful to report results here.

Cognitive/Intellectual Assessment

We usually begin this section with a nomothetic paragraph, reporting the various global scores and indicating whether they adequately represent the child's level of performance. Consistent with the example presented in Case Study 3.4, you should describe how the child's performance compares to that of the normative population for any global or factor score presented, reporting both confidence intervals and percentiles. At this point, you may wish to decide whether an additional factor score, different from those provided, needs to be calculated. For instance, if successive processing appears to be an issue, you may wish to calculate a Sequential Processing factor score. Although this paragraph focuses on global scores, it is important to conclude with a statement that they are invalid if significant subtest variability is present (Hale et al., 2016). In such a case, global scores represent so many different constructs and are confounded by so many different issues that they are conceptually meaningless (Lezak et al., 2012).

After the nomothetic paragraph, we usually write one or more idiographic paragraphs. The idiographic paragraphs represent the various clusters of subtests, broken down by the factors reported in the manual, or a unique combination of subtests based on how scores cluster together. If the global scores are valid, then you should basically describe the subtests generally, so that the reader gains an understanding of the tasks that were administered. Otherwise, idiographic analysis is demands analysis; it requires careful examination of subtest input, processing, and output demands to determine the individual's pattern of performance. Because you have limited support for your clinical interpretation at this point, it is important to qualify your interpretive statements by adding terms such as "may," "seems," "could," and the like, as we have emphasized earlier. It is important to start the idiographic paragraphs with what the child does well (i.e., strengths) before addressing his or her purported deficits. Recognizing the child's strengths not only highlights the positives for your readers, but it also helps them begin to think about how these strengths might be used for intervention purposes (Sattler, 2024). After discussing the child's possible deficits, conclude the idiographic analysis with possible reasons for the child's performance. These are the hypotheses you have generated via CHT, which are examined in the next section.

Cognitive Hypothesis Testing

Whether your results are consistent or not, CHT requires further examination of purported deficits, because most intellectual subtests are just too factorially complex to permit you to draw definitive conclusions from them (Fiorello et al., 2012; Hale et al., 2016). Support for hypotheses can come from subsequent measures, testing of the limits, observations, interviews, and rating scales. Optimally, the results of all these hypothesis-testing strategies will be presented in this section, together with support for and against your hypotheses. It is important to recognize (in our experience) that not all hypotheses generated are supported with subsequent testing/analysis; do not feel your results must match hypotheses derived from earlier data. The instruments you choose for hypothesis testing may be "neuropsy-chological" or other intellectual/cognitive subtests; the important consideration in choosing additional subtests is that the combination you choose adequately addresses your hypotheses about individual deficits.

We usually include one paragraph for each hypothesis examined, but this varies depending on the areas tapped and the relationship of hypotheses. One final consideration worth exploring has to do with your report presentation. When you are first using CHT, it is best to separate the intellectual (nomothetic and idiographic paragraphs discussed in the previous section) from the hypothesis-testing section. However, as you become more proficient at integrating assessment results, you may wish to report intellectual and hypothesis-testing data in one integrated section.

Academic Functioning

As noted earlier, it is best to administer some standardized academic achievement measures, and possibly curriculum-based measures, even if the educational diagnostician performs this task at your school. Even if another team member administers achievement measures, we recommend a similar measure to further understand how the child's cognitive and neuropsychological interpretation is related to academic performance (Flanagan et al., 2014). At a minimum, try to assess word recognition/decoding, reading comprehension, math word problems, math computation, spelling, and written language. As with the use of neuropsychological tests for hypothesis testing, you may wish to use an additional achievement measure to further your impressions, such as a pseudoword-reading subtest for a child with word recognition problems. In this section, you should discuss the similarities and differences between teacher- and/or parent-reported academic achievement and your findings. Try to ascertain the relationship between cognitive/neuropsychological and academic results, because if the child has a disability in the "basic psychological processes" this too should seem apparent in academic test results. The relationship between neuropsychological functioning and academic performance is further addressed in Chapters 5–7.

Psychosocial and Behavioral Functioning

Several childhood disorders once thought to be primarily the results of environmental determinants are now being linked directly to biological causes in the superior–inferior axis. Although these associations are becoming clear, the relationship between psychiatric disturbance and neuropsychological deficit is difficult to disentangle (Reddy et al., 2013), and examining it will require clinical vigilance on your part. For each child who presents with psychosocial or behavioral issues, we believe that you should entertain a possible genetic and neurobiological etiology for the child's problems. Even if the history, observations, and neuropsychological patterns of performance are not reflective of a biologically based psychopathology, a child's cognitive patterns may reflect a processing or an expression preference during social discourse, and this propensity could lead to social or behavioral problems. It can also reveal that the child uses certain cognitive strengths to compensate for academic or psychosocial deficits. As in Bandura's (1978) model of reciprocal determinism, the relationships among cognition, behavior, and environment are interrelated and inseparable. In this section, it is important to address both signs of internalizing and externalizing disorders, as many people consider only the latter in determining whether a child has a psychosocial problem. This section should show a clear relationship between the data collected and suspected psychopathology, as you weave a "confluence of indicators" that lead the reader to the particular emotional and/or behavior problem.

Summary and Recommendations

The report summary conveys all the pertinent information embodied in the report, synthesizing the major aspects of the child's behavior in relation to the environment. Some practitioners have questioned the utility of including a summary in psychological reports, because some readers may skip over pertinent report sections and instead read the final summary. However, busy consumers such as medical doctors need an integrative summary that captures the key findings of the evaluation. A summary should include at least one sentence covering each of the areas presented above, and several sentences related to the data. In school settings, the report summary should not include diagnostic and/or placement recommendations, but you can discuss what a child needs. Your job is not to fix the problem or label the child, but rather to offer flexibility in eligibility, placement, and intervention decisions (Sattler, 2024). Because the goal of clinical assessment is to optimize a child's development in all domains, we believe that recommendations should address all aspects of the child's life. Although report recommendations should be specific enough to be useful, they should not be mandates regarding intervention, since generating these is a team responsibility.

We prefer to offer multiple possible interventions to help parents and teachers begin the intervention-brainstorming phase of problem solving, which is addressed further in the next chapter. Some have suggested that compensatory strategies are more effective than remediation approaches, but this issue is not so straightforward. We see the compensation–remediation relationship to be directly related to age and severity of condition. For older children or those with severe deficits, a compensatory strategy should predominate, and remediation should be less prominent. However, for younger children, or those with less severe conditions, remediation should be the focus of intervention efforts. However, keep in mind our understanding of brain development, teaching to brain strengths and ignoring weaknesses only leads to more and more disparate skills, which could lead to lifelong disability (Hale et al., 2016). Whereas both strength-based compensation and/or remediation of neuropsychological weaknesses may be individualized for each child, it is important to recognize that interventions must occur within the context of academic instruction, not in isolation. Recommendations should include both instructional and behavioral components tailored to each child's unique needs, as well as classroom accommodations to help the child maintain performance in less impaired areas, as seen in Figure 3.3.

Don't think that you must know everything about intervention, or that every intervention you recommend must be implemented and effective. Traditional psychometric assessments do not provide the necessary information to facilitate intervention (Sattler, 2024), and neuropsychologists typically don't have much training in intervention; this makes your instructional and behavioral knowledge especially useful during intervention planning, implementation, and evaluation. Since you have determined the child's unique characteristics and documented these in the report summary, you now have overcome one of the greatest difficulties in linking assessment to intervention: accurate identification of the child's unique characteristics to maximize learning and/or behavioral success. Recognizing the child's strengths and needs from a neuropsychological perspective is the first important step in developing individualized interventions. Recommendations are only a first brainstorm of possible strategies that could help the child. Throughout the remainder of this book, we examine the linkages among assessment findings, recommendations for intervention, and ways to help children succeed in various academic and behavioral areas.

In the next chapter, we turn our attention to further skill development in neuropsychological assessment and intervention using the CHT approach.

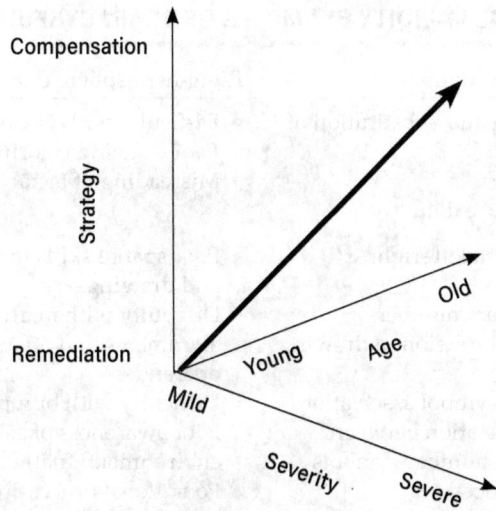

FIGURE 3.3. Tailoring teaching strategies for individual children.

APPENDIX 3.1. ECOLOGICAL VALIDITY EXAMPLES OF BRAIN DYSFUNCTION

Brain area	Left-hemisphere damage	Right-hemisphere damage
Occipital lobe	• Slow reading and substitution of letters • Poor spelling • Limited picture details	• Difficulty with visual imagery • Poor drawing/coloring • Misreading of facial expressions
Dorsal stream	• Difficulty with left–right orientation • Reverses letters/numbers • Directional confusion in drawings and writing • Poor sound–symbol association • Limited association between quantity and number symbols • Poor local processing	• Poor spatial skills in letters, words, and drawings • Difficulty with math column alignments and attention to operands • Difficulty with bumping into objects Poor awareness of self and the environment: Inattention • Poor global processing
Ventral stream	• Difficulty with recognizing and naming known objects • Poor recognition of familiar faces • Difficulty with sight-word learning and efficient reading (no automaticity) • Poor fine processing	• Difficulty with learning new objects and faces • Poor perception of facial affect • Difficulty with sight-word learning—tendency to decode everything • Poor coarse processing
Lateral/medial temporal lobe	• Difficulty with long-term memory for objects, words, and general knowledge • Poor memory for known or famous faces • Possible dislike of social studies and preference for science • Preference for abstract and flexible tasks that require creativity • Desire to explore complexities of the world, but difficulties in making decisions	• Difficulty understanding multiple perspectives and meanings of objects, words, and general knowledge • Difficulty with recognizing facial affect • Preference for routinized and specific tasks • Possible preference for reading, social studies, and language arts (especially in early grades) • Preference to avoid complexities of world for safe, predictable, and conventional behaviors
Superior temporal lobe	• Poor phonemic awareness and auditory processing • Possible "mishearing" of comments or directions • Frequent requests for repetition or clarification • Possible repetition of words that sound similar	• Poor prosody awareness and limited understanding of rate and pitch of language • Possible "mishearing" of emotional valence of words (e.g., hearing anger when speaker excited) • Possible difficulty modulating own prosody
Anterior parietal lobe	• Difficulty in grasping objects with right hand • Writing that is too soft or too dark Complaints that hand hurts when writing • Poor hand coordination in sports	• Difficulty in grasping objects with left hand • Poor bilateral motor coordination • Difficulty in catching a ball with a baseball mitt

(continued)

APPENDIX 3.1. (*continued*)

Occipital–temporal–parietal "crossroads"/ Wernicke's area	• Reliance on sight-word approach and learning math facts to automaticity because of poor sound–symbol association • Difficulty with explicit language, reading, and math comprehension • Focus on general status of relationship to understand interaction dynamics • Greater likelihood of understanding humor, metaphor, and indirect messages	• Possible use of phonemic approach to decode all words, but poor comprehension • Difficulty with implicit language, reading, and math comprehension • Focus on facts and details to understand interactions • Greater likelihood of understanding concrete, explicit, and direct messages
Posterior frontal lobe	• Difficulty with right-handed motor functions • Likelihood of ideomotor or constructional apraxia • Difficulty with drawing and writing • Difficulty with dressing or carrying out tasks requiring multiple motor behaviors in sequence • Possible ambidexterity or left-handedness • Difficulty in performing learned motor programs • Possible poor articulation	• Difficulty with left-handed motor functions • Poor learning of motor scripts • Limited motor reaction to environmental stimuli • Difficulty with bimanual motor activities • Possible poor prosody
Medial frontal lobe/ Broca's area	• Limited verbal fluency • Low mean length of utterance • Semantic and phonemic paraphasias • Halting speech and word-finding problems • Poor syntax in speech and writing	• Fluent expression and high mean length of utterance • Poor verbal prosody, mechanistic manner of speech • Semantic paraphasias due to inflexible word choice • Poor humor and overly concrete oral and written expression
Dorsolateral prefrontal cortex	• Poor encoding of new information • Preference for flexible schedules and requirements • Executive dysfunction likely, including problems with planning, organizing, sequencing, implementing, and monitoring behavior • Poor routinization of learned behavior • Poor concordant/convergent thought	• Poor retrieval of existing information • Preference for routines and detailed requirements • Executive dysfunction more likely, including problems with strategizing, evaluating, shifting, and changing behavior • Poor novel problem solving • Limited discordant/divergent thought • ADHD, inattentive type
Orbital prefrontal cortex	• Pseudodepression: Avoidance and inhibition • Negative affect • Excessive emotional regulation	• Pseudopsychopathy: Approach and impulsivity • Indifferent affect • Lack of emotional regulation

APPENDIX 3.2. BLANK BRAIN: SUPERIOR VIEW

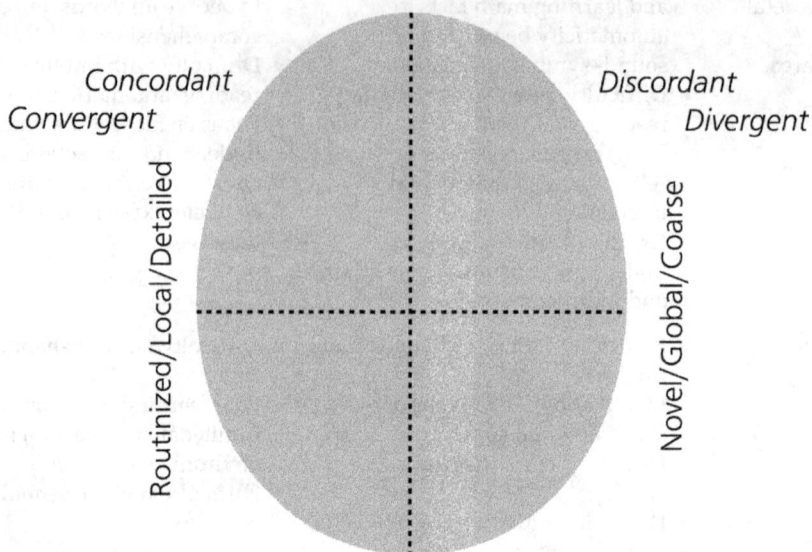

Concordant
Convergent

Discordant
Divergent

Routinized/Local/Detailed

Novel/Global/Coarse

APPENDIX 3.3. BLANK BRAIN: LATERAL VIEW

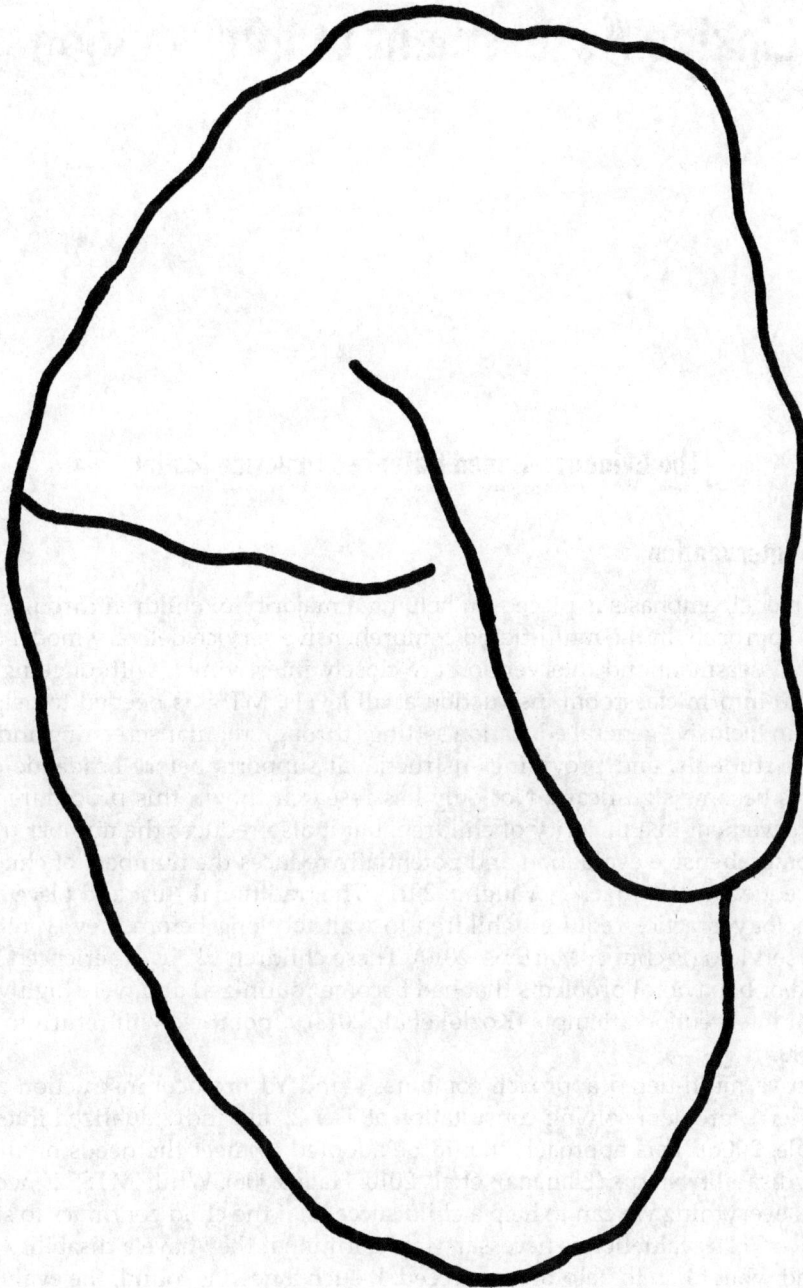

Chapter 4

Linking Assessment to Intervention

The Evidence-Based Balanced Practice Model

Response to Intervention

In our CHT model, emphasis is placed on helping a majority of children through an established MTSS approach. In the multi-tiered comprehensive service delivery model discussed in Chapter 1, assessment and intervention are closely intertwined, with ongoing data collection used to inform classroom instruction at all levels. MTSS is needed to help all children achieve in inclusive general education settings through regular screening and progress monitoring of students, and providing instructional supports before academic or behavioral problems become significant. Not only has research shown this procedure improves academic achievement in a majority of children, but it also reduces the number of referrals for formal comprehensive evaluation and potentially reduces the numbers of children who need special education (Wanzek & Vaughn, 2011). The traditional "test and place" model of school psychology practice required children to wait too long before they were provided with needed services (Erchul & Martens, 2010). These children likely experienced increased academic and/or behavioral problems that had become routinized and were highly resistant to subsequent intervention attempts (Koziol et al., 2013), a point we will return to in subsequent chapters.

An effective multi-tiered approach combines standard protocol instruction and interventions at Tier 1, problem-solving consultation at Tier 2, and individualized interventions in Tier 3 (Hale, 2006). This approach should be adopted to meet the needs of all children regardless of disability status (Flanagan et al., 2010; Hale, 2006). While MTSS is necessary to ensure we do everything we can to help a child succeed, if the child continues to struggle, a comprehensive CHT evaluation is necessary to determine if they have a disability and if so, what type and what to do to help them succeed. If such a need is found, the evaluation can assist in designing targeted interventions, consistent with legislative and legal mandates in the United States (Hale, Alfonso, et al., 2010; Wright et al., 2013). Keep in mind that even if a child is identified as having a disability and requiring an IEP at Tier 3, it doesn't necessarily mean placement outside of the general education classroom. Many children experience academic success in inclusive classrooms with IEPs and instructional accommodations.

In our multiyear study in a lower-SES community of diverse elementary children, we saw steady improvements in reading and math achievement using this combined RTI/CHT approach (Hale, Betts et al., 2010). Interestingly, every child who did not respond to Tier 1 and Tier 2, and was referred for CHT evaluation, was determined to have a disability (100% hit rate). However, only 80% of those who were evaluated in the non-RTI school were determined to have a disability resulting in the completion of more evaluations than in the RTI/CHT schools. So RTI accurately determined who needed a CHT evaluation and who had a disability. In the non-RTI school, about 20% of those children referred did not have a disability following a standard psychological evaluation, and the school psychologists completed approximately 15% more evaluations that year, requiring a lot of extra time evaluating children who didn't need time-consuming and expensive evaluations.

Before we leave these promising results, there is one last point about this study worth your consideration (Hale, Betts, et al., 2010). Some have argued that those students who are nonresponders should be considered to have a specific learning disability (SLD), largely on the basis of achievement data and lack of response to intervention (Fletcher et al., 2004). In contrast, this evidence-based balanced practice model (Hale, 2006) showed that the children should be referred for a comprehensive CHT evaluation with assessment in all areas of suspected disability as required by IDEA (2004) and U.S. Supreme Court precedent (Wright et al., 2013). Throughout this multiyear study, we found that comprehensive CHT evaluations for these struggling students showed that only some of them had SLD. Instead, many had *other* neurodevelopmental disorders requiring special education (e.g., ADHD, depression, bipolar, Tourette syndrome, and speech and language disorders). The CHT evaluation showed us what types of processing deficits these children had, and how these interfered with one or more areas of learning. With the needs for the child with a disability identified, Tier 3 special education services could be provided to develop individualized IEPs, targeted interventions, and instructional modifications/accommodations, with most children served in inclusive classrooms (Wright et al., 2013). The fact that nonresponse to intervention can suggest disability, but not the type of disability or subsequent intervention efforts necessary to help a child succeed, is but one of the reasons why the National Joint Committee on Learning Disabilities (NJCLD) has taken a position against using RTI as the sole means for identifying SLD (e.g., Gartland & Strosnider, 2020).

RTI has many benefits for helping children who struggle with learning, but nonresponse to an intervention should not automatically result in a SLD classification decision (Reynolds & Shaywitz, 2009; Gartland & Strosnider, 2020). Instead, a comprehensive evaluation guided by comprehensive cognitive and neuropsychological assessment is needed to determine *why* they didn't respond and *what* to do next to help them (Reynolds & Fletcher-Janzen, 2009). This combination of standard protocol RTI and problem-solving protocol RTI, followed by comprehensive CHT evaluations for nonresponders, uses best practices to provide all children with the best of both worlds (Hale, Wycoff, et al., 2010).

CHT in Assessment and Intervention

With their expertise in data-based decision making, school psychologists will be viewed as indispensable professionals who support the education of all children in schools. Although this is an important role and function of school psychologists, there are always children who do not respond to the interventions and supports in a MTSS model; these children need something *different* than more intensive instruction (Fiorello et al., 2012; Hale, Wycoff, et al., 2010). Clearly, more intensive instruction and arbitrary decisions regarding tier changes and interventions does not work, and can even be detrimental to student achievement, according to a large-scale, multistate, government funded study of over 20,000 students (Balu et al.,

2015). In our comprehensive model, a child who does not benefit from these initial interventions is referred for a formal CHT evaluation. The CHT evaluation is needed prior to Tier 3 special education service delivery to pinpoint areas of strength and weakness that can contribute to developing appropriate interventions, consistent with IDEA (Etscheidt & Curran, 2010) requirements and U.S. Supreme Court precedent (Wright et al., 2013). Figure 4.1 shows the cyclical nature of the CHT evaluation process, which you will note is a scientific method approach to assessment and intervention. In practicing it, you will be operating under the scientist–practitioner model of practice—a model we authors endorse without reservation.

In CHT, the referral question, history, and results of previous interventions are examined to develop a *theory* of the problem. If cognitive functioning is related to the academic or behavioral deficit areas in question, the intelligence/cognitive test is used as one of the first-level assessment tools. Using demands analysis, described later, the findings are interpreted to determine possible cognitive strengths and weaknesses. This process is where many psychologists stop. Because of time demands, psychologists in schools typically write their reports and present their findings in a team meeting; they have little contact with the child, parents, or teacher thereafter (unless individual counseling or behavior therapy is offered). *In CHT, however, we see the intelligence/cognitive test as merely a screening tool of psychological processes, not a final assessment of these skills.* Best practices and our CHT model go beyond this screening level assessment to choose additional measures to confirm or refute the intellectual test data. The results are examined in light of the MTSS data, record review, history, systematic observations, behavior ratings, and parent and teacher interviews to gain a good understanding of the child.

Completing the initial assessment is where the CHT process *begins*, not ends. Interventions are subsequently developed using the understanding of the child and the environment during collaborative consultative follow-up meetings with teachers, parents, and/or children. If a child is identified with a disability, these interventions may become part of a child's IEP, or if not, they can help inform Tier 2 problem-solving interventions, with both Tier 2 and Tier 3 service delivery preferably happening in inclusive general education classrooms. Even if a child has an IEP, we still do problem-solving consultation in Tier 3. The ideas of problem identification, problem analysis, intervention development/implementation, and intervention evaluation permeate CHT Tier 3 service delivery, but we recognize the value of cognitive and neuropsychological data in the problem analysis part. From this perspective, all data are relevant in data-based decision making.

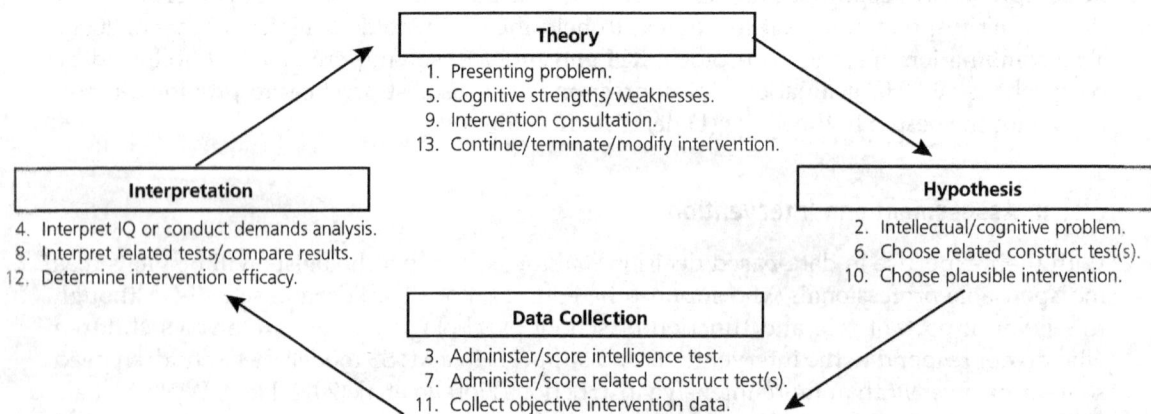

FIGURE 4.1. The CHT model.

Possible intervention strategies are brainstormed in consultation with the teacher; design, resources, and feasibility are considered; and an intervention plan likely to succeed is developed. The systematic intervention is then undertaken and evaluated to determine intervention efficacy. If the Tier 3 progress monitoring data suggest the intervention is not effective, the intervention is revised or recycled until beneficial results are obtained. We recommend using known evidence-based academic and behavioral interventions and single-subject methodology. We also use information about cognitive and neuropsychological functioning in developing and individualizing our evidence-based interventions. Understanding the child's psychological processing strengths and weaknesses in relation to his or her academic and behavioral needs allows us to truly differentiate instruction to ensure children have optimal educational outcomes (Hale et al., 2018).

Conducting Demands Analysis in CHT

Demands analysis is a core component of the CHT model. It is the key to both accurate identification of childhood disorders and to the development of interventions sensitive to individual needs. The demands analysis process that we present here is derived from two assessment traditions and modern neuroscience perspectives on brain functioning. The first tradition is the "intelligent testing" approach, which examines global, factor, and subtest scores based on clinical, psychometric, and quantitative research (Flanagan et al., 2013; Sattler, 2020). When formulating your clinical demands analysis, you must be careful to examine all relevant technical and cross-battery subtest information. As stated earlier, one cannot deny the value of a CHC-based interpretive approach, especially when there is a convergence between CHC and modern understanding of brain functions (Fiorello et al., 2008). Heavily influenced by the Lurian (1973b) approach to neuropsychological assessment, the second tradition consists of the developmental and process-oriented neuropsychological assessment approaches (e.g., Gable et al., 2015; Bernstein, 2000; Lezak, 1995; Libon et al., 2013; Poreh, 2012; Radel et al., 2017; Schneider et al., 2013). Although demands analysis may seem similar to other versions of profile analysis (Kaufman et al., 2016), the major difference is the emphasis on the neuropsychological and cognitive processes necessary for task completion.

As we noted earlier, *you will not see reference to brain structures or systems* in our evaluation reports (unless medical evidence is present in the history). We do use our *knowledge of brain structure and function help guide us in the interpretive process*. We have noted previously that the input and output demands are straightforward; they are the observable and measurable test stimuli and behavioral responses. However, research is clearly demonstrating that the underlying neuropsychological *processing demands* are essential for understanding and helping many children with their learning and behavior problems (Fiorello et al., 2012; Hale, Fiorello, et al., 2010). In other words, the key to case conceptualization, for both identification and intervention purposes, is understanding psychological processes, not input or output. This is in some ways a bane, because we can see input and output, but not processes. Only careful inferences drawn from idiographic interpretation of cognitive and neuropsychological measures can tell us about these processes in individual children, so it is both costly and time consuming. It is also a blessing because it is the clinician's understanding of psychological processes that can be critical for understanding and helping children. This dichotomy is why MTSS is essential practice, because it ensures that any child referred for a CHT evaluation is likely to have a brain-related disability that continues to interfere with academic and/ or behavioral functioning despite our best attempts at early intervention. Recall from the very beginning of the book—we have been arguing that you need to *intervene to assess* (and do both well).

For many children and most tests and subtests, a brief demands analysis should be sufficient to examine and test hypotheses about brain–behavior relationships. We have provided you with two forms (Appendix 4.1 and Appendix 4.2) to guide you in interpretative efforts. The form in Appendix 4.2 may even be more helpful as you become more accustomed to demands analysis, because this allows you to add constructs as necessary to reflect the neuropsychological processes underlying a particular subtest or if a child responds in an idiosyncratic manner.

To conduct the demands analysis, identify tests/subtests that represent the child's strengths and weaknesses. Enter them in the appropriate spaces in Appendix 4.2, and for each measure conduct a task analysis of the *input, processing,* and *output* demands. *Input* refers to the stimulus materials as well as the directions, demonstrations, and teaching items. Think about what modality or modalities are needed for the input—for example, whether there are pictures or verbal directions, whether the content is meaningful or abstract, and what other aspects of the content are relevant (e.g., level of English language used or amount of cultural knowledge required). *Processing* refers to the actual neuropsychological processing demands of the task, as discussed in Chapters 2 and 3. Think about the primary requirement of the task, but also the secondary requirements, such as the attention, executive, and working memory demands (often suggested by the test's developers and the CHC cross-battery approach; Flanagan et al., 2013). *Output* refers to the modalities and skills required for responding to the task. Is the output a complex verbal response, a simple pointing response, or a complex motoric response? If oral expression is needed, is syntax important, and is word choice an issue? How is the child's response pattern reflective of the main process demands of the tasks, and how are other processes influencing within- and between-task performances? These are some of the questions you must answer in demands analysis. Always keep in mind sociocultural differences and expectations during demands analysis, since different responses could reflect these characteristics (e.g., use of nonliteral language by indigenous populations, lower emphasis on processing speed in Latino populations).

The form we provide in Appendix 4.1 is merely a tool for you to begin thinking about underlying psychological processes on your cognitive, neuropsychological, *and* achievement tests. Yes, the neuropsychological process approach not only helps you interpret cognitive and neuropsychological tests, *but also achievement tests,* because the same brain processes both! We have included blanks in the last column for you to provide additional subtest input, processing, and output demands. Once you have listed the input, processing, and output demands for all of the child's strengths and weaknesses, it is important to look for commonalities and contradictions among the data using the CHT methodology, thereby avoiding confirmation bias as a result.

As you become familiar with processing demands and have experience in interpreting the processing differences a child demonstrates, you need not always refer to demands analyses sheets. When you are beginning the process, you may want to do it for many measures that are factorially complex (i.e., have a lot of demands at the same time). After completing demands analysis for the measures, you attempt to identify the child's patterns of performance within and between measures and attempt to verify processing strengths and weaknesses using multiple data sources. If you find that one particular processing demand is required on all low-score tests, and it is not needed for the high-score tasks, you would hypothesize that this demand is a weakness for the child. Information from your observations of the child during testing, as well as information provided by the teacher and possibly parents, should also be consistent with any definitive hypothesis to ensure concurrent and ecological validity. The weakness may be a cognitive processing weakness, but it may also be a sensory or motor weakness, a result of emotional interference, or a consequence of limited exposure or background. Enter this information on the worksheet provided in Appendix 4.3.

There is an important issue to consider before we move on. The key to this demands analysis process is generating and evaluating hypotheses. However, care is needed. You have to avoid confirmation bias in test interpretation when you look for support for your hypotheses. When teaching demands analysis, we ask students to generate hypotheses and when just learning the approach they often come up with a single probable hypothesis, because our cognitive tendency is to go to the left hemisphere to come up with the "right" answer. However, to encourage discordant/divergent thought, we say "Even if that explanation seems likely, what else could it be?" We also ask students to always include a null hypothesis, forcing them to consider that the child might not have a processing deficit or disability. This approach ensures we keep the diagnostic door open until we have convincing evidence that our understanding of the child is accurate.

Although the forms in the appendices and several interpretive texts (Flanagan, 2013; Kamphaus & Campbell, 2006; Kaufman et al., 2016; Sattler, 2020) can be helpful in conducting demands analysis, you should not be lulled into a "cookbook" approach when interpreting subtest data—a tendency that often results in erroneous interpretation. You can't have template reports where you describe a factor or subtest processes, and change the wording to reflect good, average, or poor performance on that construct. Recall that the children can use different brain areas and psychological processes to perform any given task, so you can't just say the task measures "construct A" and then change the level of performance descriptor for each child. To guard against this and to foster accurate interpretation, we have provided a checklist in Appendix 4.4. This checklist serves primarily as an aid in clinical judgment, but it could also be used as an informant rating scale.

Let's walk through a demands analysis of the WISC-V Block Design subtest to see what the process looks like. First, consider the input. The task has oral directions and is modeled for children and corrected for those who have difficulty on the first item. The stimulus materials (booklet with two-dimensional visual model and two-color three-dimensional blocks) are abstract, colored shapes, so that verbal encoding is difficult (but not impossible for those compensating for visual–spatial processing weaknesses). The task will be novel for most children (although perhaps not on re-evaluation or as the testing progresses). The processing demands are quite complex and involve both hemispheres and executive/frontal demands. Primarily, Block Design is a right-hemisphere task, since it is visual–spatial (i.e., involves the dorsal stream), is novel, and does not depend on crystallized prior knowledge. There is some bilateral processing, however, because of the bimanual sensory and motor coordination, as well as the part (directional orientation of the blocks—left parietal) and whole (gestalt/spatial—right parietal) coordination (Hain & Hale, 2010; Poreh, 2012; Swanson et al., 2013). Some children may walk themselves through this task using verbal mediation—this behavior should be noted because it might indicate that the visual–spatial skills are not as well developed as would be expected.

There are heavy frontal demands, due to the executive and motor requirements of the task. The frontal demands include planning and organization, analysis and synthesis, self-monitoring and evaluation of the response, inhibition of impulsive responding, and fine-motor and bimanual coordination. This is particularly true if the child uses a trial-and-error match-to-sample approach to the task (i.e., comparing/contrasting model to blocks, quickly flipping them repeatedly until the correct "design" is achieved). Note particularly if the child has more difficulty after the lines are removed from the stimulus book, as this may suggest difficulty with configuration or novelty. Considering the output, Block Design requires fine-motor and bilateral motor coordination, so look for problems crossing the midline or a tendency to use just one hand, or switch hands and not use them together, which suggests possible corpus callosum problems, which are surprisingly common in some neurodevelopmental disorders for which white matter development is a problem. Processing speed can also impact performance on Block Design. Look for slow performance due to overall low tone or lethargy, perfectionism, or inattention/disorganization. Also, if the child is close to completion, let the child complete the design even if time runs out. While you cannot score the design as correct, it tells you that the child's visual–spatial skills are not the problem—timing is.

Although conducting demands analysis may be helpful in understanding patterns of performance, remember that multifactorial tasks can be solved in more than one way, so that the demands analysis may differ from child to child. For instance, a child who uses good executive and psychomotor skills to compensate for a right posterior spatial problem may still do well on Block Design. It is an error if you conclude that the child had adequate visual–spatial–holistic processing skills based solely on this measure. We practitioners have often gone wrong in the past by concluding that the same subtest measures the same thing for all children. For instance, concluding that poor WISC-V Information subtest performance is due to a limited "fund of information" may not be correct if a child has retrieval problems or difficulty due to limited knowledge in just one area, such as science. Concluding that a child has adequate attention, working memory, and executive function because he or she has an average WISC-V Digit Span scaled score, but a Digits Forward score of 10 and a Digits Backward score of 2, would clearly be inappropriate (Hale et al., 2002). In addition, there can be developmental aspects of test items that influence interpretation as well; if a young child scores well on Similarities, but most items are scored 1 point, it may suggest the child has good lexical–semantic knowledge and concordant–convergent thought, but you wouldn't want to say she has good abstract verbal concept formation; whereas another child could get the same score but responds mostly with 2-point responses but the ceiling is achieved earlier. These examples bring us to a potentially disconcerting but a very real conclusion about psychological test interpretation: *the same score does not always mean the same thing for all children, even of the same age.*

Table 4.1 provides you with some sample demands analyses on a few additional subtests, so you can see how the process works. As you become more familiar with using demands analysis to task-analyze subtests, you will eventually become quite comfortable with determining the demands on any subtest. As you gain confidence, and knowledge of brain–behavior relationships, you will be surprised how easy it is to understand the psychological processes required on any task or behavior.

In our graduate child neuropsychology assessment class, we have a final exam item that requires students to do a "mystery test" demands analysis on a test they have not been exposed to in class. Though students find the thought of this daunting, and the task challenging, they typically find that they can identify the key input, processing, and output demands on the test, and this gives them incredible confidence in their budding idiographic interpretive skills. Try this activity yourself. Generalizing these skills to other measures will allow you to expand your use of demands analysis to just about any instrument you are trained to administer. It can also be generalized to almost any behavior. In another graduate school task, students pick an everyday activity (e.g., making coffee, brushing their teeth, greeting a friend) and determine the brain structures and processes involved in each of the steps. Again, this is a novel task students find daunting, but working through it helps them become more comfortable in observing overt behavior and thinking about the neuropsychological processes involved in completing it.

We now turn to a discussion of neuropsychological tests for use in the CHT model. Although many of these tests may be new to you, the demands analyses you perform on cognitive and intellectual measures apply to neuropsychological measures as well. Do not let yourself be overly concerned that these measures are "neuropsychological"; many of them are easier to administer and score than the measures you generally use. For instance, the D-KEFS Color–Word Interference Test requires approximately 5 minutes to administer, and it has brief, simple instructions. Even though it is easy to administer, this test is highly sensitive

TABLE 4.1. Sample Demands Analysis of Selected Subtests

WISC-V Block Design

Input
- Models and abstract visual pictures
- Oral directions—moderate English-language knowledge
- Demonstration/modeling
- Low cultural knowledge and emotional content

Processing
- Visual processing (spatial relations, visualization)
- Perception of part–whole relationships
- Discordant/divergent processing (analysis)
- Constructional praxis
- Bimanual coordination/corpus callosum
- Concordant/convergent processing (synthesis)
- Attention and executive demands: Moderate
- Planning and strategy use
- Inhibition of impulsive/wrong responding
- Novel problem solving: Low to moderate

Output
- Fine-motor response, arrangement of manipulatives
- Timed score with speed bonus; process score without time bonus
- Visual–motor integration

SB-5 Picture Absurdities (Levels 4, 5, and 6—Nonverbal Knowledge)

Input
- Large color pictures
- Oral directions
- Sample item
- High cultural and English-language knowledge

Processing
- Visual scanning
- Perception of objects (ventral stream)
- Crystallized ability for prior knowledge (left temporal)
- Discordant/divergent processing (analysis)
- Attention and executive demands: Low to moderate
- Persistence/inhibition of impulsive responding
- Novel problem solving/reasoning

Output
- Brief oral or pointing response
- One right answer (convergent responding)

WJ-V Visual–Auditory Learning

Input
- Brief oral directions, teaching items, feedback
- Semiabstract figures/symbols
- Moderate cultural and English-language knowledge

Processing
- Visual perception of figures/symbols (dorsal and ventral streams)
- Sound–word/symbol–rebus association

(continued)

TABLE 4.1. (*continued*)

- Working memory/learning
- Encoding and retrieval of associative/semantic memory
- Benefiting from feedback
- Inhibition of impulsive/wrong responding
- Syntax knowledge: Helpful
- Attention and executive demands: Moderate to high
- Memory: primary; novel problem solving: secondary

Output
- Brief oral response
- Oral formulation/retrieval

KABC-II NU Pattern Reasoning

Input
- Brief oral directions; sample and teaching items
- Abstract/nonmeaningful figures
- Low cultural knowledge and English-language knowledge

Processing
- Visual scanning and discrimination
- Color processing
- Visual–spatial processing (dorsal stream)
- Part–whole relationships
- Discordant/divergent processing (perceptual analysis)
- Novel problem-solving and inductive reasoning/fluid abilities
- Attention and executive demands: Moderate
- Inhibition of impulsive/wrong responding

Output
- Pointing response
- Multiple-choice format (can solve by elimination/match to sample)

to executive functions and to frontal–subcortical circuit dysfunction (particularly cingulate function), and therefore is an excellent supplement to test hypotheses generated by your initial battery. Of course, you must always remember that no one test can diagnose a specific difficulty or disability.

Assessment Tools for CHT

Fixed versus Flexible Batteries in Hypothesis Testing

One of the biggest debates in neuropsychological assessment is whether to use a fixed test battery (a standard set of tests) or a flexible battery (a set of tests chosen for an individual child) (Decker et al., 2012; Lezak et al., 2012; Riccio & Reynolds, 2013). Fixed batteries predominated early in the field's history, but flexible batteries have become increasingly popular, especially since they tend to be more time and cost effective. Fixed batteries tend to lead to more testing than is needed to address unique child characteristics. One of our biggest complaints about traditional neuropsychological assessment is that children are tested all day long on a battery of tests that may not be needed for interpretation. For instance, if explicit language skills are in the superior range on the intellectual/cognitive task, is it worthwhile to give a measure of verbal learning and memory? In addition, a fixed battery gives examiners the impression that the battery assesses all relevant neuropsychological domains, even though that is not necessarily true (Lezak et al., 2012).

We prefer a flexible-battery approach in the CHT model, because different measures and techniques can be used to address hypotheses developed after initial data gathering and intellectual/cognitive screening tool assessment. You may need one or more measures that look at a particular domain in depth. For instance, if you have a child who has handwriting problems you don't just give your intelligence test and say the child has "graphomotor" or "visual–motor integration" problems; that doesn't tell us what we need to do to help the child and there is actually no direct measure of graphomotor skills on that test! Instead, if you're interested in an apparent visual, somatosensory, motor, or integration deficit, you need to pick and choose measures that tap each of these four possible causes to get a better understanding of the problem and the direction to take for intervention. Be aware of the problem of confirmation bias, however. If you only choose tests to confirm a hypothesis, you are likely to find evidence to support it. Choose tests to disconfirm your hypotheses as well. For instance, when looking at the graphomotor problem you may be thinking about cortical problems, and sure enough you find it is largely a motor problem, but you have to think of multiple causes of motor problems, including subcortical structures such as the basal ganglia and cerebellum (Koziol & Budding, 2009). You should also ensure that you are at least screening all the major functioning areas so as not to overlook something. To further our visual–spatial example, a child may be able to copy a figure when there is a space provided for that copy (i.e., the Developmental Test of Visual–Motor-Integration), but may experience significant problems with the Rey–Osterrieth or Bender–Gestalt tests which are less structured and require the child to organize the information. These measures that are "purported"' to test the same skill, are different, and allow you to think about other aspects of the task that may be interfering with the child's performance (visual organization, attention to detail, etc.).

We are not suggesting that a fixed-battery approach should be completely avoided. Some neuropsychologists prefer a standard set of tests or published test battery, because all the children tested are administered the same tests in the same order, which increases the validity of interpretation in many practitioner's eyes, especially in many forensic settings (Kaufmann et al., 2013; Russell et al., 2005). Fixed batteries can also serve both research and practice needs. Obviously, many children who receive the same measures would be needed for a group-design research project. Missing data are the nemesis for most research projects, because many cases need to be eliminated if they are missing just one variable in a multivariate statistical analysis. Given that fixed batteries have led to many research findings, they are often recognized for strong reliability and validity, and for the use of normative data (Witsken et al., 2008). For clinicians, fixed-battery approaches not only help standardize performance expectations across children, but also allow practitioners an opportunity to develop "head norms" about child performance. It is much easier to interpret a measure after dozens of regular administrations than if it is used sparingly to test hypotheses for individual children. In addition, once demands analyses have been done on the fixed-battery subtests, they may only need to be changed slightly for children who perform them in a unique way. Finally, the use of a fixed battery does not preclude additional hypothesis testing with other instruments. Actually, using an intellectual/cognitive measure (e.g., WISC-V), a fixed neuropsychological battery (e.g., the Halstead–Reitan), and additional hypothesis-testing measures (e.g., Comprehensive Test of Phonological Processing, Second Edition, subtests) might be the ultimate approach for conducting CHT. However, it is important to remember that as the number of measures increases, the likelihood of child performance variability and of Type I error increases as well. It does no good to test a child all day, only to find his "processing deficits" occurred on the late afternoon tests. In other words, if fatigue is too great, performance deficits can be expected and not necessarily indicative of the real problem.

Intellectual Tests for Hypothesis Testing

You may be surprised to find that you are already familiar with many of the tools available for CHT—including the intelligence/cognitive tests discussed in Chapter 1. Although intelligence test subtests are typically factorially complex (Flanagan et al., 2013), there is often a wealth of information published about these measures; their technical quality can be thoroughly evaluated; and you are familiar with their scoring and interpretation. The manuals on these measures come with many statistics to support interpretation, such as reliability, standard deviations, standard error of measurement, correlations, factor analyses, and other validity studies.

To aid in your demands analysis of these and other measures, it is worthwhile to consult *Essentials of Cross-Battery Assessment* (Flanagan, Alfonso, & Ortiz, 2025), which specifies subtest technical characteristics from a Cattell–Horn–Carroll perspective, and Sattler's (2024) *Assessment of Children: Cognitive Applications* text. Similarly, CHT of the skills necessary for academic performance can utilize subtests from several achievement batteries. For instance, the Kaufman Test of Individual Achievement—Third Edition (KTEA-3) includes subtests that can be used to assess fluent retrieval of lexical–semantic information and rapid automatic naming (Associational Fluency and Naming Facility). Recall that your understanding of brain–behavior relationships is important for interpretation of all test data, and in several subsequent chapters you will get a better understanding of the psychological processes involved in academic achievement.

Although these intellectual and achievement instruments are useful in CHT, let us now examine several tests that are often considered "neuropsychological" instruments. It is important to realize that many neuropsychological tests are easy to administer and score, and that they tap many of the constructs already discussed in this book. However, some of these tasks are quite challenging to administer (especially if they tap your particular processing weaknesses). It will take some practice and/or supervised experience depending on your background before you can become proficient in their use for CHT. We do not claim to present an exhaustive list of measures here, just those that we have found to be useful in our practice of CHT. We do not suggest that these measures are better than others, or that measures not included here cannot be adopted in the CHT model. You should complete a demands analysis for measures you are not familiar with and review the extant literature on new tests before you use them. Do not automatically assume that a test measures what we suggest, or what the test authors report in the manual. Although our interpretive information is limited in this volume, you can consult the test manuals and other excellent interpretive texts to aid in your understanding of the measures (Lee et al., 2005; Lezak et al., 2012; Miller, 2019; Fletcher-Janzen & Reynolds, 2010; Riccio et al., 2010; Semrud-Clikeman & Ellison, 2009; Strauss et al., 2006). Your background, training, and experience will determine your need for individual training and supervision on these measures.

Traditional Neuropsychological Test Batteries

We begin our review of instruments by discussing two historically important neuropsychological test batteries (NTBs): the Halstead–Reitan NTB (Reitan & Wolfson, 1993) and the Luria–Nebraska NTB (Golden et al., 1985). Both have versions for children that are downward extensions of the adult batteries. Though we aren't advocating that school psychologists use these batteries, a brief description follows to familiarize you with them. These batteries are often used as "fixed" batteries, and both have a long tradition of use in neuropsychological assessment and research, so there are many supplemental resources and publications to aid in their interpretation.

Halstead–Reitan NTB

Table 4.2 provides an overview of the constructs tapped by the Halstead–Reitan NTB (Reitan & Wolfson, 1993) subtests, and of possible brain areas responsible for performance. Reviews of its empirical evidence and clinical utility can be found in Nussbaum and Bunner (2009), and Ross et al. (2013). The Category Test requires the child to view simple objects on a screen and press a button coinciding with the numbers 1 to 4. The child is not told how to perform the task, but instead receives feedback after each response. (A more recent version of the Category Test is mentioned later in Table 4.9.) For the Tactile Performance Test, the child is blindfolded and presented with an upright form board and shapes. The child places the different shapes in the corresponding holes as quickly as possible, first with the dominant hand, then with the nondominant hand, and then with both. This is an interesting task in that the input is tactile instead of visual to evaluate visual object recognition and memory. However, be aware that some children find being blindfolded disconcerting or even aversive.

The Trail Making Test is a connect-the-dots task, where the child draws a line connecting numbers in order (Trails A), and then alternates between numbers and letters (Trails B), as quickly as possible, tapping executive functions. For the Sensory–Perceptual Examination, a brief screening of visual, auditory, and somatosensory functioning is followed by three somatosensory tasks: finger touching, writing of numbers (older children) or symbols (young children) on fingers/hands, and recognition of shapes, all hidden from the child's view. The Finger Tapping test is a simple measure of motor speed and persistence.

The Halstead–Reitan provides an Impairment Index of brain dysfunction/damage, which ranges from 0 to 10. It has shown good reliability and validity for identifying brain damage,

TABLE 4.2. Characteristics of Halstead-Reitan Neuropsychological Test Battery (NTB) Subtests

Subtest	Constructs purportedly tapped	Brain areas involved
Category Test	• Concept formation, fluid reasoning, learning skills, mental efficiency	• Prefrontal area, cingulate, hippocampus, temporal lobes (associative and categorical thinking)
Tactile Performance Test	• Tactile sensitivity, manual dexterity, kinesthetic functions, bimanual coordination, spatial memory, incidental learning	• Lateralized sensory and motor areas, parietal lobes, corpus callosum, hippocampus
Sensory-Perceptual Examination	• Simple and complex sensory functions	• Lateralized sensory areas (more complex, bilateral?)
Finger Tapping	• Simple motor speed	• Lateralized motor areas
Trail Making Test, Parts A and B (Trails A and B)	• Processing speed, graphomotor coordination, sequencing, number/letter facility (Trails B also requires working memory, mental flexibility, set shifting)	• Trails A: Dorsal stream, premotor area, primary motor area, corpus callosum; Trails B: also prefrontal–basal ganglia–cingulate

and has been used for identifying strengths and weaknesses for children with learning disabilities and other disorders (Russell et al., 2005). However, the test is quite dated, having been last updated in 2004 for adults and children 15 and older (Heaton, 2004). Versions designed for children have inadequate norms (Nussbaum & Bunner, 2009) and users are cautioned about its use with children (D. C. Miller, 2019; Semrud-Clikeman & Teeter Ellison, 2009). Nonetheless, it is important to be familiar with the tests in this battery, as many of the measures have formed the basis for many more recently developed tests.

Luria–Nebraska NTB

The Luria–Nebraska NTB (Golden et al., 1985) consists of 12 scales derived from Luria's (1973b, 1980a, 1980b) approach to neuropsychological assessment, which emphasizes flexible administration and interpretation of measures. Therefore, it is not a true fixed battery per se, but practitioners may have a tendency to administer it as such. The 12 Luria–Nebraska subscales are labeled Motor, Rhythm, Tactile, Visual, Receptive Language, Expressive Language, Writing, Reading, Arithmetic, Memory, Intelligence, and Delayed Memory. The most predictive subscales are those assessing language and achievement, which are adequately assessed using more current instruments, as the norms are quite limited (Semrud-Clikeman, 2001). Although some have lauded the virtues of this battery (Golden, 2004), the traditional examination may take up to 2 days to complete (Golden, Freshwater, et al., 2001), making this instrument impractical for use in the schools, and in any case is seldom used with children anymore (Miller & Wang, 2019; Semrud-Clikeman & Teeter Ellison, 2009). It has not been updated since the 1980s, and several contemporary neuropsychological assessment tools are available (as discussed later) to assess skills similar to those tapped by the Luria–Nebraska domains, and many were designed solely for use with children. Note that A. R. Luria was not involved in the development of the measures.

Neuropsychological/Cognitive Tests for Hypothesis Testing

We now review instruments that assess multiple as well as specific areas of neuropsychological functioning. You may wish to use an entire test at times, but for the most part, you will pick and choose subtests from these batteries for CHT. They are listed in alphabetical order as to not suggest a preference for one over another for use in CHT.

Children's Memory Scale

Since we are often asked to give an indication of a child's capability of learning in the classroom, it is somewhat surprising that more educational administrators don't mandate assessment of learning and memory skills. Designed for use with children ages 5–16, the Children's Memory Scale (CMS; Cohen, 1997) was an excellent measure of learning and memory designed for clinical assessment. It was carefully standardized on a representative sample; however, its norms are now quite dated, leading us to recommend use of a more current measure. Nonetheless, it is not surprising that the CMS demonstrates adequate internal consistency for a memory measure, and comprehensive validity studies support the instrument's construct validity.

The CMS has six core subtests, two each in the Auditory/Verbal, Visual/Nonverbal, and Attention/Concentration domains; the last domain is probably the least useful in CHT. In addition, there are three supplemental subtests, one for each domain. The subtests we typically use are presented in Table 4.3. The reported subtests all have delayed portions for further examination of long-term memory retrieval—an advantage of this measure. A disadvantage is relying on the Auditory/Verbal–Visual/Nonverbal dichotomy for organizing the battery, and the norms are now quite old. For more information about the utility of the CMS, please consider these sources (Hildebrand & Ledbetter, 2001; Kibby & Cohen, 2008; Riccio et al., 2007).

Cognitive Assessment System—Second Edition

The Cognitive Assessment System—Second Edition (CAS2; Naglieri et al., 2014) retains the essential structure of the CAS, assessing cognitive functioning in children and adolescents from 5 to 18 utilizing the authors' planning, attention, simultaneous, and successive (PASS) model (Das et al., 1994). Although it is reported to be based on Luria's model of neuropsychological processing and assessment, as we have seen in Chapter 2, there is no PASS acronym in Luria's model, and the authors recommend nomothetic interpretation of PASS factors, which is essentially not a Lurian-type approach to clinical assessment. On the one hand, the authors' confirmatory factor analysis has been used to support a four-factor model, but cross-battery analyses of the first edition have raised doubt about the model, with findings suggesting that the Planning and Attention factors should be combined (Georgiou et al., 2020; Keith et al., 2001). On the other hand, Planning and Attention have differential predictive validity of outcome, supporting the authors' model. This model would certainly fit with Luria's (1973b) theory, as attention and executive functions are intimately related to the integrity of the third functional unit or frontal lobes (except for cortical tone, which would be the responsibility of Luria's first functional unit). The separation of planning and attention leads to different recommendations, supporting the treatment validity of the PASS model (Das et al., 1996). In addition, the CAS has been shown to have construct validity and diagnostic utility for children with ADHD (Canivez & Gaboury, 2016) and the factor scores predict achievement well (Naglieri & Rojahn, 2004) and have been shown to be related to intervention (e.g., Iseman & Naglieri, 2011).

TABLE 4.3. Characteristics of Children's Memory Scale (CMS) Subtests

Subtest	Constructs purportedly tapped
Auditory/Verbal	
Stories	• Auditory attention, semantic long-term memory encoding and retrieval, sequencing/grammar, verbal comprehension, expressive language
Word Pairs	• Paired-associate task; auditory attention, learning novel word pairs
Word Lists	• Selective reminding task; long-term memory encoding, storage, and retrieval of unrelated words
Visual/Nonverbal	
Dot Locations	• Visual–spatial memory encoding and retrieval (dorsal stream), susceptibility to interference
Faces	• Visual–facial memory encoding and retrieval (ventral stream)
Attention/Concentration	
Sequences	• Rote recall of simple information followed by mental manipulation/ executive function items

We like several of the CAS2 subtests for hypothesis testing (albeit the CAS2 authors would not support such use in actual practice). The scale was adequately normed, and most subtests show good technical characteristics. In addition, the test authors have provided us with the first substantial treatment validity studies of any cognitive measure, presented in the PASS Remedial Program (PREP; see Das et al., 1997). The PREP has focused primarily on reading, with training of successive and simultaneous skills leading to improved word recognition and decoding skills. There is also evidence that strategy-based instruction can improve mathematics achievement in students with poor planning skills. We do not think, however, that the CAS2 should be used to measure global intellectual functioning, even though it provides a Full Scale standard score (SS). Absent from the CAS2 is a measure of crystallized intelligence (Gc). Although the lack of Gc measurement makes the CAS2 a fairer test for people of linguistic and cultural difference than most other intellectual/cognitive measures, it doesn't adequately tap left-hemisphere processes as a result. Therefore, though we feel that the CAS2 is not adequate as a baseline measure of global functioning for most children, it is a good tool for hypothesis testing.

We present the CAS2 subtests that we recommend in Table 4.4. Note that our interpretation is somewhat different from that presented by the test authors. Naglieri and colleagues have conducted some useful intervention research with the original version of the CAS showing the link between PASS processing strengths and weaknesses and intervention choice, and linking assessment to intervention that leads to improved outcomes (Goldstein et al., 2011; Haddad et al., 2003; Iseman & Naglieri, 2011; Naglieri 2002; Naglieri & Johnson, 2000; Tomporowski et al., 2008). This is noteworthy given our earlier complaints about test publishers not examining the treatment validity of their measures

Comprehensive Test of Phonological Processing, Second Edition

The Comprehensive Test of Phonological Processing—Second Edition (CTOPP-2; Wagner et al., 2013), is a unique measure of the cognitive constructs most commonly associated with reading and language disorders. Designed for use with children and youth aged 4–24, it measures phonological awareness, phonological memory, and rapid automatized naming, which have been linked with word recognition, word attack, and other basic reading skills (Wolf, 2001). The CTOPP-2 is composed of 12 subtests, several of which we find useful in CHT. It was normed on a large representative sample, and subtests have good to excellent technical characteristics. Validity studies show the phonological awareness and rapid naming tasks have strong relationships with reading skills.

Table 4.5 outlines the CTOPP-2 subtests and what they measure. The Nonword Repetition subtest is an interesting task that taps phonemic processing and expression skills for nonsense words (e.g., "lidsca"), similar to other visually presented pseudoword tasks for comparison purposes. However, it includes an auditory model (so the child hears the nonword first) and an auditory working memory component (because the child has to recall what he or she heard). This task can be combined with the Blending Nonwords (e.g., "raq" + "di") subtest to help determine whether the phonological breakdown is occurring at the individual-phoneme level or the phonological assembly level. One concern with the CTOPP-2 is the limited assessment of rapid naming. Including rapid naming of more complex letter combinations (e.g., digraphs, diphthongs) and simple words presented two grades below reading level would have been helpful. Although phonological processes have been linked to left temporal lobe functions, rapid naming is typically associated with temporal lobe and frontal–subcortical circuits, as well as cerebellar functions. Further information about brain functions and reading competency are discussed in Chapters 2 and 5. The first and second editions of the CTOPP have been used extensively in research, attesting to its value in

TABLE 4.4. Characteristics of Cognitive Assessment System, Second Edition (CAS2) Subtests

Subtest	Constructs purportedly tapped
Planning	
Planned Number Matching	• Sustained attention, visual scanning, psychomotor speed, noticing pattern and figuring out appropriate strategy
Planned Codes	• Similar to WISC-V Coding, but format allows for strategy use (e.g., filling in by code rather than in order)
Planned Connections	• Substitute for Halstead–Reitan Trails A and B (see Table 4.2), but no separation of scores
Attention	
Expressive Attention	• Substitute for Stroop Color–Word Test (see Table 4.9); inhibition of automatic response (reading words) to name ink color of printed word
Number Detection	• Cancellation task; sustained attention, visual scanning, visual discrimination, inhibition, psychomotor speed
Simultaneous Processing	
Nonverbal Matrices	• Typical *Gf* measure of inductive reasoning; multiple-choice format
Verbal/Spatial Relations	• Receptive language, verbal working memory, grammatical relationships, visual scanning/discrimination
Figure Memory	• Similar to DAS-II Recall of Designs (see Chapter 1, Table 1.2); visual perception, spatial relationships, visual memory, graphomotor reproduction, constructional skills, figure–ground relationships
Successive Processing	
Word Series	• Word span; rote recall of unrelated words
Sentence Repetition	• Rote recall of meaningless sentences; grammatical structure important (ages 4–7)
Sentence Questions	• Similar sentence stimuli to Sentence Repetition, but child answers questions (e.g., "The brown is purple. What is purple?" Answer: "The brown.") (ages 8–21)
Visual Digit Span	• Rote sequential memory using visual stimuli

understanding the relationship of its measures to brain function, reading competency, and even treatment response (Conant et al., 2013; Foorman et al., 2015; Hutton et al., 2020; Kovelman et al., 2012; Lonigan et al., 2009; Leitão & Fletcher, 2004; Marshall et al., 2013; McNorgan et al., 2013; O'Brien et al., 2013; Park & Lombardino, 2013; Pollitt & Harrison, 2021; Pugh et al., 2013; Saygin et al., 2013; Toste et al., 2020).

Delis–Kaplan Executive Function System

No one has inspired and transformed the field of neuropsychology like Edith Kaplan, who could be considered the founder of the neuropsychological process approach (Oscar-Berman & Fein, 2013). Kaplan attempted to bring process assessment into the mainstream by developing

TABLE 4.5.   TABLE 4.5. Characteristics of Comprehensive Test of Phonological Processing, Second Edition (CTOPP-2), Subtests

Subtest	Constructs purportedly tapped
Phonological Awareness	
Elision	Phonological perception, segmentation, individual phonemes
Blending Words	Phonological assembly
Sound Matching	Phonological perception, segmentation, individual phonemes
Phoneme Isolation	Phonological perception, segmentation, individual phonemes
Blending Nonwords	Phonological assembly
Segmenting Nonwords	Phonological perception, segmentation, individual phonemes
Phonological Memory	
Memory for Digits	Rote auditory memory
Nonword Repetition	Phonemic analysis, assembly, auditory working memory
Rapid Naming	
Rapid Color Naming	Naming automaticity, processing speed, speed of lexical access, verbal fluency
Rapid Object Naming	Object recognition, naming automaticity, processing speed, speed of lexical access, verbal fluency
Rapid Digit Naming	Number automaticity, processing speed, speed of lexical access, verbal fluency
Rapid Letter Naming	Letter automaticity, processing speed, speed of lexical access, verbal fluency

measures that were both clinically useful and had psychometric integrity (Libon et al., 2013), which is not an easy feat. She will be terribly missed but her legacy and contribution to the field of neuropsychology continues. Her trainees carry on her tradition which is very similar to Luria's approach to clinical assessment and testing of limits to understand brain structure, function, and implications.

One of her legacies is the Delis–Kaplan Executive Function System (D-KEFS; Delis et al., 2001). While it is a prominent measure of executive functions, mediated primarily by the prefrontal cortex, largely the dorsal system that deals with planning, organization, strategizing, monitoring, evaluating, and shifting behavior (Hale et al., 2013), the norms are becoming outdated. A revised version, the D-KEFS Advanced, which will be all-digital, is expected to be available in 2025. The original test was developed and normed on a large representative national sample to assess ages 8–89. Unlike many neuropsychological measures, the D-KEFS has extensive information about technical quality presented in the manual, which facilitates interpretation. Any of the specific tests can be administered separately, making it ideal for use in CHT. Of particular interest is the trail-making task, which allows the examiner to parse out sequencing, executive, and motor demands. It is also the only tool that has a tower task normed with other executive measures. Many of the tasks are versions of tasks with rich histories in neuropsychological assessment, and research supports the validity of the measures (Delis et al., 2004). A great deal of research has explored the psychometric characteristics (e.g., Sevadjian et al., 2011; Fine et al., 2011; Latzman & Markon, 2010), with evidence of both concurrent brain function and clinical utility examined (e.g., Berninger et al., 2008a,

2008b; Corbett et al., 2009; Figueras et al., 2008; Latzman et al., 2010; Lin et al., 2012; Poretti et al., 2013; Strong et al., 2010; Vasilopoulos et al., 2012). Table 4.6 describes the individual D-KEFS tests and the constructs purportedly assessed by each.

NEPSY—Second Edition

The NEPSY—Second Edition (NEPSY-II; Korkman, 2007) is the updated edition of the first *truly* developmental neuropsychological measure designed for children. This latest edition is for children ages 3–16. There are 32 subtests designed to provide a comprehensive evaluation of six functional domains: Attention and Executive Functioning, Language, Memory and Learning, Sensorimotor Functions, Social Perception, and Visuospatial Processing. However, unlike its predecessor, the NEPSY-II does not give factor or index scores, so it is ideal for use in hypothesis testing, and this was the reason the test publisher did not provide a method for calculating global scores. The NEPSY-II subtests and flexible administration format are primarily based on Luria's (1973b, 1980a, 1980b) model. This allows the examiner to pick and choose a subtest to test a specific hypothesis. Since this process requires the user to have enough understanding of brain–behavior relationships to recognize the processes tapped, some beginning practitioners might not consider the NEPSY-II, but we find some measures incredibly useful in CHT.

Although the test is based on a Lurian approach, the test does not break tasks down into primary, secondary, or tertiary skills; nor does the manual readily identify the relationships between subtest performance and the first, second, and third functional units. With many years in development, the NEPSY-II has all the advantages of being published by a major test developer, including an adequate normative sample, subtest technical quality, and ample validity studies. Not all of the NEPSY-II subtests show comparable technical quality, however, so Table 4.7 presents the subtests we have found to be most beneficial in CHT. In addition, though the Language subtests serve as a measure of *Gc*, the NEPSY-II does not adequately measure *Gf* or novel problem-solving skills. Both versions of the NEPSY have sufficient evidence of its use as a measure (e.g., Hayes & Watson, 2013; Horska & Barker, 2010; Schwartz et al., 2013).

TABLE 4.6. Characteristics of Delis–Kaplan Executive Function System (D-KEFS) Subtests

Subtest	Constructs purportedly tapped
Sorting Test	Problem solving, verbal and spatial concept formation, categorical thinking, flexibility of thinking on a conceptual task
Trail Making Test	Mental flexibility, sequential processing on a visual–motor task, set shifting
Verbal Fluency Test	Verbal fluency
Design Fluency Test	Visual fluency
Color–Word Interference Test	Attention and response inhibition
Tower Test	Planning, flexibility, organization, spatial reasoning, inhibition
20 Questions Test	Hypothesis testing, verbal and spatial abstract thinking, inhibition
Word Context Test	Deductive reasoning, verbal abstract thinking
Proverb Test	Metaphorical thinking, generating versus comprehending abstract thoughts

TABLE 4.7. Characteristics of NEPSY-II Subtests

Subtest	Constructs purportedly tapped
Attention/Executive Functions	
Auditory Attention and Response Set	Sustained auditory attention, vigilance, inhibition, set maintenance, mental flexibility
Design Fluency	Visual–motor fluency, mental flexibility, graphomotor responding in structured and unstructured situations
Animal Sorting	Ability to formulate basic concepts and to transfer those concepts into action
Clocks	Planning and organization and visual–perceptual and visual–spatial skills
Inhibition	Ability to inhibit automatic responses
Statue	Motor persistence and inhibition
Language	
Phonological Processing	Similar to WJ-IV *Ga* subtests (see Chapter 1, Table 1.6); auditory attention, phonological awareness, segmentation, assembly
Comprehension of Instructions	Receptive language, sequencing, grammar, simple motor response
Repetition of Nonsense Words	Auditory presentation of nonsense words; phonemic awareness, segmentation, assembly, sequencing, simple oral expression
Oromotor Sequences	Oromotor programming
Speeded Naming	Rapid semantic access
Word Generation	Verbal productivity
Memory and Learning	
List Memory	Remember list of unrelated words over multiple learning trials; one delayed trial after interference list
Memory for Designs	Visual-spatial memory; also requires maintenance of rules
Memory for Faces	Select previously viewed photo from an array
Memory for Names	Learn the names of line drawings of children's faces over multiple trials
Narrative Memory	Recall of orally presented narratives; recall of details and inferential comprehension
Sentence Repetition	Rote auditory recall; grammatical knowledge
Word List Interference	Rote repetition of unrelated words, with each set of two followed by recall of both sets; working memory
Social Perception	
Affect Recognition	Matching photos expressing the same feeling: happy, sad, fear, anger, disgust, neutral
Theory of Mind	Understand how others are feeling, understand false beliefs; also requires verbal comprehension and memory
Sensorimotor Functions	
Fingertip Tapping	Simple motor speed, perseverance
Imitating Hand Positions	Visual perception, memory, kinesthesis, praxis

(continued)

TABLE 4.7. (*continued*)

Visual–Motor Precision	Visual–motor integration, graphomotor coordination without constructional requirements
Manual Motor Sequences	Motor imitation
Visual–Spatial Processing	
Design Copying	Visual perception of abstract stimuli, visual–motor integration, graphomotor skills
Arrows	Spatial processing, visualization, line orientation, inhibition, no graphomotor demands
Block Construction	Similar to WISC-V Block Design (see Tables 1.5 and 4.1)
Geometric Puzzles	Mental rotation, visual–spatial analysis, and attention to detail
Picture Puzzles	Visual discrimination, spatial localization, spatial localization, and visual spanning
Route Finding	Visual-spatial relations and directionality

Process Assessment of the Learner—Second Edition: Test Battery for Reading and Writing and Test Battery for Mathematics

The artificial distinction between "ability" and "achievement" in SLD identification led us down a clinical path that ignored their interrelationship. To look in more detail at the processes involved in reading and writing, the Process Assessment of the Learner—Second Edition: Test Battery for Reading and Writing (PAL-II RW; Berninger, 2007b) is available to complement regular standardized achievement testing. Individual subtests can be administered and interpreted, making this test ideal for CHT. There are also intervention materials available for both individual and classroom implementation based on Berninger's extensive research findings. The PAL-II RW includes measures of phonological processing; orthographic coding; rapid automatized naming; phonological decoding; and integration of listening, note taking, and summary writing skills. Although the PAL-II RW is used for examining academic skills, it focuses on the psychological processes associated with these skills, making it especially useful for linking assessment to intervention.

The Process Assessment of the Learner—Second Edition: Test Battery for Mathematics (PAL-II Math; Berninger, 2007a) measures the development of cognitive processes that are related to math. The PAL-II Math includes measures of numeral writing, numeric coding, quantitative working memory, spatial working memory, rapid naming, and graphomotor integration. Like the PAL-II RW, the PAL-II Math's user guide contains resources and recommended interventions based on the assessment results.

Berninger is one of the most accomplished researchers in the field, and has used an extensive evidence base to establish the validity of the PAL-II (e.g., Abbott et al., 2010; Altemeier et al., 2008; Berninger et al., 2006; Berninger et al., 2010; Berninger & Dunn, 2012; Berninger et al., 2013; Berninger & O'Malley May, 2011; Berninger & Niedo, 2012; Berninger & Richards, 2010; Niedo et al., 2013; Brooks et al., 2011; Richards et al., 2009). Not only does the work cited here show her impressive work to highlight the validity of the PAL-II, but she also documents its utility with research in the field and laboratory, showing changes in brain functioning after intervention. Not only is the PAL-II a useful test for use in CHT, this depth of literature across disciplines is worth reading to help you understand the relationship between test data, brain functioning, classroom achievement, and brain-based treatment response.

Feifer Assessments of Reading, Mathematics, and Writing

Well known in the school neuropsychology field, Steven Feifer has developed a family of instruments designed for the neuropsychological assessment of processes underlying achievement. These relative newcomers are well designed from a acomprehensive view of the neuropsychology of learning. Unfortunately, the norms are grade-based, making direct comparison to other measures that are mostly age-based (as we recommend) difficult, but the excellent coverage of processing components makes them very useful for CHT. The Feifer Assessment of Reading (FAR; Feifer, 2015) has several subtests assessing each of phonological skills, fluency, and comprehension. The more unique and therefore most useful subtests for CHT assess visual perception, orthographic processing, semantic concepts, print knowledge, and morphological processing. The Feifer Assessment of Mathematics (FAM; Feifer, 2016) has sections assessing verbal retrieval and linguistic components of math, procedural knowledge, and semantic components. The semantic index, in particular, includes many useful subtests for CHT, including measures of number sense, magnitude representation, visual–spatial and conceptual components of math, and high-level problem solving. The Feifer Assessment of Writing (FAW; Feifer, 2020) assesses graphomotor skills with several subtests, two measures of spelling contributing to a dyslexia index, and an executive index. As you will see in later chapters, writing is one of the most cognitively complex tasks we undertake, and the executive component is considerable. The FAW subtests will be useful in CHT for students with writing difficulties.

Test of Memory and Learning—Second Edition

The Test of Memory and Learning—Second Edition (TOMAL-2; Reynolds & Voress, 2007) is in many ways a more comprehensive measure of learning and memory than the CMS. The current edition has been normed for children and adults ages 5–59. (Note that the TOMAL-3 is being normed as this book is being written.) The TOMAL consists of eight core and six supplemental subtests, and two delayed-recall subtests. It was carefully standardized, and the norms are representative of the U.S. Census population. Reliabilities tend to be quite strong across ages, especially for the composite scores. However, further support for its use in memory assessment can been found in subsequent studies reported in the literature. Table 4.8 provides an overview of the TOMAL-2 subtests we find useful in CHT. The Delayed Recall Index includes delayed recall from the Memory for Stories, Word Selective Reminding, Facial Memory, and Visual Selective Reminding subtests. As with the CMS, one of the difficulties with the TOMAL-2 is its breakdown into verbal and nonverbal memory domains. It is not surprising that the second edition has strong technical quality and evidence of clinical utility (e.g., Brooks & Iverson, 2012; Dehn, 2010; Fuentes et al., 2012; Lajiness-O'Neill et al., 2010; Sutton et al., 2011; Meekes et al., 2013; Riegler et al., 2013; Thaler et al., 2012; Thaler et al., 2010; Till et al., 2013).

Wide Range Assessment of Memory and Learning—Third Edition

The Wide Range Assessment of Memory and Learning—Third Edition (WRAML-3; Adams & Sheslow, 2021) was the first child memory scale on the market, having been first developed in the 1980s. Like the other measures reviewed here, it examines verbal and visual memory, and includes an attention/concentration index score. Additional examination of delayed recall, working memory for children nine and older, and recognition are possible. For verbal memory, rote, sentence, and story memory are tapped. For visual memory, both abstract and meaningful memory are assessed. These tasks are challenging yet interesting for children,

TABLE 4.8. Characteristics of Test of Memory and Learning, Second Edition (TOMAL-2), Subtests

Subtest	Constructs purportedly tapped
Verbal Memory Index	
Memory for Stories	See CMS Stories (Table 4.3 lists this and other CMS subtests)
Word Selective Reminding	Similar to CMS Word Lists, but no interference task
Paired Recall	See CMS Word Pairs
Digits Forward	Auditory rote memory, sequential recall, attention
Digits Backward	Similar to WISC-V/WJ-IV versions; more demands on attention, working memory, executive functions than Digits Forward
Letters Forward	Auditory rote memory, sequential recall, attention
Letters Backward	Working memory, attention, executive functions
Nonverbal Memory Index	
Facial Memory	See CMS Faces; good ventral stream measure
Visual Selective Reminding	Visual analogue to word selective reminding, with dots; dorsal stream, visual–motor coordination, praxis without visual discrimination
Abstract Visual Memory	Visual discrimination of abstract symbols, recognition memory
Visual–Sequential Memory	Visual discrimination of abstract symbols, sequencing, praxis
Memory for Location	See CMS Dot Locations; good dorsal stream measure
Manual Imitation	Short-term visual–sequential memory, praxis
Object Recall	Visual and verbal presentation of objects with verbal recall over multiple trials.

making the WRAML-3 a possible alternative to the CMS and TOMAL-2. It is fairly easy to administer and score. It has a large normative sample and adequate technical characteristics. The WRAML-3 is a popular test and well-liked by children taking it. The Third Edition is much improved in terms of its psychometric characteristics and clinical utility was established in the second edition (e.g., Atkinson et al., 2008; Burton et al., 2012; Goldstein et al., 2014; Lajiness-O'Neill et al., 2013; McKnight & Culotta, 2012). Given this is a new measure, it will be important to see how well it fares in independent research.

Supplemental Neuropsychological Measures for Hypothesis Testing

Table 4.9 presents a number of other neuropsychological measures we have found useful in CHT. Although some are specifically for use with children, others listed in this table have a long history of use in neuropsychological assessment of adults, and most have been adequately extended downward for use with children. These instruments measure a variety of cognitive or neuropsychological constructs, and many have been found to be sensitive to brain functions and dysfunctions. They can be used to test initial hypotheses or validate hypotheses derived from previously discussed measures. Some measures, such as the Rey–Osterreith Complex Figure (a visual–spatial–graphomotor task) and the California Verbal Learning Test—children's version (a language task), could be listed under other table subheadings. We have put the measures in the domains that are most likely to serve our CHT purposes.

TABLE 4.9. Supplemental Measures for Hypothesis Testing

Subtest	Constructs purportedly tapped
Attention Memory/Executive Function	
Children's Category Test (Boll, 1993)	See Halstead–Reitan Category Test (Table 4.2)
Wisconsin Card Sorting Test (Heaton et al., 1993)	Executive functions, problem solving, set maintenance, goal-oriented behavior, inhibition, ability to benefit from feedback, mental flexibility, perseveration
Tower of London (Shallice, 1982)	Planning, inhibition, problem solving, monitoring, and self-regulation
Stroop Color–Word Test (Golden et al., 2002)	See CAS-2 Expressive Attention (Table 4.4)
Rey–Osterrieth Complex Figure (Meyers & Meyers, 1995)	Visual–motor integration, constructional skills, graphomotor skills, visual memory, planning, organization, problem solving
Conners Continuous Performance Test 3 (CPT-3; Conners, Sitarenios, & Ayearst, 2018)	Computerized measure of sustained attention, impulse control, reaction time, persistence, response variability, perseveration, visual discrimination
Hale-Denkla Cancellation Task (Hale et al., 2009)	Attention, concentration, visual scanning
California Verbal Learning Test—Children's Version (Delis et al., 1994)	Verbal learning, long-term memory encoding and retrieval, susceptibility to interference
Comprehensive Trail-Making Test—Second Edition (CTMT2; Reynolds, 2020)	Attention, concentration, resistance to distraction, cognitive flexibility/set shifting
Behavior Rating Inventory of Executive Function, Second Edition (BRIEF2; Gioia et al., 2015)	Parent and teacher rating scales of behavioral regulation, metacognition; includes clinical scales assessing inhibition, cognitive shift, emotional control, task initiation, working memory, planning, organization of materials, and self-monitoring; includes validity scales assessing inconsistent responding and negativity
Tests of Variable Attention (TOVA; Leark et al., 2008)	Computerized measure of sustained and selective attention
Sensory–motor/Nonverbal skills	
Developmental Test of Visual–Motor Integration, Sixth Edition (Beery & Beery, 2010)	Visual–perceptual skills, fine-motor skills, visual–motor integration
Purdue Pegboard (Tiffin & Asher, 1948)	Fine-motor skills, bimanual integration, psychomotor speed
Grooved Pegboard (Kløve, 1963)	Complex visual–motor–tactile integration, psychomotor speed (compare to simple sensory–motor integration)
Judgment of Line Orientation (Benton & Tranel, 1993)	See NEPSY-II Arrows (Table 4.7)
Language Measures	
Oral and Written Language Scales, Second Edition (Carrow-Woolfolk, 2011)	Listening comprehension, oral expression, written expression; not limited to single-word responses
Comprehensive Assessment of Spoken Language, Second Edition (Carrow-Woolfolk, 2017)	Language processing in comprehension, expression, and retrieval in these categories: lexical/semantic, syntactic, supralinguistic, pragmatic *(continued)*

TABLE 4.9. (*continued*)

Clinical Evaluation of Language Fundamentals—Fifth Edition (CELF-5; Wiig, Semel, & Secord, 2013)	Assesses receptive and expressive language with the core subtests, but also allows assessment of language structure, language content, and memory; includes standardized observations in the classroom and assessment of pragmatic language skills, in addition to individual assessment
Test of Language Development—TOLD-5, Primary and Intermediate; Newcomer & Hammill, 2019)	Primary version assesses phonology, semantics, and syntax; Intermediate version assesses semantics and syntax
Receptive auditory/Verbal skills	
Wepman Auditory Discrimination Test—Second Edition (Wepman & Reynolds, 1987)	Auditory attention, phonemic awareness, phonemic segmentation, phoneme position (primary/medial/recent)
Peabody Picture Vocabulary Test, Fifth Edition (PPVT-5; Dunn & Dunn, 2018)	Receptive vocabulary (visual scanning/impulse control); conormed with EVT-3 (see below)
Token Test for Children, Second Edition (TTFC-2; McGhee et al., 2007)	Receptive language, auditory working memory, direction following without significant cultural content
Expressive auditory/Verbal skills	
Controlled Oral Word Association Test (Spreen & Benton, 1977)	See NEPSY-II Verbal Fluency (Table 4.7)
Boston Naming Test (Goodglass & Kaplan, 1987)	Expressive vocabulary, free-recall retrieval from long-term memory versus cued-recall retrieval (semantic/phonemic)
Expressive Vocabulary Test, Third Edition (EVT-3; Williams, 2018)	Expressive vocabulary (picture naming); conormed with PPVT-5 (see above)

Behavioral Neuropsychology and Problem-Solving Consultation

Utilizing Assessment and Consultation Skills

Now that we have reviewed the assessment part of our model, let's integrate it with consultation. Notice the heading above. Isn't *behavioral neuropsychology* an oxymoron? No, because we believe that these two orientations should be seen as integrated, not as antithetical. In the past, consultation was seen as something a school psychologist would do before a comprehensive evaluation, or instead of a comprehensive evaluation. In contrast, we see consultation as an integral part of everything you do in all the tiers! Data collection is important in consultation too, and the fact that you are doing standardized assessments doesn't mean you can't also do problem-solving consultation. Data collection is important for understanding and serving children, but how you use it is probably even more important for your practice of neuropsychology. We are suggesting that these two functions of school psychologists can be combined to make both stronger. You can bring assessment data into the consultation data-gathering phase when this is appropriate, linking interventions to the child's strengths and needs. The CHT emphasis on *ecological validity* and *treatment validity* is what sets our model apart from other test interpretation models, which have largely focused on testing for identification or diagnostic purposes. As Miciak and Fletcher (2020) recommend, assessment data should lead to intervention, a point we wholeheartedly agree with—your testing is not only about *understanding*, but it is also about *doing*—linking assessment data to intervention to improve outcomes for all children is best practice.

Most referrals for problem-solving consultation concern academic problems, and most of those academic problems are reading difficulties. Although general consultation on reading instruction may be helpful, combining this knowledge with information about the multiple determinants of the child's problem can have important effects on the intervention you and the teacher choose, and on the success the child experiences as a result of your efforts. Consultation is intended to be a collaboration between equals, but the fact that the consultant is there to help the consultee solve a problem has the potential to make the power relationship unequal. We have to guard against a traditional mental health consultation approach that does not work well in schools. There's a tendency for consultees to defer to the "expert" neuropsychologist consultant, agree with the consultant during meetings, but then not feel ownership of the interventions developed during consultation. The problem-solving collaborative consultation approach must be an equal partnership because without consultee ownership many of these interventions will not be fully implemented or implemented with integrity (Erchul & Martens, 2010). We believe that the power issues within the consultative relationship must be acknowledged and dealt with directly. Both school psychologists and teachers feel that expertise and informational power are essential in making changes with teachers (Owens et al., 2018). You are using your expertise and knowledge to help solve a problem, influence a teacher to make changes, and support and develop the teacher's skills (Erchul & Martens, 2010). By gaining knowledge and skills in instructional leadership, systems issues, collaborative team building, and academic and behavioral interventions, you can be an important source for the consultee, and guide him or her toward solutions without being coercive.

Consultation begins with the premise that the consultant works with the consultee (usually the classroom teacher) to solve a client's (the teacher's student's) problem. It is also assumed that both professionals have specific expertise to bring to bear on the problem. In our view, your knowledge of neuropsychological and cognitive functions, neuropsychological assessment, the academic and behavioral interventions literature, and intervention-monitoring methodology should be the core of expertise that you bring to the relationship. The teacher's knowledge of the student's classroom performance, awareness of effective and ineffective teaching techniques for the child, and professional experience as a teacher form the core of his or her expertise as the consultee. Fully acknowledging the expertise of the consultee is one part of building rapport. This consultee's expertise is also necessary if an appropriate problem solution is to be found. An intervention plan that takes into account available resources and the interventions the teacher is already trying should have greater applicability and effectiveness (Miller et al., 2019).

The following problem-solving consultation model is a summary of content and skills presented by several experts combined with our CHT model (Erchul & Martens, 2010; Brown-Chidsey & Andren, 2012). This model is especially relevant in the Tier 2 approach (problem-solving RTI approach) in an attempt to serve children before comprehensive evaluation is ever considered, and in Tier 3 following comprehensive CHT evaluation. The only difference is that in Tier 3 the cognitive and neuropsychological processing characteristics are also considered in problem analysis.

Stages of Problem-Solving Consultation

Problem Identification

During the initial interview, the consultant (you) and the consultee identify a target behavior for intervention. The behavior must be defined in an observable, measurable way. It is typical for teachers and parents to report summative judgments ("He's depressed") rather than an operational behavior that is related to that summative judgment (slow in completing work, does not interact with peers). Information is needed about how often and when the behavior occurs, so information about frequency, duration, and severity need to be considered. To do this well, you often need to consider multiple behaviors before choosing the target behavior. It is important to list and operationalize all behaviors, and then hierarchically order them from most to least significant in the eyes of both the consultee and consultant. Many models suggest picking the most significant problem, but in reality this may not be feasible or appropriate. It is sometimes more important to pick a target behavior that is readily changeable so both the child and consultee experience success. It does no good to pick a significant problem that is so routinized that change is unlikely or very difficult, thus discouraging all those involved in the process. Instead, you should consider task-analyzing (breaking the problem behavior into subcomponent parts), and then using a shaping process (reinforcing successive approximations of target behaviors) to encourage success before taking on the more significant problem. In addition, consultation and behavioral research have shown us that if we just suppress a behavior it will manifest in another way, so we also need a positive replacement behavior we want to increase. The main idea here is you want to punish (extinguish) problem behaviors, and reinforce positive replacement behaviors. To do this, we need to think about strategies such as differential reinforcement of alternative (DRA), differential reinforcement of incompatible (DRI), or differential reinforcement of other (DRO) behaviors. As a reminder, DRA involves decreasing an unwanted behavior while at the same time reinforcing an alternative, more acceptable, behavior. DRI is when a behavior that is incompatible with the target behavior is reinforced. For example, a child who pulls out her hair is instead engaged in squeezing a stress ball, which is reinforced. This gives the child a distraction which requires her to use her hands for something else besides hair pulling. DRO is simply reinforcing the behavior that you wish to shape, while ignoring or extinguishing the problem behavior.

CHT problem identification is somewhat more complex than in other problem-solving models. CHT includes data collected from MTSS interventions, observations, interviews, and cognitive, neuropsychological, academic, and behavior assessment results. As noted previously, it is important that the teacher be consulted to determine that your findings have concurrent and ecological validity.

Problem Analysis

Even if you have conducted a CHT evaluation, a more in-depth study of the target behavior is made during problem analysis, possibly including a functional behavioral assessment (FBA) and/or curriculum-based measurement (CBM). A handbook for conducting a functional assessment in schools, such as Steege et al. (2019) will be helpful at this stage. For assistance with academics, the work of Hosp et al. (2016) is a useful resource. An FBA should include a review of the prior intervention data collected, and an interview with the teacher to identify possible causes, antecedents, and consequences of the behavior. Most functional assessments focus on obvious causes for the behavior, such as stimuli that precipitate problem behavior, or consequent events such seeking attention or escaping from a task. Although discussing functional behavior analysis would seem counterintuitive in a school neuropsychology book, this is hardly the case since the environment plays an important role, not only in determining the antecedent and consequent events associated with a given behavior, but also in how these interact with brain function.

The CHT process will provide information about the student's cognitive processing strengths and weaknesses to use in developing working hypotheses, such as processing difficulties, memory problems, language deficits, or difficulty with unstructured situations. As part of the problem analysis, a review of interventions that have already been attempted and their effectiveness is also helpful. Although CHT includes functional analysis in this stage, it relies on much more information from numerous data sources and integrates these sources with our understanding of the child's individual neuropsychological strengths and weaknesses.

While considering an FBA for academic problems is potentially useful if the problem is a performance deficit instead of a skill deficit, in many cases a skill problem is important to identify. If the child does not have the skill to complete the task, then that skill should be taught first. Both survey and specific level assessments can be useful in determining the level and pattern of academic skills deficits, especially using the validated CBM tools discussed later in this chapter. Your CHT evaluation may have adequately linked the processing deficits associated with the achievement problem, but the CBM can give you a more fine-grained analysis of the problem. What CHT acknowledges, which is absent in the either/or perspective regarding skill or performance deficit, is that an executive problem (a skill deficit) can look like a performance deficit, because the child does the skill sometimes and not others, due to poor executive control. A more detailed explanation of academic error patterns can be found in Chapter 5 (reading), Chapter 6 (mathematics), and Chapter 7 (written expression). Recall that error analysis is the key to understanding academic skill deficits, and when linked with your understanding of brain function, you can design individualized interventions for children, which is the next problem-solving step.

Plan Development/Implementation

Following the problem analysis step, a working hypothesis needs to be developed conjointly by the consultant and the consultee as a basis for the intervention. In our experience, this can be a very challenging stage for many beginning consultants and even advanced consultees. School psychologists may be better versed in interventions such as cognitive-behavioral therapy (e.g., Kendall, 2011) or social skills interventions (Gresham, 2016) than academic interventions. One of the things we recommend is that every school psychologist buy special education books for teachers, such as *Students with Learning Problems* (Mercer & Pullen, 2010) or *Positive Behavioral Supports for the Classroom* (Scheuermann, Hall, & Billingsly, 2011). These books are useful for two reasons; they give you a good idea of what teachers are exposed to in their training, and they also give you a lot of great ideas for evidence-based interventions to pull out during the consultation process, and subsequently to address the child's needs.

During this phase, the consultant and consultee recognize there are multiple factors associated with intervention development and implementation that require careful consideration. This process begins with a good operational definition and specification of the goal, which includes the behavior objective (also written in problem identification), content, materials, conditions in which the behavior will occur, and the criterion for acceptable performance. The plan takes into account the student's characteristics and behavior, the classroom ecology, the resources available, and the teacher's style and preferences. Working together, the consultant and consultee brainstorm many possible interventions, and then choose the intervention that is likely to be effective and can be plausibly implemented. Based on the child, consider instructional or intervention strategies and modifications, evaluate resources for implementation, and consider reinforcers or consequences to increase the student's behavior or performance. For instance, some reinforcers like social interaction may be best for some students, but others may prefer video game time.

Be sure to write these intervention plans with extensive behavioral detail, and data collection methods. Whenever possible, using extant rating scales or academic probes for data collection is a good choice, but on many occasions you may have to develop your own. Finally, determine how long it might take for the child to show significant improvement. The length of intervention in relation to the severity of the problem is a difficult consideration. If the problem is significant, and the intervention period is too short, the intervention will not be successful. If the problem is mild and a long intervention period is considered, the child and teacher can become frustrated as improvement is so gradual and the intervention may be terminated prematurely. Feasibility is a key variable here. In our experience teachers get excited about the intervention effort, and sometimes pick strategies or measurement systems that may not be feasible. For instance, teachers may want to do a frequency count of a target behavior by marking every time it occurs on a sheet during the class, but this often is not feasible. Instead using an intermittent count may be more helpful.

Finally, consider how to ensure the intervention is implemented with integrity and how you will evaluate it. Even though the consultant attempts to work with the teacher to develop the plan, it may need recycling because any of the details just noted might not have been feasible. What is the best intervention for children with academic or behavioral needs? The answer is simple: The best intervention is the one that works.

Plan Evaluation/Recycling

The key to successful interventions is ensuring fidelity of interventions and treatment integrity (Harn et al., 2017). Several times during the intervention it is important for the consultant to "check in" with the consultee to see how the intervention is progressing and review the data collected. These repeated informal connections help identify if more formal consultation meetings are needed, and they ensure the interventions are implemented with integrity. Periodic checks and data collection/graphing can help the consultant and consultee evaluate intervention effectiveness (i.e., data collection/analysis and data interpretation) and determine when changes are needed. There are numerous methods for evaluating interventions via within-subject experimental designs, several of which we will review later in the chapter. If the intervention is successful, either the intervention is extended, or it is discontinued if the target has been reached.

If minor revisions appear necessary, the consultee makes them at this time, and he or she decides on an additional meeting to evaluate the revised intervention. If different or more intensive interventions appear necessary (i.e., a new working hypothesis), a new intervention can be attempted, or additional special education support services may be needed. This evaluation process is also important as the instructional supports begin to be removed and the child begins to function completely within his or her natural environment with natural consequences. In most instances, however, there are minor and on occasion even major revisions during recycling. Recall it is the consultee who takes ownership of the intervention, and so the consultee may need to recycle the intervention several times before we get a good response. The theory–hypothesis–data collection/analysis–data interpretation cycle continues until the problem appears to be under natural stimulus–consequence control. As you can see, the CHT model is not really about testing per se; it is about a way of practice that combines the best techniques of problem-solving consultation with comprehensive evaluations and multiple data sources.

Practicing Behavioral Neuropsychology

Since we are suggesting that you combine neuropsychological assessment with behavioral methods, In-Depth 4.1 and Table 4.10 review the basics of behavioral interventions for those readers who may not recall the details. As part of the problem-solving model, you need to recognize that antecedent and consequent actions affect the child's learning and behavior

(Crone et al., 2015), and also that cognitive and neuropsychological processes interact with these determinants. Having this understanding allows you to use what cognitive psychologists have called *stimulus–organism–response* (S-O-R) psychology, in which stimulus and response are still important, but the organismic variables (i.e., child neuropsychological processes) help you determine what the best intervention is and how to carry it out. This is not unlike Bandura's (1978) reciprocal determinism model, where one considers the behavior, cognitions, and environment in both understanding the child and in developing interventions that meet the child's needs. The behavior techniques become especially useful in designing the intervention, determining intervention efficacy, and managing contingencies.

IN-DEPTH 4.1. Review of Behavioral Psychology Principles

RESPONDENT CONDITIONING TECHNIQUES

Respondent conditioning is a method of eliciting behavior by manipulating a stimulus. An example of a conditioned stimulus is the teacher's turning on and off the light to cue a child's transition behavior. Behavioral examples might include anxiety about tests or speaking in class, or fear when the teacher raises his or her voice. Common interventions, including relaxation training and systematic desensitization, may be used to treat anxiety responses in students. However, more broadly conceived, variations in stimuli can lead to different behaviors (e.g., varying spacing or size of letters during reading, using simultaneous visual and auditory teacher instructions, using an adapted pencil for sensory problems for writing, tapping on a desk to cue on-task behavior, etc.). Modeling and discriminative stimuli designed to elicit operant behaviors, though not considered respondent techniques, can both be related to stimulus–response psychology.

OPERANT CONDITIONING TECHNIQUES

Operant conditioning is a method of affecting behavior by manipulating the consequences of that behavior. Behaviors that are followed by reinforcing consequences (either presentation of something positive or removal of something negative) will tend to recur. Behaviors that are followed by punishing consequences (either presentation of something negative or removal of something positive) will be less likely to recur, as indicated in Table 4.10. One of the best uses of operant technology is the "Premack principle," in which a less reinforcing behavior is reinforced by a more reinforcing one (e.g., providing computer time after a certain level of reading accuracy is obtained). Positive reinforcement can include natural consequences (these are preferable) or secondary ones (e.g., tokens, points). A good use of negative reinforcement is reducing the workload if a child demonstrates mastery on an assignment.

People are often confused about the difference between *positive reinforcement* (presenting something positive) and *negative reinforcement* (removing something negative). Why do children have tantrums? Not only because they are positively reinforced for having tantrums, but also because their parents are negatively reinforced—they get peace and quiet by giving in to the children. Most interventions in school should use *positive reinforcers*, and these can even be used to teach children *not* to do something, so (we hope) you don't have to use punishment. You identify an alternative behavior, preferably one that is incompatible with the negative behavior, and reinforce that behavior (i.e., differential reinforcement of other, alternative, or incompatible behavior). For example, Taniqua is always running in the halls. Instead of punishing her for running, reinforce her for walking. In some cases, a child may not be able to do the target behavior. In these situations, reinforcing successive approximations of target behaviors, or "shaping," is what we have to do with academic and behavioral deficits.

Is there a place for punishment in the schools? If a child is always being punished at school, it becomes aversive, something to avoid; it may even eventually lead him or her to drop out. A particular teacher who, or a subject that, is punishing may also be seen as aversive. There is another problem with punishment, though: The child isn't actually learning a replacement behavior. We prefer to use school interventions to teach children how to do something, rather than just to suppress negative behavior. If you must use punishment, we recommend that you use negative punishment that involves taking away something positive (either *time out from reinforcement* or *response cost*) combined with differential reinforcement. For example, if Kyle is aggressive on the playground, you can use negative punishment by having him sit on the sidelines and miss 5 minutes of recess, but you must also use positive reinforcement when you see Kyle playing nicely.

As you will recall from training, the schedules of reinforcement influence how a skill will be learned and maintained. Continuous reinforcement is good for skill acquisition, but this acquired skill will also be extinguished quickly, so intermittent reinforcement on a variable-ratio or interval scale is more appropriate. Think about slot machines; infrequent payoffs can maintain betting behavior for a long time. The same thing can happen in a classroom. If a teacher slips and accidentally reinforces an unwanted behavior, that behavior will be maintained longer.

Developing and Evaluating Interventions

After cycling through the first eight steps of CHT evaluation and refining a theory as to what will help the child, the next step is to utilize behavioral strategies that are combined with specific empirically supported instructional methods to help the child learn—through either remediation, accommodations, or both. In Chapters 5–7, we offer a number of interventions for academic skills problems. Some problems transcend academic domain boundaries, and the comorbidity among academic learning and other disorders is quite high. To help you understand the relationship between neuropsychological functioning and academic domains, we have provided a worksheet in Appendix 4.5. This worksheet may be useful in your examination of the academic issues associated with a child's neuropsychological functioning. This ensures that when you identify the cognitive pattern of performance, you are relating it to the academic pattern of performance seen on testing and in the classroom, which should help guide intervention planning and implementation. Taking what you know about the child's current level and pattern of performance, academic interventions, problem-solving consultation, and behavioral techniques, you can design, implement, and evaluate an intervention for him or her.

In CHT, we recommend using single-subject (within-subject or single-case) research

TABLE 4.10. Reinforcement and Punishment

	Provide	Remove
Positive consequence	Positive reinforcement	Negative punishment (response cost)
Negative consequence	Positive punishment	Negative reinforcement

Note. Shaded boxes *increase* the preceding behavior; unshaded boxes *decrease* the behavior.

designs to evaluate the effectiveness of interventions. We believe that practitioners should collect child performance data on a regular basis to ensure that interventions are effective. In this way, progress monitoring in the MTSS model permeates all parts of the balanced practice model and CHT process, so you are truly a data-based problem solver (Burns & Gibbons, 2013). We recommend that similar models be used to evaluate any intervention, whether it is behavioral, academic, cognitive, or socioemotional. These interventions must be individualized based on the teacher, student, and classroom.

In the next section, we review the most useful designs for evaluating school-based interventions, illustrating each intervention model with examples. Keep in mind that we are presenting the ideal research designs to demonstrate the effectiveness of an intervention scientifically; in real life, you may have to modify these designs to be more acceptable and less cumbersome, even if doing this provides less experimental control. Graphing behaviors is an excellent way of demonstrating progress to teachers and students, though, so we do encourage you to use them in progress monitoring. Nothing speaks louder than data in our opinion, and since psychologists are often the data management specialists in schools, this is a good role for you to take on. These visual illustrations show teachers, parents, and administrators the fruits of your intervention efforts. In addition, since graphing can be time consuming, some children can learn to graph their own behavior, and research supports their accuracy in doing so.

Research Designs for Evaluating Interventions

All of the research designs we discuss require two basic concepts. One is that you must have some way of *measuring the outcome* you want. Behaviorists generally call this "taking data," but you can think of it as "progress monitoring" or "checking up on the intervention." You can't simply say, "Jimmy's doing better"; you must have some way to *show* that the child is doing better. The outcome measure you choose depends on the target behavior and the goal of the intervention. Data might include information that the teacher already collects (i.e., authentic data—homework completed, spelling test score, office referrals or detentions, absences, etc.). You might collect information as part of the intervention itself (e.g., math worksheets, CBM probes of reading fluency, flashcards placed in correct and incorrect piles). Students can also collect and chart their own data, which reduces the load on the teacher, as described next.

During consultation, you and the teacher can also develop a data collection plan that interferes very little with the teacher's routine (e.g., child self-monitoring, using a wrist counter, completing end-of-the-period or end-of-the-day checklists). If it is too demanding, the likelihood of successful implementation is unlikely. For behavioral interventions, rating scales can be useful, but in some cases systematic observations can be used to evaluate progress by observing the target behavior directly, using event, duration, latency, and partial- or whole-interval recording. With observational data collection, it is important to use a randomly selected peer at baseline to establish a discrepancy with the target child. Finally, scatterplots are effective for teachers if they are recording behaviors (e.g., recording a + or − for a class period) themselves. Finally, students can take their own data, such as marking a checkmark on a sheet of paper, usually for either occurrence or nonoccurrence of the behavior. Table 4.11 presents some suggestions for outcome measures that can be useful in the classroom.

The second basic concept is that you must have a *baseline* measurement, in addition to measuring the behavior during the intervention. Teachers are generally familiar with just measuring the outcome of teaching, such as giving a test at the end of a chapter. In order to

TABLE 4.11. Examples of Outcome Measures for School-Based Interventions

Outcome area	Possible measures
Several behaviors	• Pre- and post-ratings on a brief behavior rating form. • Daily report card with ratings for day. • Systematic observation using event, duration, latency, partial- or whole-interval recording.
Negative classroom behavior (e.g., calling out, getting out of seat, yelling, aggression)	• Measurement of rate via tally marks, golf wrist counter, or pennies/paper clips transferred from pockets. • Student self-monitoring of behavior on sheet or card.
Serious negative behavior	• Count of office referrals or detentions.
Positive classroom behavior (e.g., raising hand, giving correct answers)	• Measurement of rate or student self-monitoring as above. • Observational data as above.
Attention, on-task behavior	• Periodic classroom observations. • Child self-monitoring of skills.
Academic work completion	• Worksheets or other permanent products. • Measurement of accuracy, rate, or both.
Homework completion	• Completed homework. • Daily report card signed by parent and/or teacher.
Academic skills accuracy	• Correct–incorrect flashcards kept in separate piles by student or peer. • Worksheets graded in percentages correct and recorded in grade book.
Academic skills fluency (speed and accuracy)	• Progress monitoring probes (e.g., DIBELS, AimsWEB).
Academic skills comprehension	• Pre- and posttest with alternate forms.

evaluate the effectiveness of an intervention, you have to measure the child's performance at the start (without the interventions), and then keep measuring as you implement the intervention to see how the child's performance changes. Without having a baseline for comparisons, you won't know whether the child's improvement is really due to the intervention. In describing some of the intervention models that follow, we use the letter *A* to refer to the baseline condition. The other letters (i.e., *B*, *C*) represent whatever interventions you implement.

ABAB/ABAC Designs

The ABAB design is used when you have picked one intervention and you want to see if it works better than the baseline condition (i.e., better than what the teacher would normally do). It is also sometimes called a "reversal design," because you do the intervention, then reverse to baseline for a short while, then do the intervention again. While this is a good way to show that the intervention is really what is affecting the child's performance, and can be published in behavioral journals, it doesn't work well for a situation where your intervention actually teaches the child something new. For example, if you teach a child to break a word into syllables to sound it out, you can't "unteach" that for the reversal phase. It also is not appropriate to do a reversal phase if the behavior you are trying to reduce is harmful to the child or others. For instance, if you are using time-out to reduce hitting, it would be unethical to do a reversal phase. As a result, this design is best for situations where you want to change the *rate* at which a child does something that he or she already knows how to do. For an example of an ABAB design, please see Case Study 4.1 and Figure 4.2.

The ABAC design allows you to compare two different interventions to see whether they are different from the baseline, and to see which is better at changing the child's behavior. Similar to the ABAB design, you first collect baseline data, then implement the first intervention (B), then reverse to baseline, and finally implement the second intervention (C). For instance, after taking baseline data on multistep math addition item accuracy (A), you can determine whether a child is more accurate if he or she draws lines between columns (B), or follows a step-by-step algorithm sheet on how to complete the problems (C). Case Study 4.2 and Figure 4.3 provide an example of an ABAC design.

Multiple-Baseline Design

A multiple-baseline design is useful when you expect the child's learning to be cumulative, so you don't want to reverse success. This design can teach children to display target behaviors across settings, people, or behaviors. For instance, if staying on task is the target behavior, you first seek on-task behavior in one class, then another, and so forth. In this design, you

---

Case Study 4.1. Jared's Impulsive Calling Out

An 8-year-old boy diagnosed with ADHD, Jared, was described by his teacher as extremely impulsive. The behavior that she identified as most problematic was Jared's calling out in class. Systematic observation data suggested that the teacher typically accepted Jared's answer when he called out, but then she often reminded him to raise his hand the next time. After discussing the baseline data with the teacher, we decided that she would use a wrist counter to count whenever Jared called out during whole-group instruction.

Figure 4.2 presents the results for the ABAB intervention designed to reduce his inappropriate call-out behaviors. During the first week, the teacher collected the baseline data. She counted Jared's call-outs without doing anything different about them, and this information was charted. The next week, the teacher continued to count Jared's call-outs, but she ignored him immediately after each call-out, practicing negative punishment. She only acknowledged Jared if he raised his hand first and did not call out, which is differential reinforcement. Notice that, at first, Jared's call-outs increased. This is called an *extinction burst*—a very common finding when a previously rewarded activity is being ignored. After that, Jared's call-outs began to decline. The teacher then returned to baseline for a short time (accepting call-out answers and reminding him to raise his hand), and the call-outs became frequent again. After a few days of this, the intervention was reintroduced. As you look at Figure 4.2, you should notice a few things. Each phase is separated by lines and labeled, so the baseline and intervention phases are clear. Within the baseline phase, Jared was calling out very frequently; the average was about 20 times per day. During the first intervention phase, his call-outs increased at first and then began to decline. As soon as the reversal to baseline took place, they increased again to about 20 times per day. During the second (and final) intervention phase, call-outs declined to an average of only 8 times per day. You can clearly see that the intervention was what was affecting Jared's behavior (this is called *establishing functional control*), because every time the intervention was implemented, he changed his behavior.

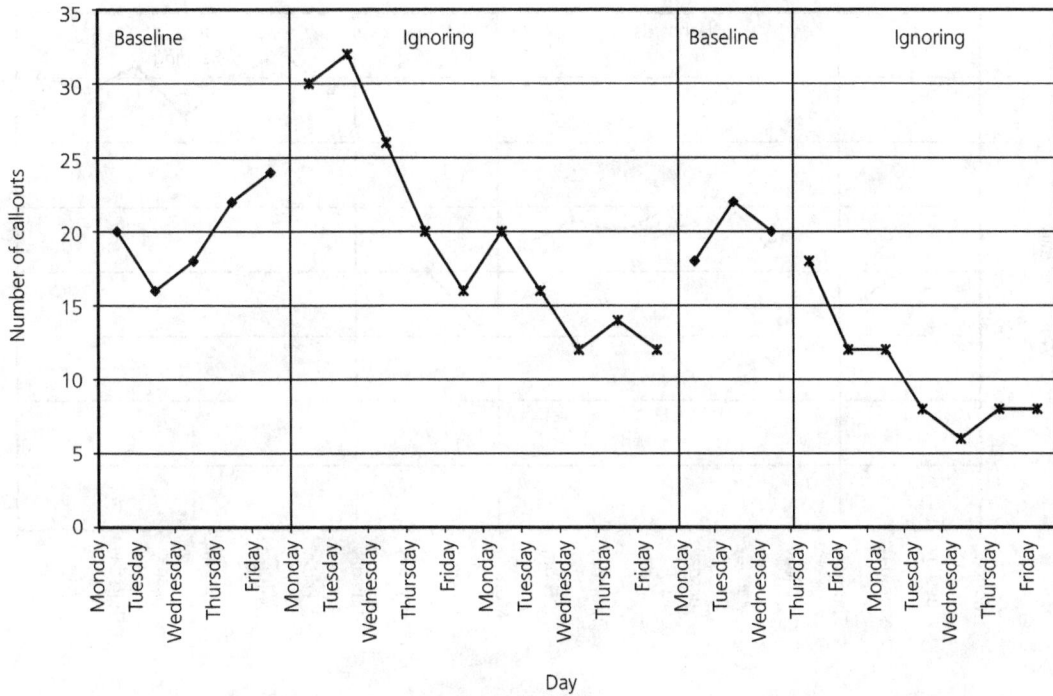

FIGURE 4.2. Jared's calling out.

Case Study 4.2. Increasing Mia's Reading Speed

Mia was a 9-year-old girl who was pleasant, cooperative, and hardworking. However, she was a slow, choppy reader, and her teacher sought support in helping Mia to read more fluently. Mia was in a small reading group with three other children, and the teacher worked individually with her for 15 minutes every day, but she was still struggling. The teacher now had an aide in class and wanted to know what the aide could do with Mia. Based on the CHT evaluation information, one of us (Hale) found that Mia had good phonemic awareness skills, and her phonemic segmentation and blending were not problems, but her word finding and rapid naming skills were quite poor. Hale met with the teacher, and they thought of two possible interventions for Mia: one where the aide would use flash-cards to improve Mia's speed at identifying words, and one where the aide would read orally with Mia to increase the fluency of her reading. They decided that CBM of reading fluency, using daily 1-minute probes, would be a good outcome measure. As can be seen in Figure 4.3, her fluency was quite low at baseline (A). During the first intervention phase (B), the aide pronounced each word for Mia; Mia repeated it; Mia and the aide then practiced with the flashcards for about 10 minutes; and they finished with another 1-minute CBM probe. After this intervention, the teacher returned Mia to the baseline condition (A), but the aide continued to take CBM probes during this time. Finally, the second intervention phase was introduced (C). This intervention involved the aide's reading the passage to Mia one time with expression and fluency, and then their reading it together in tandem for about 10 minutes. Again, the sessions ended with another 1-minute CBM probe. As you can see from looking at Mia's chart, the flashcard drill improved her fluency over baseline, but the tandem reading was much more effective. This is not to say that tandem reading is a better intervention for all children; it just appeared to be better for Mia.

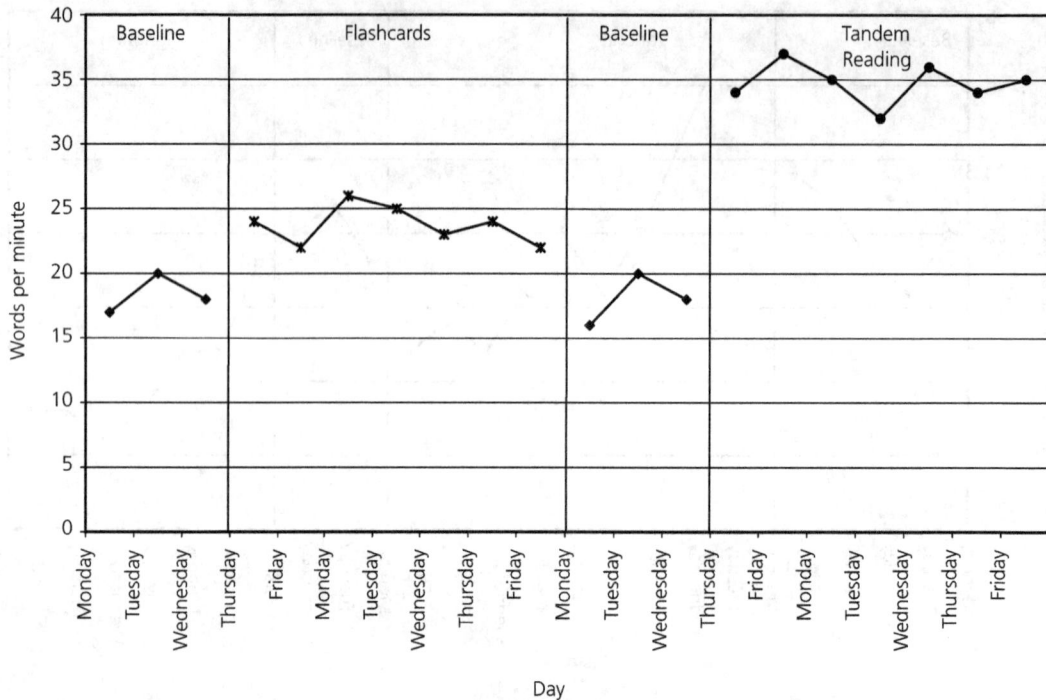

FIGURE 4.3. Mia's reading fluency.

collect baseline data in two or more subjects or at two or more times during the day. Then you start the intervention in one subject or at one time during the day, while continuing to take baseline data at the other time(s). Later, you introduce the intervention in the other subject or at the other time. If the child's performance changes in each setting only when the intervention is in place, you will know that the intervention is responsible for the change. An example of this design can be found in Case Study 4.3 and Figure 4.4.

Pre- and Posttest Design

A pre- and posttest design is useful when the teacher, student, or you can't collect data every day, but you want to measure the effectiveness of an intervention via direct observation, test, or rating scale. Although it is more difficult to establish functional control of the behavior at any given time, it is an easier method of data collection and is more likely to be acceptable to teachers. Keep in mind that if the intervention or data collection methods are too difficult or time consuming, they are unlikely to happen with integrity. Additionally, some data are better than no data, so a pre–post design may be optimal in some situations where resources are limited. For this design, it is important to choose a test (preferably one with alternate forms) or a rating scale that can be given repeatedly with minimal practice effects. There is increasing evidence that direct behavior ratings, including daily report cards, are a reliable and valid way to frequently assess behaviors in school (Miller et al., 2019). The pretest results become your baseline, and then you test again after implementation of the intervention to judge its effectiveness. Observations and brief rating scales can be used repeatedly if you choose to gather multiple data points during the intervention. Case Study 4.4 and Figure 4.5 provide an example of how to use a pre- and posttest design.

Case Study 4.3. Ellen's Accuracy Problem

Ellen was a 7-year-old girl who presented as a fast, careless worker. She reportedly completed her seatwork as fast as possible, without worrying about the accuracy of her responses. One of us (Fiorello) met with Ellen's teacher, and we decided to try to increase Ellen's accuracy by using rewards for correct responding. The teacher used Ellen's number correct on her seatwork papers to measure the outcome. She made sure that there were exactly 10 questions on each worksheet in math and spelling, and noted in her grade book the number correct for each day. For the first week, the teacher collected baseline data in both subjects for each day, and these data were charted on a multiple-baseline graph (see Figure 4.4). After collecting a week of baseline data, the teacher explained to Ellen that she could earn 1 point for each spelling word she copied correctly during seatwork, and the points could be traded for free time at the end of the morning classes. At the same time, Ellen's math work was kept in the baseline condition, with no rewards offered. As you can see from Ellen's chart, her spelling accuracy improved when rewards were added, but her math remained inaccurate. The next Monday, the teacher explained that the point system would apply to math as well, and as you can see from the figure, Ellen's accuracy in math improved thereafter.

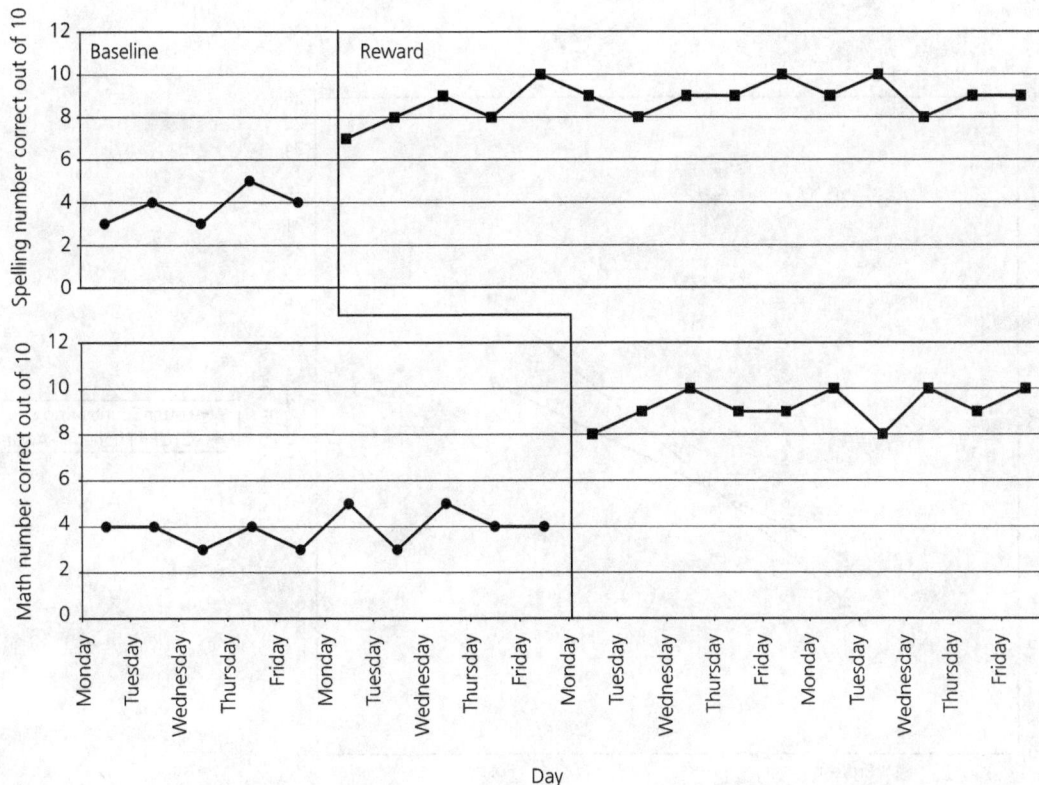

FIGURE 4.4. Ellen's accuracy.

Case Study 4.4. Herman's Auditory Processing

Herman was a boy with a common problem: a history of frequent ear infections (otitis media) and poor auditory processing. He was having difficulty learning the letter sounds in his kindergarten class. His teacher referred him to the reading specialist, who arranged for Herman to complete a 6-week computer-based auditory processing and phonics program. Before Herman began the program, one of us (Fiorello) was called in to develop a method for monitoring the efficacy of the program. We agreed that Fiorello would administer the CTOPP-2 and CBM of the alphabet sounds and would chart his scores, as depicted in Figure 4.5. After 6 weeks, Fiorello administered both tests again. Since the CTOPP-2 has age-based SSs, you can see that Herman's auditory processing improved over the course of the program. In addition, charting his improvement in letter sound knowledge helped the teacher compare Herman to other children, to guide her expectations for his curricular progress.

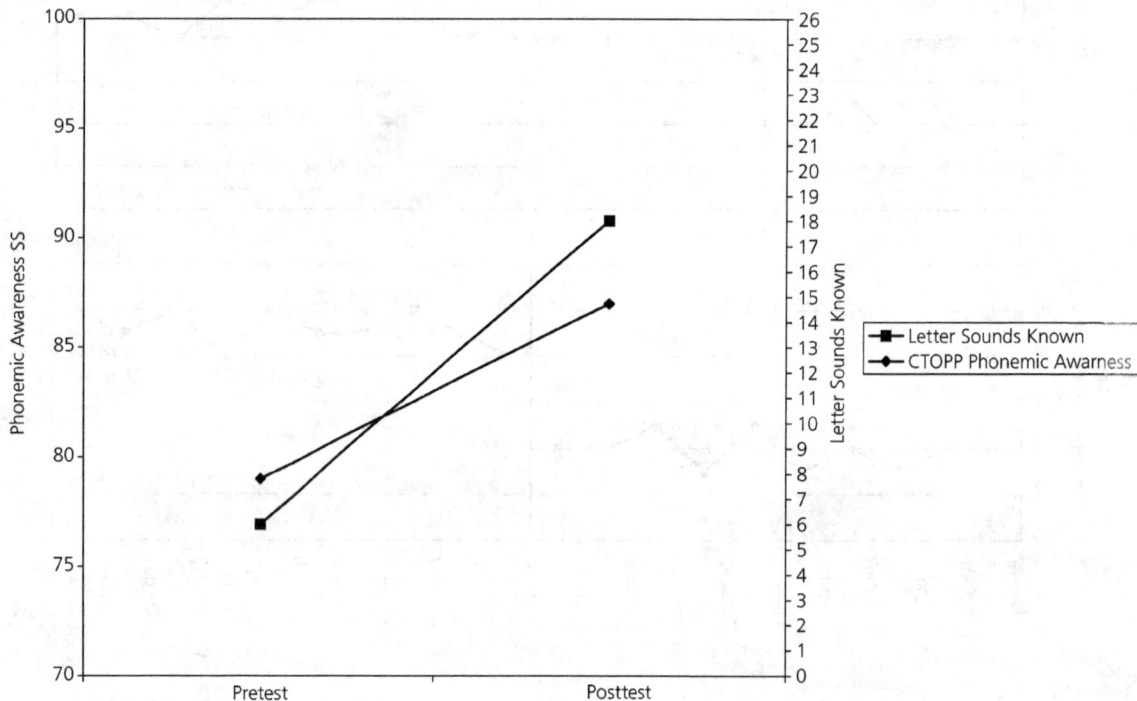

FIGURE 4.5. Herman's auditory processing and letter-sound knowledge.

CBM Progress Monitoring

CBM is useful for evaluating the effectiveness of instructional interventions on reading, mathematics, and writing. A brief probe is completed for several days during baseline, and then repeated every 1–2 days following the intervention session. To use this method, you have to determine the performance discrepancy (the child's functioning relative to peers), the goal for intervention (where you want the child to be after a period of time–usually where peers will be at that time), and the length of the intervention, all of which are somewhat subjective and dependent on a number of factors, including the severity of the child's problem and the cognitive functioning of the child.

CBM data are plotted to gauge progress over time, hence the name progress monitoring of performance. An *aimline* is drawn between the current functioning and the goal that has been set for the student. The beginning of the line is determined by the child's baseline performance or behavior; the end of the line is determined by where the child should be, compared to his or her peers, and how long it will take for the child to "catch up" once the intervention is in place. Unfortunately, there are no explicit guidelines for "how long it should take." For instance, if the child is 2 years behind, saying that he or she will make it up in a month is unrealistic, and would produce a very steep slope, ensuring in essence they would not respond to the intervention. Conversely, it is inappropriate to give a child too long to catch up, even though it might make them look like a responder throughout the process. After you establish an aimline, a *trendline* is drawn and recalculated regularly. The trendline shows the rate of improvement over time. If the trendline is below the aimline for several data points, the intervention should be adjusted or changed, or possibly you have set too high a goal for the child. Case Study 4.5 and Figure 4.6 highlight the use of CBM progress monitoring.

Case Study 4.5. Beverly's Limited Expressive Language

When one of us (Fiorello) was called in to consult with Beverly's teacher, Beverly was having considerable difficulty with expressive language, primarily because she spoke very little during conversations with her teacher and peers. CHT results revealed difficulty with word retrieval, oral fluency, and expressive syntax. Data collection with an audio recorder began, and Beverly's oral fluency at baseline was found to be only 23 words per minute on average (see Figure 4.6). Her teacher set a goal of 45 words per minute, and the teacher and Fiorello decided that a peer tutoring program would be implemented. The teacher picked a child who was not only friendly with Beverly, but also talkative, social, caring, and supportive. Each time the two children would get together, they would discuss a topic of interest. To facilitate this process, the teacher brainstormed possible topics with them before the intervention. As you can see, the peer tutoring improved Beverly's oral fluency at first, but on Days 10, 11, and 12, Beverly's fluency scores fell below the aimline. When three data points fall below the aimline, a decision point is reached. This means that it is time either to adjust or change the intervention, or to readjust the aimline. In Beverly's case, this ensured that goals would be set at a level where they could realistically be attained, while still ensuring that Beverly was making appropriate progress. It was decided that Beverly's goal might have been a little ambitious; however, she was making progress in the program and was developing a good relationship with the peer.

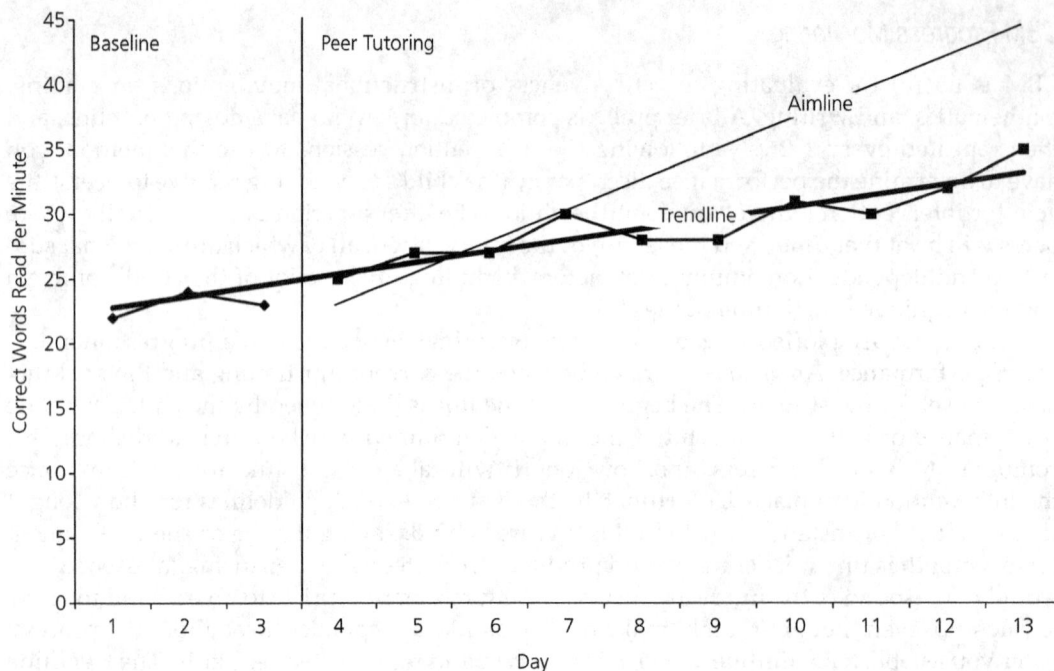

FIGURE 4.6. Beverly's CBM chart.

Multiple-Intervention Design

Before we leave our section on behavioral neuropsychology and problem-solving consultation, it is important to recognize that not all intervention designs discussed will fit nicely
with the needs of a child, teacher, or parent. Certainly you want experimental control and
good outcome data, but beyond that, you have to be sensitive to the needs of all parties, or
the intervention effort will not be effective. Interventions that are easy are preferred, but they
may not be effective. Others may be labor-intensive and have good experimental control,
but because they are so cumbersome, treatment adherence or integrity is limited. This is
where you, as the consultant, must work with the consultee to take into account the nature
of the problem, the environmental determinants of the problem, and the resources available
to affect behavior change. Schools that are implementing MTSS may already have progress
monitoring procedures in place; in other cases, you will have to develop a data collection
system that is not intrusive. We have found that pretest–posttest designs, and ongoing monitoring using direct behavior ratings or CBM probes, are the most acceptable to teachers. Case
Study 4.6 and Figure 4.7 provide an example of alternative treatments for a child who does
not respond easily to interventions.

Linking Assessment to Intervention: A Case Study

Considerations and Caveats

Now that we have given you a good understanding of assessment practices and measures,
brain–behavior relationships, and consultation and intervention techniques, the next step

Case Study 4.6. Coping with Gary's OCD

Gary was a student diagnosed with OCD. His classroom teacher's main concern was Gary's incessant questioning about assignments during seatwork. Gary typically asked for clarification of the directions, and the meaning of individual items. The teacher wanted to decrease Gary's questioning and increase his on-task behavior. She agreed to count Gary's questions with a wrist counter during the seatwork period in her class. As can be seen in Figure 4.7, Gary's baseline average was a little over 10 questions per period. We decided to try a number of interventions, starting with the easiest to implement and gradually adding more intrusive ones. This called for a variation on the ABAC design, where the interventions were cumulative (it might be called an A-B-BC-BCD design). First, the teacher developed a checklist for completing seatwork, and she taught Gary to use it to answer his own questions. She then laminated it and let him check off each item for himself. During this intervention, Gary's questions decreased slightly, to an average of about eight per period. The next intervention added was a set of five tokens that Gary had to use to ask questions. He would turn in one token every time he asked a question; any question after that would not be answered. Gary's questions decreased again, eventually settling at five per period. At this point, the teacher added one more intervention: She provided Gary a reward—a choice of activity during the last 5 minutes of class—if he had one token left at the end of the period. This lowered Gary's questions to four immediately. If the teacher had felt that even fewer questions would be allowed (based on what was normally acceptable in class, perhaps one or two), she could have gradually increased the number of tokens necessary for a reward.

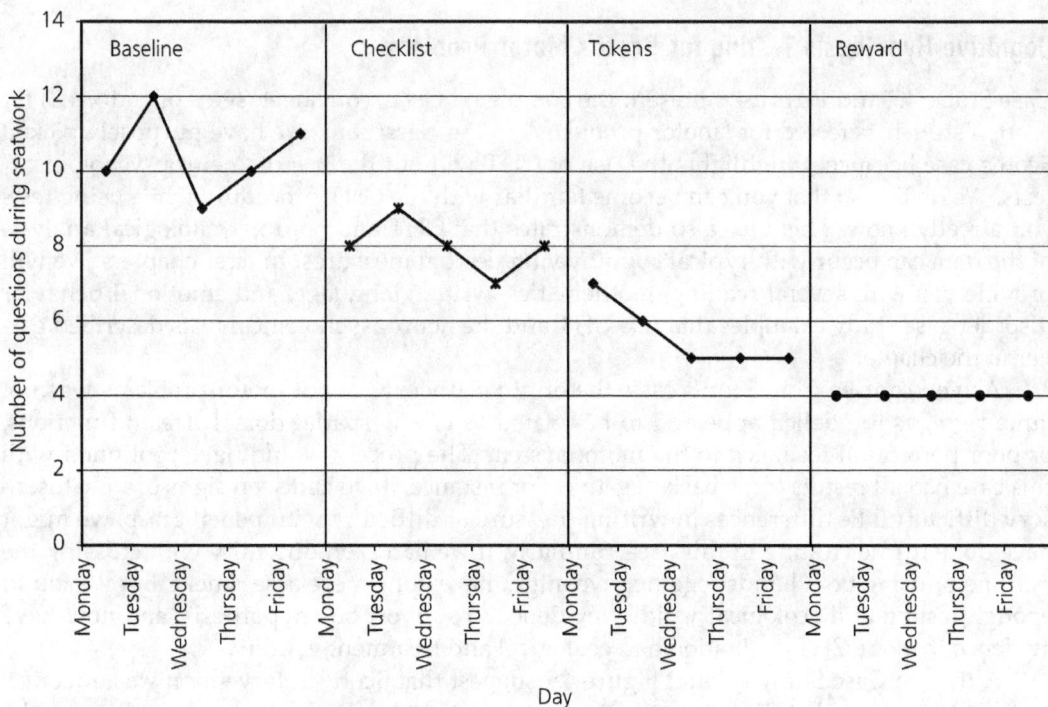

FIGURE 4.7. Gary's teacher questions.

is to bridge the gap between these apparently disparate areas of psychology. We provide you with one more case study, and detailed information in Chapters 5–8, in an attempt to make assessment information meaningful for individualized interventions for children with unique assets and deficits. You may be disappointed to find that we don't offer you diagnostic–prescriptive advice in the following chapters. We feel that this is where the early researchers on aptitude–treatment interactions went astray: Not all children learn the same way, even if they show similar neuropsychological profiles, so we don't oversimplify by saying, "If you have this disorder, then do this intervention." There is no guarantee that the first attempt at intervention will be successful, even with CHT, because most times we need to recycle or "tweak" the intervention until response is achieved. That is the thing about CHT, its recursive scientific method approach ensures hypotheses are generated and tested using data, with new hypotheses developed, and data collected and evaluated, until response is achieved.

To paraphrase an old adage, some interventions work for some children some of the time, but no interventions work for all children all of the time. You may feel confident that you have a good understanding of a child's psychological and neuropsychological strengths and weaknesses, but if you don't have ecological and treatment validity, then your results are of questionable value. Even if you have a good handle on the problem and the findings have ecological validity, the intervention you and the teacher choose may be ineffective. Don't dismiss the original findings; rather, try to understand why the intervention the teacher thought would be effective was not, and try to modify it or try another intervention. This recycling of interventions is necessary, whether you use a CHT approach or a regular behavioral consultation method. We provide you with assessment and intervention information about various learning and behavior disorder subtypes, but it is up to you to use CHT with the techniques presented in this chapter to individualize interventions for the children you serve.

Cognitive Hypothesis Testing for Scott's Motor Problem

Case Study 4.7 and Figure 4.8 present the completed CHT worksheet (see Appendix 4.3) for Scott, a student referred for "motor problems" in the classroom. We have purposely picked Scott's case because it highlights the use of CHT without the use of "neuropsychological" tests. We do this so that you can become familiar with the CHT procedure while using tests you already know. This case also demonstrates that CHT and neuropsychological analysis of the data can occur with typical cognitive/intellectual measures. In later chapters, we will provide you with several reading, mathematics, written language, and emotional/behavior disorder case study examples that use CHT and the neuropsychological tests described earlier in the chapter.

As you can see from Scott's case, the original "theory" about motor problems was not quite right, as the deficit appeared to be related to visual–spatial dorsal stream functions, or poor perceptual feedback to the motor system. The process would have continued with this case had all results come back negative. For instance, if we had seen signs of somatosensory difficulty, like differences in writing pressure or difficulty with pencil grasp, we might have done further testing in this area. Similarly, if we had seen difficulty with crossing the midline or using both hands together, we might have done more assessment. But we found enough testing and ecological validity evidence to support our hypothesis, and now have evidence that our CHT evaluation had ecological and treatment validity.

Although Case Study 4.7 and Figure 4.9 suggest that Scott's intervention was effective, it should be noted that Scott was receiving occupational therapy during this time, so the positive results could have been related to this intervention. Obviously, as time went on, both interventions may have had a positive and complementary effect. This is not a good empirical practice per se, as we don't want two interventions going on at the same time. But in real life, students will be receiving multiple interventions, and it may not be feasible to evaluate the effectiveness of each individually. The bottom line is that we need to help children, and if they get better and we have data that shows it, we are better off as a result. It might not get our case study published in the *Journal of Applied Behavior Analysis*, but it will lead to successful outcomes, and that is why this is a practitioner book, not a research one. Now that we have the methods to link assessment to intervention in multiple tiers of service delivery, the remainder of this book will focus on the neuropsychological aspects of specific academic and behavior problems experienced by the children we serve, and the interventions to help them achieve success.

Case Study 4.7. CHT for Scott's Motor Problem

Scott, age 9, had attention, social, and handwriting problems. The teacher referred him for "fine-motor problems," because his work was always messy, and there were many erase marks and smudges on the work he turned in. His poor alignment of columns resulted in many math calculation errors on multistep problems. After prereferral strategies were unsuccessful at improving the quality of this work, he was referred for a comprehensive CHT evaluation. As can be seen in Figure 4.8, the initial assessment with the WISC-V suggested strengths in auditory working memory, and three possible weaknesses: spatial visualization, visual–motor coordination, and/or visual memory. Having developed a theory as to what was difficult for Scott, one of us (Fiorello) needed to test my hypotheses one by one to see which ones were correct.

To examine these possible problems, Fiorello wanted to use untimed visual processing tasks that did not require motor output. She picked the WJ-IV Spatial Relations and Picture Recognition subtests to look at spatial visualization and visual memory. Then she decided to choose a task measuring motor coordination and speed without significant visual processing to look at motor functioning. For this, she picked the motor portion of the Beery Developmental Test of Visual–Motor Integration (VMI). Based on the overall profile and results of these hypothesis testing subtests, only the Spatial Relations subtest was impaired; this suggested that Scott's difficulty was more of a dorsal stream problem than a ventral stream or frontal motor problem.

However, these findings would be considered tentative until Fiorello checked to make sure that the results had ecological validity. The information from the teacher interview and ratings, classroom behavior observations, and work samples provided the necessary confirmation that Scott had difficulty with spatial processing and perceptual feedback to the motor system. At this stage, it is important to remember to check for possible alternative explanations to the hypothesis, in order to avoid confirmation bias. For Scott, you will notice that work samples showed problems with spatial organization on the page and poor column alignment in math. In addition, the teacher interview indicated that Scott had problems during recess and gym with respecting peers' personal space. As a result, these apparently disparate findings were entered in the ecological validity section.

At this point, Fiorello felt she had a fairly clear understanding of Scott's strengths and weaknesses. Her understanding of neuropsychology helped to clarify why Scott was having attention and social problems as well, since right parietal lobe dysfunction can lead to neglect of self and environment. She now had a "theory" as to why Scott was having problems with learning and social functioning, and could meet with the teacher to discuss interventions, developing hypotheses about what interventions might work, implementing the most probable one, and determining whether it was successful.

To begin this process, Fiorello completed the assessment of academic skill problems and cognitive weaknesses. Next, she examined resources available and cognitive strengths for possible use in the intervention. For Scott, the team referred him for occupational therapy, and made classroom recommendations to improve his current academic functioning. She met with the teacher, and we decided to focus on his messy work/handwriting problem. The teacher liked the idea of using graph paper, and we decided that Scott would be rewarded for staying within the lines on his writing assignments first, and on his math assignments second. After completing his assignments, Scott completed a checklist that indicated how many times his writing went outside the prescribed lines. For each word or problem Scott stayed within the lines on, he received a token reinforcer that could be traded in at the end of the day for a computer time reward. This setup called for a multiple-baseline design as described earlier. In Figure 4.9, notice how Scott showed some improvement in writing, but math difficulties were still prominent. After the intervention was implemented during math class, Scott began to improve in both areas.

Student's name: _Scott_____ Age: _9-9___ Grade: _4_____

Reason for referral: _Messy written work, poor handwriting_____

Preliminary hypotheses—Based on presenting problem and initial assessment, the following cognitive strengths and weaknesses are hypothesized:

Strengths:

Auditory working memory

Possible weaknesses:

Spatial visualization
Motor coordination
Visual memory

Hypothesis testing—Follow up with related construct tests:

Areas of suspected weakness:

Spatial visualization
Motor coordination
Visual memory

Follow-up tests:

WJ-IV Spatial Relations
Beery VMI inc. motor section
WJ-IV Picture Recognition

Strengths/weaknesses:

Spatial relations on WJ-IV well below average—Weak spatial visualization
Motor coordination on VMI average—No motor weakness
Picture recognition on WJ-IV average—No visual memory weakness

Associated with academic and/or behavior problems?:

Yes—Spatial visualization weakness can lead to poor handwriting (spacing and letter formation) and messy work layout on page.

(continued)

FIGURE 4.8. Completed Cognitive Hypothesis Testing Worksheet.

Ecological validity—Information from observations and teacher ratings:

Strengths:
Participating in class discussion

Possible weaknesses:
Spatial organization—layout on page, trouble aligning columns in math, difficulty with peers in recess and gym re: "space"

Evaluation summary—Based on analysis of all evaluation information, the following cognitive strengths and weaknesses are identified, and concordance or discordance is calculated if necessary:

Cognitive strengths:
Oral language
Auditory memory

Concordant with academic and/or behavioral strengths?:
Yes—class discussion relies on oral language and auditory skills.

Weaknesses:
Spatial visualization and organization in space

Concordant with academic and/or behavioral weaknesses?:
Yes—spatial visualization is related to work layout, handwriting, and interpersonal space issues.

Discordant with cognitive strengths?:
Yes—spatial visualization is mediated by right occipital lobe, while oral language and auditory memory is primarily mediated by left hemisphere.

(continued)

FIGURE 4.8. (*continued*)

Summary of evaluation information for intervention development	
Academic/behavioral presenting problems: Messy work Poor handwriting	**Cognitive weaknesses:** Spatial organization and processes
Resources for intervention in environment: Consultant available Special education and OT consult and materials	**Cognitive strengths:** Oral language Auditory memory
Potential interventions: Use paper with raised lines and graph paper for written work. Allow dictation for lengthy written assignments. Teach keyboarding skills. Work with psychologist on interpersonal space issues.	

FIGURE 4.8. (*continued*)

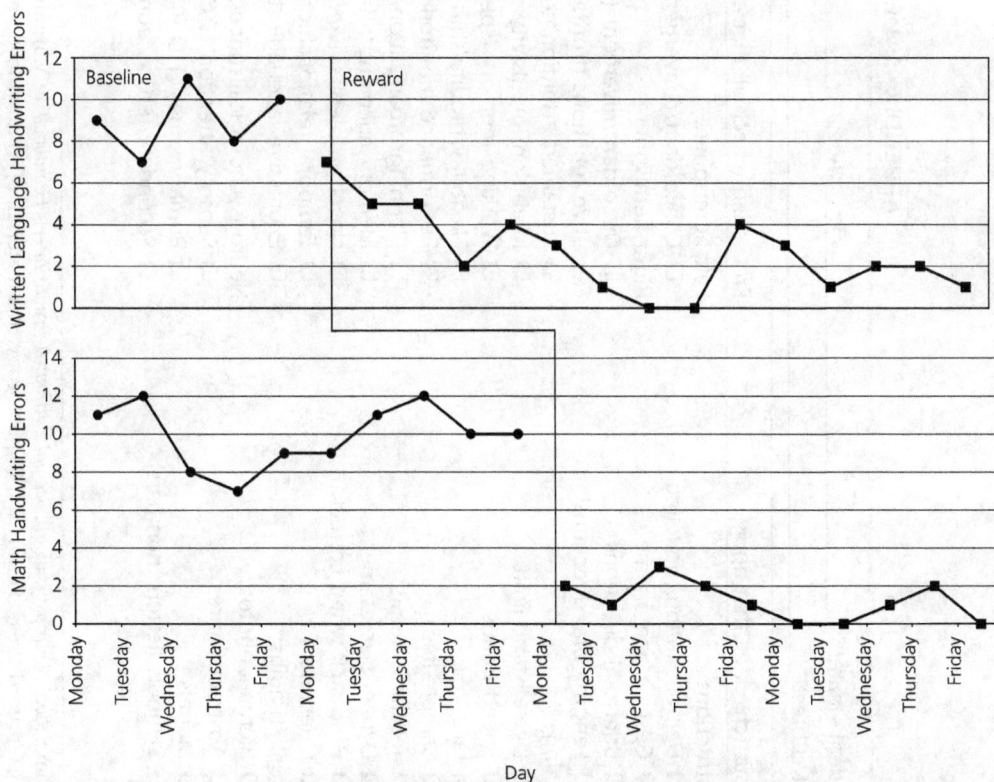

FIGURE 4.9. Scott's graph paper intervention.

APPENDIX 4.1. DEMANDS ANALYSIS

Student's name: _____ Age: _____ Grade: _____

Test/subtest

Input (check all that apply)	Processing (check all that apply)	Output (check all that apply)
Instructions ☐ Demonstration/modeling ☐ Gesture/pantomime ☐ Brief oral directions ☐ Lengthy oral directions **Timing** ☐ Overall time limit ☐ Speed bonus **Teaching** ☐ Sample item ☐ Teaching item(s) ☐ Dynamic assessment ☐ Feedback when correct ☐ Querying **Visual stimulus** ☐ Pictures/photos ☐ Abstract figures ☐ Models ☐ Symbols (letters, numbers)	**Left hemisphere** ☐ Concordant/convergent ("explicit") **Right hemisphere** ☐ Discordant/divergent ("implicit") **Executive functions (frontal–subcortical circuits)** ☐ Sustained attention/concentration ☐ Inhibition/impulsivity ☐ Working memory (specify _____) ☐ Flexibility/modify/shift set ☐ Performance monitoring/benefit from feedback ☐ Planning/organization/strategy use ☐ Memory encoding/retrieval ☐ Novel problem solving/reasoning ☐ Temporal relationships/sequential processing ☐ Expressive language (L R) **Neuropsychological functional domains** ☐ Sensory attention (T O P) (L R) ☐ Primary zones (T O P) (L R) ☐ Secondary/tertiary zones (T O P) (L R)	**Oral** ☐ Brief oral ☐ Lengthy oral ☐ Report of strategy use **Motor** ☐ Fine-motor–point ☐ Fine-motor—graphomotor ☐ Fine-motor—manipulatives (e.g., block pictures) ☐ Visual–sensory–motor integration ☐ Gross motor **Written language** ☐ Brief written response ☐ Lengthy written response **Response format** ☐ Open/free-response ☐ Constrained/multiple choice

☐ Written language
☐ Large–small
☐ Color important
Auditory stimulus
☐ Brief verbal
☐ Lengthy verbal
☐ Spoken
☐ Audio recording
  (headphones used? Y N)
☐ Background noise
Content
L M H Cultural knowledge
L M H English-language knowledge
L M H Emotional content

☐ Prior learning/long-term memory
☐ Sensory–motor coordination
☐ Multimodal integration
☐ Dorsal stream (occipital–parietal)
☐ Ventral stream (occipital–temporal)
☐ Receptive language (L R)
CHC abilities and narrow abilities
Higher-level processing
☐ Gf—fluid reasoning
☐ Gl—long-term storage and retrieval____
☐ Gr—retrieval fluency____
☐ Gv—visual processing
☐ Ga—auditory processing
Lower-level processing
☐ Gs—processing speed____
☐ Gwm—working memory capacity____
Acquired knowledge and achievement
☐ Gc—crystallized intelligence____
☐ Grw—reading/writing
☐ Gq—quantitative ability

Other
Input: _____
_____
_____
Processing: _____
_____
Output: _____
_____
Comments: _____
_____

In the "Input" column: Y N, yes or no ; L M H, low, medium, or high. In the "Processing" column: L R, left or right ; T O P, temporal, occipital, or parietal ; CHC, Cattell–Horn–Carroll.

APPENDIX 4.2. BRIEF DEMANDS ANALYSIS

Student's name: _____ Age: _____ Grade: _____

Test/subtest	Input	Processing	Output
Strengths			
Weaknesses			

APPENDIX 4.3. COGNITIVE HYPOTHESIS-TESTING WORKSHEET

Student's name: _____ Age: _____ Grade: _____

Reason for referral: _____

_____

_____

Preliminary hypotheses—Based on presenting problem and initial assessment, the following cognitive strengths and weaknesses are hypothesized:

Strengths:

Possible weaknesses:

Hypothesis testing—Follow up with related construct tests:

Areas of suspected weakness:

Follow-up tests:

Strengths/weaknesses:

Associated with academic and/or behavior problems?:

(continued)

Ecological validity—Information from observations and teacher ratings:

Strengths:

Possible weaknesses:

Evaluation summary—Based on analysis of all evaluation information, the following cognitive strengths and weaknesses are identified, and concordance or discordance is calculated if necessary:

Cognitive strengths:

Concordant with academic and/or behavioral strengths?:

Weaknesses:

Concordant with academic and/or behavioral weaknesses?:

Discordant with cognitive strengths?:

(continued)

APPENDIX 4.3. *(page 3 of 3)*

Summary of evaluation information for intervention development	
Academic/behavioral presenting problems:	**Cognitive weaknesses:**
Resources for intervention in environment:	**Cognitive strengths:**
Potential interventions:	

APPENDIX 4.4. NEUROPSYCHOLOGICAL ASSESSMENT OBSERVATIONS CHECKLIST

Student's Name: _____ Age: _____ Grade: _____

1. Pays close attention to task.	1 2 3 4 5	Has difficulty with selective or sustained attention.
2. Attention is consistent despite distraction.	1 2 3 4 5	Is easily distracted by external stimuli.
3. Shows good impulse control.	1 2 3 4 5	Is overly impulsive.
4. Shows appropriate activity level.	1 2 3 4 5	Has inappropriate activity level (specify: low or high).
5. Affect/mood is appropriate.	1 2 3 4 5	Affect is not appropriate (specify:).
6. Works quickly when appropriate.	1 2 3 4 5	Pace is too slow.
7. Can hold information in working memory to respond to questions.	1 2 3 4 5	Has difficulty retaining information in working memory to answer questions.
8. Can switch easily from one task to another.	1 2 3 4 5	Has difficulty switching tasks.
9. Plans/organizes before responding.	1 2 3 4 5	Responds without planning or organization.
10. Evaluates performance/modifies behavior.	1 2 3 4 5	Does not evaluate performance or modify behavior.
11. Comprehends orally presented information.	1 2 3 4 5	Does not comprehend orally presented information.
12. Follows directions or answers questions without repetition.	1 2 3 4 5	Requires frequent repetition of directions and questions.
13. Has adequate syntax and grammar.	1 2 3 4 5	Has difficulty with syntax and grammar.
14. Completes directions with one or more steps.	1 2 3 4 5	Has difficulty with sequential processing of directions.
15. Expresses self fluently.	1 2 3 4 5	Has difficulty expressing self fluently.
16. Does not exhibit word-finding difficulty.	1 2 3 4 5	Has word-finding difficulty.
17. Verbalizations are logical and organized.	1 2 3 4 5	Verbalizations are rambling and tangential.
18. No difficulty with nonliteral, metaphoric, or figurative language.	1 2 3 4 5	Language is overly literal and concrete.
19. Articulation is clear.	1 2 3 4 5	Has poor articulation or phonemic paraphasias.
20. Can easily recall information from long-term memory.	1 2 3 4 5	Has difficulty recalling information from long-term memory.

(continued)

APPENDIX 4.4. *(page 2 of 2)*

21. Learns new material without repetition.	1 2 3 4 5	Needs many repetitions to learn new material.
22. Can learn new associations with few errors.	1 2 3 4 5	Makes frequent errors when learning new associations.
23. Can perceive and differentiate colors.	1 2 3 4 5	Appears to be partially or completely color-blind.
24. Easily discriminates/perceives visual stimuli.	1 2 3 4 5	Has poor visual acuity or visual perception.
25. Perceives visual stimuli throughout visual fields.	1 2 3 4 5	Has visual neglect. (Side? _)
26. Easily understands body language.	1 2 3 4 5	Has difficulty understanding body language.
27. Perceives spatial/holistic/global relationships.	1 2 3 4 5	Does not readily identify spatial/holistic/global relationships.
28. Shows no spatial configuration breaks.	1 2 3 4 5	Shows configuration breaks.
29. Shows no directional confusion.	1 2 3 4 5	Has directional confusion/orientation problems/reversals.
30. Perceives objects and faces.	1 2 3 4 5	Has difficulty perceiving objects and faces.
31. Can easily perceive auditory stimuli.	1 2 3 4 5	Has difficulty perceiving auditory stimuli in the R _ and/or L _ ear.
32. Hears and uses prosody effectively.	1 2 3 4 5	Has difficulty with receptive or expressive prosody.
33. Perceives tactile stimuli well.	1 2 3 4 5	Has difficulty discriminating tactile stimuli.
34. Handles materials smoothly.	1 2 3 4 5	Is clumsy when handling materials.
35. Has good pencil control/graphomotor skills.	1 2 3 4 5	Has poor pencil control/graphomotor skills.
36. Has established handedness (side? __).	1 2 3 4 5	Has not established handedness.
37. Has good bimanual control.	1 2 3 4 5	Has difficulty with bimanual control or crossing the midline.
38. Has good gross-motor skill.	1 2 3 4 5	Has poor gross-motor skill (clumsy or awkward).
39. Has good balance.	1 2 3 4 5	Has poor balance.
40. Has good muscle tone.	1 2 3 4 5	Has tone problems (too floppy, too rigid).

APPENDIX 4.5. PSYCHOLOGICAL PROCESSES WORKSHEET

Client's name: _____ Date of birth: _____

Clinician's name: _____ Date: _____

Identify the psychological processes associated with the student's identified learning deficits with a (–) sign, and the strengths with a (+) sign. Remember that more than one psychological process should be involved for identified deficits.

Attention and Executive Frontal Lobe Processes

	Basic reading	Reading comp.	Basic math	Math reasoning	Spelling	Written lang.	Oral exp.	Listening comp.
Sustained attention								
Selective attention								
Overall tone								
Planning								
Strategizing								
Sequencing								
Organization								
Monitoring								
Evaluation								
Inhibition								
Shifting/flexibility								
Maintenance								
Change								
Motor overactivity								
Motor underactivity								
Constructional apraxia								
Ideomotor apraxia								
Ideational apraxia								
Visual scanning								
Sensory–motor integration								
Expressive language								
Long-term memory retrieval								
Working memory								
Perseveration								
Grammar								
Syntax								
Math algorithm								
Problem solving								
Fluency/nonfluent aphasia								
Dysnomia								

(continued)

APPENDIX 4.5. *(page 2 of 3)*

Attention and Executive Frontal Lobe Processes *(continued)*

	Basic reading	Reading comp.	Basic math	Math reasoning	Spelling	Written lang.	Oral exp.	Listening comp.
Paraphasia								
Circumlocution								
Confabulation								
Concept formation								

Comments: _____

Concordant/Convergent Left-Hemisphere Processes

	Basic reading	Reading comp.	Basic math	Math reasoning	Spelling	Written lang.	Oral exp.	Listening comp.
Sensory memory								
Discrimination								
Perception (meaningful)								
Phonemic awareness								
Phonemic segmentation								
Phonemic blending								
Sound–symbol association								
Morpheme comprehension								
Lexicon/word comp.								
Sentence comprehension								
Literal/concrete/explicit comp.								
Math fact automaticity								
Long-term memory								
Declarative memory								
Automaticity								
Simple/rote sensory–motor integration								
Detail perception								
Sight-word recognition								
Local/part/fine processing								
Dysphonetic								
Convergent thought								
Concordant thought								
Fluent aphasia								
Paraphasia								
Neologism								
Left–right confusion								

Comments: _____

(continued)

APPENDIX 4.5. *(page 3 of 3)*

Discordant/Divergent Right-Hemisphere Processes

	Basic reading	Reading comp.	Basic math	Math reasoning	Spelling	Written lang.	Oral exp.	Listening comp.
Sensory memory								
Discrimination								
Perception (abstract)								
Spatial processing								
Perceptual analysis								
Visualization								
Ambiguity								
Asomatognosia								
Prosopagnosia								
Agnosia								
Neglect								
Object visual perception								
Spatial visual perception								
Grapheme awareness								
Sensory integration								
Complex sensory–motor integration								
Constructional apraxia								
Prediction								
Inference								
Metaphor/idiom/humor								
Nonliteral/figurative/implicit comp.								
Social perception/judgment								
Prosody								
Word Choice								
Holistic/global/gestalt processing								
Whole/coarse processing								
Novelty/new learning/encoding								
Pragmatics								
Facial/body gestures								
Problem solving								
Dyseidetic								
Divergent thought								
Discordant thought								
Fluent aphasia								
Paraphasia								
Neologism								

Comments: _____

Chapter 5

The Neuropsychology of Reading and Reading Disorders

Reading and Brain Functioning

The Word Recognition Emphasis and Missed Opportunities

In the early 2000s, most of the empirical reading research focused on single-word reading, because reading decoding or word recognition skills were often cited as the major prerequisite for reading comprehension (Lerner & Johns, 2015). In fact, some have argued that underlying all reading competency is word reading, with phonological awareness the most important predictor of word-reading skills. It was thought that the identification of reading disorders (RDs) could be largely simplified to a common processing deficit—with phonological awareness at the core (Demonet et al., 2004; Ehri et al., 2001; Vellutino et al., 2004). This led to large-scale studies designed to improve basic reading skills. For example, the 13-state, 243-school U.S. Department of Education study (Balu et al., 2015) used an MTSS and RTI framework in an attempt to improve reading competency.

As a result of this work, the majority of RD research has largely focused on single-word reading—to such an extent that the term "dyslexia" became synonymous with word recognition deficits due to phonological processing delays. If this assumption were true for all children, then those who respond to phonics instruction and read single words better would do better in all areas of reading, including reading fluency and comprehension. Although it is true that fluent word recognition skills are a prerequisite for reading comprehension, automatic word recognition skills and word attack/decoding skills are not the same thing, and as we will discover, are mediated by different neurocircuitry. The assumption that good word recognition skills and reading fluency are sufficient for adequate reading comprehension is a simplistic understanding of a very complex process. Much has changed in the past 25 years in our understanding of reading competency, beginning with the identification of the five pillars of reading instruction, phonemic awareness, phonics, fluency, vocabulary, and comprehension, laid out in the National Reading Panel Report (NICHD, 2000). A more complex model, the reading rope (Scarborough, 2001), indicates that skilled reading derives from increasingly automatic word recognition (phonological awareness, decoding, and sight recognition) together with increasingly strategic language comprehension (background knowledge, vocabulary, language structures, verbal reasoning, and literacy knowledge). This model has become the basis of a movement referred to as "The Science of Reading" (Snowling et al., 2022).

Children have reading problems for a variety of reasons, some of which may be instructional in origin (Vellutino et al., 2004). For instance, evidence suggests that phonics instruction is crucial for early reading skills, so those who are not provided with this fundamental learning experience are more likely to struggle with all aspects of reading (Ehri et al., 2001). Despite this apparently clear finding, reading is similar to other academic skills in that numerous processing weaknesses can lead to RDs. In addition, children with RDs try to use compensatory strategies that may be successful in the short term, but these strategies may fail them as literacy demands increase.

Children who struggle with reading try their best to read words any way they can, and that is why you sometimes see a child who has a very different comprehension score when they read silently versus reading aloud (a point we will return to later). What neuroimaging has taught us is that children with processing weaknesses typically compensate by using different areas of the brain to process reading than a typical child does, although such differences dissipate with remediation (e.g., Shaywitz et al., 2003; Simos et al., 2007; Temple et al., 2001). But are all causes of RD the same and do they require the same intervention? What if a child reads words accurately, but reads by sounding out or decoding each word without displaying adequate word recognition (sight-word) skills? What about a child who reads all words by sight, but cannot sound out or decode words?

We have encountered children who display these and other patterns in the early elementary grades. Children with these patterns can attain average word-reading scores on standardized testing, only to struggle later on as the curriculum and comprehension demands change. For a beginning reader, reading comprehension largely entails left hemisphere "correct" answers—facts and details that can be found directly in the text. However, as one progresses into middle grades and beyond, comprehension questions require an element of right-hemisphere function, as students need inferential thinking, fluid reasoning, implicit understanding, and use of context clues to decipher more sophisticated prose, skills that are not readily tapped when the child reads in the early grades.

As is the case with other academic competencies we will discuss, a *comprehensive analysis of error patterns* will be essential for making differential diagnoses and conducting individualized interventions that will lead to effective reading outcomes. We want to make sure when we do our evaluations we don't miss a child who is struggling with basic reading skills because this struggle may be an early sign of a learning disability in reading. These missed opportunities for identifying and serving children in early grades is often linked to later problems in reading and learning. Interventions are most effective when begun prior to the age of 9. If we use a MTSS approach, and are sensitive to patterns that could lead to RDs, we can intervene early and potentially diminish the severity of RDs in some children. Examining patterns of performance is critical for those with clear RDs as well. When we do these fine-grained analyses, we realize there are multiple causes of word-reading RD, reading fluency RD, and reading comprehension RD. Surely, it is common to have all three in the same child, because impaired word reading causes poor fluency and limited comprehension, but the interrelationship of these important components of reading competency is essential to consider in neuropsychology practice. It is also possible to have difficulty with reading comprehension when adequate knowledge of phonics and good word attack skills are present. This difficulty often stems from problems with working memory as it is difficult to understand what has been read when one cannot remember what came earlier in the sentence (Potocki & Laval, 2019). With effective neuropsychology practice comes an important opportunity to serve all children who struggle with reading, not just those with RDs. It wasn't until one author (Hale) was in the trenches trying to teach children with reading and other problems that he realized the old adage "one size fits all" does not apply to children with learning disorders (LDs; see In-Depth 5.1).

Previous research has suggested that RD may be comorbid with mathematics disorder (MD). For some children this may be true (see Chapter 6). Some studies have found that students do not experience severe LDs across reading and mathematics domains (Dirks et al., 2008), with phonological deficits at the core of RD and numerosity at the core of MD (Moll et al., 2015), whereas other studies show the comorbidity to be as high as 65%, with language deficits presumed to be the core for both RD and MD (Snowling et al., 2021). In the Dirks et al. study, only 7.6% of the sample was found to show comorbid RD and MD while 8.0% showed specific word-reading LD, and 5.6% showed math LD. Additional studies using genetic analysis have found that decoding fluency and mathematics may stem from independent genes which, in turn, suggests different pathways responsible for RD and MD (Hart et al., 2010). Still, even children with "pure" RDs can have RDs for different causes and comorbid symptoms are more likely with some subtypes than with others. Application 5.1 gives you an idea of why the subtype issue is important in identification and intervention of disorders. We'll discuss subtypes at greater length later in the chapter.

APPLICATION 5.1. Differential Diagnosis and Comorbidity

Why is differential diagnosis important to you as a practitioner? You certainly can recognize the danger of categorizing and stereotyping children, and we have all learned that children can develop a self-fulfilling prophecy as a result of being labeled. So why not just say that they need help? This might work if all children learned the same way. However, because they do not, labels and diagnoses help us understand the types of help children need. We can't ignore the facts that children have different learning and behavior patterns, and that different disorders and subtypes of disorders exist. Since we firmly believe that differential diagnosis of educational and psychopathological disorders is a critical component of developing effective interventions, you must remain ever vigilant in your exploration of individual differences. But at the same time, every child is ultimately a single-case study. You must not attempt to make children "fit" the category to which they "should" belong; you must see them as individuals, with unique strengths and needs. This is true even if they meet the criteria for only one particular disorder. In this and the remaining chapters of this book, this comorbidity of disorders is highlighted, and some information will be redundant because of the shared neuropsychological characteristics of many disorders.

Why the Word Recognition Emphasis?: The Historical Perspective

Samuel T. Orton (1928) was one of the first brain researchers to bring widespread attention to what he thought was a cause of congenital word blindness, with his notion of strephosymbolia or "twisted symbols" leading many to suggest poor visual processing of letters was the cause of RD. He found that many children with RD either had letter reversals or poor letter order when reading. Orton's writing suggested it was the association of the visual image of letters with spoken words that was the problem for a majority of children with word-reading RD.

Consistent with Orton's assumptions about cerebral organization, early brain researchers focused on abnormal lateralization patterns in RDs; they found that individuals with RDs were less lateralized for receptive language (Bryden, 1988) and showed smaller left planum

IN-DEPTH 5.1. Lessons in Learning: The Teacher's World

In the beginning, one of us (Hale) was a teacher—a good starting place for a psychologist practicing in the schools. He became a teacher because he wanted to help children with special needs experience academic and psychosocial success. When Hale began his student teaching, he thought he had a good understanding of the knowledge base and the tools necessary to teach children with and without disabilities. He had just finished a dual-certification preparation program in learning disabilities and behavior disorders—one that had given him the confidence to teach in his cross-categorical seventh- and eighth-grade classroom. His strong belief in operant techniques had been codified by professors. He also began his experience with a good understanding of classroom management strategies, as well as of direct instruction (e.g., advanced organizer, demonstration, modeling, guided practice, independent practice), learning strategies (e.g., self-monitoring, evaluation), and social skills (e.g., conversation skills, problem solving) curricula.

As is the case for many children with LDs, reading was a major problem in Hale's classroom. He decided to collect baseline data on word recognition and reading rate with the Informal Reading Inventory (IRI) and to complete some curriculum-based probes of comprehension skills. Hale determined appropriate goals based on each child's current level of functioning, developed a reinforcement menu for each one, and then set out to improve reading skills. His interventions included direct instruction with flashcards to increase word recognition/semantic knowledge (definitions on backs of cards). When students reached instructional level for these words (90% accuracy), each child read a passage that included the practiced words. Word recognition and reading speed were measured, and the students charted their own progress. However, in the months to come, it became clear that some children had trendlines well above their aimlines, while others had the opposite pattern. Some children also comprehended the passages quite well, but others had considerable difficulty, and these patterns did not appear to be consistently related to word knowledge (semantic meaning), word recognition (accuracy), or reading speed (fluency). To find out why, Hale tried systematically manipulating schedules of reinforcement, instructional design, and measurement systems, one at a time, and still came up with different results for different children.

Hale remembered a lecture from graduate school about the "process–product paradigm" in teaching. The professor asked, "Is the learning process or the learning outcome more important?" Because Hale's program was largely behavioral, he believed that outcomes or products should be his focus. Process was nebulous and intangible, and couldn't be measured effectively. But then it dawned on him: Could the process be influencing the product in the classroom? That was what his professor had concluded during her lecture. This teaching experience, combined with many others, led Hale to two questions:

- Why don't all children learn the same way?
- If they don't learn the same way, how do we teach them differently so they can all be successful?

When Hale started his doctoral program in psychology, he knew that behaviorism was an essential component of successful learning experiences. He has since also discovered that behaviorism is not the panacea some professors made it out to be. Thus, Hale became a reformed radical behaviorist—one who believes that process *and* product are important. People often asked him, "What made you change?", and the reply was always the same: "Children did." They taught him that no two children with LDs are alike. There is no "one size fits all" when it comes to serving this diverse population.

temporal regions than is typical (Galaburda et al., 1985; Hynd & Semrud-Clikeman, 1989). The Geschwind and Galaburda (1985) model suggested that the path for reading begins in the occipital lobe, then proceeds to the angular gyrus, and then to Wernicke's area for interpretation, before it moves to Broca's area via the arcuate fasciculus for oral expression.

The Geschwind–Galaburda (1985) model certainly makes sense, given what we knew at that time about the structure and function of these areas, but subsequent research has revealed that reading competency is far more complex than auditory- or visual-processing problems. In fact, this focus on visual processing in RD led researchers, clinicians, and teachers down the wrong path for helping many children with RDs (Snowling, 2012). For typical readers, visual–spatial processing apparently contributes little to our understanding of reading competency, at least at the word-reading level (Siegal & Mazabel, 2014). However, what is true of typical readers may not be true for those with RD, given the amount of right-hemisphere activity associated with their word-reading performance (Hung et al., 2018; Pugh et al., 2001; Simos et al., 2007).

The Geschwind–Galaburda (1985) model has only an indirect relationship with language processes—specifically, phonological processing, which we know today is highly related to reading competency and language development (Melby-Lervag et al., 2012). With the advent of neuroimaging and well-designed studies, we have found that many processes are involved in reading, so RD cannot be caused by just one deficit but by several, and these can occur separately or more often together, even in the same child. The evidence is fairly clear that children with RDs can have phonological (i.e., superior temporal lobe), orthographic (i.e., occipital lobe), naming speed (inferior temporal lobe) (Semrud-Clikeman, Guy, et al., 2000), working memory (frontal lobe), and executive functioning deficits (Fiorello et al., 2006; Semrud-Clikeman, 2005) before one even considers the higher-level language systems such as pragmatic speech and abstract, figurative language. Table 5.1 highlights these regions. A meta-analysis of functional neuroimaging studies in dyslexia found that several cortical and subcortical regions are involved in word reading alone, clearly showing that not one sole psychological process is involved (Maisog et al., 2008). When one adds meta-analytic findings about the regions associated with lexical–semantic (e.g., meaning) processing (Binder et al., 2009), the whole process of reading competency becomes quite complex. Table 5.2 highlights these regions according to these two seminal meta-analytic studies.

Basic Components of Word Reading

There are several components to successful word reading. At the word recognition level, it is important to realize that words are just symbols representing our own personal reality. The symbols mean something to us. As a result, the development of symbolic thought is critical to developing both oral and written language. Although symbolic representation can occur in infancy through the use of gestures, it is not until later that the posterior tertiary cortical regions (e.g., zones of overlapping) can easily associate the sounds of language with the associated symbols (letters), which is an essential prerequisite for all reading skills. However, as we will see, there are numerous interdependent psychological processes which must converge to yield accurate word-reading skills.

Oral language requires processing of phonemes (sounds), whereas written language requires recognition of graphemes (symbols), and children must learn to associate the two for successful reading (Ashkenazi et al., 2013). The term orthography is often used to indicate the letters that represent graphemes, but these terms are not interchangeable. For instance, the vowel digraph "ou" is one grapheme but has two letters, so there isn't necessary a one-to-one correspondence between orthography and graphemes. Beyond simple

TABLE 5.1. Cortical Areas Implicated in Reading

- Striate and extrastriate cortex for word processing
- Perisylvian areas for phonological processing
- Angular gyrus and supramarginal gyrus in deciphering written words
- Wernicke's area for comprehension
- Broca's area for articulation, production of language, and syntax
- Dorsolateral prefrontal cortex for executive planning, organization, production, and evaluation of language output

phoneme–grapheme correspondence, readers must also learn structural analysis to recognize morphemes, which are the smallest grammatical units in words. Some words have one morpheme (e.g., *ball*—a free morpheme), while others have several (e.g., *mean-ing-ful*—bound morphemes). Words that sound orally like the same word but are spelled differently (e.g., *let us* and *lettuce*) can be quite confusing for a child, especially if English is their second language. The correspondence between phonemes and graphemes can be inexact in English relative to other languages (e.g., Italian, Spanish), with many rule exceptions present, making the learning of English sound–symbol association difficult for English learners (ELs). However, research suggests this challenge is not the primary source of RDs in this population (Lipka et al., 2005).

When the brain areas associated with phonemes, graphemes, and morphemes in their "triple-word form" approach to understanding reading competency and RD were explored, it was confirmed that phonological, orthographic, and morphological components of reading are interrelated, but are represented in different areas of the brain (Richards et al., 2006). This complex interrelationship is made clearer, albeit more difficult, in understanding that children can read some words by using phonetic analysis or word attack skills (e.g., *b-e-s-t*), while other words are necessarily sight words (e.g., *taught*), and some can be read using both part (word attack) and whole (sight) relationships (e.g., *f-u-n-c—tion*). In the word *function* a child can sound out the first part, but then must recognize the suffix *-tion* acts as a single morpheme and is pronounced "shun" instead of "t-i-o-n." Finally, syllabication is breaking a word into its component parts, whereas phonological analysis and assembly are important for putting word parts together into a whole word. This process can occur at the phonemic, graphemic, and/or morphemic levels, attesting to the complexity of these critical skills. Since both require manipulation of words, auditory sequential and working memory processes play a role in the manifestation of these advanced skills.

When one thinks of the complexity of the English language, where there are many exceptions to the rules, it is no wonder many children have difficulty mastering the phoneme–grapheme–morpheme relationships necessary to read correctly. Using both standardized norm-referenced tests (NRTs) and criterion-referenced tests (CRTs) to examine error patterns during oral reading can help shed light on the nature of a child's reading problems. As a result, we do our best to not only elicit correct responses, but also error responses, because the *errors displayed tell us more about the child's reading skills and strategies* then correct responses. That's why we often discourage children from saying "I don't know" and tell them instead to "give it a try, I want to see if you can get it." It is the *pattern* of word reading error responses that help us understand how to help children learn to read better, not the correct responses. We may not know why the child got an item correct, but we can surely see how a strategy failed during an error response.

TABLE 5.2. Brain Regions Associated with Reading Comprehension and Semantic Processes

Study	Cortical region activated					
	AF	IF	MF	ST/MT	IP	IO
Beauregard et al. (1997)		•	•		•	
Bookheimer et al. (1995)		•			•	•
Braze et al. (2011)			•			
Damasio et al. (1996)		•				•
Hasson et al. (2007)	•	•				
Herbster et al. (1997)						•
Howard et al. (1992)				•		•
Kapur et al. (1994)		•				
Moss et al. (2011b)	•					
Petersen et al. (1989)		•	•			
Price et al. (1994)				•	•	•
Pugh et al. (1997)	•	•				
Vandenberghe et al. (1996)		•		•	•	•
Yarkoni et al. (2008)	•	•				
Xu et al. (2005)	•	•	•			

Note. A, anterior; I, inferior; M, middle; S, superior; F, frontal; T, temporal; P, parietal; O, occipital.

As noted in Chapter 4, both level and pattern of performance are important to consider in differential diagnosis and developing interventions for children with disabilities. Although some may consider NRT and CRT/CBM practices antithetical, they have served complementary purposes in education for some time. For instance, a NRT can be used as a Survey-level Assessment to get at a general idea of how a child compares to the norm (e.g., levels of performance), whereas a CBM CRT test can be used as a Specific-level Assessment to help identify errors (e.g., patterns of performance), and this information can help guide instruction.

A good way to determine the types of errors observed during a child's oral reading is to perform an error analysis, and this can occur on both NRTs and CRTs. Your job is to determine the phonological, orthographic, graphemic, and morphemic error pattern(s) observed, and to link these patterns with cognitive functioning and interventions. This is no easy task of course, but it is better to do this then to just add all the 1-point responses and get a normative score for a child. For instance, if a typical child gets the pattern 1, 1, 1, 1, 1, 0, 0, 0, 0 (the ceiling) and you discontinue the test, they get a raw score of 5. This pattern is much different than a child who gets a 1, 1, 0, 1, 0, 0, 0, 1, 0, 1, 0, 0, 0, 0, even though both yield raw scores of 5. It is your job as the practitioner to find out why the second child got the error pattern they did, and error analysis is critical not only for assessment, but intervention as well. For the first child it is likely that they hit their "ceiling" and had no further skills to demonstrate. The second child may have problems with foundational skills, which can be due to lack of school experience, development of splinter skills, and possible lack of development of foundational skills. One would want to examine the child's school attendance, experience in the class, and to follow up with further testing of basic phonological, orthographic, or morphemic skills.

Here are some common error patterns during oral reading to consider. These patterns (with abbreviations that you can use when taking notes) include the following:

- Articulatory problem (AP)—Child does not enunciate clearly, often due to poor auditory perception of phonemes at early age (e.g., repeated ear infections); other likely causes are oral–motor difficulties or a central auditory processing disorder.
- Omission (OM)—Child leaves out words, skips words, or asks for help.
- Insertion/addition (IA)—Child adds letters or words.
- Pause/repetition (PR)—Child delays or repeats words, suggesting limited automaticity.
- Sequencing/reversal (SR)—Child reverses word order or parts of words.
- Phonemic substitution (PS) or paraphasia—Child substitutes letters within words, can change word meaning in some cases; different from articulation problem as errors are pronounced clearly.
- Semantic substitution (SS) or paraphasia—Child substitutes whole words, often meaningful ones, showing text comprehension.
- Configuration substitution (CS)—Child uses initial letters or whole-word configuration to provide meaningful substitution (which can violate context of sentence).
- Syntax error (SE)—Child ignores or adds punctuation by pausing, changing, or omitting inflection.
- Metacognitive (executive) correction (MC)—Child automatically corrects word, either immediately or after reading additional text.

The Neuropsychology of Word Recognition

What parts of the brain are responsible for the components of word recognition? Views of the neuropsychological basis of word recognition and related RDs have undergone several speculative phases—from early beliefs that word recognition was largely a visual process and a right-hemisphere deficit (e.g., Orton's strephosymbolia), to more recent beliefs that it was largely phonological, to current beliefs that many areas of the brain are responsible for accurate word recognition (Richards et al., 2006). Growth-curve analyses reveal developmental trends in typical readers, with phonological, orthographic, and morphological skills developing throughout the elementary grades (Berninger et al., 2010; Galushka et al., 2020). Clearly, there is not just one neuropsychological process involved in word-reading competency.

Words must not only be read accurately but also quickly. This introduces the neuropsychological process of rapid automatic naming and its importance in reading fluency, which is another cause of RD (Bowers & Wolf, 1993; Vukovic & Siegel, 2006). Research confirms that children with deficits in both phonological processing and rapid naming are at greater risk of reading failure and are more difficult to remediate (Miller et al., 2006), with as many as 49 to 79% of children with RDs having this double-deficit problem (Lovett et al., 2000). When phonological, orthographic, and rapid naming deficits all occur in the same individual (Plaza & Cohen, 2007), the need for intervention is substantial, even if higher-level neuropsychological processes required for reading (such as working memory, receptive language, and expressive language) are intact. Similarly, if attention is problematic in conjunction with rapid naming problems, then the child will show even more significant reading difficulties (Semrud-Clikeman, Guy, et al., 2000), as frontal systems presumed to be deficient in ADHD (Jagger-Rickels et al., 2018) can lead to difficulty with sequential processing, working memory, and efficient retrieval from long-term memory (e.g., Hale et al., 2011).

Phonological Processes

Auditory processing, phonological awareness, language competency, and word-reading skills are strongly related (Pennington & Bishop, 2009; Scarborough, 2009; Segal & Petrides, 2013). After the visual causes of RD were largely dismissed, phonological processing deficits were considered to be the core deficit in RDs (Pennington & Bishop, 2009). Although we no longer simplistically think that children with RDs represent the lower end of a normal distribution of reading due to these phonological processing problems, it is clear that phonological processes are the single most important predictor of reading competency (Melby-Lervag et al., 2012).

In a comprehensive examination of phonemic awareness (Hoien et al., 1995), three phonemic, syllabication, and rhyme factors were extracted, with the phoneme factor showing the most variance in predicting reading achievement, and some additional variance explained by the rhyme factor. Phonological analysis relies heavily on detecting changes in sound frequency and amplitude (Berninger et al., 2010). Critical for developing good phonological skills, sound frequency modulation accounts for a substantial amount of variance in nonword reading (Huslander et al., 2004); thus it is not surprising that frequency modulation is difficult for many children with RDs, and that poor frequency modulation combined with poor amplitude modulation is likely to lead to significant phonological deficits and RDs.

This most common RD subtype, caused by auditory processing deficits that lead to poor phonological awareness, is often called phonological dyslexia. Although many children with phonological RD may have a genetic cause (Galaburda et al., 2006), a child may also have an environmental cause for their phonological RD. Sometimes children of this subtype may have a normal audiological examination, but may have a history of chronic ear infections that result in poor phonological processing skills. They may also have problems with speech articulation as a result (McGrath et al., 2008), so it is important to ask about ear infections and oral articulation errors when assessing phonological and/or word-reading deficits.

Early skills that are important for reading involve word-level reading, and these skills later move into a focus on decoding of multisyllabic words. In order to decode these words it is necessary to have strong working memory skills (Compton et al., 2012). These skills allow the child to hold in mind the letters and sounds which allow the child to tie together these skills while also comprehending the material. Research has now found that working memory, as a concept, is more strongly related to reading decoding and reading comprehension compared to IQ, phonemic awareness, and general language skills (Ouellette & Beers, 2010). In addition, another neuropsychological aspect that is crucial for reading skills is that of processing speed. Processing speed affects how quickly lower-level skills (i.e. phonemic processing, rapid naming) are executed. Slower speed has been linked to difficulty applying foundational skills when higher-level processing is required (i.e., reading fluency and comprehension) (Compton et al., 2012). These findings strengthen the theory that underlies this volume in that the unexpected underachievement seen in LD is best conceptualized in terms of strengths and weaknesses (Fuchs et al., 2008). Most recent studies have found that children with word-reading LD show more difficulty on working memory tasks and language skills with relative strength in processing speed (Compton et al., 2012). They were also found to be relatively stronger on applied mathematical problems and reading comprehension. In contrast, children with reading comprehension LD were found to have more difficulty in language, particularly with abstract language concepts, with relative strength in processing speed. These children were also found to show a relative strength in mathematics calculation.

If there are childhood hearing problems due to early ear infections, the informed reader may wonder why a phonological processing problem persists even if hearing is no longer a problem. The answer can be found in our discussion of neuroanatomy in Chapter 2. Recall that primary cortical regions register stimuli, but association cortical areas (secondary and tertiary zones) learn to interpret that input. So the reason why phonological problems persist even when hearing is no longer a problem is that the association cortex learned to hear phonemes wrong (and still hears them wrong even after the hearing problem has been corrected). This condition speaks to the importance of parents and other caregivers recognizing ear infections in their children, and intensive intervention for children with repeated ear infections, including surgically implanting tympanostomy tubes in severe cases.

Not only do children with phonological dyslexia have problems with auditory processing and, as a result, with receptive language, but they also have difficulty with basic word attack skills and perform poorly on pseudoword tasks (e.g., reading nonwords such as "hesrid"). A majority of children with dyslexia have repeatedly been found to have difficulty on phonological and pseudoword tasks, so it is important to examine phoneme–grapheme correspondence on these tasks even if word reading is within normal limits. This finding may be largely because these children do not have good sound–symbol awareness, which is caused by poor metalinguistic understanding that words can be broken into their phonological parts (Fletcher, 2012). In severe cases, these children may be better taught using sight-word approaches that stress their strength rather than building on a weakness, though with younger students or less severe cases, phoneme–grapheme correspondence (e.g., phonics) remediation should be emphasized first (Hale et al., 2016).

Neuroimaging Findings in Phonological RD

In order to be an accomplished reader, it is necessary to recognize simple words quickly, and several brain networks are required for fluency (Wandell et al., 2012). The ventral systems, which are implicated in orthography, are strongly connected to the phonological (dorsal) systems with the left inferior frontal gyrus and temporoparietal regions also strongly involved (Schlaggar & McCandliss, 2007). The circuits of the left ventral occipital temporal cortex (an area that processes visual material) along with the left frontal gyrus have been found to change over development as reading skills improve (Wandell et al., 2012). These structures work collaboratively to process letter strings but are also strongly connected to phonological and semantic systems involved in fluent reading (Schlaggar & McCandliss, 2007). These structures and pathways are also intimately connected to Broca's area (oral reading) and the frontal gyri in the left hemisphere (Koyama et al., 2011). However, the separation of frontal and posterior systems, in both input and output reading processes, provides for parallel processes more sophisticated than this linear description (e.g., Dehaene, Cohen, Morais, & Kolinsky, 2015).

Several cortical areas have been implicated in reading problems with a phonological processing basis, particularly the perisylvian temporal regions (primary and association auditory cortex), middle temporal gyrus, Wernicke's area, angular and supramarginal parietal gyri, striate and extrastriate cortex, and frontal lobe, especially in the left hemisphere (see Figure 2.1; Dehaene et al., 2018; Pugh et al., 2013; Richards & Berninger, 2008; Segal & Petrides, 2013). Consistent with the literature cited in Chapters 2 and 3, the brain does not work in isolation on any cognitive skill. Rather, there are networks that connect right and left, anterior–posterior, and anterior–inferior axes that are integral for the reading process. Thus, reductions in left temporal lobe gray matter in children with phonological dyslexia are not specific to the perisylvian region (Wandell et al., 2012), which could account for the strong relationship among reading, receptive language, and crystallized/convergent/concordant processing deficits. Difficulties with mapping of orthography to the phonological language system are likely related to deficits in the rapid processing of speech sounds (Golestani et al., 2007), which could be cerebellar in nature (Schwartze & Kotz, 2016), while deficits in the temporoparietal cortex are related to problems with phonological storage and retrieval (Vigneau et al., 2006). Thus, network deficits in mapping phonological and orthographic stimuli are consistent with problems with RDs (Newman & Joanisse, 2011). Disruptions to this basic reading circuit compromise the basic processes that are needed for fluent reading and these disruptions are present early on and continue into adulthood (Richlan et al., 2011).

The connection between sound (superior temporal lobe) and symbol (extrastriate cortex) is largely a function of inferior parietal lobe in an area called the angular gyrus (Pugh et al., 2013). As noted in Chapter 2, the left angular gyrus has been implicated in RD, as this multimodal convergence zone serves to connect visual (occipital) and auditory (superior temporal gyrus) language processes. It is not surprising that children with this type of RD show decreased fMRI or PET activation in response to phonological tasks in the left temporal and parietal regions (Pugh et al., 2013; Richards et al., 2006; Richards & Berninger, 2008). Conflicting findings have indicated hypo- and hyperactivation in the inferior frontal gyrus (Hoeft et al., 2007), hyperactivation in the left (Richlan et al., 2011) or right (Hoeft et al., 2011; Maisog et al., 2008) insula but not the inferior frontal gyrus. Further study is needed to clarify the differential role of these prefrontal regions in reading. What is known is that children with RDs have less efficient functional circuits (Casanova et al., 2010; Vourkas et al., 2011). Some studies have found more activation and greater functional connectivity in responders to intensive reading remediation (Farris et al., 2011; Hoeft et al., 2011). Existing evidence suggests that these inefficient functional circuits can normalize with appropriate intervention (Aylward et al., 2003). In fact, normalization of the inferior parietal regions associated with response to phonics instruction separates responders from nonresponders (Odegard et al., 2008).

Researchers have found that, compared to controls, individuals with phonological RD showed lower levels of activation in the left-hemisphere areas associated with competent readers (Pugh et al., 2013; Simos et al., 2007). They also showed lower activity during phonological assembly tasks in the superior temporal gyrus, angular gyrus, and striate and extrastriate visual cortex (Pugh et al., 2013). A comparison of correlations between these regions of interest showed that they were highly connected (correlated) for the typical group, but functionally disconnected for the group with phonological RD, supporting the notion that the alphabetic principle—the ability to make sounds into letters—may represent the core deficit in word RD (Berninger, Richards et al., 2015).

Reduced gray matter volume has been found in the left temporoparietal (Hoeft et al., 2007), ventral occipito–temporal cortex (Silani et al., 2005), and cerebellum (Laycock et al., 2008). Diffusion tension imaging (DTI) allows for the visualization of white matter tracts that are utilized for a task. Findings from DTI indicate a strong importance of the arcuate fasciculus, superior longitudinal fasciculus, optic radiation, and callosal fibers for general reading with abnormalities in these tracts found in children with RDs (Frye et al., 2011; Wandell et al., 2012). Similar to the circuits identified by fMRI, reversal of these tract abnormalities has been found following intervention (Keller & Just, 2009).

In sum, as a result of this disconnection of sound and symbol, children with alphabetic principle deficits tend to rely on compensatory processes for reading (Dehaene et al., 2018; Pugh et al., 2013; Simos et al., 2007), using a sight-word approach and guessing at words based on their general configuration. This finding would account for the greater occipital–temporal lobe activity found in children with phonological dyslexia, who may use memory-based strategies for word recognition (Shaywitz et al., 2004). For instance, they may say "loud" for the stimulus word "lost." Because they make many decoding errors and may have both receptive and expressive language deficits, these children are likely to be recognized by parents and teachers as having a learning problem. Interestingly, those with phoneme–grapheme correspondence problems (i.e., superior temporal–inferior parietal problems) may use the occipital–temporal area differently, depending on whether they successfully compensate for their deficits.

Could children with phonological RD be attempting to use a different pathway (i.e., the ventral stream) for word recognition? Certainly they could rely on a more ventral stream (i.e., sight word) path for word recognition (Ashkenazi et al., 2013), and this process could possibly explain superior temporal–parietal underactivation and disconnection during word recognition tasks. However, as we will see later, fMRI studies of typical children also fail to show angular gyrus activation on some reading tasks, so this is not a clear-cut picture. Perhaps expert readers don't use the angular gyrus because they have automatized word reading, so the ventral stream automatically processes the words quickly and efficiently. As these findings suggest, the left posterior brain structures are functionally different in children with phonological RD (Segal & Petrides, 2013). Therefore, determining whether it is an auditory (superior temporal), visual (ventral occipital–temporal), or integration (angular and supramarginal gyrus) problem is an important distinction to make during your evaluation, as suggested by Case Study 5.1.

Grapheme/Morpheme/Orthographic Processes

We can now recognize how auditory processing skills affect phonological awareness and the acquisition of sound–symbol associations, but shouldn't visual deficits also lead to RDs? Intuitively, you know that RDs can't always be the result of auditory processing deficits because reading is a visual task, so at some level visual processes must be required. However, after early research suggested that phonological processing deficits lead to RDs, the role of vision in reading was neglected for some time. Visual processing of words at the cortical level has been touched on briefly in the preceding section. Not only are these cortical areas implicated in this type of RD, but so are frontal and subcortical structures. Research has confirmed that orthographic skills are related to reading speed independent of phonological

---

Case Study 5.1. Paul's Phonological Processing Deficit

Paul was an 8-year-old boy who had difficulty learning the alphabet and could not read even basic sight words, despite 2 years of remedial support. Paul was pleasant, compliant, and hardworking during the evaluation. However, some expressive language issues, including articulation problems, were noted. A review of the history revealed several instances of otitis media (ear infections), but his audiological examination was fine. For word reading, Paul read a few words correctly (e.g., "as," "then") but he had many letter reversals (e.g., reading "b" for "d"). Paul did not pass any pseudoword-decoding items. It seemed as if Paul had the classic signs of a phonological processing disorder; surprisingly, however, he had no difficulty on visual or auditory processing tasks, so further hypothesis testing was necessary. Paul made several block design orientation errors (i.e., reversals and rotations). He also had left–right confusion, as well as poor handwriting notable for uneven pencil pressure. An examination of spatial and motor skills found few problems in these areas, so what was Paul's problem? Paul apparently had difficulty with sound–symbol association, somatosensory feedback, and directional orientation—all characteristic of left parietal lobe dysfunction. Providing Paul with phonological awareness instruction wasn't the key to helping him, since he heard phonemes and saw letters just fine; he needed help with integrating sounds and symbols.

skills (Berninger et al., 2010) and that these skills are strong predictors of reading competency by the middle elementary grades.

The RD subtype that involves difficulty with grapheme/morpheme problems due to impaired orthography is often called *orthographic dyslexia*. Children with orthographic dyslexia have little difficulty with words that make phonemic sense, but they often read in a slow, laborious manner. These children tend to have problems with reading sight words that are irregular; for instance, they can read the word "grand" quite well, but have problems with "right," probably saying "rig-hut." These children have also been found to have difficulty in the striate, extrastriate, and inferior parietal lobe areas. Neuroimaging studies have shown that the left ventral stream (primarily the striate, extrastriate, lingual, and fusiform areas) is important in orthography, whereas morpheme recognition and fluency are related to posterior temporal–parietal areas and Broca's area (Aylward et al., 2003).

Although these cortical areas have been implicated in reading, children with this type of RD could have deficits that result from dysfunction of early visual processes. In their review of these processes, J. F. Stein (2001) and M. I. Stein (2014) note that children with orthographic RD have impaired magnocellular functioning (see the discussion of the M pathway in Chapter 2), directly affecting the dorsal visual pathway from the occipital lobe to the parietal lobe. Some have suggested that children with dyslexia have difficulty with processing visual information that has reduced contrast; that is, they are not sensitive to the difference in contrast between the letters and the background. In addition, children with dyslexia were found to have problems with motion discrimination, which are skills modulated through the magnocellular pathways. Difficulty with processing rapid stimuli has been found in children with dyslexia in both the visual and auditory modalities leading to a conclusion that there is a dysfunction of temporal resolution in the magnocellular pathways (Demonet et al., 2004). This difficulty can be related to other problems seen in children with dyslexia, including attention and eye movement differences. In fact, meta-analyses support the notion that motion perception is a strong group difference between children with RD and typical readers. These findings seem to support a magnocellular deficit as a partial but not full explanation for dyslexia, at least for some individuals with RDs.

The magnocellular deficit theory of dyslexia is controversial as findings seeking to replicate this type of difficulty in children with dyslexia have been equivocal. For example, the visual deficits seen in children with dyslexia move beyond the frequency domain (which is specific to magnocellular functions) to also include deficits in the processing of slowly evolving events (Amitay et al., 2002). Others suggest that no clear account has been proposed as to how this magnocellular pathway, which originates in the retina and projects to the primary visual cortex via the magnocellular layers of the lateral geniculate nucleus of the thalamus, leads to problems with reading acquisition (Skottun, 2000). Several studies have not found problems with contrast sensitivity or with movement leading to a questioning of this theory (Ben-Yehudah et al., 2001; Skottun, 2000). Further study is needed to determine the contribution this pathway makes to orthographic dyslexia. One more recent study found that the RD subjects had perceptual deficits on both visual and auditory tasks that were not consistent with a magnocellular deficit (Amitay et al., 2002). The children who performed the poorest on all of these tasks showed a broad deficit in all perceptual areas. Those who performed similarly to those in the control group showed visual and auditory perceptual difficulties that were unrelated to magnocellular functions. These studies do not fully refute the magnocellular theory of dyslexia; rather they suggest that it may explain the crucial role of the timing for information that is problematic for some children with dyslexia. It has been theorized that it isn't how fast the information is presented but rather the interval that is present between the stimuli.

Eye Movements in Reading

Eye movements are another area that has been studied in RD. For typical readers of languages that are read left to right, the normal span is 3 to 4 spaces to the left and 14 to 15 spaces to the right (Bellocchi et al., 2013). When tasks are more difficult, the perceptual span is smaller. When the text requires quite a bit of processing, then the perceptual span is generally 7 to 8 spaces. Eye movements (saccades) are related to attention, particularly visual–spatial attention, and attention will modulate how big the region is that is attended to (Rayner et al., 2010). Research findings indicate that there is an optimal preferred viewing location that is generally in the beginning and middle of the word which assists in word identification and shortening the recognition time (Li et al., 2011). Successful reading requires good visual attentional and sequential processes (Ruffino et al., 2010). In addition, eye movement fluency has also been implicated in RD. One thing to ask students with presumed visual tracking problems is why they struggle with reading and then watch them read. Their eyes will often go back and forth when reading, suggesting limited "fluent pursuit" of the gaze during reading. They will often complain that the letters or words "jump around" on them when reading. By using a penlight, and asking the student to track the light in all visual fields, this phenomenon can be documented in some cases. As elaborated on in In-Depth 5.2, deficits in motion sensitivity could explain why many of these children complain that letters and words move. When reading fluently, the child must be able to segment the word and letter strings, and then shift attention from one segment to the next one. This process allows the child to fixate on letters and not to become distracted by letters above or below the selection (Ducrot & Grainger, 2007).

Preschoolers who show stronger visual–spatial attention have been found to show better reading skills by second grade (Franceschini et al., 2012) and children with ADHD have more difficulty with visual tracking and convergence insufficiency (Granet et al., 2005), which could possibly account for the RD–ADHD comorbidity. Difficulties in eye movements of children with dyslexia have found that a smaller number of words elicit fixation, more words omitted, and more multiple fixations which results in poor reading, longer reading pace, and difficulty with whole-word recognition (Hawelka et al., 2010). Bellocchi et al. (2013) suggest further study is needed on the link between faulty eye movements and reading problems but the initial findings suggest that eye movements which do not promote fluent

---

IN-DEPTH 5.2. The Moving Target

How could motion sensitivity be related to RDs, given that the eyes are what move, not the words? Recall that the dorsal stream is responsible for spatial and motion processing, and for self-direction of movement. Although the problem could be related to the coordination of the receptive system with the frontal eye fields (which guide and control eye movements) and the cranial nerves, as discussed in Chapter 2, much of the focus has been on the difficulties with motion processing. Tracking of visual stimuli works both ways: As the eyes move across the page, the letters must be instantly encoded and at the same time integrated, with poorly coordinated eye movements related to "movement" of the letters in working memory. Consistent with these arguments, motion sensitivity predicts orthographic skills better than phonemic skills, and accounts for 25% of the variance in reading (Stein, 2001). Although visual and motion processes are certainly important in the reading process, some researchers have suggested that phonological and orthographic deficits could reflect the same underlying pathology—a hypothesis we explore later in this chapter.

reading (skipping letters, fixating too long on specific letter strings) are related to visual–sequential processing and also to reading fluency. However, it should be noted that interventions designed to facilitate visual tracking and reduce convergence insufficiency have generally not been supported for most children with RD (McGregor, 2014; Vellutino et al., 2004), even though they may influence some of these children (e.g., Caldani et al., 2020).

Fluency, Timing, and Retrieval Speed Processes

The study of fluency, timing, and retrieval speed has been an increased area of inquiry into the deficits associated with RDs. Fluent reading is rapid, smooth, and automatic, without attention paid to reading mechanics such as word attack skills or decoding (Pikulski & Chard, 2005). Reading fluency is directly related to naming speed—a skill needed for making the transition from slow, laborious reading to quick, efficient, accurate reading (Santoro et al., 2008). Because articulation speed, naming speed, and processing speed are related to reading accuracy and speed (Parrilla et al., 2004), it is important to look for expressive speech and language characteristics, retrieval difficulties, and/or slow psychomotor or processing speed in the children you test. Children with RDs who have good phonemic and poor rapid automatized naming (RAN) skills are likely to be better at decoding, but tend to read slowly, to make more spelling errors on tests of orthographic accuracy, and to have more difficulty with attention (Volkmer et al., 2019).

The factors affecting reading fluency include the following (Hudson et al., 2013):

- Proportion of words recognized as morphemes or orthographic units
- Speed variations in sight-word processing
- Processing speed during novel word identification
- Use of context clues to facilitate word identification
- Speed of semantic access of word meanings

Notice how phonology is *not* one of the factors associated with RAN and reading fluency, and research supports the distinction (Wolf et al., 2002). However, the associated "double-deficit hypothesis" or phonological and rapid naming deficits are common among children with RDs, and some suggest they are not distinct (Vukovic & Seigel, 2006). Obviously, if you can't read a word, you can't read quickly (Thomson et al., 2013).

The cerebellum's role in dyslexia is even less well understood. It has been hypothesized that the cerebellum is important for the automatization of reading and writing skills. Along this line, balance and motor-coordination disorders have been found to be present in children with dyslexia particularly when the child is straining the attentional system (Nicholson et al., 2001). The cerebellum is also important for higher cognitive processes (reading, inferential thinking, executive functions), particularly when procedural memory is required (Berninger et al., 2017). Difficulty with timing and automatization of tasks has been linked to cerebellar dysfunction and dyslexia (Demonet et al., 2004). While the cerebellum certainly contributes to procedural memory, it is not sufficient for these skills and many other cortical, subcortical, and some cerebellar areas are important for skill learning. Thus, deficits in any of these pathways can contribute to problems with reading speed and fluency. The role of the cerebellum in attention pathways is the most likely link to poor automatization (Bledsoe et al., 2009).

If the frontal lobes are important for understanding temporal relationships, and the left hemisphere is the detailed, local, parts hemisphere, then the left–frontal combination for reading makes good sense. Poor temporal–sequential relationships can lead to problems with auditory–sequential processing; skills which are important in receptive language.

Orthography, including the visual word-processing areas (fusiform and lingual gyri) also appears to be rate-dependent (Ziegler & Goswami, 2005). This explanation makes good neuropsychological sense, as executive processes are responsible for the sequential organization of responding, which occurs within a temporal framework (Berninger et al., 2010). An additional finding is that the brain areas associated with articulation during silent reading are used by readers with dyslexia during word attack (S.E. Shaywitz et al., 2003). Frontal processes even extend beyond this framework, as highlighted in In-Depth 5.3.

Although frontal lobe and executive problems seem to be part of the picture, it is important to consider that supporting structures, such as the cingulate and cerebellum, may also play a role in reading fluency. Researchers have recently found greater support for the cingulate's role in executive functions (especially the online monitoring of performance) (Semrud-Clikeman, Fine, et al., 2013). The dorsal cingulate has been implicated in cognition particularly for error detection while the ventral cingulate has been found to be important for emotional processing with lesions causing emotional instability (Bush et al., 2000). A study of the relation between the anterior cingulate cortex (ACC) volume and reading found that reading achievement was strongly related to the left anterior cingulate cortex particularly in rate of reading (Ripamonti et al., 2014). This finding is intriguing as it suggests the reading circuit needs to include the ACC as part of the feedback loop to assist in reading fluently and error free.

What brain areas could affect reading speed and fluency? Thinking back to Chapter 2, we would predict the subcortical areas associated with cortical tone; the frontal lobes, for regulation of attention, sequencing, retrieval, and temporal relationships; the cingulate, with its anterior–posterior pathway; and the cerebellum, because of its involvement in timing and skill routinization. Indeed, with the exception of the cortical tone areas, all these areas have been implicated. These areas include the thalamus and M pathway (as described earlier), the cerebellum, Broca's area, and the dorsolateral prefrontal cortex. How does one see and read a word? First, the letters are registered in the occipital cortex. The right-hemisphere–visual holistic processing of the gestalt determines whether there is a sight-word reading potential, with the left and right ventral streams working side by side via the corpus collosum to attempt a sight-word reading. If a sight word can be retrieved from the left ventral stream, the word is read before the next word is considered. However, if not recognized, the left dorsal stream is activated to decode the sound–symbol word relationship.

Left- and Right-Hemisphere Processes

Before we discuss word-reading interventions, you will note that most of the information discussed earlier has primarily focused on the left-hemisphere and subcortical areas involved in reading. Does this mean that word reading is a left-hemisphere task and has little to do with the right hemisphere? The answer is, of course, yes and no. Many of the fMRI and PET studies reported here showed activation primarily in left-hemisphere areas; however, unlike patient studies, these neuroimaging studies have provided convincing evidence of bilateral processing during reading in dyslexia, even at the word recognition level (Shaywitz et al., 2006). Since reading is a visual task, shouldn't it be a right-hemisphere activity? The assumption most researchers have made is that there are two interconnected routes: the faster, automatic *semantic route*, which relies on the visual system to retrieve whole words (i.e., sight words), and the slower *phonological route*, which depends on auditory mediation to process words (i.e., word attack skills) as well as working memory to retain and recover sounds which have been previously heard (Jobard et al., 2003). We know that with beginning readers the right hemisphere is more activated because initial letter and word calling are a "novel" task and hence the province of the right hemisphere. As reading becomes more automatic, the task moves

IN-DEPTH 5.3. The Executive Reader

How are executive functions related to RDs? Many authors have found that working memory is important in effective word reading (Breznitz, 2001), and that children with RDs have deficient executive function skills. As discussed earlier, there is considerable overlap between RDs and ADHD, possibly because frontal dysfunction may be involved in a subset of children with RDs. Studies have shown high overlap between the conditions, but children with the inattentive type of ADHD would appear to be more at risk for RDs than children with the hyperactive–impulsive type (Willcutt & Pennington, 2000). Consistent with these findings, symptoms of inattention appear to predict rapid automatic naming and orthographic processing, but hyperactivity has no significant relationship to either phonological or orthographic processes (Berninger et al., 2001). However, it is unclear whether these ADHD-like symptoms suggest comorbidity, or are primarily the result of one disorder or the other (Pennington et al., 1993; Swanson et al., 1999).

---

to the left hemisphere. From Shaywitz's seminal neuroimaging work, we now know that children with reading problems do not make the switch from right to left hemisphere. In this case, reading continues to be a novel task. Similarly, for experienced readers, the slow and fast routes are often used simultaneously. In this view, the visual word form area processes known words as a whole as well as graphemes, syllables, and morphemes. When a word is presented, the experience of the reader with the word comes into play and it is accessed through the direct route (semantic route). If the word is not familiar, then the word is segmented visually by letter combinations or by the use of simple graphemes. For example, the segment "tion" is frequently found in English words and is generally processed as a whole. Similarly, the blend "ch" is often found and also processed as a whole. In less skilled readers, these segments are not as readily chunked or read and thus require additional processing by both the right and left hemispheres. Recall our novel (right-hemisphere)–routinized (left-hemisphere) distinction discussed in Chapter 2; that model again explains why word recognition skills are primarily lateralized to the left hemisphere, even when they are retrieved as sight words. Neuroimaging findings support these routes and suggest more strongly that reading is not solely a right–left process but rather an anterior–posterior process as well that is generally in the left hemisphere in accomplished readers.

As we have seen in Chapter 2, right-hemisphere processes are required during ambiguous and novel problem-solving situations, so it is not surprising that when children are first learning sound–symbol associations, right-hemisphere activity is relatively high. When infants initially process language, we have seen that the right hemisphere is important during language acquisition and, sure enough, these right-hemisphere processes do predict reading skills at age 8 (Molfese et al., 2012). But as we have seen, the left hemisphere is responsible for categorizing information and developing routinized codes. Since reading decoding is related to forming new associations between phonological and orthographic representations, children with RDs have difficulty forming these associations and view these as novel events. Thus, processing of even previously learned material is more effortful and requires cognitive resources that could be better used for other tasks.

Children with phonological dyslexia have been found to rely on the right inferior occipital region for letter and word recognition leading to right temporal and then left temporal lobe semantic activation, and finally to phonological output in Broca's area (Castles & Coltheart, 2004). Since these children may be less automatized in their reading performance, we would expect them to have considerable difficulty when they cannot recognize a word by using visual memory skills. Because they can't access visual–verbal connections quickly (Clements et al., 2006), children with RDs are likely to require more effort when reading, and to be less efficient readers than their nondisabled peers. It has also been found that there are sex differences, with males showing more left lateralization for reading than females for phonological tasks and females utilizing more bilateral structures. In contrast, the males showed greater bilateral functioning completing a visual–spatial task while the females were more left lateralized. Such differences are intriguing and suggest that males (who have a higher incidence of reading problems) are more lateralized than females—it is possible that having the ability to bilaterally process phonological tasks is protective against developing a reading problem.

If efficient (i.e., fluent) reading requires ventral stream sight-word reading, then why not teach all words by sight? Some teachers even say that children should "guess" if they don't at first recognize the word, fostering ventral stream reading guessing to respond based on general or initial letter configuration of the word, often as part of "whole language" or "three-cueing system" reading instruction (Moats, 2000). Why, then, does this fail readers? The answer is simple. While early on in reading, words are commonly both heard and seen in print, as the lexicon is small for young children. If one has a good visual memory, this recognize–guess word-reading approach might work well. But as the lexicon expands from dozen to thousands of words, we know many more words through oral language (hearing) than we do by sight (reading), so when encountering an unknown word we need to switch back (via the vertical occipital fasciculus) to the dorsal stream to read it, and repair sentence level comprehension errors that would occur if we just guessed. Although guessing would work when young, the more one guesses wrong at words, the more comprehension will be impaired. Take for instance the word "stethoscope." Since we are exposed to this word early in life and have even seen it used, we know what one is. But the reality is we almost never see the word stethoscope in print. It is easy to see if we guess at the word, reading, "The doctor used a *stegosaurus* (guessing by initial letter configuration) to listen to the heart" we would obviously not comprehend the sentence.

What is important to understand from this description of psychological processes involved in word reading is that what is true for the average reader may not be the same for a child with a word-reading RD. Again, the one size fits all approach to understanding reading competency and other disorders is often oversimplified by only discussing typical learners, perhaps in an effort to focus phonics instruction, which is crucial for all individuals regardless of brain functional area involved in the disorder (Galuschka et al., 2014).

The Neuropsychology of Reading Comprehension

Components of Reading Comprehension

Marcus reads well in class, so why doesn't he understand what he's reading? Reading comprehension is much less studied than word recognition, because it is assumed by some that accurate, fluent reading leads to good comprehension, although the path may be more complex and indirect. Reading comprehension has been defined as the ability to construct and extract meaning from a text and requires the coordination of phonemic and phonological awareness as well as analyzing the context of the word (Sencibaugh, 2007). Difficulties with reading comprehension appear to be rooted in problems with associating meaning with words, recognizing and recalling details, making inferences, and drawing conclusions—all of which could be related to executive function deficits (Cutting, Materek, et al., 2009). These skills are generally believed to be higher level processes that are typically addressed in mid-elementary grades and increase with age/grade. Could it be that poor readers are limited by lower-level processes, and we never really get to higher-level instruction to determine whether comprehension is a problem? And what about children who show no lower-level problems, only higher-level comprehension problems—such as children with "nonverbal" learning disorders (Semrud-Clikeman, Walkowiak, Wilkinson, & Christopher, 2010)?

Certainly, higher-level reading skills such as word and text comprehension require accuracy and proficiency in the lower-level processes, but they also require integration of prior knowledge, suggesting that personal experience interacts with text information to create a unique interpretation of the text. Thus, prior learning and familiarity with the subject (a left hemisphere function) are always at play in comprehension tasks. Comprehension also requires working memory in order to keep the content in mind while reading the passage, while also performing higher-level skills that enable the reader to interpret text meaning and draw conclusions about passages. It has been found that the executive functions of working memory, planning, and organization play a large role in reading comprehension but not typically in word reading once attention, fluency, and vocabulary are controlled for (Sesma et al., 2009). Similarly, in a large-scale study comparing children who were developing typically with those with general RDs and those with reading comprehension disorder, it was found that RD groups had difficulty with word fluency and oral language (Cutting, Materek et al., 2009). In addition, it was found that the children with reading comprehension deficits showed prominent weaknesses in executive functioning. These studies highlight the relation between working memory, planning, organization, and reading comprehension.

We have already explained that a basic level for reading is the word recognition process. Moving beyond these lower-level constructs, word meaning, which is derived from semantic knowledge of morpheme root words, prefixes, and suffixes, is quite important. Understanding word relationships requires examination of objects and of actions, and of interactions among objects, actions, and events. Semantics is related to both individual words (vocabulary knowledge) and sentence structure or word order. Indeed, word knowledge and use are intimately related to syntax or grammar; syntax is the system of rules for word order and combinations and for sentence organization, and results suggest Broca's area is important for ordering ideas during comprehension. Good semantic and syntactic knowledge is likely to lead to comprehension competency. The relationships among words and structuring of text may be explicit (requiring literal comprehension—more a left-hemisphere function) or implicit (requiring inferential comprehension—more a right-hemisphere function).

In addition to all of these skills, the child must also be able to retrieve the meaning of words from his or her lexicon. This skill requires frontal lobe coordination with the association areas in the back of the brain, the hippocampus, and posterior cingulate to retrieve a meaning. When children have difficulty with this process it is called *word-finding difficulties*. You may have experienced this phenomenon when you try to remember a name or object but cannot retrieve that information. This often happens in children with ADHD, who struggle with working memory, thereby affecting memory retrieval (see the hemispheric encoding/retrieval asymmetry [HERA] model; Habib et al., 2003). Imagine what it is like for a child to have the same problem throughout reading and still be expected to "comprehend" the passage.

In addition to right-hemisphere comprehension of implicit or figurative reading passages (e.g., poetry), such as interpreting text that is nonliteral, metaphor, humor, sarcasm, inuendo, indirect meanings, and multiple meanings, the right hemisphere is also responsible for pragmatics, which is the purpose, meaning, or gist of the text. This final aspect of reading comprehension is difficult to define and measure. It is best described as the function of the message conveyed, and is often used to describe communicative competence or social discourse in oral language. It is by its very nature based on personal experience and values, so in reading comprehension this area is often referred to as comprehension evaluation or "critical reading."

Neuroimaging Findings in Reading Comprehension

Compared to research on word reading, research into the neuropsychological basis of reading comprehension has been limited. Although the results of these studies vary, depending on the tasks administered and comparison tasks used, some general findings emerge. Most neuroimaging studies of semantic processing of categorical and semantic information have implicated the left temporal lobe, both inferior and anterior to the sections described in connection with phonological processing (Landi, 2013). This finding is consistent with our earlier arguments that the left temporal lobe serves as a warehouse of long-term memory for explicit information Gazzaniga et al., 2013), with animate objects/verb knowledge more likely anterior and inanimate objects/noun knowledge more posterior in this region (Tyler et al., 2001). To build upon this distinction, nouns appear to be more a temporal lobe function, whereas verbs include frontal language areas (Carota et al., 2017; Horowitz-Kraus, Vannest, Gozdas, et al., 2014).

Not surprisingly, frontal lobe activity is also required for semantic judgment and comprehension of text, although some studies show bilateral activity, and others show primarily left-hemisphere involvement during comprehension tasks. A number of researchers have shown that children with RDs have problems with executive functions (or, in cognitive–educational parlance, "metacognition"), which result in difficulty with monitoring, adjusting, and regulating cognitions (Cutting et al., 2006). It has been suggested that for reading comprehension, executive functions such as working memory and metacognitive skills are more likely to differentiate adolescents and older readers with RDs from controls than lower-level reading processes, such as phonology and morphology, which are automatic in older typical readers (Swanson et al., 2006).

As suggested in the previous discussion, comprehension deficits due to executive dysfunction appear to be independent of the phonological/articulatory functions subserving word recognition (Cutting, Eason, et al., 2009). In a direct comparison of prefrontal and posterior measures, children with RDs were found to have greater executive deficits, including problems with selective and sustained attention, inhibition, set maintenance, flexibility, and phonemic production (Pham et al., 2011). Thus, the role of the dorsolateral frontal–subcortical circuit—not a typical "language" structure—attests to the relevance of executive deficits leading to reading comprehension problems in the absence of lower-level phoneme–grapheme or rapid naming problems (e.g., Follmer et al., 2017; Klaus & Schutter, 2018).

Neuroimaging studies have identified several key areas associated with reading comprehension. Obviously, the word recognition areas described previously play a role in reading comprehension—but possibly to a lesser extent than one would think. This may be due to other factors affecting comprehension as opposed to simple reading decoding or word recognition. Many studies implicate strong bilateral activation in the occipital lobe fusiform and lingual cortices (ventral stream) in both word recognition and semantic processing. Structures that are generally activated during sentence-level comprehension were also activated during narrative reading comprehension. These include the middle and superior temporal gyri and inferior frontal cortex as well as the anterior temporal lobes (Hasson et al., 2007). What is most important is the finding that the dorsomedial prefrontal cortex is more highly activated for reading comprehension than for other types of comprehension (Yarkoni et al.,

2008). This finding strongly suggests that there is a network that is active in reading comprehension that is specific to this process and includes anterior systems and, to a lesser extent, posterior regions (Xu et al., 2005). While most of these structures were found to show stronger activation in the left hemisphere, when the material is abstract and requires substantial processing, there is more bilateral activation particularly in the dorsomedial prefrontal cortex (Hasson et al., 2007; Yarkoni et al., 2008), which is involved in self-referential thinking. Thus, metacognition or "thinking about your thinking" is relevant not only for self-control of learning but also for understanding what is read and the meaning one creates from it.

In addition to the findings just noted, the role of memory for what has been read has also been evaluated using neuroimaging. The posterior parietal region has been found to be involved in the reading of individual words and translating letters to words. It is also important for updating the changes in stimuli from letters or sounds to words. In contrast, the temporal lobe structures are important for updating the task comprehension through pairing of words to meaning, with explicit understanding more a left-hemisphere function, an implicit understanding more right hemisphere in nature (Bryan & Hale, 2001). Memory plays an important role in both hemispheres, making implicit comprehension both a right- and left-hemisphere function, with an intact corpus callosum allowing for information flowing between the hemispheres. Memory functions have been found to be important for analysis of the whole of the narrative task in contrast to the comprehension of single sentences (Yarkoni et al., 2008).

The Role of the "Default Mode" Network in Reading Comprehension

As we've seen, the role of the right hemisphere in reading comprehension has become quite clear in recent years. However, narrative comprehension is a bilateral task and not solely a right-hemispheric one (Ferstl et al., 2007; Yarkoni et al., 2008). Analysis of fMRI activation in children who were exposed to scrambled sentences versus stories found that both hemispheres showed increased activation over time spent reading, which predicted recognition and comprehension on tests administered after the scan was completed (Yarkoni et al., 2008). When looking at comprehension of coherent versus incoherent written materials, it was found that the dorsomedial prefrontal cortex is most activated for reading comprehension and this activation is bilateral (Xu et al., 2005). Similarly, the areas of the dorsomedial prefrontal cortex, the angular gyrus and the precuneus of the parietal lobe work together as a network and are considered a "default mode" network; this network is activated when a person is not actively working on a task (Buckner et al., 2008). This network has been implicated in a child's ability to engage in self-referential processing and the forming of mental images by retrieving and integrating information (Hassabis & Maguire, 2007). Because comprehension requires such reconstruction of content, the activation of this default network is reasonable as the child reading works at obtaining meaning from what has been read.

It is important to differentiate between narrative text and expository text. Narrative text tells a story and requires inferential thinking and "theory of mind"—that is, the ability to think about what is being read and how it applies to previous experiences of the reader. Thus, there is an element of orbital functioning in narrative comprehension involving discourse to understand the gist of the communication (Hale & Fitzer, 2015; Jacoby & Fedorenko, 2020). In contrast, expository text explains a situation and frequently uses technical ideas and terms that may be unfamiliar to the reader (Graesser et al., 2004). To support this hypothesis, in one study participants were asked to read, paraphrase, and self-explain different texts during fMRI. Brain areas associated with executive function and comprehension were activated during these tasks with the anterior prefrontal cortex most activated when learning from text was involved (expository reading) (Moss et al., 2011b). This area may serve as a link between the ability to externally represent the idea presented in the text and the internal representation of what has been read. The latter incorporates memory and linkage of what was read to previous experience, thus activating the default network. Requiring the child to explain what has been read to him or her improves reading and also is associated with this default network as well as the executive attention network (Moss et al., 2011a; Sen, 2009).

There are also similarities and differences between comprehension of orally presented information and visually presented information. Oral comprehension provokes increased activation in the superior temporal gyrus (Braze et al., 2011), while reading a word shows increased extrastriate activation and greater left lateralization (Constable et al., 2004). In summary, the differences with words versus sentences versus paragraphs and oral versus written communication are qualitative in nature. In most cases, similar networks are present but depending on the task presented, different parts of the brain are activated differentially. This is why we admonish practitioners to understand task demands when evaluating test results or accommodations taken by classroom teachers. When asked if a student had reading comprehension problems during a teacher interview, the teacher replied, "No, he doesn't have problems; when I read the text out loud in class, he comprehends just fine." While this tells you there is a dissociation between listening and reading comprehension, it tells you little about why there is a difference. That is why your CHT approach to assessment has to understand the *processes* underlying a deficit, and not just solely rely on the input and output demands, or what the CHC-factor categorization suggests. Needless to say, not all comprehension problems are the same.

Neurodevelopment plays a role in our understanding of reading comprehension, too. Similar to increased phonics knowledge, as well as word recognition skills, the brain areas involved change with age. For reading comprehension, activation of the right inferior and superior frontal gyri has been shown to decrease with age with improved comprehension abilities (Meyler et al., 2007), suggesting comprehension is less novel and does not require problem solving to comprehend as one ages. This shift does not occur for children with reading problems. The difference in activation has also been found with adults (Plante, Ramage, & Magloire, 2006) and with dyslexics from Germany (Kronbichler et al., 2006). This finding is similar to that of Shaywitz (2003) where disabled readers had difficulty making a shift from right- to left-hemisphere processes in beginning reading, following the novelty-routinization dichotomy presented in Chapter 2. However, as one interprets more complex prose in the later grades, such as content presented in poetry, the right hemisphere becomes more engaged again to understand the implicit meaning associated with the content (Beeman & Chiarello, 2013; Horowitz-Kraus, Vannest, Gozdas, et al., 2014).

With such a complex system, it is reasonable to speculate about why children can experience difficulty at any level in the reading process. Please consider the following question: Is it possible to have a reading comprehension problem without a word-reading problem? From what we've already learned, the answer is undeniably yes—depending on the task requirements involved as well as the child's ability to reread, paraphrase, or infer information from the materials. The outdated belief that fluent word reading is the only skill needed for reading comprehension is not supported by the behavioral reading data or neuroimaging studies.

You can see that multiple brain areas and neuropsychological processes are involved in reading comprehension. Not only are the basic psychological processes of word recognition included in reading comprehension, but several other higher-level skills associated with left- and right-hemisphere tertiary areas are required as well. As has been proposed by some researchers, adequate word recognition and fluency skills are important, but not sufficient, for adequate reading comprehension (Castles et al., 2018), which requires many systems not tied directly to reading or language, such as executive and right-hemisphere functions.

Empirical Studies of Psychological Processes in RD Assessment and Intervention

Although a thorough review is beyond the scope of this book, we would like to share with you some important evidence to further your understanding of the relevance of psychological processes for reading assessment and intervention. There has been considerable CHC theory-driven research that attests to both the value of a "pattern of strengths and weaknesses" (PSW) approach to assessment and its relevance for intervention. One extremely valuable source has been compiled by Kevin McGrew and colleagues over the last 25 years. Although this chapter emphasizes the differences between typical reading and those who have processing deficits that lead to RDs, this research group has focused on typical CHC achievement relationships, with limited distinction between typical learners and those with RD.

In the original work by Evans (2002) and McGrew and Wendling (2010), CHC relations with reading achievement showed strong relationships between CHC factors of crystallized intelligence (*Gc*), long-term memory/retrieval (*Glr*), processing speed (*Gs*), and working memory (*Gsm-WM*), and appear to be most related to basic reading skills and reading comprehension. Whereas the influence of *Gs* and *Glr* decreased with age, *Gc* and *Gsm-WM* influences increased with age, suggesting the switch from basic skill development (e.g., associative learning, naming speed) to more language-based and prior knowledge constructs necessary for later reading. For reading comprehension, there was an element of auditory processing (*Ga*) and, of course, *Gc* and *Gsm-WM*, but fluid reasoning (*Gf*) also played a role in older children, suggesting higher-level comprehension requires maintaining content in working memory to solve novel (or more complex) comprehension questions.

In their updated work (Cormier et al., 2017), the researchers found that reading achievement was most predicted by *Gf, Gc, Gwm,* and *Ga*, which is consistent with the literature. Although *Gs* was a strong predictor of reading fluency, as expected, *Gf* and *Gc* also showed modest relationships, as was the case with their prediction of reading comprehension. However, some interesting findings emerged, such as the fact that *Gc* was related more to reading fluency than to reading rate. This is likely due to the nature of the task, since reading fluency requires reading and comprehending simple sentences, and deciding if they are true/false, so reading fluency is just part of what this test measures. The strong *Gf* relationship, in post hoc analyses, revealed most of the variance was related to Number Series, which requires detecting numerical–sequential relationships to recognize the pattern among the numbers, attesting to the importance of sequential processing and novel problem solving when reading passages to decipher their meaning. In an attempt to address the limitations of applying standardization sample results to different populations, Hajovsky et al. (2020) used quantile regression using a large sample ($N = 3,891$) to show how relevant cognitive-achievement relations differed depending on outcomes, but that these relationships were stronger for those at the lower end of the achievement distribution. They found *Gc* and *Ga* to be strong predictors of reading comprehension achievement, even when the influences of word reading and sentence reading fluency were included in the equation.

There have also been numerous studies that show the value of a PSW approach in understanding individual differences in reading, many of them conducted using the C-DM model of SLD identification described in Chapter 1. These references focus on different processing characteristics of those with RDs, as well as typical learners, furthering the argument about the relevance of PSW research in differential diagnosis or identification of children with RDs. For instance, Fiorello et al. (2006) found four subtypes of RDs, including a global RD, fluency-comprehension RD, phonological RD, and orthographic RD, consistent with the literature presented here. These findings were further elaborated on in our chapter on the relevance of the WISC-IV for Assessment and Intervention (Hale, Fiorello et al., 2008), where different CHC predictors of achievement outcomes for children with RDs were established. For instance, while *Gc* was a strong predictor of both word reading and reading comprehension for both samples, it was higher for the RD group. In contrast, *Gsm-WM* was more important for word reading in the typical group, but considerably more important for reading comprehension in the RD group. Notably, the shared variance among all four factors was only 10% for word reading and 11% for reading comprehension in the typical readers, but only .7 and 2%, respectively, in explaining these reading domains for children with RDs, attesting to the importance of going beyond general intelligence for those with RDs. We then discuss the relevance of CHC processes for assessment of RDs on the DAS-II (Elliott, 2008), with differences found between the typical and C-DM determined population of children with RDs. Interestingly, over 42.5 and 45.7% of the word-reading variance was predicted by CHC factors in the typical and RD groups, respectively. While CHC predictors accounted for 48.9% of reading comprehension variance in the typical group, they only accounted for 29.7% of this achievement area for children with RDs. Regardless, these are substantial amounts of variance, attesting to the value of cognitive CHC processes in reading achievement. In addition, different patterns were found for both groups, with *Gc* (.39), *Gf* (.18), *Gsm-WM* (.22), and *Ga* (.29) found to predict word reading, but for children with RDs, the pattern was different. Consistent with neuroimaging findings, *Ga* (.59), *Gv* (.26), *Glr* (.30), and *Gs* (.22) predicted word reading for the RD group, suggesting compensatory right-hemisphere mechanisms attempt to compensate for poor phonological awareness.

Others have found similar results supporting the many psychological processes that are important for differential diagnosis of RDs, several using methods similar to those just described. For instance, a special issue of *Learning Disabilities: A Multidisciplinary Journal* was devoted to the relevance of PSW approaches to understanding SLD using the C-DM model (Mather & Tanner, 2014). In the Carmichael et al. (2015) study, no SLD, left-hemisphere SLD, right-hemisphere SLD, working memory SLD, processing speed SLD and Executive SLD subtypes were found. However, they did find the WM and EX SLD subtypes to be more impaired than the PS SLD group on Number–Letter, the LH group more impaired on Story Memory, and the RH group more impaired on Design Memory. One article in particular was related to reading (Feifer et al., 2015). They found differences in predictors of word reading, reading fluency, and reading comprehension for their No SLD, Associative Learning *SLD, Gf-Gv, Gc,* and *Gs* subtypes, again demonstrating that children with RDs are a diverse, heterogenous group, with different processing strengths and weaknesses accounting for their deficits.

Fiorello et al. (2014), in their summary paper for the *Learning Disabilities* special issue, note that as evidence emerges into the numerous causes of SLD, including RDs, practitioners can see the relevance for PSW in their assessment and intervention practices. Their paper argues for a merging of neuropsychological theory and CHC-based practice, with a Lurian model serving as a meaningful template for the intersection of science and practice (Hale, Fiorello et al., 2010; Schneider et al., 2013). Clearly, while CHC-based research helps guide interpretation efforts, the cognitive differences between typical learners and those with RDs make it clear that more careful analysis of patterns of PSW be considered when conducting assessments and interventions for children with RDs (Decker et al., 2013). While the treatment efficacy of findings has been limited thus far, results suggest that understanding cognitive-achievement relationships could foster more tailored or specific intervention efforts for those who struggle with SLD (Fiorello et al., 2008; Fuchs et al., 2011; Hale, Fiorello, et al., 2010).

Instructional Strategies for Children with RDs

Individual Differences and Intervention

Now that we have a basic understanding of the neuropsychological bases of word recognition and reading comprehension, let us turn briefly to intervention. As stated in the previous chapters, we feel that a majority of children can be helped by using prereferral strategies, and for those who cannot be, comprehensive evaluation and individualized intervention are in order. With the information on the neuropsychological bases of RDs described in this chapter, you can develop an assessment protocol designed to examine each child's unique characteristics, develop and test hypotheses about his or her strengths and weaknesses, and provide recommendations for intervention that are uniquely tailored to the child's needs. As stated in previous chapters, this is merely the *beginning* of linking assessment to intervention. Building upon your shared knowledge with the teacher, you can work collaboratively with him or her to brainstorm instructional strategies, develop data-based interventions, and evaluate the efficacy of your intervention. The continuation of the CHT model beyond the initial classification or diagnosis is what allows you to be sure that interventions are effective for each child, and that your assessment results have true treatment validity. It also allows for the information to be conveyed in a therapeutic manner; that is, not just presenting scores but clarifying what the scores actually mean for the student you evaluate.

As a result, we do not offer you a "diagnostic–prescriptive" model in this or the remaining chapters. There are too many systems involved in reading, especially comprehension, to choose a 1:1 association between processing deficit(s) and a single intervention. The early attempts to find aptitude–treatment interactions (ATIs) failed largely because researchers had poorly constructed measures of cognitive processes and little understanding of how the brain actually works; they also relied on interventions that were not designed to meet the unique needs of individual children (Hale, Wycoff, et al., 2011). If you develop large-group ATI designs and put heterogeneous children in each group, it is not surprising that the overall results will be insignificant. This is what largely happened with a massive failed RTI study where the only defining feature was more "intense" reading instruction (Balu et al., 2015). However, we cannot accept the null hypothesis about ATI—that there is no relationship between neuropsychological functioning and educational and psychosocial outcomes. We must instead continue to explore individual ATIs at the single-subject level, but this cannot happen if we fail to recognize each child's unique pattern of neuropsychological performance (Hale et al., 2013). We have provided a model of neuropsychological functioning along with reliable and valid measures to tap those constructs. It is now up to you to establish concurrent, ecological, and treatment validity for each individual child.

Interventions for Word Reading and Reading Comprehension

Given the caveat stated above, let's explore the major interventions for word reading and reading comprehension. In addition to the ideas presented here and in Appendix 5.1, which lists several of the recommended interventions for word recognition cited in the literature, you may wish to purchase one or more general texts on special education or specific reading interventions. We make no claims as to the efficacy of these evidence-based interventions, and further consultation with the sources will be necessary before you undertake any one intervention. These interventions should be beneficial for addressing many of the reading deficits described in this chapter, but always keep in mind that programs must be tailored to the child's individual needs. In addition, recall that the use of compensation, remediation, or both is dependent on the child's age and the severity of his or her problems, as noted in Chapter 3.

Linking Assessment to Intervention

The complexity of these issues is highlighted in the following case report, where we take you from assessment to intervention with a boy who appeared to have attention problems only, but who was found to have significant problems with reading. Case Report 5.1 shows that recommendations for children similar to John need to be made using a systematic CHT approach.

Case Report 5.1. Summary of Neuropsychological Evaluation

Name: John C

Reason for Evaluation

John C is a 7-year, 11-month-old, right-handed, Caucasian male, referred for a complete neuropsychological evaluation. He attends a Montessori School and receives an Individualized Education Plan (IEP) under the primary category of Developmental Delay. He is currently in second grade. John's father reported that John has continued to exhibit significant fine-motor difficulties, despite receiving intervention. John also has demonstrated academic difficulties, such as having trouble learning to read.

Behavioral Observations

John was cooperative with requests and followed directions. Rapport with John was easily established and maintained. John exhibited a neutral to happy mood and congruent affect. John responded best to concrete, specific questions.

Impressions

John's current neuropsychological evaluation revealed significant variability within his performance on indices of cognitive functioning ranging from average scores to significantly below average ability. Specifically, his skills in many key areas measured were within the average range of functioning and consistent with age expectations. For example, his ability to learn new associations was in the average range, such as associating new names with pictures, both immediately after presentation and after a time delay. Additionally, his verbal reasoning and knowledge skills were in the average range. In contrast, John demonstrated a distinct area of weakness within the cognitive measure, as he had significant struggles with tasks that measured simultaneous processing skills. This finding means that he had difficulties with nonverbal reasoning tasks, which involve the integration of nonverbal information to solve problems, such as completing a block pattern or completing an incomplete figure with the correct configuration. These findings do not support a diagnosis of a developmental delay or of intellectual impairment.

John's ability to read a short passage and respond to questions about the passage was in the impaired range. He was able to identify single letters accurately (such as the letters "f," "h," and "w"); however, he was unable to read or sound out any of the required words. Teacher ratings also indicated that John exhibits learning problems in the school environment. Additionally, John's performance on reading tasks is significantly discrepant from his cognitive abilities and is consistent with a diagnosis of a Specific Learning Disorder, With Impairment in Reading (also referred to as *dyslexia*). Additionally, John's academic skills in writing and mathematics were not evaluated within the current evaluation as he was quite fatigued following the measures that were administered. Upon completion of an academic achievement test in the school evaluation, it is recommended that his educational team consider whether John meets criteria for a specific learning disorder in written expression and/or mathematics, based upon the achievement data in these domains.

Additionally, John has a history of speech/language difficulties, which were evident in informal language samples throughout the evaluation. John's phonological processing skills were assessed in the current evaluation, and his performance was in the average range and consistent with his previous results. Parent ratings of John's overall adaptive skills of daily living indicated that his communication skills are below average, with a particular weakness noted within his expressive communication. Teacher ratings endorsed that John demonstrates mild weaknesses within his functional communication skills at school. Further testing of John's speech/language skills is deferred to the speech/language pathologist at his upcoming school evaluation.

John's attention and executive functioning skills were also evaluated. Executive functioning refers to a set of skills including the child's ability to monitor thoughts and behaviors in order to achieve a goal or complete a task. John showed several difficulties with inhibition, working memory, verbal fluency, and planning and organization. Parent and teacher reports also indicated that John exhibits significant symptoms of inattention and mild symptoms of hyperactivity in the home environment.

Given the cluster of learning, executive functioning, and attentional problems that he is exhibiting, John's brain appears to be compromised in a manner consistent with a diagnosis of static encephalopathy. Static encephalopathy is a general impairment in brain development and is nonprogressive. This diagnosis captures the manner in which John's specific problem areas, including learning, attention, and executive functioning, are apt to be related to brain-based difficulties regarding functioning and development. It remains very important to continue to monitor John's attention and executive functioning as he progresses, and to pursue re-evaluation if his struggles in these areas persist or exacerbate despite supports and interventions.

John demonstrates several weaknesses on tasks of fine-motor skills, including speed and dexterity, despite receiving an additional year of occupational therapy services and supplemental opportunities to practice fine-motor skills in the home environment. The cluster of difficulties he continues to exhibit with fine-motor control is consistent with a diagnosis of dyspraxia. His history of articulation difficulties can be associated with dyspraxia as well, given the motor demands involved in exhibiting proper articulation of words. Continued consultation and intervention with the occupational therapy team within John's school district is warranted in light of his profile of fine-motor skills difficulties.

Recommendations

The following are recommendations to foster John's progress in the home, school, and community environments. For ease of reference, recommendations that were provided during the prior evaluation and that remain relevant to John's functioning are listed. There are also new recommendations included, based on the current pattern of strengths and weaknesses demonstrated by John.

School/Academic Recommendations

1. We recommend that John's parents share the results of this evaluation with John's school so that the information may be incorporated into his upcoming re-evaluation for special education services via an Individualized Educational Plan (IEP). Consideration of the educational categories of Specific Learning Disability and/or Other Health Impairment is warranted. As noted above, it will be important for his educational team to obtain information regarding John's current level of academic achievement as compared to his cognitive functioning. His educational team is encouraged to implement proactive accommodations that will help to continue to facilitate his strengths while accounting for his difficulties with areas such as learning/academics, executive functioning, and speech/language skills.
2. Additionally, John's educational team is encouraged to consider his eligibility for Extended School Year (ESY) services to allow John to continue to improve and make progress in academics throughout the summer and to reduce potential for a delay or decline in skill acquisition.
3. John is currently at a key period of his development, particularly within the academic/educational context. It is essential for John to receive intensive intervention services during this window of opportunity to foster his growth and progress. For example, he exhibits noteworthy difficulties with learning how to read. Reading permeates the academic environment, particularly as a child becomes older. It is very important for John's educational team to incorporate reading interventions into his daily school programming, in order to foster his foundational skills in this area. Upon

further evaluation of his academic achievement skills, his educational team is also encouraged to consider his eligibility for daily intervention in the core subjects of mathematics and written expression.

4. It is highly recommended that his educators implement teaching strategies so that John can learn new information via multiple modalities, such as combining visual aids with spoken narrative. For example, he is apt to respond best to learning a new math concept with the use of tangible examples (such as blocks or small tokens) in addition to didactic explanation of the math processes.

APPENDIX 5.1. WORD RECOGNITION INTERVENTIONS

Reference	Intervention description
Denton et al. (2011)	Phono-graphix program used and improvement seen on decoding as well as on fluency and comprehension
Fawcett & Nicholson (2001)	Automaticity instruction using direct instruction, task analysis, and mastery
Lindamood (2004)	LiPS: The Lindamood Phoneme Sequencing Program for Reading, Spelling, and Speech
Oakhill & Cain (2012)	Reading accuracy improved with intensive intervention with phonemic awareness and processing
Orton-Gillingham & Stillman (1973)	Highly structured multisensory approach, focusing on 48 English phonemes and rules for consonant and vowel combinations
Weiser (2013)	Integration decoding and encoding activities in early grades fosters improved word recognition skills in later grades

Chapter 6

The Neuropsychology
of Mathematics Disorders

Characteristics of Children with Mathematics Disorders

Is Math Different?

Much more is known about reading disorders (RDs) than about mathematics disorders (MDs) and other types of learning disorders (LDs), even though epidemiological studies suggest they may actually occur at comparable rates. The MD prevalence is estimated to be at 6 to 7% (Geary, 2004) and at 17% with a combined RD and MD (Dirks et al., 2008). Because there is so much emphasis on reading in teacher-training programs, teachers find themselves struggling with mathematics computation, fluency, and word problem instruction, especially when children have difficulty in these areas. These math problems are frequently identified later than those with reading, furthering the problem with underidentification of MD (Toll et al., 2011). It has also been found that these difficulties translate into significant problems in mathematics unless addressed in the early elementary school years (Mix & Cheng, 2012), when the opportunity to learn basic math skills is crucial. Many children with math problems also have problems in reading and written language (up to 65% in one study; Snowling et al., 2021) and in these cases there may be similar neuropsychological explanations for their difficulties in these subjects. Some children are quite anxious when it comes to math skills; others take great pleasure in learning math concepts and computation skills. Some children with MDs have significant psychosocial concerns, while others seem to be well adjusted. The reasons for their differential presentation can be environmental, biological, cognitive, or in all likelihood a combination of all of the above (Geary et al., 2012).

Some argue that MD is essentially the lower end of the normal distribution of math achievement, but the use solely of low achievement definitions for MD likely leads to overidentification of minority and disadvantaged children, or those with behavioral—not academic—concerns (McDermott et al., 2006). In addition, global cognitive scores obscure important math performance differences for children of racial/ethnic difference (e.g., Ortiz et al., 2014). Research criteria for classifying children with an MD have included math scores below the 11th percentile (Mazzocco et al., 2013). Children scoring between the 11th and the 25th percentile are considered to be low achievers in mathematics, but the causes of low achievement differ between children with MD and typical math learners (Hale, Fiorello, Dumont et al., 2008).

248

The use of a percentile score to delineate an MD is a rather crude way of diagnosing a deficit in the basic psychological processes affecting math performance, so it should be no surprise that the CDM PSW approach is preferred by Hale et al. The C-DM approach may be more helpful in differentiating math delay and MD. Findings have suggested that children with an MD show an underlying significant problem with novel problem solving that interferes with learning of mathematics concepts with accompanying weaknesses in working memory (Swanson et al., 2018). Particular weaknesses in MD, but not math delay, include the ability to have a mental representation of a number line and to be able to reject answers that are improbable (Geary, 2013). It was also found that reading skill, particularly reading comprehension, was very poor for children with an MD versus those with a math weakness (Willcutt et al., 2013). This literacy demand likely affects math problem-solving/word problems skills, at least for some children with MD. As we will see, math word problems tap frontal executive and left-hemisphere language processes in addition to traditional calculation skills, so the differentiation of the skills associated with math calculation alone is warranted.

Certainly, math difficulty, whether due to low achievement or MD, is of concern to children, teachers, and parents alike. As was the case with RDs, recognizing how children with MDs solve math problems, and what types of errors they commit, can provide us with an understanding of how to remediate or compensate for their deficient math performance. As we have stressed throughout this book, each child's MD is unique in some way, a combination of processing weaknesses and prior learning influencing the child's performance on outcome measures. A thorough neuropsychological investigation may reveal different underlying causes for difficulties, as can be seen in Case Study 6.1.

Basic Components of Math Competency

To understand the underlying neuropsychological processes required for math competency, it is important to recognize how math skills develop. What do children need in order to learn math skills? In his discussion of concrete operations, Piaget (1965) taught us about several important underlying concepts critical for math competency, including one-to-one correspondence, classification, seriation, and conservation. While you may think these basic cognitive-developmental processes seem too far removed from math competency to warrant your attention, you should recognize that preschoolers' understanding of an approximate number system is at the core of subsequent math achievement (Libertus et al., 2011), with inadequate number sense a major determinant of MD (Jordan et al., 2007). Just as phonological awareness and the alphabetic principle are important for considering RD, the poor understanding of magnitude and quantitative relationships are key problems found in MD.

When children are learning about quantity and operations (especially addition), teachers often use concrete objects at first and then move to representing quantity using numbers. From these basic skills, students learn addition, subtraction, multiplication, division, and fractions typically in a hierarchical fashion. Most researchers recommend introduction of word problems early during this sequence, if not at the very beginning (Toll et al., 2012). More advanced areas, such as geometry and algebra, are not always taught in the same order or in the same grade, with these associated math competencies being introduced at earlier grades than was the case in the past. Although a review of math scope and sequence charts suggest that math instruction is fairly predictable, it is important to examine each child's curriculum and exposure to different math concepts before determining whether the child has a math deficit based on standardized and/or curriculum-based tests. As many children will tell you, one reason they can't do a particular math operation is "We haven't done that yet." This is also why ability–achievement discrepancy is easily seen in some children with above

Case Study 6.1. Lessons in Learning: Making Math Count for Maria

Maria, an 8-year-old girl, was referred for a comprehensive evaluation because of her persistent difficulty with math computation and word problems (the latter was especially problematic). During the teacher interview it, was reported that no matter how hard Maria tried, "she just didn't get it." Although Maria's teacher, Ms. Sollem, was hard-pressed to provide details, she said that Maria's homework wasn't too bad, but that she couldn't remember how to do the work during board time (when children did problems at the board) or on tests. Ms. Sollem suspected that Maria's concerned mother was helping her complete her homework, which took "hours" every night. The same pattern emerged upon reading Maria's file: fairly good homework performance and abysmal test scores. It was found during the evaluation that there was difficulty with retrieval of information and processing speed difficulties, but these findings were inconsistent. The CHT did not sufficiently support these deficits, and again findings were inconsistent. Maria did much better on multiple-choice than on free-recall tasks, consistent with retrieval problems; however, her language skills and verbal fluency were intact. In addition, Maria did fine with math computation, had greater difficulty with word problems, and performed quite poorly on a math fluency subtest. Maria's math problems were a neuropsychological mystery.

When there appears to be no consistent pattern of performance borne out during CHT, it may be because there are no real neuropsychological deficits, and you should look for psychosocial explanations. The personality/behavioral evaluation results revealed signs of anxiety, withdrawal, depression, and isolation. Maria also had low self-esteem and unresolved attachment issues. In addition, Maria reported during the interview that she had always hated math, became nervous when she had to work at the board, and froze during the math tests. She felt "stupid" when it came to doing math, and "sick" when it came time to take tests. As you will see in Chapter 9, there is a strong interrelationship between psychosocial and neuropsychological functioning, and Maria's case seemed to be a prime example of this. After the evaluation was completed, it became clear that Maria's problems were largely related to psychosocial issues. The examiner and the teacher developed an intervention to increase Maria's sense of math self-efficacy, enhance her test-taking skills, and improve her peer relationships. This was combined with anxiety management strategies (systematic desensitization, relaxing breaths, and progressive muscle relaxation). Strategies were also suggested to improve the mother–daughter relationship and decrease homework completion time. Maria's performance began to improve over the following months, and eventually she gained confidence in her math skills. Soon thereafter, Maria began to do just as well in class and on tests as she had during her homework sessions, and her homework only took a half hour every night.

---

average cognitive functioning—these children typically cannot achieve beyond what they've been taught in the classroom, hence their scores may be mathematically discrepant.

As noted in Chapter 5, part of linking assessment to intervention requires an examination of the types of cognitive and achievement errors a child displays during testing. As is the case with reading error patterns, it is important for you to identify the child's math error patterns during your comprehensive CHT evaluation. This cannot always be ascertained by looking at the child's final answers, so if error types are found, it is often helpful to have the child verbalize the algorithm steps as he or she completes the problem. Take, for example, the following verbalization from a child named Lucy as she solved a problem:

$$\begin{array}{r} 64 \\ + \underline{13} \\ 14 \end{array}$$

64   *"First I look and see if it is addition or subtraction. OK, addition, so you always*

+ 13   *go top to bottom and left to right. So I add 6 + 4, and that equals 10, and then*

14   *1 + 3 equals 4, and then I add them together, top to bottom, 10 + 4 equals 14."*

As you can see, what at first seems to be a random response, or a poor attempt at sub-traction, becomes clear from Lucy's commentary regarding her faulty algorithm. Her simple addition is OK, but she has little concept of place value or of the algorithm she needs to respond successfully to such two-digit addition problems. Look for these and other error patterns when you are conducting CHT evaluations for children with MDs. The following error patterns (with abbreviations that you can use in making notes) are frequently found in children with various types of MDs:

- Numeracy error (NE)—Child has not learned quantitative knowledge, does not recognize number magnitude or relationships among quantity.
- Math fact error (FE)—Child has not learned math facts or does not automatically retrieve them from long-term memory.
- Operand error (OE)—Child performs one operation instead of another (e.g., performs $6 + 3$ for $6 - 3$ problem – common in children with attention problems).
- Algorithm error (AE)—Child performs steps out of sequence or follows idiosyncratic algorithm or pattern of solving problem (e.g., subtracting smaller from larger number, regardless of position: $123 - 87 = 164$; that is, $7 - 3 = 4$; $8 - 2 = 6$; $1 - 0 = 1$).
- Place value error (PE)—Child carries out the steps in order but makes a place value error (which could be due to visual–spatial processes, but also to algorithm problems).
- Regrouping error (RE)—Child regroups when not required, forgets to subtract from regrouped column during subtraction, or adds regrouped number before multiplication.
- Executive error (EE)—Child loses track of steps in the problem, does not incorporate previously solved part of problem, or misses steps in the problem.
- Spatial error (SE)—child misaligns columns and arrives at incorrect solution or has difficulty transposing a horizontal problem

$$2 + 4 = 6$$

to a vertical problem

$$\begin{array}{r} 2 \\ +4 \\ \hline 6 \end{array}$$

Difficulties in Math Related to Age

Difficulty with mathematics can show up at an early age. The earliest signs of difficulty are present in young children in learning to count, problems recognizing numbers, difficulty understanding quantity, difficulty understanding the relation of the numeral to number of items, problems with organization, and difficulty discriminating shapes. For elementary aged children problems with learning math facts is a primary area of concern. This difficulty later translates into difficulty mastering more advanced classes in applied mathematics and later in high school in classes such as algebra and calculus. In a recent evaluation, when asked to do a multistep math problem, the student had no problem saying, "We don't learn how to do these problems by hand, give me a calculator and I can do just fine." Although this commonly used "accommodation" is touted by many math teachers, the bottom line is the brain learns by *practicing* math, not by providing a calculator to do the math for the children.

Difficulty with remembering math algorithms and functions also emerges in elementary aged children. Similarly, problems can arise with understanding measurement, money, and time. By adolescence and adulthood, difficulties are present with estimation, budgeting, applying math facts to word problems, problems with balancing the checkbook, and difficulty approaching a problem from more than one perspective. Today's "modern math" approach, which emphasizes concept formation and problem solving, may work well for those who have acquired basic math facts and calculation skills; however, for those with rudimentary understanding of basic math skills, the idea of solving problems that require those skills is largely absent. I often will ask students, "Quickly, tell me which answer is more 87 − 74 (answer 13) or 22 − 5 (answer 17)?" Without a good number sense and understanding of quantitative relationships or estimation skills, the answer is not easily obtained.

Children entering kindergarten who later display MDs generally are found to show poor number aptitude upon entry into school and poor sight-word vocabulary (Geary et al., 2012). In this study, difficulties with number aptitude have been found related to poor fluency in understanding numerals and quantity while the poor sight-word vocabulary was due to slow rapid automatized naming. In addition, children with MDs displayed problems with long-term memory for facts, working memory, and attention—difficulties that spanned from kindergarten through fifth grade. Of particular interest are the neuropsychological functions of attention, working memory, and automaticity that are implicated with MDs. An intervention remediation study of kindergarteners who performed below the 50th percentile on a numeracy test found that those who were between the 25th and 50th percentile responded well to direct teaching of numeracy, but those below the 25th percentile did not show similar improvement (Toll & Van Luit, 2012). Children who had stronger verbal working memory skills showed more academic increases from the intervention in their mathematics skills. This finding strongly suggests that working memory is an important component in numeracy and in early mathematics mastery. It also supports the hypothesis by Andersson (2008) that in order to provide a comprehensive and useful assessment of mathematical achievement, it is very important to assess early number sense as well as working memory abilities. A recent meta-analysis of cognitive factors involved in math learning disabilities (Kroesbergen et al., 2023) revealed that number sense, working memory, and rapid automatized naming (a measure of fluency of retrieval from long-term memory) were lower in people with MD.

CHC Theory and Math Achievement

Much of the CHC research has been conducted using normative samples, and so focuses on typically developing students rather than those with identified MDs. Although students with MDs may process information differently, an overview of the basic research linking cognitive processing with math will be helpful as a starting point.

A great deal of research focused on CHC theory has been conducted by Kevin McGrew and his research team. A systematic review of the CHC cognitive processes and their links to achievement (McGrew & Wendling, 2010) discusses both basic math skills and math reasoning. The broad abilities of fluid reasoning (*Gf*), crystallized ability or verbal comprehension and knowledge (*Gc*), and processing speed (*Gs*) are linked to basic math skills. Narrow abilities also predict basic math skills. Phonological processing (*Ga-PC*) is a significant predictor for ages 6 to 13 and is linked to fact fluency deficits in children with MDs, perhaps because speech sound processing is involved in counting and solving problems. Within processing speed, number facility (*Gs-N*) and perceptual speed (*Gs-P*) are important predictors of basic math skills, perhaps as a function of rapid retrieval of math facts and subitizing ability, which are key deficits in students with MDs. Working memory (*Gwm-MW*) is significantly and highly linked to basic math skills in individuals of all ages and has been identified as a core deficit in people with MDs.

Math reasoning or math problem solving depends in part on basic math skills, but cognitive processes contribute as well. McGrew and Wendling (2010) identify fluid reasoning (*Gf*) as a strong predictor of math problem solving, consistent with prior research. In addition, fluid reasoning is often a key deficit in individuals with MDs. Comprehension and knowledge (*Gc*) predict math problem solving with increased significance over the developmental period, which may reflect the linguistic processing required for more complex math problems. Processing speed (*Gs*) is also a contributor to math problem solving, most notably perceptual speed (*Gs-P*), linked to counting speed and rapid processing of numbers. Working memory (*Gwm*), including memory span, working memory capacity, and visual memory, are important to math problem solving. As with basic math skills, phonological processing (*Ga-PC*) shows some significant links to math reasoning, especially at younger ages.

In a study comparing students with no LD to students demonstrating an MD defined two different ways (one based on low achievement alone and one based on IQ–achievement discrepancy with low achievement), Tolar and colleagues (2016) found cognitive ability differences between the two groups of students with LD. The discrepancy-identified MD students showed poorer working memory and word problem solving than the low-achieving MD students. A comparison of the low-achieving MD students with low average math achievers shows differences in fluid reasoning and working memory, with the MD students performing worse on both. Although these authors did not evaluate as many cognitive abilities, their findings are consistent with previous work, confirming that working memory and fluid reasoning are critical to identifying MDs.

Students with a nonverbal learning disorder (NVLD) were compared to students with no identified LD in a small study (Mammarella et al., 2013). The NVLD group, which showed an MD, also displayed poor visual–spatial working memory as assessed with complex span tasks. This study focused on geometry difficulties, highlighting the importance of visual–spatial working memory.

Although Naglieri's PASS theory is not entirely compatible with CHC theory or the neuropsychological model of cognitive functioning, his concept of planning is one part of what we call executive functions. Students who exhibit difficulties in mathematics and who are poor in planning have been shown to benefit from strategy-based instruction (Naglieri & Johnson, 2000).

Comorbidity Disorders and Math Difficulties and Disorders

As noted in Chapter 5, the overlap of MD and RD can be substantial (65%; Snowling et al., 2021). The historical emphasis on RDs but not MDs, is misguided as prevalence rates indicate that RDs and MDs are each found in about 6% of the population (Geary, 2004). A large epidemiological study found MD rates ranged from 5.9 to 13.8%, with many of these children (35 to 57%) *not* having comorbid RD (Dirks et al., 2008). These findings suggest there may be distinct explanations for reading and math LDs, at least in some children, but for others, a core deficit might explain both RD and MD.

Not surprisingly, there is some debate as to the nature of MDs in relation to RDs and other LDs. Whereas some have suggested that MDs can be unique LDs, others suggest that MDs are due to more generalized LDs, as they frequently co-occur. In one study (Swanson, 2012) that addressed this interrelationship, children with MD scored lower than those with RD on visual–spatial and visual working memory measures, but scored higher on measures of motor speed and random word generation. In contrast, children with MD, RD, and low achievement all scored lower than those functioning in the average range on random word generation, motor speed, and verbal working memory measures. Similarly, RD and MD have been found to show overlap in some neuropsychological and psychosocial deficits, with phonological and naming speed deficits unique to RD and a set shifting deficit unique to MD (Willcutt et al., 2013). As such, MDs and RDs may share some of the same underlying neuropsychological difficulties such as working memory, processing speed, and verbal comprehension (Willcutt et al., 2013), with comorbidity rates high not only among LDs, but also between MD and ADHD (Mayes & Calhoun, 2006). A common link often cited is working memory deficits for MD and ADHD (Geary et al., 2012; Willcutt et al., 2005). Although this could suggest a common underlying deficit associated with MDs and RDs, others are quick to point out that poor instructional techniques and textbooks could take the blame for some math problems (Watson & Gable, 2012). Because math instruction is sequential and hierarchical (Fuchs, Powell, et al., 2010) students with math learning problems may quickly fall behind their peers, making subsequent instructional efforts less likely to lead to academic success. If more intense instruction in an MTSS model is not successful, we shouldn't give them more of the same, but instead find out how best to help the student overcome their MD.

ADHD and MD

As discussed earlier, children with MDs often have difficulty with visual working memory (Toll et al., 2016), which is thought to be one of the deficits found in children with ADHD (Young et al., 2011). Children with ADHD have similar difficulties with working memory as well as with attention, planning, and organization. Solving arithmetic problems requires adequate attention to detail as well as the ability to maintain and manipulate information in working memory. Some have suggested that the problems children with ADHD have with mathematics are due to these difficulties and not due to MD (Preston & Carter, 2009). Studies have found an overlap of approximately 11 to 26% of MD and ADHD (Monuteaux et al., 2005). Another study found an overlap of 20% of MD and ADHD (Capano et al., 2008). The presence of MD and ADHD was not found related to gender or age (Shalev, 2004). When MD and ADHD co-occur, more difficulties are found in general learning and academic achievement likely related to difficulties with working memory, language, and lower IQ (Capano et al., 2008). In comparison, children with ADHD and without MD were not found to show similarly poor performance in these areas. Twin studies have found genetic factors accounting for comorbidity of these disorders (Polderman et al., 2011). Findings of a stronger relation between attention and MD compared to hyperactivity and MD suggest a unique genetic contribution apart from IQ or reading abilities (Greven et al., 2014). Peterson et al. (2017) studied a large community-based sample of twins ages 8 to 16. Processing speed was found to show a strong contribution to difficulty with attention and mathematics but not to reading difficulties. Visual working memory was also found to be associated with problems with mathematics while inhibition was found to be more related to attentional problems than to mathematics. Conclusions from this study were that it is important to identify these children early, and that children with attention deficits but not hyperactivity are at higher risk for mathematics problems. Finally, weaknesses in processing speed need to be considered a strong risk factor for difficulty with mathematics. While this study found that mathematical difficulties continue through childhood and adolescence, some mathematic skills emerge only in later teen years and thus serial evaluations are strongly recommended for children with ADHD.

Anxiety and MDs

Mathematics anxiety has been defined as a negative emotional reaction to mathematics where a person actively avoids math (Carey et al., 2016). Girls are reported to have higher anxiety toward math than boys generally at the high school level (Hill et al., 2016). Two dimensions have been described for mathematics anxiety: cognitive (worry) and affective (nervousness, tension) (Dowker et al., 2016). Mathematics anxiety is not a diagnostic category but rather a description. Two models have been suggested (Carey et al., 2016): the debilitating anxiety model and the deficit theory. The deficit theory suggests that anxiety is based on poor mathematics performance while the debilitating theory is where a person has high mathematics anxiety that interferes with learning. Some studies have found that children with MD show higher rates of math anxiety than children without MD (Lai et al., 2015). While the deficit theory has roots in MD, it has not been posited that the debilitating anxiety accounts for MD (Ma & Xu, 2004). In a large study of children with MD, Devine et al. (2018) found a moderate negative correlation between MD and anxiety. It is important to note that almost 80% of this sample of children with MD did not show higher anxiety, which means that 20% did show higher anxiety, particularly around mathematics. Similar to the findings in the general population of higher anxiety toward math in girls than in boys, girls with MD also showed higher levels of anxiety, with girls reporting lower self-efficacy toward mathematics, particularly in secondary school levels. Interventions that have addressed anxiety toward mathematics, as well as teaching mathematical constructs, have been found to be more successful than those that concentrate solely on mathematics (Ramirez & Beilock, 2011).

Turner Syndrome/Fragile X and MDs

Given that the genetic disorders of Turner syndrome and fragile X syndrome influence white matter functioning, it is not surprising that children with these disorders also experience MDs at a higher rate than typically achieving peers (Mazzocco, 2001). However, there appears to be a dissociation for the two disorders, with those with fragile X syndrome showing more difficulty with visual–spatial relationships (presumably right parietal) than those with Turner syndrome showing more object recognition delays and better math achievement (Mazzocco et al., 2006). Thus, visual–spatial aspects of mathematics cognition, and executive-mediated visual working memory, as opposed to the relationship with visual object recognition, explain this difference (Murphy et al., 2010).

Defining and Differentiating MD from Other Math Problems

In Search of the Core Processing Deficit in MD

How can you tell whether a child has an MD or not? You may be thinking that we will provide you with a "red flag" test predictor. Unfortunately, as was the case with RD, MD can be caused by multiple problems, with no consistent finding for all children with MD or consistent factor that discriminates children with MD from those who are low math achievers. Adding to the confusion is that the term *MD* has been used interchangeably with the neuropsychological term *dyscalculia*, a specific impairment in math computation or concepts frequently present after a CNS event (a stroke, etc.) but it can also occur developmentally as well.

As we have discussed earlier, however, the likelihood of a "pure" MD in the children you see is unlikely, but it does occur. Some argue that basic processing of numbers, or understanding of quantitative relationships, underlies all MDs (Landerl et al., 2013). Those with MD do not appear to develop the prerequisite approximate number system that reflects the essence of quantitative relationships (Mazzocco et al., 2011). When one considers the hierarchical and sequential nature of math instruction, it should not be surprising this foundational skill underlies math competency, with failure to understand numeracy being the cause of many MDs. Geary (2004) notes that subitizing (size differences), ordinality (< or >), and serial counting are necessary prerequisites for developing basic math skills. That is, in essence, an element of math that is perhaps different from other academic subjects, in that quantity *in relation to another quantity* explains the essence of math skill development. Children who master the foundational skills of reading numerals, counting, number line concepts, and mental addition will attain sufficient numeric processing competency to achieve higher-level mathematics (Mazzocco & Thompson, 2005).

There is evidence that the ability to represent space as a mental number line begins in early childhood extending to adulthood (Noles et al., 2005). When this ability does not develop, the children frequently have significant problems with understanding quantity and basic mathematics facts. An intriguing finding is that people can more quickly identify small numbers with their left hand than with their right hand, which has been termed the SNARC (Spatial Numerical Association of Response Codes) effect; it involves representing quantities linearly using the body as the midpoint (de Hevia & Spelke, 2009; Lourenco & Longo, 2009). When these basic skills do not develop, children experience significant problems with mathematics, and some suggest that like reading, there is a double-deficit hypothesis in MDs, which includes deficits in both number sense and nonverbal working memory (Toll et al., 2016).

Included with visual–spatial processing is the ability to engage in spatial reasoning, or the manipulation of spatial content for problem solving. There has been a link between spatial ability and mathematics ability in the literature for quite some time (Geary et al., 2007; Rasmussen & Bisanz, 2005). Neuroimaging studies have confirmed that similar areas are activated when children are required to process spatial and number tasks with increased activation in the tertiary parietal lobe areas for both skills (Umilta & Zorzi, 2009). In addition visual–-spatial working memory has been linked to several mathematics skills such as counting (Kyttala et al., 2003), estimation (Geary et al., 2007), and overall mathematics performance (Alloway & Passolunghi, 2011; Meyer et al., 2010). Similarly performance on visual–spatial tasks such as the Wechsler Block Design subtest is also found to correlate significantly with math achievement from the grades of kindergarten to 12th grade (Jordan et al., 2009; Lachance & Mazzocco, 2006; Markey, 2010).

Given its hierarchical nature during instruction, it is not surprising that early intervention has been seen as crucial for mathematics (Jordan et al., 2009). Although numeracy is clearly critical for mathematics competency, there are different cognitive and neuropsychological causes of MD reported in the literature, with alternative intervention strategies offered based on the type of MD. Clearly, one of the problems with most research in mathematics is that children who are achieving well in mathematics are compared with low achievers and those with MD, but how one defines these groups may affect intervention choice and outcomes. As was the case with RDs, increasing our understanding of math deficits by utilizing assessment of specific mathematical problems will improve our ability to provide appropriate interventions.

MD Subtypes Beyond the Core Numeracy Deficit

Collateral evidence can be found to support looking at different underlying deficits in MD, suggesting the presence of specific deficits rather than global delays (Geary et al., 2012). Research had initially suggested three subtypes of MDs: the semantic memory, procedural, and visual–spatial subtypes (Mazzocco & Myers, 2003). The *semantic-memory subtype* is characterized by poor number–symbol association and math fact automaticity. This subtype often has comorbid RDs and language disorders. The *procedural subtype* often involves poor strategy or algorithm use, and has been associated with ADHD and other executive function deficits, which could also affect problem solving during math word problems given the high executive demands required (Prabhakuran et al., 2011). Finally, the *visual–spatial* subtype includes problems with column alignment, place values, operand adherence, and a mental number line. This is the subtype most often associated with Rourke's (1984) NVLDs. We use the term *nonverbal* for continuity with the literature, despite the fact that this is a misnomer, since those with white matter right-hemisphere dysfunction also display deficits in higher-level implicit language skills (Bryan & Hale, 2001), a point that Rourke readily acknowledged. These subtypes have also been found in our research involving the right-hemisphere visual–spatial subtype, fluid/quantitative reasoning, executive/working memory, and numeric quantitative knowledge subtype (Hale, Fiorello, Dumont, et al., 2008). We also found a subtype characterized by presumed left-hemisphere dysfunction, suggesting affected individuals would have similar symptoms to what is known as Gerstmann syndrome—thought to be a left parietal lobe problem (Menon, 2016).

While these classifications have been useful in the past, more recent research has turned to looking at skills for subtype analysis. Using a PSW approach, specifically our concordance–discordance model, Kubas and colleagues (2014) identified a number of subtypes of math disabilities. It should be noted that this study identified the children using a purely psychometric approach, as opposed to using a full CHT model. Nonetheless, a comparison of children with no LD and MDs based on calculation, fluency, or problem-solving scores can be made. Students who showed an MD based on poor math fluency showed a significant weakness on WISC-IV Coding, a test of processing speed that also depends on learning associations between numbers and symbols. They performed relatively strongly on measures of reasoning. Students who displayed an MD based on poor math calculation tended to also score poorly on math fluency as well as on Coding and measures of auditory working memory. Students identified with an MD based on poor applied problems (math problem solving) scored poorly on most measures of achievement, most notably in all areas of math but also reading comprehension. Their cognitive profiles indicated weaknesses in processing speed and working memory but generally average performance otherwise.

In their chapter about the neuroscience of math disabilities, Lindbergh and Brown (2018) identify a number of cognitive processing difficulties underlying math disabilities. The first is number sense, where students with MDs may have deficits in the mental representation of magnitude. Next is fact retrieval, which may indicate difficulties in memory retrieval (*Gr*), working memory (*Gwm*), and processing speed (*Gs*). Fact retrieval difficulties were also identified by de Chambrier and Zesiger (2018) as key in identification of math disabilities. Of course, fact retrieval depends on learning to fluency, which means that ruling out a lack of instruction is particularly important for this ability. Working memory is critical to math performance (Lindbergh & Brown, 2018). Students with MDs also show delays in procedural development and have difficulty with fractions and proportional reasoning.

The understanding of fractions is critical to higher math instruction (Booth & Newton, 2012) and is often specifically difficult for students with MDs (Berch, 2017). Students with MDs often have difficulty even accurately reading decimals and translating the written Arabic numerals into oral language. Translating or understanding the equivalencies among different representations of fractions (decimals, ratios, graphs, etc.) is even more difficult.

In a longitudinal study, Geary (2011a) identifies intelligence, but also processing speed and working memory, specifically the central executive and visual–spatial skills as early predictors of later math achievement. Number sense, here defined as fluency in processing and manipulating set size, numerals, and placements on a number line, was a unique predictor.

In a review of the literature, Cragg and Gilmore (2014) focus on the role of executive functions in math achievement. They identify working memory, inhibition, and shifting as critical components in the development of math proficiency. They posit that working memory predicts facility with math facts and procedures and that shifting predicts proficiency with procedures and concepts, and inhibition predicts all three.

The semantic memory subtype has been broken into three separate subtypes in our new working model. The first subtype is described as a *core deficit in processing quantity* (Butterworth, Varma, & Laurillard, 2011) and *number sense* (Piazza et al., 2010), which lead to difficulty with numerical reasoning and problem solving. These children experience significant problems with quantity estimation (Mazzocco et al., 2011), thought to be a right-hemisphere function. The second subtype is a *weakness in symbolic processing* where children experience weaknesses in the association between a number and a quantity have the but an ability to understand the association between size and quantity (Rubinsten & Henik, 2006). These children have difficulty understanding the difference between numbers (9 is 3 times larger than 3) but can demonstrate this difference when using tangible objects (Rousselle & Noel, 2007). This symbolic number deficit may be bilateral, given the left parietal lobe's involvement in symbolic number representation (L. Kaufmann et al., 2011).

The third subtype combines the procedural subtype and visual–spatial subtype. Children with this math difficulty show *deficits in attention, working memory,* and *visual–spatial reasoning* that are causative of MD instead of a strict number processing deficit (Ashkenazi & Henik, 2010; Toll et al., 2011). These children experience difficulty with the procedures involved in mathematics (similar to the procedural subtype) but not deficits in number sense. Difficulties with visual–spatial and working memory are present (similar to the visual–spatial subtype) (Swanson et al., 2006), attesting to frontal–parietal task positive network activity during math computation. These children demonstrate adequate quantitative knowledge and quantity–symbol associations, but their computation and strategy use are characterized by difficulties with attention, working memory, processing speed, and inhibition (Szucs et al., 2013), which lead to many calculation errors (Chong & Siegel, 2008). As a result, these children tend to rely on immature strategies such as SUM or MIN (see In-Depth 6.1) to solve problems (Geary, 2004). This has been linked to problems with mental computation and processing efficiency and likely affects mathematics problem solving in general. A major difference between the first two types of MDs and the third subtype is related to attention and executive function in the third subtype, with cognitive assessments demonstrating that children with this subtype have considerable difficulty manipulating information in working memory (Geary et al., 2012).

Although multiple executive functions can be implicated in this subtype, working memory has been found to predict mathematical skills better than any other executive function deficit in MDs (Toll & Van Luit, 2012). Working memory has been linked to difficulties with the updating of information as a problem is solved mostly because the storing and manipulation of information during problem solving is disrupted (Andersson, 2008). Other executive functions such as inhibition and shifting have not been linked to MDs (Andersson, 2008; Talairach & Tournoux, 1988; Toll et al., 2011), at least in young children. However, shifting and inhibition may come into play as the complexity of mathematical problems becomes more advanced in later grades. Other executive deficits, such as limited cognitive flexibility, sequencing errors, and difficulty with maintaining information in working memory may be present (Willcutt et al., 2010). Given this evidence suggesting that children with the *working memory/attention* subtype of MD are more likely to experience attention and executive function deficits, you should not be surprised to find that MDs have been associated with the inattentive type of ADHD (Ashkenazi & Henik, 2010) or if hyperactivity and impulsivity are present, the combined type presents due to executive control deficits (Friedman et al., 2018).

IN-DEPTH 6.1. Developmental Progression of Basic Arithmetic

Most children learn initial quantitative relationships by simply counting, using a one-to-one correspondence. As the developmental progression advances, a typical sequence of quantitative knowledge and computation skills is observed. As Geary and colleagues (2000) describe, children gradually shift from counting on fingers, to verbal counting, and then to using what these authors call the MIN (counting on), MAX, or SUM (counting all) procedures until memory-based strategies are used. For the MIN procedure, children usually take the larger addend as a starting point, and then count the quantity necessary to reach the smaller number total (e.g., 7 + 3 = 7, 8-9-10). In the SUM procedure, the child starts at 1 and counts both numbers (e.g., 1-2-3-4-5-6-7, 8-9-10). The MAX procedure starts with the smaller addend, and then counts up from there (e.g., 3, 4-5-6-7-8-9-10). Developmentally, after finger and verbal counting, SUM and MAX are typically used, but MIN is the last procedure to emerge prior to obtaining math fact automaticity. Not only are children with MDs (especially those with comorbid RDs) more likely to use SUM and MAX procedures, but they continue to use these strategies when their peers have attained automaticity of basic math facts (Geary et al., 2000).

The final combined procedural and visual–spatial subtype is a group of children who have the most severe type of MD in that they have difficulty with representing and manipulating numbers on an internal number line and in working memory (Ashkenazi et al., 2013; von Aster & Shalev, 2007). These children have frequent comorbid RDs even though the problem is more right-hemisphere lateralized, and problems with oral and/or written language are common. It would be interesting to see if children with this subtype have more problems with implicit language than explicit language. Similar to the symbolic relationships discussed in connection with word recognition, number processing requires translation of verbal to Arabic numbers, so sound–symbol (number) association is important in math as well. Quantitative concepts are similar to other semantic knowledge, and the quantity–number–symbol association is similar to the sound–letter–symbol association found for reading. The child must learn to map numbers onto quantity (Geary et al., 2012), just as they have to do with mapping phonemes onto graphemes when decoding words. Children gradually learn to associate concrete, semiconcrete, and then abstract representations of this quantitative–symbolic relationship, as highlighted in In-Depth 6.1.

Not surprisingly, children with this subtype of MD have difficulty with learning and/or retrieving basic math facts from memory. Retrieval or math fluency appears to be etiologically distinct from math computation deficits, and it has been suggested that it is largely a genetically determined cause of MD (Petrill et al., 2012). Individuals with this MD type take longer amounts of time to retrieve facts, and their retrieval accuracy and fluency is typically poor, but this problem can also found in low math achievers (Geary et al., 2012), suggesting it has limited discriminative power. In fact, Geary (2011b) suggests children with MDs and their low achieving peers have deficits in understanding and representing numerical magnitude, difficulties retrieving basic arithmetic facts from long-term memory, and delays in learning mathematical procedures, making the key difference that separates MD from low math achievement being largely due to working memory in the former.

Children within this subgroup frequently have poor visual–spatial–organizational, psychomotor, tactile–perceptual, and concept formation skills, but adequate rote, automatic, and verbal skills. They also show semantic problems when verbal information is complex or novel, which can lead to comprehension deficits. As you can see, children with this MD subtype have numerous nonverbal and verbal problems. Children with these difficulties have been found to show particular difficulty on visual–spatial, visual–motor, and fluid reasoning measures compared to children with ADHD or high-functioning autism (HFA) (Semrud-Clikeman, Walkowiak, Wilkinson, & Christopher, 2010). It has also been found, relative to typically developing children and children with ADHD, children with NVLD experience more difficulty in executive functioning (Fine et al., 2012; Semrud-Clikeman, Walkowiak, Wilkinson, & Butcher, 2010). These findings suggest that there is a separate type of MD that is also associated with problems with social functioning and well as executive functioning, confirming theories proposed by Rourke (Rourke et al., 2002). While some researchers specializing in NVLDs have required an MD for a diagnosis (Rourke, 2000; Semrud-Clikeman, Walkowiak, Wilkinson, & Butcher, 2010), others have subdivided an already small population into children with NVLD + or – MD (Davis & Broitman, 2011; Forrest, 2007), so the relationship is neither simple nor uniform. It is important to note that an MD is not sufficient for a diagnosis of NVLD and for some theorists it is not necessary for a diagnosis. Clearly, there are MDs that do not show visual–spatial problems as is the case with Gerstmann syndrome, thought to be a largely left parietal lobe problem that leads to finger agnosia, dyscalculia, dyspraxia, and left/right confusion (Ardila, 2020; Menon, 2015b).

This subtype is also likely to have comorbid literacy problems and RDs (Swanson et al., 2009), which affects number comprehension and production (Geary, 2011). As the name of this MD subtype suggests, cognitive assessment indicates that these children have problems with lexical–semantic memory, which may be important to consider in addition to the working memory problems, which may be more indicative of the procedural MD subtype (Geary et al., 2012). Drawing upon their extensive research findings, children with comorbid MDs/RDs and those with only RDs have difficulty encoding and retrieving information from long-term memory or crystallized abilities (Willcutt et al., 2013); this difficulty affects quantitative knowledge, number concepts, counting, arithmetic, and cognitive functions beyond the influence of global intelligence.

Neuroimaging in Mathematics

While "dyscalculia" has been associated with damage to the left parietal region (Menon, 2015a), recent research has implicated several areas of the brain with math competency, and that disruption to one or more of these regions can lead to MDs. Note that MD is a developmental disorder but it can also be an acquired disorder due to brain damage or compromise. MD is thought to arise basically from a problem with understanding quantity, which requires multiple cognitive processes. These processes include the ability to represent and retrieve symbolic information, attention to the task, working memory, and cognitive control (Ashkenazi et al., 2013). Because mathematics (and reading) requires so many cognitive skills, the brain areas involved in these skills are widespread and not localizable to the right or left hemisphere. Rather, networks are involved and are most important for conceptualizing how we solve mathematical problems, and how dysfunctional networks can lead to MDs.

Some basic questions can be posed before we discuss neuroimaging findings with MDs. Are there subtypes of disability that relate to different structural regions? What is the relation between particular deficits in MD and neuropsychological functioning? How do neuroimaging findings inform the professional when trying to understand a particular child? More importantly, how do we tailor interventions to a child's particular educational needs? While at this time there is no empirical evidence to link neuroanatomical/neurofunctional

Case Study 6.2. Jerry's Nonverbal Learning Disorder

We were asked to do a re-evaluation of Jerry, a child with a "nonverbal learning disorder," who had been diagnosed with Asperger syndrome and an MD by a clinical psychologist 3 years prior to his evaluation. At the time, he was in a resource room setting for math and written language instruction, and was receiving social skills instruction and counseling. The special education teacher, Lisa, reported Jerry was doing well with his math calculations, but he was having difficulty with word problems and still had difficulty with peer and adult interactions. She said that drawing lines to ensure column alignment had worked well, but he had never really had a problem with writing his numbers or letters, and his written language problems involved ideas and organization rather than handwriting. For word problems, Jerry couldn't seem to sort the relevant from the irrelevant information, or to turn the verbal information into written equations. The school psychologist, Fred, reported he was teaching Jerry to recognize facial and verbal affect by labeling different pictures and voices with emotions. Jerry reportedly had done so well with this affect recognition intervention that Fred was thinking about discontinuing the service, until he talked with Lisa about Jerry's continuing social problems. Fred thought that maybe Jerry just needed additional instruction, so that he could generalize the skills he had learned to the classroom environment.

Review of the previous psychological evaluation showed a tell-tale WISC-V Verbal Comprehension–Perceptual Reasoning split, which was 22 points. Jerry also had relative difficulty with Arithmetic and Comprehension compared to his other Verbal subtests, but these scores were well above his Performance subtest scores, and Digit Span (both Digits Forward and Digits Backward) was fine. Surprisingly, his score on the Developmental Test of Visual–Motor Integration was pretty good and in the low average range. Rating scale data generally showed social and attention problems. A CHT evaluation was conducted with the Woodcock–Johnson IV (WJ-IV) as the screening intellectual/ cognitive instrument. Jerry's *Gv* (visual–spatial) and *Gs* scores were just fine. He had some relative difficulty with the *Gsm* subtests (measures of attention, working memory and executive function), but these processes did not appear to be impaired. Where were Jerry's nonverbal deficits that were seen on the WISC-V? They were there all the time, but assuming they were related to visual–perceptual difficulties had led the special education teacher and the school psychologist down the wrong intervention path. It was the *Gf* (fluid reasoning) subtests that were impaired on the WJ-IIV, and this was confirmed with the Differential Ability Scales–II (DAS) Nonverbal Reasoning subtests. What Jerry needed help with were anterior right-hemisphere functions (novel problem-solving skills), not the posterior ones the teacher and school psychologist were addressing with their generic "nonverbal LDs" interventions. Although these would be excellent interventions for children with posterior right-hemisphere problems, they would not meet Jerry's needs.

---

data to interventions, there is some anecdotal and case study information. Case Study 6.2 highlights one child with some of these difficulties.

Neuroimaging Findings in Mathematical Processes

Mathematical cognition requires the activation of multiple distributed brain structures. Approximate quantities are represented in the bilateral intraparietal sulcus and dorsal region of the parietal lobes (Feigenson et al., 2004; Rosenberg-Lee, Chang, et al., 2011). The intraparietal sulcus has also been implicated in the ability to maintain attention and integrate multisensory processes. In addition, the left fusiform gyrus plays an important role in a variety of numerical tasks (Arsalidou & Taylor, 2011; Feigenson et al., 2004). The left fusiform gyrus has been implicated in orthographic processing (Binder et al., 2006), but it is perhaps the direct pathway for accessing math facts in the inferior temporal lobe, similar to what is seen in reading sight words. However, subtle distinctions in mathematics and linguistic semantics have been noted in the literature (Amalric et al., 2017).

Multiple cognitive networks are called into play for more complex mathematical processing. Particular higher-level systems involved in mathematics include executive functions and visual–spatial working memory (Ashkenazi et al., 2013), implicating the (largely right) dorsolateral–parietal task positive network; skills you will recall that are involved in at least two of the mathematics subtypes described earlier. In these cases, the prefrontal cortex is activated for mathematical processing, particularly dorsal and middle frontal regions dedicated to managing effort and retrieval as well those utilized for working memory when performing multistage calculations (Zago et al., 2008). (See Figure 2.6, which shows these structures.)

Another important network is that of the bilateral anterior cingulate. This network is important in error monitoring (Kerns et al., 2004) and becomes activated when children are solving numerical problems (De Smedt et al., 2010). In addition, the language areas in the left temporoparietal cortex and the left inferior frontal gyrus become significantly activated as the child retrieves well-memorized math facts (Prado et al., 2011; Rosenberg-Lee, Barth, et al., 2011). It is important to note here that brain regions involved in mathematics differ between adults and children, with adolescents falling somewhere in the middle. As experience and learning take place and skills become more automatized, the prefrontal cortex and left intraparietal sulcus may become less involved (Ansari & Dhital, 2006). There are also changes that occur quickly at specific times of childhood. For example, between grades 2 and 3 significant brain response and connectivity changes have been found (Rosenberg-Lee, Barth et al., 2011). Similarly during development, numerical understanding and processing become more automatized and less effortful with continued efficiency of brain networks continuing to develop through childhood and adolescence (Blair et al., 2011). In addition, visual–spatial working memory can be a specific source of difficulty for children with MDs related to higher activation in the prefrontal cortex rather than the posterior parietal systems used by adolescents and adults when solving mathematical problems (Dumonthell & Klingberg, 2012).

Finally, we would be remiss in presenting evidence of the neuropsychology of MD without specifically talking about brain similarities and differences on math reasoning/word problems in comparison to computation skills. This is where the language and mathematics brain areas clearly interact with one another, but of the cognitive predictors of performance on math problems, a fluid reasoning subskill called *quantitative reasoning* plays an important role (Green et al., 2017; Naglieri & Otero, 2017). Take for instance the following word problem: "Liam had 7 apples. He ate 3 apples and gave 2 apples to his friend. How many apples does Liam have now?" A student solved this problem by giving the answer "6." Upon questioning, though, he did the math correctly. He had 7, then ate 3 (7 – 3 = 4), so "ate" was correctly equated with subtraction. However, the student then did 4 + 2 = 6. Why? Because he read "gave two apples to his friend" as an addition statement, deciphering "gave two apples" as an addition requirement, instead of another subtraction requirement.

In addition to language demands, why is fluid reasoning so important for math word problems? Fluid reasoning or novel problem solving requires analysis and synthesis, two key tasks required in math word problems. When a word problem is processed, the first thing that must be attended to is lexical–semantic and syntactic relationships among the words. Then one must analyze the content to determine those words that reflect quantity and the relationship among quantitative words to perform the calculations. Once the calculation equation is established, and carried out using typical math skills, the answer can be determined, and then translated back into a verbal response. Thus, while a student may be good at calculation, their poor language processes and/or limited fluid reasoning skills can undermine performance on math word problems (Daroczy et al., 2015; Green et al., 2017). Obviously, a key component is interhemispheric transfer of information via the corpus callosum, with bilateral activity likely given the complexity of math word problem task demands.

Functional Neuroimaging Studies of MDs

Many of the fMRI studies have concentrated on the skills underlying the ability to compare numbers. Numbers that are closer together (e.g., 2 and 3) take more time to compare and show more errors than those farther apart (e.g., 2 and 10). The intraparietal sulcus (IPS) in the parietal lobe has been found to be particularly sensitive to these types of comparisons. Reduced activation in this region has been found in children with MDs with the right IPS showing reduced activation for nonsymbolic and symbolic number comparison tasks and during numerical ordering (Kucian et al., 2011; Mussolin, Meijas et al., 2010). In addition to these differences, decreased activation in the ventral occipitotemporal cortex, superior parietal lobule, and prefrontal cortex was found in children with MDs while doing basic number comparison tasks (Ashkenazi et al., 2013). The bilateral middle frontal gyrus and right middle cingulate gyrus also showed reduced activation when the child was asked to compare how far apart two sets of numbers were (2 and 4 vs. 4 and 10) (Mussolin, DeVolder, et al., 2010). These findings consistently found lower activation in the IPS, prefrontal cortex, and frontal and middle frontal gyri in children with MDs. Although spatial ability is clearly related to math skill, meta-analyses suggest its association may be more due to logical analysis of content than specifically to mathematics skills (Hawes et al., 2019), yet this hypothesis would be considered controversial given the preponderance of evidence.

Another area that has been studied is the retrieval of arithmetic facts. Math fact instruction has been deemed by some to be irrelevant, but as we argue here it is crucial to develop math fact automaticity for higher-level math problem solving. In typically developing children during grades 2 and 3, a shift is made from effortful calculation to direct retrieval of previously learned material. Children with MDs use finger counting and other tangible devices for skills that should have become automatic by this time with atypical activation in the IPS and premotor cortex and middle frontal gyrus (Aaron, 2003; Ashkenazi et al., 2012; Davis et al., 2009). In addition, Ashkenazi et al. (2012) analyzed response patterns and found that brain activation to complex and simple problems was not modulated in children with MDs particularly in the bilateral IPS. These findings strongly suggest that children with MDs show underactivation in key mathematical processing regions and they do not modulate the brain activity to accomplish mathematical calculation efficiently. Simple problems are just as complex for these children as more abstract ones, due to the lack of math fact automaticity. This lack of automatization makes all mathematical tasks effortful, increasing demands on working memory. If you recall from Chapter 3, automatization of foundational skills frees the brain to do more complex tasks and thus to be more efficient in managing cognitive resources. It is this very reason why using calculators for math facts and calculations should be avoided, except in severe situations of dyscalculia (e.g., bilateral parietal lobe damage).

Another method for evaluating brain function in mathematics is comparing key structures and networks between children with MDs and those who are typically developing. Two methods have been utilized for these studies: structural MRI, which looks at various structures volumetrically, and DTI, which looks at the integrity of white matter tracts that connect the right and left hemispheres, superior–inferior regions, and anterior–posterior regions. A structural MRI study of children with MD compared to controls found decreased gray matter volume in the right IPS, left inferior frontal gyrus, bilateral middle frontal gyrus, and the anterior cingulate. You will recall that these are similar structures that had been identified with fMRI (Rotzer et al., 2008; Rykhlevskaia et al., 2009). In addition, right-hemispheric white matter projection tracts were found in the inferior frontal–occipital fasciculus and inferior and superior longitudinal fasciculus (Molko et al., 2002; Rotzer et al., 2008; Rykhlevskaia et al., 2009). These emerging empirical findings show volumetric differences in the brains of children with MDs as well as the white matter tracts that connect these structures. Such network analysis strongly suggests that there are deficiencies in connectivity in white matter and thus likely a white matter deficit that lies at the root of many problems with mathematics. Further study is needed to clarify these findings and to also determine what effect interventions will have on these fiber pathways.

As suggested previously, a distinction between math computation and math word problem skills is relevant here. Although at first glance the differences appear to be dramatic, research has shown that both tasks require similar parietal regions (posterior parietal, intraparietal sulcus), whereas word problems also utilize the traditional areas for receptive (Wernicke's area) and expressive (Broca's area) language (Newman et al., 2011). However, executive frontal lobe activity is greater during math reasoning tasks (Prabhakaran et al., 2001), which could be in part due to increased working memory demands for math reasoning. However, the structure of the task and its consistency with the operation determines the degree of prefrontal involvement (Ng et al., 2021). Study differences may be in part due to those who visualize versus those who verbalize content during problem solving.

Given our understanding of the neuropsychological processes involved in math computation and word problems, you can begin to formulate ideas about a child's processing strengths and weaknesses, and to determine which brain areas are involved during math performance. However, recall that different brain areas may be involved as a child ascends some computational hierarchy, and that children with MDs may use different problem-solving routes when completing their math assignments and tests. This can help you develop individualized interventions designed to meet the needs of children with MDs, several of which are presented in Appendix 6.1.

Instructional Strategies for Children with MDs

Now that you have a basic understanding of the cognitive and neuropsychological characteristics of children with MDs, intervention becomes an important aspect for work with children with MDs. Interventions for math problems have received a great deal of attention by investigators, but as you can see in Appendix 6.1, most programs are not tailored for individual strengths and weaknesses. Recognizing the reason why a child is struggling with mathematics is an important first step for tailoring empirically based instructional approaches to individual needs. Using the information described in the preceding section, you should be able to recognize where the breakdown is in the child's learning, complete an error analysis of failed responses, and then compare the errors to correct responses. First, look for types of error responses in permanent products from the classroom. Error responses, not simple yes – correct, no – incorrect coding of responses helps you learn how to teach the child with MD. Having a child talk out loud or use the think-aloud technique to tell you the steps he or she uses during computation can be extremely helpful. This additional information cannot be obtained from standardized measures, which should really be considered as math screening measures (Fuchs, Geray, et al., 2010), so it might be helpful to ask the child's teacher for some math computation worksheets to further examine the pattern of performance.

It's important to help a student identify where he or she succeeds and where he or she struggles in mathematics. Doing so not only empowers the child but also provides training in metacognition (executive functioning) to help the child monitor performance. For mathematics, repeated practice using different types of stimuli can also be quite helpful—utilizing computer applications as well as providing different avenues for intervention allows the child or adolescent to begin to generalize skills. The use of graph paper for students who have problems aligning numbers or who experience problems with organization is a useful strategy we have successfully used for individuals with visual–spatial problems. Helping a child look at problems from more than one perspective can also be helpful, teaching direct relations among numbers and their manipulation. On an addition problem, teach counting up from the larger number rather than from the smaller number (e.g., MIN procedure). If the problem is 12 + 17, starting from 7 rather than 2 is easier—so 7 plus 2 is 9 rather than 2 + 7 is 9. Use estimation skills and teach this directly to children with visual–spatial/presumed right-hemisphere dysfunction. If memorization of math facts is difficult, then direct exposition on how numbers relate can help the child recall the facts. For example, if $2 \times 5 = 10$ then if 10 is doubled to 20, 4×5 must equal 20. Use concrete examples or tangible objects (i.e., Cuisenaire rods) so the child begins to learn relations among numbers and quantities. For math word problems, try direct instruction of mathematics terms. For example, "How many more?" always means to add and "How many less?" always means to subtract. There are many other mnemonics that can be used to add the child in recalling items. Greater than and less than signs can be the alligator eating the number for less than and pushing the number for more than.

Direct teaching of mathematics concepts, numerosity, and terms has been found to be the most successful intervention (Compton et al., 2012). Similarly, training in spatial ability has also been linked to improvement in mathematics. Children with visual–spatial difficulties and the mixed subtype have the most difficulty with direct mathematical problem-solving skills. There have been a few studies that looked at training children on a mental rotation task to determine whether gains would be found in mathematics. Calculation skills have been found to improve following direct training in mental rotation in a group of early elementary children with learning problems in mathematics calculation (Mix & Cheng, 2012). This research, while promising, is in its infancy and further study is needed before spatial training can be verified as legitimate intervention.

After you have conducted these initial steps, you will have a better understanding of the reason why the child is having problems in math. For example, in preparation for your consultation meeting with Mike's teacher, ask yourself the following questions. Is the problem related to prior learning and/or difficulty with retention/retrieval of math facts? Does Mike find math difficult because it is boring or too abstract for him, or does anxiety lead to inefficient processing and poor task completion? Mike seems to have difficulty with algorithm understanding or use; is this because he has difficulty following the sequence of steps? Does he show attentional concerns, failing to recognize the operands at times? Does he have difficulty with the spatial characteristics of multistep math problems and show poor handwriting? Or is the solving of novel problems, especially word problems, difficult for him? Is the severity great enough that you should suggest a compensatory technique, or is remediation sufficient? Has Mike tried these techniques without success for too long, or is he still young enough to make good progress through systematic intervention designed to reduce error responding? These questions must be asked as you begin to work collaboratively with the teacher to brainstorm appropriate intervention strategies and formulate a plan to evaluate the efficacy of your intervention.

Math Case Study: Linking Assessment to Intervention

The complexity of these assessment and intervention issues is highlighted in the Case Study 6.3, where we take you from assessment to intervention with a boy who appeared to his teacher to have problems with math secondary to a NVLD or ADHD. As you can see from Matt's unique pattern of performance, he did immediately seem to fit well into a "category" of MD; however, even though he did seem to show characteristics of the procedural subtype of MD, assuming that this pattern was automatically associated with ADHD would have been problematic. As we emphasize throughout this book, if we are to truly serve the needs of children like Matt, we must not make recommendations based on initial teacher referral questions or even preliminary test data. Instead, we can only make recommendations for such children after we understand the complexities of their cognitive profiles, and the ways they use those cognitive processes to solve math problems.

Case Study 6.3. Matt and Math

One of us (Hale) was called into a local school to consult with a fourth-grade teacher, Rita, who was perplexed about Matt's poor math performance. Matt had a history of fairly adequate math performance until last year, when his math grades started to deteriorate. In addition, although his reading skills were excellent, his comprehension began to fail as well. Rita described Matt as a "good kid" who was never disruptive, but he seemed somewhat inattentive and withdrawn. His mother wanted to put Matt on medication for what she called "ADD," but the school-based support team suggested that he should have a psychological evaluation first. At the team meeting, the school psychologist concluded that Matt had test anxiety, particularly in the areas of math and comprehension. This hypothesis was also invoked to explain his attention problems in the classroom. Matt did not qualify for special education services because the team adhered strictly to the discrepancy model, and his WISC-V Full Scale IQ was in the average range and his KeyMath scores were only low average. The team recommended Americans with Disabilities Act/ Rehabilitation Act counseling accommodations for Matt's anxiety problem.

Rita agreed that Matt would tense up at times, but she didn't really see Matt as an anxious child. She remembered reading something about NVLD and MD, so she decided to do some research. She read several learning disability subtype studies from the Windsor Taxonomic Laboratory (see Rourke, 1994). In these studies, children with math problems were found to have good reading/spelling skills and poor mechanical arithmetic performance. They also tended to have a characteristic WISC-V Verbal Comprehension > Perceptual Reasoning IQ split, suggesting possible right-hemisphere dysfunction. Because Rita had some knowledge of brain–behavior relationships, she easily understood the assumption that children with math disabilities must have deficient visual–spatial, nonverbal, and graphomotor skills. These perceptual deficits would lead to problems with spatial processes and column alignment in math calculation. She also agreed that Matt showed some of the socioemotional signs of NVLDs, as he was somewhat "peculiar" and socially reticent.

Returning to Matt's student file and his permanent products (e.g., worksheets, tests), Rita looked at the data for evidence of this pattern. She was surprised to find that Matt didn't have this Verbal–Performance split at all, but she noticed significant WISC-V subtest scatter. Matt did have problems with Block Design and Coding, which brought down his Performance score, but he was still in the average range. He also had a low average Arithmetic and Comprehension score, but the Digit Span subtest was average (although Digits Forward was significantly better than Digits Backward). Other than a low average Bender–Gestalt score, there were no other cognitive data available. Achievement test results revealed inattention to signs or operands, and messy, disorganized work, but little other evidence of a math deficit. Matt's classroom math papers and tests did not show any column alignment errors in multistep problems, but he did show several algorithm and apparently some math fact retrieval errors. Matt rarely completed his math assignments on time, and he missed many points on tests for the same reason. The only psychosocial evaluation data available were the Bender–Gestalt score interpreted from a projective approach (not recommended!) and a score on a Conners Rating Scale, which was significant for attention problems. When everyone sat down to discuss the case, they first explored changes in home or classroom that could have accounted for Matt's deteriorating performance. There seemed to be nothing out of the ordinary going on in the home, but Rita commented that she wasn't sure whether Matt's mom was a reliable informant. When questioned about this comment, Rita said, "Sometimes it seems like she's not all there"—that is, as if the mother were distracted by something.

Our initial hypothesis was that an attention problem could explain the computation errors, and that Matt might have ADHD, inattentive type (consistent with executive dysfunction), with comorbid anxiety. However, the history obtained from the mother and Rita revealed other interesting facts, including a possible birth trauma and a family history of psychiatric problems. When Hale began his assessment, he decided that he would collect more information on Matt's personality and behavior, including mother, teacher, and self-report forms. Hale began his evaluation by using the DAS as my screening tool, to see whether Matt indeed had "adequate" nonverbal skills, and to compare nonverbal reasoning to visual–spatial skills. The following data were obtained (the General Cognitive Ability [GCA] and clusters are in standard scores [SSs], subtests are in *T* scores):

<u>General Cognitive Ability (GCA) = 95</u>

Verbal Ability = 87	Nonverbal Reasoning Ability = 93	Spatial Ability = 106
Word Definitions = 45	Matrices = 48	Recall of Designs = 52
Similarities = 40	Sequential and Quantitative Reasoning = 45	Pattern Construction = 56

Consistent with the WISC-V results, Matt's scores on measures of visual–perceptual skills were adequate, and nonverbal reasoning skills, while in the lower end of the average range, were not impaired. Matt was often perseverative and inflexible on these measures, but never disinhibited or impulsive. So far, the results appeared to be consistent with ADHD, inattentive type. However, after the CHT theory was developed, they had to test the hypothesis that attention and executive problems were the source of Matt's problems. They decided to use the repeatable ADHD drug trial battery in preparation for a possible drug trial (recall that Matt's mother wanted medication for "ADD"), supplemented by additional executive function measures (most results are converted to SSs, with higher scores = better performance).

Task	Variable	SS	Raw score
Hale Cancellation Task	Correct	95	
	Time	82	
Selective Reminding Test	Long-Term Storage	85	
	Consistent Retrieval	80	
Go–No Go Test	Correct		29/30
Conners Continuous Performance Test II	Omissions	90	
	Commissions	110	
	Reaction Time	65	
	Reaction Time Block Change	88	
	Reaction Time ISI Change	80	
Stroop Color–Word Test	Interference	78	
	Errors		8
Trail Making Test, Part B	Correct	95	
	Time	79	
Test of Memory and Learning	Digits Backward	85	
Wisconsin Card Sorting Test	Errors	88	
	Perseverative Responses	80	
	Perseverative Errors	86	
	Categories		5
	Failure to Maintain Set		0
	Trials to First Category		18
Controlled Oral Word Association Test (COWAT)	Letters (F/A/S)	96	
	Category	68	
WJ-III	Planning	87	
Developmental Neuropsychological Assessment (NEPSY)	Tower	75	
	Design Fluency	92	

Certainly the test results and environmental data pointed to ADHD, inattentive type. The test data were all suggesting that Matt's dorsolateral prefrontal cortex and/or cingulate circuits were impaired, but something didn't quite fit. Was it just psychometric "noise"—a very real possibility, given the number of measures and different norm groups? Why the low Comprehension score on the WISC-V? Why was his COWAT Category score so low, and the Letters score so high? Why did he have such slow psychomotor speed on some tasks but not others? Why were his graphomotor skills adequate, but his drawings disorganized and perseverative? Why were his nonverbal skills adequate when these skills are often difficult for children with ADHD? The reported classroom behaviors and family psychiatric history made Hale consider an additional possibility: thought disorder. Sure enough, through further examination of the behavior ratings and of Matt's self-report, Hale felt comfortable suggesting that Matt's math and comprehension problems were probably due to executive and attention problems. Hale added that he thought these problems did not constitute a "primary" attention deficit (one that would benefit from stimulant treatment), but were "secondary" to Matt's "internal distraction" and "unique way of thinking about and solving problems." In other words, it seemed that evidence was emerging that Matt had a thought disorder. During the feedback, Hale discussed these concerns with the teacher and mother. Both confirmed that Matt displayed idiosyncratic and "peculiar" (both actually used this word!) behaviors in the classroom and at home. He also had a rich fantasy life that he claimed was "real" at times. In addition, the family history of psychiatric problems included an incarcerated uncle who had "lost it" and was "on lots of medication."

Why was this differentiation important? First, they discovered that the apparent reasons for Matt's math and comprehension problems were attentional and executive in nature, not due to anxiety or NVLD. Systematic desensitization would not really help Matt, but metacognitive instruction designed to foster self-structure and evaluation during academic tasks could help him. He was taught to use a checklist to ensure that he double-checked the operand and his math facts after completing each problem. He was also given extended time for math and other language-based subjects. Furthermore, they wouldn't waste time trying to teach spatial skills, column alignment, or graphomotor skills in an attempt to overcome NVLD. Finally, it is true that all of these decisions could have been made with the finding of attention and executive function deficits, regardless of the underlying pathology— but they might not have recognized the psychosocial issues as such, because Rita reported that Matt was a "good kid" (as we will see in Chapter 9) internalizers are always seen as "good kids"). In addition, if a pediatrician or psychiatrist were to read the report and conclude that Matt had ADHD, they might have treated Matt with a dopamine *agonist* (e.g., Ritalin), which could have a detrimental effect on a child with a thought disorder. What he needed was counseling, social skills training, help with peer interactions, and careful psychiatric monitoring to ensure that a dopamine agonist wasn't needed.

APPENDIX 6.1. MATHEMATICS INTERVENTIONS

Reference	Intervention description
Fuchs et al. (2008)	Strengthening attention and processing speed improved computation skills. Problem-solving difficulty related to problems with language. Problem-solving skills were also related to race and poverty issues.
Fuchs, Geary, et al. (2010)	The program Pirate Math provided word problem tutoring improving both calculation and procedural calculation.
Fuchs et al. (2011)	Preventative tutoring of problem-solving skills with sessions 3 times per week 30 minutes per session improved mathematics skills in 3rd graders particularly when focus was on direct teaching of problem types as well as improving skills in reading relevant information in charts, graphs, and pictures.
Maccini et al. (2007)	For secondary students in math strategies using mnemonic strategy instruction, graduated instruction, cognitive strategy instruction that involved planning, schema-based instruction, and contextualized videodisc instruction were found to be very helpful and increased math achievement.
Mong & Mong (2010)	Math to Mastery and Cover, Copy, and Compare interventions effectively improved mathematics fluency with Math to Mastery showing the best response to intervention.
Slavin et al. (2009)	Cooperative learning improved math performance significantly while computer-assisted learning was not found to be a significant contributor to improved math achievement.
VanDerHayden et al. (2012)	Directly teaching math and math procedural fluency improved overall mathematics performance.

Chapter 7

The Neuropsychology
of Written Language Disorders

The Complexity of Written Language

From a neuropsychological perspective, written language is by far the most difficult academic skill and one that is an important marker for a child's overall development (Wiznitzer & Scheffel, 2009). Unfortunately, written language has received relatively little empirical attention, and formal classroom instruction in written expression is often limited. The old belief that writing is a natural extension of oral language may have something to do with it. This belief, long held by the educational establishment, that if you provide children with a pencil and handwriting instruction, they will be able to convey their thoughts on paper as easily as they do when speaking is long outdated and clearly inaccurate. As empirical evidence emerges that oral and written language are dissociable, the basis of this belief is slowly being eroded and there is renewed emphasis on written language instruction in the classroom. We now know that there are many cognitive processes associated with written language achievement; dysfunction in one or more of those areas can lead to a written language disorder (WLD).

Unlike the other academic domains discussed so far, written language is the only academic skill that is primarily an output task. Written language depends on the input system for memory and feedback to the output system, but it is more of a "frontal" skill than other academic domains. Written language depends on many of the executive functions managed by the prefrontal cortex because it requires planning, organization, strategizing, monitoring, evaluating, and changing the writing product, so we would predict that the dorsolateral prefrontal and anterior cingulate would be important for writing success. When writing, the child must first brainstorm ideas, and then plan the writing process. He or she has to organize the ideas into sentences and paragraphs, retrieve words from long-term memory to convey meaning and link ideas, use graphomotor skills to write and spell words, evaluate the accuracy of the draft product, and edit/rewrite as necessary until a satisfactory final product is achieved. In fact, the executive or critical analysis of the written language product may be the single most important determinant of writing success (Yoshimasu et al., 2011). Unfortunately, the executive skills of planning, organizing, evaluating, and revising written language products are seldom used by children with WLDs (Fayol et al., 2012), perhaps because of the limited (or even the absence of) instruction in these metacognitive executive skills.

Writing requires the child to have a plan for what he or she will write. It requires mental flexibility and an element of fluid reasoning to brainstorm ideas and develop the content that will be written. Executive demands are high as the child forms the idea for the writing, accesses prior knowledge and experiences to develop the written material, utilizes spelling and grammar rules, and obtains somatosensory and spatial feedback to direct the hand during handwriting. Spelling and handwriting are prerequisite skills, which are subsumed under the broader, more complex skill of written language. As is the case with basic reading and math skills, fundamental spelling and handwriting skills are important precursors or predictors of fluent written expression in young children (Kim et al., 2011). WLDs can occur because of problems in any of these areas. Although difficulties with spelling and handwriting can be overcome using a computer-based compensatory technique, we will discover that using keyboards and automatized spell checks can undermine achievement, not only in written expression but in reading as well. It is the complexity of the written language process that has probably dissuaded researchers and practitioners alike from allotting the necessary time and resources to examine this important academic domain thoroughly. Teachers tend to be inconsistent or eclectic when providing written expression instruction (Cutler & Graham, 2008), leaving many children inadequately prepared to convey their thoughts in writing, especially if they have a WLD.

Prevalence and Comorbidity of WLDs

Given the paucity of research into the nature and causes of WLDs, it is not surprising to find limited information about their prevalence and comorbidity with other disorders (Grigorenko et al., 2020). Because writing skills require many of the same cognitive processes required for other academic and psychosocial functioning, especially executive deficits, it is not surprising that WLDs co-occur with other disorders. WLDs rarely occur in isolation, and are typically comorbid with many other language disorders and language-based learning disorders (Berninger et al., 2008b), as well as with ADHD (Yoshimasu et al., 2011), and with other neurodevelopmental disorders such as bipolar disorder, autism, anxiety, and depression (Mayes & Calhoun, 2007). Given that executive deficits in WLD are common, individuals with comorbid LD have poorer adjustment and school functioning than those with a single disorder (Martinez & Semrud-Clikeman, 2004).

Epidemiological studies using absolute criteria cutoffs have revealed prevalence rates for WLDs to be quite high. A population-based birth cohort study found that approximately 6.9–14.7% of children were found to have a WLD depending on how the disorder was defined (Katusic et al., 2009). Moreover, 25% of the cases had a WLD without an RD. Within the above study, boys were found to be 2 to 3 times more likely to have a WLD compared to girls independent of how a WLD was defined. Of even more concern was that the discrepancy between writing skills for boys and girls increases with age with larger increases found at the secondary level (Berninger et al., 2008a). While this study found that boys are more impaired in orthography than girls, there were no gender differences in spelling skills. Finally, myths about the low prevalence of WLD have been rewritten, with WLD found to be the *most* common RD (92% of children with RD) in a large clinical population (Mayes & Calhoun, 2007). When studying a large clinical neuropsychiatric sample, Mayes and Calhoun (2006) found WLD to be twice as common as RD or MD, suggesting it is grossly unrecognized or a poorly classified type of learning disability in the schools.

Many aspects of brain functioning are embedded within the written language task. Written language requires eye–hand coordination, spatial perception, and graphomotor coordination for handwriting (Penner-Williams et al., 2009). It also requires good conceptual and linguistic skills as well as executive functions of working memory, organization, and evaluation (Berninger et al., 2008a). Developmentally, written language skills typically begin with a focus on mechanics instruction (letter formation, handwriting, spelling) and then move on to the ability to communicate ideas and thoughts in an organized and fluent manner (Berninger et al., 2008a; Brooks et al., 2011). Deficits in written composition may continue into adulthood even when other aspects of reading and writing difficulties have been remediated (Schulte-Körne et al., 2007), perhaps because of the limited focus on and/or measurement issues associated with formal instruction and evaluation of written expression.

Children with WLDs tend to write fewer words and sentences, have more spelling errors, and write fewer words per minute compared to age-matched peers (Gregg et al., 2007), thereby limiting analysis of their writing strengths and weaknesses. Poor spelling and slow, laborious writing is frequently seen in children with WLDs which in turn constrains the quality of the composition particularly for younger children (Wagner et al., 2011). A child who experiences difficulty with spelling and processing of information will have slow handwriting due to these problems (Sumner et al., 2013). The problems with composition appear to stem from the strain on cognitive resources as the child attempts to recall or retrieve the appropriate spelling, which burdens working memory, a critical executive function for the writing product.

Thus, it is important to evaluate whether problems with handwriting, spelling, language, organization, and evaluation are each contributing to the child's problem with learning to write effectively. Similar to reading, if a child is not fluent in written expression prerequisites (i.e., proficient at handwriting and spelling), the writing task becomes that much more difficult and effortful. However, a majority of students have more difficulty with executive components of written expression than the underlying mechanics. Just because they can show good spelling and handwriting does not mean they are good writers, even if oral expression is adequate. The next sections will talk about each of these areas of written language.

WLD and Brain Function

Spelling

Spelling is an integral part of written language, but it is a seldom-studied academic domain, especially when it comes to brain–behavior research. One of the difficulties for children in learning to spell in the English language is that English is a morphophonemic orthography (Nunes & Bryant, 2006); that is, it requires phonology (sound units), orthography (spelling units including one- and two-letter groups), and morphology (word parts that relate to meaning and grammar), mirroring Richards et al. (2006). Spelling difficulty has been identified as a reliable indication for dyslexia in English with variable sound-symbol relationships (Berninger et al., 2008b) as well as in languages such as German which has predictable spellings based on phonics (Rabiner & Malone, 2004). Thus, it is important to identify a child's phonologically accurate and inaccurate spellings and contrast this performance with misspellings on words that cannot be spelled phonetically (e.g., sight words).

Developmentally, children learn the difference between writing and drawing prior to kindergarten as they learn street signs (e.g., stop signs) and other common signs (e.g., McDonald's restaurant). The ability to spell improves as phonological awareness is developed in the early school grades. Being aware of the different sounds within a word is a prerequisite for learning what letters those sound correspond to (c-a-t means cat). The child learns that phonemes can be translated into graphemes, and spelling skills are developed as the child masters important alphabetic principles. Thus, as the child matures, he or she learns patterns that are present in irregular and regular words (i comes before e except after c, etc.). English is a particularly difficult language to learn to spell because it is orthographically inconsistent, as noted earlier. That means the same letter can have different sounds (the *c* in *magic* vs. the *c* in *magician* or the *k* in *milk* vs. the *k* in *knight*) (Galuschka et al., 2020).

Spelling difficulties continue throughout life and have been linked to a locus on chromosomes 15, 1, and 6 (Rabiner & Malone, 2004). In contrast, genetic linkage for dyslexia has been identified with at least 20 possible loci for dyslexia including chromosomes 15 and 6 as well as linkage to other chromosomes (Schmacher et al., 2007). An additional study utilized a genome scan for spelling ability in families with a proband with dyslexia. Spelling was found to have a model that included 4 genomic regions (Rubenstein et al., 2011). When the Verbal IQ (VIQ) was adjusted, evidence was present for a linkage of spelling to chromosomes 2q, 9q, and 15p with weak evidence of linkage to chromosome 6 (q is the long arm of the chromosome and p is the short arm; see Chapter 11). When the VIQ was not controlled, the linkage to chromosome 6 was stronger. Whereas irregular word reading is most related to chromosome 4p15, irregular spelling is related more to chromosome 17p13, suggesting reading and spelling are at least genetically dissociable but related causes of both (Bates et al., 2007). These findings, taken together, indicate that spelling has some relation to the genetic underpinning of dyslexia, but they are not synonymous.

Development of Spelling Skills

As with other academic skills, students move through developmental stages in acquiring spelling competency. Recognizing the developmental progression of spelling stages can help you determine whether a child's spelling errors are developmentally appropriate. Learning to spell requires the child to learn the phonological codes in spoken words as well as the orthographic codes in written words (Berninger, Raskind, et al., 2008). Embedded within these skills is working memory to keep track of the spelling as it occurs. Working memory is important for spelling, as the child has to switch between the phonological loop (hearing how a word sounds) and the orthographic loop (letter; visual–symbolic) for writing the corresponding letters (Berninger, Winn, et al., 2008). The phonological loop coordinates the phonological and orthographic units of the word, which is related to the inferior parietal regions. The writing of the letters is associated with the orthographic loop and requires the ability to rapidly and automatically retrieve the letter forms (Berninger, Abbott, & Garcia, 2009). Coordinating the phonological and orthographic loops is a key aspect for spelling as well as when spelling difficulties arise (Garcia et al., 2010).

As is the case with other academic domains, it is important to look for error patterns within the developmental context. As noted earlier, always consider phoneme–grapheme correspondence error (phonetically accurate) versus sight-word errors (phonetically inaccurate), which requires more visual memory. While young children frequently use invented spellings or show letter reversals, this practice is uncommon in older children (Chamberlain et al., 2019), likely due to parietal lobe maturation during early childhood. Severe spelling errors can cause the reader to miss the point that the child is trying to convey or to actually discount the worth of the writing even though the ideas are excellent (Graham et al., 2011). Thus, poor spelling is as detrimental to written composition as problems with phonics are to reading (Graham et al., 2018). The most common error patterns in children with spelling difficulties are:

- Letter additions
- Letter omissions
- Letter reversals
- Sequencing errors

- Consonant substitutions
- Vowel substitutions

Given that phonological awareness is an important prerequisite for both reading and spelling, it is not surprising that children with reading problems tend to have spelling problems as well (Garcia et al., 2010). In many ways spelling is more difficult than reading, because it requires many of the skills that word recognition does, but also requires visual–motor coordination and graphomotor skills to produce written words, and executive skills to compare produced spellings to visual memory of those words. We will return to the importance of handwriting in the next section of this chapter. In addition, spelling requires detailed information about all of the letter forms within the word (a high-quality orthographic representation); reading can be successful using only a partial cue to recognize a word (e.g., *output* vs *input*) (Galuschka et al., 2020). Thus, the substantial difference between spelling and reading is that the former requires orthographic retrieval, whereas the latter requires only recognition of graphemes and morphemes. Although it has been suggested that spelling words and reading words develop comparably in typical peers, with some suggesting spelling shouldn't be taught or assessed, the reality is we often don't assess or teach typical peers, so if spelling and reading are different, the astute clinician should ask why.

There are only 26 letters in the alphabet, but over 500 spellings used in representing the 44 phonemes in the English language (Berninger et al., 2013). To cover that much ground, children must think of unique ways to order the letters to produce the desired product. On top of this, add the irregular sight words—those words that do not follow standard orthographic–phonemic rules—and it is easy to see why so many children have difficulties with spelling that persist even after their reading decoding skills have improved. In addition, children with dyslexia have been found to pause more often when writing to check their spelling rather than having explicit handwriting difficulties (Sumner et al., 2013).

CHC Theory and Cognitive Processes Linked to Basic Writing Skills

In a study of basic writing skills in children, which included spelling as well as punctuation and capitalization, Floyd et al. (2008), found that the contribution of different cognitive processes varied over time. Comprehension–knowledge (*Gc*) was moderately associated with basic writing skills for ages 7 to 9, and strongly thereafter. This is not surprising, considering the knowledge of letters, morphemes, and words needed for correct spelling of English. Processing speed (*Gs*) and working memory (*Gwm*) were also moderate contributors throughout the age range. Processing speed was assessed through paper-and-pencil tasks, and therefore may be related to graphomotor skills and the fluency of handwriting. Working memory is important for holding the word and its spelling in memory as writing progresses. Interestingly, phonemic awareness (*Ga-PC*) showed negligible effects on basic writing skills, suggesting that the sound–symbol association was not important for spelling. This may be an artifact of the inconsistent spelling of sounds in English, and it would be interesting to contrast this to the learning of spelling in a phonetically regular language. This study was completed using the normative sample for the Woodcock–Johnson III, so keep in mind that children with WLDs may use different processes than typical children.

The Neuropsychology of Spelling

Spelling requires both memory for the word (lexical) and memory for phonological rules (sublexical) and simultaneous processing of these skills. The child must understand how to spell words that follow phonological rules (e.g., *bottle*) as well as irregular words (*the, was, right*) that must be memorized. Regular words follow grapheme–phoneme rules while irregular words do not. Lexical processes allow for automaticity of reading while sublexical processes require retrieval of previously learned phonological units or morphemes (i.e., *tion*) to match to the word. As has been suggested throughout this book, error analysis is key to understanding where the spelling process is breaking down. Not only can it tell you about spelling, but by comparing and contrasting word-reading errors, you can help the child improve both skills.

Spelling errors have been found to be more related to phonology problems than orthography problems (Bernstein, 2009). Inaccurate vowel substitutions are the most common mistake found in poor spellers and in those with dyslexia. Bernstein (2009) studied phonological deficits (*lain* for *lane*), alphabetic errors (*cr* for *car*), and phonological errors (*han* for *hen*). In addition, phoneme misclassifications were evaluated with words that sound similar (*han* for *hen*) versus those which are far different from the target (*crusp* for *crisp*). For most children with spelling problems the phonological errors were predominant with vowel mistakes being the most common type of error. You can see why spelling can be so difficult—if a child does not have the vowel sounds automatized, then it is very difficult to spell the word correctly and quickly. If the child has not automatized the vowel sounds, it is difficult to write fluidly and correctly. Interestingly enough, the children in the Bernstein study (2009) were able to correctly identify the vowel sounds but their difficulty lay in the ability to translate these vowels into written form.

It is not surprising that neuropsychological studies of spelling suggest that spelling depends on a network of relatively independent, albeit interconnected, cognitive processes and several different brain areas (Hillis et al., 2002). One way of thinking about this is that there is a working memory buffer in the brain that holds the sequence of the letters while the child is writing. This region is linked to the left frontal and parietal lobes (Cloutman et al., 2009). Neuroimaging has also found that there is a specialized region of the brain that is important for visually processing the word form, which is part of the ventral visual system (Szwed et al., 2011). This region is activated preferentially for words compared to objects. This region develops with experience and age and connections anteriorly are formed with experience with word forms (Glezer et al., 2009) and with the development of higher order thinking abilities (Price, 2010). Further studies have found that the visual word form region, and a region just lateral to this area, are specifically activated for spelling but not for reading (Purcell et al., 2011). The addition of graphomotor skills when spelling words, and the fact that spelling is a production rather than a recognition task, also make it different from reading.

Neuroimaging has found that when participants have less accurate and slower processing of irregular words, more neural networks for processing are required, including the left inferior frontal gyrus, and bilateral middle temporal gyrus. For regular words, activation was most pronounced in the left posterior superior temporal gyrus, right precentral gyrus, and right fusiform gyrus (Norton et al., 2007). Thus, dual processing is required depending on the type of word: frontal lobe functions, as well as left sensory–motor areas, are needed to carry out the act of handwriting. These findings have important implications for education in that both skills need to be addressed. In a recent comparison, only the graphemic/motor frontal area, thought to be the allographic representation of motor memories, was unique to spelling. Thus, while both reading and spelling share many posterior brain regions, only sensory–motor processing was unique to written spelling (Planton et al., 2019).

Clinically, it is important to recognize how children's spelling skills relate to their word attack skills. Is there a tendency to use sight-word approaches and spell from memory (ventral stream)? Do children use sound–symbol association skills to spell words phonetically (temporal–parietal)? Do they make the same or different types of error, and when they make errors, do they recognize and change them (frontal monitoring/evaluation)? Do they have problems with letter ordering (frontal) or reversals (parietal)? Recognizing these error patterns will provide you with a better understanding of each child's spelling and word recognition skills, leading to more effective interventions as a result.

Interventions for Children with Problems with Spelling

Spelling difficulties can significantly interfere with writing and with clarity in what is written. While spelling difficulty itself is not generally diagnosed as a learning disability, it can pose significant problems in understanding what the student is attempting to present in their written work. Often children with RD have difficulty with spelling due to phonetic deficits. Thus, Appendix 7.1 lists some of the major teaching strategies for spelling instruction. Although many of the techniques for developing sound (phoneme)–symbol (grapheme) association listed in Chapter 5 (see Appendix 5.1) apply to spelling instruction, the additional importance of visual memory retrieval in spelling is worth recognizing. As we have noted, spelling by its very nature is an output or production task, whereas reading is a recognition task. In reading, children have the correct word in front of them, but having the auditory representation (e.g., "I want you to spell the word *comprehensive*") requires a systematic search (frontal executive) for visual word images (ventral stream). This information must be translated into a sequential representation of the motor plan for writing the word (frontal and supplementary motor cortex), then there is sensory–motor integration for handwriting (left somatosensory–motor cortices), and finally there is evaluation of response and modification as necessary (frontal). We can't just assume that because Olivia can read well, she can also spell, because there are many more processes involved in the spelling; it requires a complementary but different network than reading.

As we can see from Appendix 7.1, several interventions require multiple steps and recommend a multisensory approach. The spelling interventions described in this appendix offer you some idea of what has been effective in the literature. The combination of your knowledge about cognitive patterns of performance, your familiarity with successful strategies reported in the literature, and your effective collaborative consultation meetings with teachers will help you to develop, implement, and evaluate interventions for children with SDs. More recent studies have found that teaching memorization strategies to improve spelling is not as successful as directly teaching the skill required for the task at hand.

We believe that researchers will begin to establish that interventions are not uniformly or equally effective for all children with special needs. A meta-analysis of spelling interventions found that spelling interventions need to incorporate phonics, orthography, and morphology to be effective (Galuscka et al., 2020). Thus, a spelling program really needs to be comprehensive for most children with spelling problems. If the child has excellent phonics, then of course, the program should build on that skill; similarly, if the child is good in orthography, then build on that strength to support phonics.

Here is a final point regarding handwritten and oral spelling versus computer-assisted spelling. Sometimes we see children with spelling problems given a keyboard and spell-check program as an accommodation. This is unfortunate, even if the end result is a correctly spelled word. Why? Because through the white matter pathways, the frontal lobe (Broca's/Exner's) area can help make sound–symbol associations in the posterior parietal region, so remediating handwritten spelling can actually improve reading decoding/word attack skills, as has been shown in the work by Virginia Berninger and colleagues (Berninger, Richards, et al., 2015). By giving the student a keyboard, one can actually undermine the potential of handwritten or oral spelling (front of brain) to assist sound–symbol associations (back of brain). Recall from Chapter 2 the interconnected nature of the frontal with posterior regions and the interdependence of these anterior–posterior systems known as the "axis" model.

You may be asking yourself if there is other evidence that spelling instruction helps develop reading and writing skills? In a meta-analysis designed to answer this question, Graham and Santangelo (2014) found formal teaching of spelling leads to better spelling than informal or no instruction in spelling, with moderate to large effect sizes found. These gains were not only translated into improved spelling, but the new skills were maintained over time, and improved spelling generalization to the written expression product. In addition to better writing, formal spelling instruction also improved phonological awareness and reading skills, consistent with the arguments we've presented in this section.

Handwriting

Handwriting is often a problem for children with learning disabilities, particularly children with WLDs and NVLD. This difficulty can certainly affect written language or conveying one's thoughts and words in writing, often referred to as *dysgraphia*. If Sophia doesn't like to write because it hurts her hand (due to poor somatosensory–motor coordination), takes too much time (due to poor processing speed), or her writing is illegible (due to visual–motor integration problems), then she is less likely to write, even though she may have good ideas. Sophia may readily discuss her ideas and provide you with a coherent oral narrative, easily telling you about the people, actions, and outcome of her story. However, as we saw early in the chapter, oral and written communication are not synonymous, and it is frustrating to hear of teachers scribing for students' oral discourse and calling that their written language performance. No matter how good at oral expression Sophia is, if she sits down to write about the same topic she easily conveys orally, she struggles, becomes frustrated, and shuts down. When reviewing her writing sample, we see Sophia's product lacks fluency and clarity; she produces only three short sentences, and these are disconnected and flat. How could this be? Although there are several possibilities—one that we have already discussed (spelling), and another that we will discuss later (written language)—many children with LDs have difficulty with writing tasks simply because of their poor handwriting. Some observers have questioned the use of handwriting at all, suggesting that keyboarding has become the skill to learn, but as we suggest here and earlier, *handwritten expression* is not equivalent to keyboard written expression, especially when we are considering neurodevelopment of academic skills.

Approximately 2.7–5% of children with WLDs have problems with handwriting, while 4–13% have spelling problems (Katusic et al., 2009). Graphomotor skills are developing during the elementary school years and can affect spelling competency. Poor visual–somato-sensory–motor coordination could be due to a lack of practice or poor pencil grip. However, if the problem extends beyond these basic functions, a thorough neuropsychological evaluation is needed. In addition, the evaluation shouldn't only be related to written expression. If graphomotor skills are evident during handwriting, they should also exist in other areas requiring fine-motor control, such as drawing, putting a cap on a bottle, and buttoning clothes. Your job is to determine whether poor graphomotor skills are due to a visual–somatosensory–motor problem, and if this cognitive deficit is interfering with the writing process or with accurate letter reproduction. It does no good for us to test a child with messy handwriting and in our report say, "He has a graphomotor problem." We already knew that! Instead, we need to use our understanding of neuropsychological processes to get to the bottom of the graphomotor problem, so that we (or the occupational therapist) can provide the appropriate intervention.

Development of Handwriting Skills

Handwriting is an important skill that involves fine-motor control, bilateral and visual–motor coordination, motor planning, hand dexterity, visual attention, and finger sensory awareness (Feder & Majnemer, 2007). It has been estimated that school-age children spend 31–60% of their time completing handwriting tasks and that approximately 10–30% of school-age children have difficulty with the mechanics of writing. Handwriting generally develops quickly during grade 1, reaches a plateau by grade 2, and by grade 3 should be an automatic skill (Karlsdottir & Stefansson, 2002). Children with handwriting difficulties frequently experience significant problems with the volume of written work and poor handwriting is often judged more harshly compared to the same ideas presented in good handwriting. In addition, children with poor handwriting are often judged negatively concerning their motivation and abilities, which leads to frustration and emotional difficulties for these children (Connelly et al., 2006). If handwriting is the difficulty, remediation has been found helpful and includes direct instruction in perceptual–motor/visual–motor control and individualized exercises (Schoemaker et al., 2005).

Children with WLDs tend to show poorer letter formation, spacing, and size, and their overall spelling and written language output is lower than that of their same-age peers (Parush et al., 2010). Are the graphomotor skill problems inherent in WLDs, or are they comorbid? They certainly seem to require different brain areas, so we would expect to see a dissociation between WLDs and graphomotor problems. Returning to previous neuropsychological material in Chapters 2 and 3, we need to know if the child has constructional apraxia (as opposed to ideational or ideomotor apraxia), for it is this type of apraxia which signals a fine-motor coordination problem that must be remediated by the teacher or occupational therapist.

The notion that poor graphomotor skills interfere with spelling and writing competency has been hotly contested, with researchers arguing both for and against the dissociation of letter representations and sensory–motor processes. In addition, as is the case with spelling, determining whether handwriting is interfering with written language, math computation, or other skills requiring visual–somatosensory–motor integration (e.g., art) is a critical part of any comprehensive CHT approach to serving children with LDs.

Several areas of written language should be considered during your evaluation of a child with an LD, handwriting problems, and poor visual–motor integration skills. In addition to looking for signs of constructional (apraxia) problems and poor psychomotor speed, it is important to look directly at the quality of handwriting either produced by the child during testing or gathered informally. This can help you determine whether the difficulty is a visual–spatial (dorsal stream), somatosensory (tactile and kinesthetic feedback to motor system), motor (primary or secondary motor areas), or integration (corpus callosum) problem.

Handwriting begins to develop with early scribbling that, with time, becomes letters and words (Feder & Majnemer, 2007). Learning to print begins with the ability to draw vertical and horizontal strokes at about age 2 and circles by age 3. Drawing then progresses to integration of vertical and horizontal strokes (a cross) to squares and circles by age 5. Children who are able to complete the cross are able to cross the midline and also are able to copy significantly more letters as well as items on the Developmental Test of Visual-Motor Integration (VMI) (Feder & Majnemer, 2007). According to Mercer and Pullen (2010), the following attributes should be examined in your handwriting assessment:

- Letter shape (letter slant/changes)
- Letter size (large, small, not uniform)
- Letter spacing (crowding, too much)

- Letter alignment (not online)
- Line quality (slant/directional issues)

One study found that overall legibility predicts handwriting performance during copying while speed and legibility predicted handwriting performance during dictation (Parush et al., 2010). There is some debate about the print (manuscript)–cursive (script) distinction in handwriting: Printing is easier to read, but cursive is less likely to produce reversals or interfere with the flow of thought. Cursive is also easier for children with significant fine-motor difficulties as it does not require the child to pick the pencil up after each letter. Certainly there are similar neuropsychological processes associated with both, so let's briefly explore them before we move on to written language. Given the benefits of cursive writing, especially for children with LDs, it is surprising that many schools don't even teach cursive anymore. Switching to keyboarding to compensate for graphomotor deficits, or as a substitute for handwritten cursive expression altogether, appears to undermine development of frontal–parietal regions (Beers et al., 2018), consistent with the arguments presented above.

The Neuropsychology of Handwriting

More neuroimaging studies of hand movements and handwriting have been completed than studies of spelling and written language. Before we review them, let's review the processes we think should be involved in visual–somatosensory–motor integration for handwriting— such as copying notes from the board. Recall that constructional abilities typically require bilateral visual perception, so the frontal eye fields coordinate eye movement with the cranial nerves to receive the image in the retina. This is transferred to the subcortical thalamus and the superior colliculi structures en route to the striate or primary visual cortex. From there, the dorsal stream is probably needed, as this area is important for directionality, symbolic representation, part–whole relationships, and visual–spatial processing.

This receptive information must be translated to the left premotor and/or supplementary motor area (e.g., Exner's area), which then directs the left primary motor cortex (in right-handed people) to carry out the motor act, with somatosensory (tactile and kinesthetic) feedback provided by the left anterior and superior parietal lobe. Let's not forget that the corpus callosum may be needed if new learning or holistic perceptual and/or motor processes require right-hemisphere involvement. This seems simple enough, but let's see whether this generalizes to handwriting, and also whether involvement of the corpus callosum varies based on whether the task is novel or routinized. In fact, research suggests after controlling for reading, handwriting shares a great deal of variance with written expression (67% of the variance), and automaticity of handwriting separates those with and without written expression difficulties (Jones & Christensen, 1999).

For handwriting competency, a meta-analysis of the most recent neuroimaging studies found that the left superior frontal and middle frontal gyrus, the left intraparietal sulcus/superior parietal area, and right cerebellum were structures intimately involved in handwriting (Planton et al., 2013). Areas involved in nonspecific motor actions included the left primary motor and sensorimotor cortices, the supplemental motor cortex, the thalamus, and the putamen. The linguistic portion of handwriting was found to be centered in the left ventral premotor cortex and the left posterior–inferior temporal cortex. These studies have been able to isolate handwriting from nonspecific motor movements and the linguistic processes involved in writing. Thus, the important information to note here is that the frontal area is important for working memory to direct how the letters are formed while the parietal lobe and cerebellum provide support for the smooth motor movements needed to put letters to paper.

Consistent with our novel–automatic distinction, studies demonstrating prefrontal effects often examine new motor learning, with the right frontal region activated during initial stages, and later learning associated with left frontal activation (Muller et al., 2002). Prefrontal activity also seems to be most prevalent during new learning, and as tasks become routinized, more posterior activity is likely (Staines et al., 2002). Not surprisingly, handwriting and motor program studies have implicated the frontal–subcortical circuits, and the subcortical structures receiving attention have included the hippocampus, thalamus, basal ganglia, and cerebellum (Haslinger et al., 2002). Even Broca's area has been implicated in handwriting and fine-motor skills, as suggested in In-Depth 7.1. The involvement of subcortical structures including the caudate and its connections to the frontal lobe is likely the reason why there is a high rate of comorbidity between ADHD and fine-motor problems, since the basal ganglia is involved in both (Hale et al., 2011). And it could account for improvements in handwriting found for children with ADHD treated with methylphenidate (Flapper et al., 2006). However, some evidence suggests that while 50% of children with ADHD have fine-motor coordination problems, some neuropsychologists see them as related but distinct (Goulardins et al., 2015).

With our recognition that the angular gyrus is involved in sound–symbol associations, and our knowledge that left-hemisphere dysfunction leads to Block Design reversals, could the parietal association cortex be responsible for both the letter reversals seen in RDs and in left–right orientation problems? Certainly, the available evidence would point to this plausible explanation for why children with LDs experience so many related deficits in disparate academic and linguistic areas. Recognizing these interrelationships may hold the key to effective interventions for children with handwriting problems, as is suggested in Case Study 7.1.

IN-DEPTH 7.1. Broca's Area and Handwriting

When you think of Broca's area, you often think of nonfluent or expressive aphasia, affecting oral language or speech production. However, unilateral or bilateral activity in Broca's area has also been reported during handwriting and fine-motor activity (Haslinger et al., 2002; Muller et al., 2002); at first glance, this is somewhat surprising, considering that this is the expressive speech area. Since Broca first described his aphasic patients, it has been a basic tenet of neuropsychology that damage to Broca's area leads to expressive aphasia. Although no one disputes this finding, some have questioned whether this area is solely responsible for expressive language. If we think back to our arguments presented in earlier chapters, could it be that the psychological processes are more important than the (verbal) output? Instead of thinking that Broca's area is responsible for verbal functions, many have noted that expressive language is a motor skill. It just so happens that Broca's area is responsible for producing detailed motor responses within time (Schubotz & von Cramon, 2001) or sequence, and so it is a likely candidate for both oral and handwritten language skills. Since this activity is sometimes bilateral during learning of motor behaviors, the right and left Broca's areas are working together to fine-tune motor movements to form a synchronized motor (verbal or nonverbal) pattern. This could account for the high comorbidity rate of aphasias and apraxias (Liepmann, 1908), with the underlying psychological processes affecting both types of output.

Case Study 7.1. Nathaniel's Handwriting Problem

Nathaniel was a 7-year-old boy who was originally evaluated and classified as having a LD 2 years prior to consultation with his teacher. He had been receiving resource room services for reading problems and speech–language services. A review of existing records and evaluations revealed that Nathaniel had a classic "double-deficit" RD and both receptive and expressive language delays. In addition to his linguistic deficits, the psychological and educational evaluations said that Nathaniel had "visual–spatial" problems because his graphomotor skills were poor. Test results confirmed difficulty with graphomotor skills, processing speed, and visual–motor integration, but nonmotor visual–perceptual skills appeared to be adequate. The resource room teacher reported that Nathaniel had made much progress in the visual–spatial area, as he easily discriminated simple and complex visual stimuli, recognized spatial relationships, and identified part–whole relationships. But Nathaniel still had difficulty with his handwriting. An examination of his handwriting confirmed that he had difficulty in this area. Although Nathaniel did not have a full CHT evaluation, the hypothesis-testing approach was used to look at his visual–motor functioning. Sure enough, Nathaniel's visual–motor integration skills were poor; however, his visual processes were intact, whereas motor skills were significantly delayed. He also had particular difficulty with learning and replicating motor sequences. In other words, Nathaniel showed classic signs of apraxia secondary to left-hemisphere dysfunction, consistent with his aphasic symptoms, and no amount of visual training would remediate his apparent motor problems. With this information, the teacher began helping Nathaniel sequence motor actions and coordinate graphomotor skills, using templates and tracing guidelines to improve his handwriting. But the focus was now on the motor action, not on the nonexistent visual–spatial problems thought to be present during his evaluation.

Interventions for Children with Handwriting Disorders

Now that you have a good idea about the brain–behavior relationships involved in handwriting, it is important to think about whether the intervention can be handled by you, the teacher, the parent, an occupational therapist, or some combination of interested parties. One important decision you must make is related to whether the problem is uniquely a graphomotor problem that causes difficulty with handwriting, or a more severe developmental coordination disorder (apraxia) requiring an occupational therapy evaluation and treatment plan. As in many of the disorders we discuss, there is probably a continuum spanning adequate, delayed, and deficient psychomotor and graphomotor skills. Thus, you will require an understanding of both fine-motor development, in general, and the child's unique profile of handwriting and other fine-motor skills.

As is the case with deficit types in reading, it may be important to determine whether a child has a single, double, or triple fine-motor coordination deficit (i.e., sensory, motor, and/or frontal–subcortical); the more severe the condition, the more likely the need for occupational therapy assessment and/or intervention. The distinction is dependent on many factors, including how severely affected the child is in each area, how old he or she is, and whether remediation has been successful in the past. That is why the CHT approach we advocate can be so important. Look at somatosensory skills (e.g., finger agnosia, astereognosis) without the need for motor skills. Examine left- (i.e., right-hemisphere) and right- (i.e., left-hemisphere) handed motor skills (e.g., finger tapping, pegboard) to see if there is a difference. Examine visual–spatial relationships (e.g., NEPSY-II Arrows) in the absence of significant sensory or motor demands. Finally, look at visual–motor integration (e.g., VMI), to see if the problem is one of interhemispheric or interlobule communication.

Written Language

In the preceding two sections, you have developed an understanding of how two technical skills, spelling and handwriting, can contribute to written language problems. When you also consider the cognitive demands of expressive language and executive skills required in written language, it is easy to see why some children have difficulty developing, writing, and editing their writing assignments. Although prevalence rates vary, some studies have suggested that as many as 6.9 to 14.7% of school-age children have a significant writing problem in one of these areas (Katusic et al., 2009). The comorbidity rates of neuropsychiatric disorders, given their frontal–subcortical circuit and hemispheric involvement, is quite high (Mayes & Calhoun, 2007). Written expression can be seen as the pragmatic extension of the posterior–anterior and inferior–superior axes, with the anterior-superior overlap readily evident in both LDs and psychopathology (Hale et al., 2018).

What makes one child a good writer while another struggles? Obviously, spelling and handwriting are at play for some children. It is easier to pick a word that you know how to spell (e.g., visual memory of word–ventral stream) versus one for which you need phoneme–grapheme correspondence to spell letter by letter (e.g., dorsal stream). Similarly, if handwriting is challenging and uncomfortable, it is easier to write fewer sentences and fewer words per sentence. But when it comes to actual written expression, some children readily enjoy putting their ideas on paper. They easily develop their ideas before writing, write flexibly and with ease, monitor and evaluate their drafts, and then revise their prose for a good product. Other children may struggle with the writing process—planning little before starting, writing very little in an attempt just to get something on the paper, and then failing to check the paper for understanding, grammar, or legibility (Grigorenko, 2007).

Given that many children experience written language problems, it is somewhat surprising that the study of written expression has lagged behind that of other academic domains (Berninger et al., 2010). While children with WLDs may show improvement in language and reading skills, their written language deficits may persist into adulthood and affect their vocational skills (Grigorenko, 2007). Compared to peers, children with WLDs tend to write fewer long sentences; produce more fragments; use fewer advanced vocabulary words; and have higher rates of spelling, capitalization, and punctuation errors. They do not develop their ideas well and organize them poorly in writing, often failing to develop a coherent theme (Carter & Sellman, 2013). The contribution of visual–spatial and visual–motor coordination skills make written expression distinct from reading, and math to a lesser extent (Carlson et al., 2013), so these core skills should always be considered for a child with written expression problems.

CHC Cognitive Processes in Written Expression

As we would expect, comprehension knowledge (*Gc*) was found to have a moderate effect on written expression from ages 7 to 10, and strong thereafter (Floyd et al., 2008) in a normative sample. Processing speed (*Gs*) showed moderate to strong effects, probably through the graphomotor fluency of handwriting, as we've discussed above. In addition, working memory (*Gwm*) was moderately related throughout the age span. Working memory is important at both the basic (remembering the letter formation and word spelling needed) and the advanced (remembering what you intended to say) levels. Automaticity of basic writing skills frees up working memory capacity for more complex written expression. Auditory processing (*Ga-PC*) was important at age 7 and at ages 15 through 17, possibly related to figuring out how to write new words whose spelling is not known. Fluid reasoning (*Gf*) became moderately involved at ages 15 and 16, possibly reflecting the greater planning necessary for longer, more complex writing tasks. Again, this study used a standardization sample, and may not reflect how children with WLDs process information.

Neuropsychology of WLDs

In addition to the spelling and handwriting components of written language that we just discussed above, executive functions and semantic knowledge are required, both of which require memory processes (i.e., long-term and working memory). The most important components of executive functioning for written language include working memory, sustained attention, inhibition of competing responses, and self-monitoring (Feiffer, 2011). Working memory is important to keep information in mind while constructing a sentence and paragraph. Sustained attention allows for attentional resources to be used in order to have "flow" to the writing and persistence to ensure the product is complete. The writer must inhibit responding to other ideas as the main idea is being discussed. Finally, the writer must self-monitor the writing to make sure that the thoughts logically follow one another and that there is an organization to what is written. Writing requires the ability to generate full sentences, to evaluate and revise accordingly, and to switch attention among the various functions to produce a good sample. So when you think about what we called executive functions in Chapter 2 (planning, organizing, strategizing, shifting/switching, monitoring, evaluating, and modifying behavior) you have a definition of written expression. All these executive skills are needed for good written expression (plus working memory, which is also an executive function), so it is not surprising that the comorbidity of executive-based disorders like ADHD are highly comorbid with WLD (Yoshimasu et al., 2011).

Writing can become problematic when these functions are interrupted or don't develop in the manner to be expected. In addition, recall that one of the executive circuits is the motor circuit, hence the overlap between impaired handwriting skills and WLD. Proficient writers spend a great deal of time planning what they will write and then focusing attention on the prose as they make revisions; these skills that are not found in writers with learning problems (Graham & Perin, 2007). Good writing also requires planning and organization of thoughts. The child must retrieve words from lexical–semantic memory and organize these words into a cohesive whole sentence. These skills develop over time particularly as the lexicon increases. Uhry and Clark (2005) estimate that first graders have an expressive language vocabulary of approximately 2,600 words and a receptive vocabulary of 20,000 words. By high school graduation, this lexicon increases to over 45,000 words. For most children the lexicon is stored in an organized fashion with networks of concepts connected through experience and practice (Gazzaniga et al., 2013). The types of words matter. Nouns appear to be more related to temporal lobe functioning (long-term memory storage for lexical–semantic information), while verbs are more frontal lobe (action related) in origin (Cappa & Perani, 2003), although the simplicity of this distinction has been challenged and is more nuanced (Crepaldi et al., 2011). In addition, the left inferior frontal gyrus is important for morphological and syntactical control (Matchin & Hickok, 2020), not just the expressive language component of written expression.

Children with WLDs most frequently show problems with orthographic, phonological, and morphological coding; storing and processing spoken and/or written words; and with executive functioning (Berninger & O'Malley May, 2011). Writing requires the coordination of many processes including handwriting, spelling, phonological coding, orthographic coding, and executive functions (particularly working memory), so difficulty in any of these areas can create a WLD. As a result, any student who has written expression problems should receive a thorough executive function assessment in all of these areas. While intensive instruction may improve these skills, the child, and later adult, will always have a susceptibility for written language difficulties due to the underlying genetic disposition (Berninger, 2008) and writing may always be an effortful task because these tasks are not fluent, especially if prerequisite skills of spelling and handwriting are also impaired.

Subtypes of WLDs

Empirical studies have looked at various ways of identifying subtypes of WLDs. A linguistic formulation of written expression was used to determine subtypes of writers in late elementary school (Wakely et al., 2006), including both good and poor writers. These researchers defined four types of poor writers: low semantics, low grammar, low spelling–reading, and poor text quality. The low semantics and low grammar groups were considered to have more general language deficits. The low spelling–reading group had difficulty with reading and spelling. The poor text quality group was characterized as having executive function difficulties, including poor planning, organization, self-monitoring, and metacognition.

In a study using our concordance–discordance model of LD (see In-Depth 1.2) using a referred sample, Fenwick and her colleagues (2016) identified several subtypes of writing difficulties. All students with writing deficits demonstrated spelling difficulties, confirming that this is a base-level skill for written expression. Students with left-hemisphere difficulties, those with processing speed deficits, and those with executive functioning difficulties all showed significant weaknesses in writing fluency. Further neuropsychological testing revealed that working memory was a significant weakness for students with executive functioning deficits, as expected. Verbal learning with delayed recall was particularly difficult for students with left-hemisphere difficulties and processing speed problems. Meaningful memory was poor for students with left-hemisphere difficulties. Crystallized verbal ability and verbal memory are critical for identifying students whose difficulties with writing stem from general linguistic deficits. Motor sequencing and motor speed were poor for students with processing speed deficits, not surprising given that the WISC-IV Processing Speed subtests were used. Executive measures, including working memory, were poor for students with executive functioning deficits, as expected, and also those with right-hemisphere difficulties.

Differential Diagnosis of WLDs

Because WLDs are, by definition, complex and interrelated with other disorders, differential diagnosis of WLDs requires careful examination of multiple subcomponent processes. Your job is to examine the written language process and products beyond spelling and handwriting to determine the problematic areas for subsequent intervention. Developmental influences on executive functions, visual–spatial processes, and language processes can all have an impact on written language competency.

Feifer and Defina (2002) suggest conceptualizing written language difficulties on the basis of executive function problems.

- Difficulty beginning a project
  - Few ideas generated
  - Unfocused writing
  - No beginning framework developed
- Difficulty persisting on a project
  - Problems with sustained attention
  - Begins but doesn't finish
  - Sentences disjointed—poor transitions among subjects

- Difficulty with inhibition
  - Pulled easily off-task with content so that paragraphs don't flow
  - Problems with spelling with letters added inappropriately
- Difficulty shifting topics
  - One topic predominates the writing
  - Poor writing from dictation
  - Perseverates on the same issue
  - Same (often simple, with fewer clauses) sentence structure for passage
- Difficulty organizing information
  - Main idea is not clearly present throughout the essay
  - Messy desk and messy paper
  - Sentences seem to jump from one topic to another without a cohesive whole
- Difficulty discussing events/situations
  - Poor verbal fluency
  - Poor transitions
  - Limited topic or conclusion sentences, or content inconsistent with these
- Difficulty with editing
  - Careless spelling and grammar
  - Poor punctuation
  - Careless errors
  - Sloppy work
  - Resistant to reviewing work and rewriting

Clearly, we are seeing that written language expression is by far the most difficult academic subject, requiring virtually every part of the brain to work concertedly toward a final product. Obviously, many more cognitive processes are required for written language competency than for other academic skills. It requires brainstorming, planning, and organization skills; choosing appropriate words and phrases; putting together a coherent sequence of words and sentences; adherence to grammar and syntax conventions; handwriting and spelling; and monitoring, evaluating, and changing the written product. Determining where a child is having difficulty can help you understand how to help that child, so the child may effectively communicate ideas in both oral and written form.

Hemispheric Differences in Written Language and WLDs

Finally, let's examine the left- and right-hemisphere processes in written language. As noted in Chapter 2, our model of hemispheric functioning suggests that the left- and right-hemisphere processes can be characterized by local–global, fine–coarse, and concordant/convergent–discordant/divergent distinctions. While the hemispheres are working together in a complementary rather than segregated way during writing, the left hemisphere may be utilized to access the lexicon, while the right hemisphere will contribute to the linguistic complexity of the output (Feiffer, 2011). Children with left-hemisphere dysfunction may then have difficulty adhering to grammatical rules and structured responses. It is important to note whether these syntactic problems are more anterior (e.g., Broca's area/inferior frontal gyrus) or posterior (posterior temporal-parietal crossroads) (e.g., Matchin & Hickock, 2020). These are the children who may need separate grades on their writing assignments: one for content and another for grammar.

Similarly, an anterior to posterior gradient is also likely in written language. Left frontal regions are very important for working memory and other executive functions as well as for the graphomotor skills needed to write a letter for right handers (Longcamp et al., 2003). Posterior regions are important for forming letters as well as for orthographic knowledge (Rapp & Lipka, 2011). Letter formation and visual perception have been tied to the occipital–temporal regions (visual word form area), as well as cerebellar functioning (James & Gathier, 2006; Richards et al., 2011).

Children who have difficulty with abstract or complex language writing and instead produce literal, concrete writing products will often not be identified until the late elementary or middle school years, when these demands increase. During the early school years, these children are likely to produce grammatically correct sentences that obey conventional syntactic rules, but they are less likely to produce complex syntactic structures (Rourke, et al., 2002), which are not required until later grades. For lexical–semantic use in writing, they may produce straightforward sentences using common words, but may have more difficulty thinking of alternative words to represent their ideas. Thus, their writing is rather straightforward but does not utilize a more complex and expository output. This writing is often pedantic with closely related words, single interpretations, and semantic integration (Richards et al., 2011). These writers may be overly focused and literal, missing the ultimate objective of their writing assignment. They would especially struggle with creating visual imagery in writing, writing poetry, and creative writing in general.

NEUROIMAGING

Neuroimaging has found that good writers show more brain activation in the following regions compared to poor writers: left precentral, left postcentral, left inferior parietal, and left cerebellar vermis (Richards et al., 2011). In contrast to good writers, poor writers were found to activate the following regions: the left occipital regions (calcarine and cuneus), left temporal regions (fusiform and lingual), left superior parietal and posterior cingulate. On the right, the cuneus and cerebellar vermis were activated (Richards et al., 2011). Areas activated for poor and good writers generally include the left occipital region and the right and left cerebellar vermis on the midline. These findings indicate that poor writers activate more brain regions than good writers, showing that the neural distribution for the writing process is more widespread than that for good writers, attesting to our basic tenet of automaticity—less brain does more in proficient writers (as is the case with reading and math). Such widespread activation generally results in poorer performance as well as a more effortful way of completing work. Research into this area is just beginning and further information is needed to determine what developmental and treatment effects there may be for children with WLDs. The reason why children with WLDs are so exhausted by writing is they may not have achieved automaticity in spelling, handwriting, or written expression. This lack of automaticity is why practice in writing is so critical for children with writing problems or WLDs.

ADHD AND WLD

It has been strongly suggested that children with ADHD are more susceptible to WLD compared to other diagnoses. Problems with visual–motor integration and motor coordination, deficits commonly seen in ADHD, interfere with writing skill development (Cole et al., 2008). Similar to the earlier discussion of the contribution of working memory to WLD, many children with ADHD also have working memory as well as organizational and planning problems. Studies have found that difficulties with handwriting quality and written language are pronounced in children with ADHD (Racine et al., 2008; Re et al., 2007). A population study found a strong association among children with ADHD and WLDs with 64.5% of boys and 57.0% of girls showing WLDs (Yoshimasu et al., 2011). In contrast for children without ADHD, 16.5% of boys and 9.4% of girls showed WLDs.

Yoshimasu et al. (2011) also found that the risk of being diagnosed with WLD was similar for boys and girls when RD did not co-occur. When RD did co-occur, the risk was higher for girls than for boys. Boys with a diagnosis of ADHD and WLD showed more complex written language difficulties compared to boys with WLDs and without ADHD. These studies suggest that ADHD is a complicating factor for WLD. These written language difficulties extend into college and adulthood (Semrud-Clikeman & Harder, 2011), making college-level and even occupational writing activities very difficult. Thus, ADHD has a long-standing effect on WLD and suggests that children with ADHD should be fully evaluated for a possible WLDs at all ages.

Interventions for Children with WLDs

As we have discussed regarding spelling intervention, written expression requires all of the visual memory, graphomotor skills, and executive functions that spelling does. However, the executive demands are what set written expression apart from all other achievement activities, at least the level of executive control required. As we've seen, writers need to brainstorm and retrieve ideas; develop a plan; organize their ideas into a sequence; develop a strategy for writing and integrating information; monitor their writing at the word, sentence, paragraph, and whole-product levels; remain flexible to change their ideas, words, or sentences; and evaluate the clarity of their content. Even if they do this well, they still must focus on the mechanics, such as proper spelling, punctuation, capitalization, and grammar. It is no wonder that many children with LDs have problems with written language, especially if comorbid psychopathology is noted (Hale et al., 2018). As with other academic areas, you must first attempt to recognize a child's cognitive pattern of performance, link this information to the written language product (both formal and informal assessment data), and then work collaboratively with the teacher to develop an effective intervention. However, because written language is so complex, there may be more than one problem area, so it is important for you and the teacher to remain flexible and open to exploring multiple strategies and interventions. Again, the key is the use of progress monitoring and recycling to ensure intervention efficacy.

It is important to recognize that few, if any, of the interventions in Appendix 7.2 were developed with the knowledge we now have about brain–behavior relationships. Therefore, even a very good strategy may be individually effective for some children, but not for others. It is essential that you design interventions for each individual child during the collaborative problem-solving meeting with the teacher(s) and/or parents. For instance, some children really struggle with knowing what to write and generating ideas that support their product. Once they write the first sentence, the writing is more fluid. In cases like this we've had children make free associations of words/ideas not written as sentences, from which they build sentences thereafter. If this is also a challenge, we often suggest (if visual–spatial skills are good), that the child draw a picture or series of pictures, and then use these pictures to generate the writing passage.

The intervention ideas presented in this chapter are merely suggestions to help you generate ideas in the problem-solving interview. Even an intervention that works for most children may need to be tailored to the child's unique characteristics so that it may be even more effective. Your ongoing intervention monitoring, evaluation, and recycling will be the key for ensuring the treatment validity of your evaluation and maximizing individualized instruction practices in written language.

Written Language Case Study

The study that follows (Case Study 7.2) presents an interesting case of a child with a WLD that wasn't quite what it seemed. As is the case with oral language, written language competency is related to both the fluency and the quality of the response. As we can see in Elise's case, she didn't really seem to have good ideas at all (of course, it depends on how you define "good"). The case again highlights how referral questions, histories, and observations are limited in helping you understand written language problems. If it weren't for our CHT evaluation, there were several interventions we might have considered, but few would have been related to the actual cause for Elise's writing problems.

Case Study 7.2. Elise's Ideas

Elise was an 11-year-old girl referred for a psychological evaluation because of parental concerns about her writing. She reportedly had good ideas, but couldn't seem to convey them on paper. Elise was described as a polite, cooperative, and reserved girl who was slow to warm up, but could be quite talkative with her best friend and family. Elise was hardworking and conscientious about her schoolwork, and had earned above-average grades for most of her schooling. Socially, Elise was best friends with Debbie, but she had few other friendships. She seemed to get along well with others, sometimes talking extensively about a particular book or topic she was interested in. However, Elise was somewhat isolated and teased by others, and one of Elise's teachers, Bert, couldn't seem to pinpoint why. Bert said that sometimes Elise seemed awkward in social situations. Sometimes Elise would get angry when others were joking around, and would say things that were unrelated to the conversation; other than that, however, she seemed fine. Bert said that Elise was an avid reader, preferring reading to any other activity, and often remained in the periphery during social situations.

The social studies teacher reported that Elise had no difficulty with objective exams; she just had problems with essay exams. She also had difficulty with both expository and creative writing in English, often writing little during creative writing exercises. Examining her writing, one of us (Hale) found that her handwriting was fairly good (she had big loops on some curved letters, though), and she had adequate capitalization and punctuation for the most part. The sentences mostly followed the same subject–verb–object pattern, however, and ideas were seldom connected. Overall, the longer samples had very limited organization, and the paragraphs didn't seem to flow well. Despite her reported reading skill, Elise tended to answer comprehension questions that asked her to retrieve facts and details from assignments.

A CHT evaluation was undertaken, using the Differential Ability Scales (DAS II) as the screening tool. The following results were obtained:

General Cognitive Ability (GCA) = 94

Verbal Ability = 108	Nonverbal Reasoning Ability = 86	Spatial Ability = 90
Word Definitions = 59	Matrices = 39	Recall of Designs = 37
Similarities = 52	Sequential and Quantitative Reasoning = 45	Pattern Construction = 52

Recall of Digits = 55

Recall of Objects—Immediate = 41

Recall of Objects—Delayed = 47

Speed of Information Processing = 48

From this evaluation, it appeared that Elise had adequate skills in many areas, and that verbal areas appeared to be a strength—an uncommon finding for children with WLDs. Her nonverbal reasoning or fluid abilities seemed to be somewhat low, and there was a large difference between the two DAS Spatial Ability subtests, with Recall of Designs much poorer than Pattern Construction. This finding leads to the hypothesis that something about Elise's visual–motor integration or constructional praxis could be affecting handwriting, but Recall of Designs also taps memory, so memory problems were another possibility. The diagnostic subtests were largely adequate, but Elise's memory for objects was low. Interestingly, the Immediate score on Recall of Objects was worse than the Delayed score, suggesting that once she had these word–object associations in memory, she was fine. Obviously, there was nothing in the data that would suggest a writing problem, so some detective work was necessary. Could Elise be a child with an NVLD affecting a "verbal" skill such as written language? In an attempt to examine this possibility, Hale looked into nonverbal or fluid reasoning, visual memory, and nonliteral language as possible causes for her difficulties. Given the history of problems with organization and flexibility, I also thought it would be important to look at executive functions as well. The following were the results of the hypothesis-testing stage (all scores are converted to standard scores):

NEPSY	Test of Memory and Learning	Cognitive Assessment System (CAS)
Tower = 95	Memory for Location = 100	Nonverbal Matrices = 95
Design Fluency = 85	Object Recall = 85	Planned Connections = 105
Verbal Fluency = 95		Expressive Attention = 100
Design Copy = 105	Wisconsin Card Sorting Test (WCST)	Woodcock–Johnson IV
Arrows = 100	Errors = 92	Concept Formation = 86
Memory for Faces = 85	Perseverative Responses = 85	
Narrative Memory = 105	Perseverative Errors = 88	
	Categories, Trials to First Category, Failure to Maintain Set > 16th %ile	

Comprehensive Assessment of Spoken Language (CASL)

Antonyms = 106	Grammatical Morphemes = 104	Nonliteral Language = 75
Synonyms = 114	Sentence Comprehension = 89	Meaning from Context = 87
Sentence Completion = 92	Grammaticality Judgment = 108	Inference = 82
Idiomatic Language = 102		Ambiguous Sentences = 80
		Pragmatic Judgment = 92

The hypothesis-testing results revealed that Elise did not appear to have significant difficulty with nonverbal reasoning and fluid ability, but as these tasks became less structured, she had more difficulty; she performed best when given a multiple-choice format. Similarly, her attention and executive functions appeared to be good, but she was somewhat perseverative on the WCST, an unstructured, self-directed task. She also seemed to have more difficulty on the last items of the CAS Planned Connections subtest (consistent with Trails B difficulties), making several errors. On the NEPSY, there was an apparent dissociation between her Verbal Fluency, which was fine, and her Design Fluency, which was low average; this suggested that maybe the visual nature of this task or the graphomotor skills required were causing her difficulty. However, her skill at drawing designs according to a model was intact, and other dorsal or visual–spatial–memory skills appeared to be adequate. Elise's memory for object–word associations and facial memory were limited, pointing to possible ventral stream problems. The CASL results appeared to confirm that Elise had language difficulties associated with right-hemisphere temporal lobe dysfunction. She had difficulty with non-literal language, gaining meaning from context, drawing inferences, and deciphering ambiguous sentences. She performed adequately on the CASL Idiomatic Language subtest, which is some-what surprising at first glance. But an examination of this subtest reveals that the idioms are fairly straightforward and commonly used. This is why the CASL's author placed the Idiomatic Language subtest in the Lexical/Semantic category. Consistent with this assumption, Elise easily recognized these simple idioms by using her good rote memory skills, and she had no problem providing the appropriate definition of each.

The results of the CHT evaluation confirmed the hypothesis that Elise apparently had a "nonver-bal" LD affecting written language. Subsequent to the CHT, Hale worked with the teacher to develop some written language strategies designed to increase Elise's brainstorming of ideas prior to writing, her flexibility in interpretation and production of language, her consideration of multiple word choices and meanings, and her skill at linking ideas and concepts; she was encouraged to provide details only after the concepts were developed and associated. The teacher also came up with a great strat-egy—namely, using poems to work on Elise's skill at interpreting multiple meanings of words. Finally, we offered counseling to help Elise read facial and vocal affect and recognize colloquial language during conversation.

APPENDIX 7.1. SPELLING INTERVENTIONS

Reference	Intervention description
Berninger, Winn, et al. (2008)	Spelling taught through the use of direct teaching of strategies such as Photographic Leprechaun and Proofreader's Trick.
Berninger et al. (2013)	Spelling intervention using grapheme–phoneme correspondences and orthographic spelling strategies.
Berninger et al. (2002)	Alphabet principle and teacher scaffolding.
Chapleau & Beaupre-Boivin (2019)	Morphemic strategies worked more quickly with children with dyslexia compared to alphabetic or orthographic strategies.
Dymock & Nicholson (2017)	Comparing look, say, cover, write, check with phonological spelling strategies.
Galuschka et al. (2020)	A meta-analysis of the efficacy of spelling interventions found that memorization strategies were not effective. Treatment approaches using phonics, orthographic, and morphological instruction were found to be most effective.
Mercer & Mercer (2001)	Cover and write method: Looking and saying word, writing word while looking, covering word and writing it, and uncovering to see if correct.
Salas (2020)	Nonphonological strategies were found to be more useful in teaching spelling compared to morphographemic strategies. Morphological and lexical strategies were harder for children.
Schiff et al. (2017)	Children with training in metacognitive strategies plus metalinguistic instruction significantly outperformed children who only received metalinguistic instruction.
Williams et al. (2018)	Spelling interventions using direct teaching (such as cover–copy–compare) and technological assistance were most helpful for children with LD or EBD.

APPENDIX 7.2. WRITTEN LANGUAGE INTERVENTIONS

Reference	Intervention description
Berninger et al. (2006)	Teaching of orthographic free motor activities and motor-free orthographic activities improve accuracy and legibility of writing while visual cues and verbal mediation also improve rate of writing and word reading.
Berninger, Winn, et al. (2008)	Direct teaching of strategies for planning, writing, reviewing/revising of narrative and expository texts improved production and composition as well as spelling.
Berninger & O'Malley May (2011)	Interventions that are developmentally appropriate and include training in executive functions, letter writing, orthographic coding, finger sequencing and phonological coding.
Berninger (2009)	Use of a writer's workshop approach outlined for 16 sessions.
Graham & Perin (2007)	Utilizing writing strategies (summarizing, sentence combining, prewriting, inquiry activities, process-writing approach, study of models, writing for content learning).
Scott (2020)	Language sample analysis was used with children. It involves analyzing writing at word, sentence and text levels. This analysis allows for the development of an intervention that specifically targets the areas of difficulty the child is experiencing in writing and thus improves writing skills.
Spencer & Peterson (2018)	Oral presentation of material improved writing quality for young students. Groups received oral narrative instruction over 2 weeks and then wrote their own stories. Stories improved in terms of structure and language complexity.

Chapter 8

The Neuropsychology of Autism Spectrum Disorder, Nonverbal Learning Disorder, and Attention-Deficit/Hyperactivity Disorder

The neurodevelopmental disorders most frequently seen in neuropsychology clinics and by school psychologists are autism spectrum disorder (ASD), attention-deficit/hyperactivity disorder (ADHD), and nonverbal learning disorder (NVLD). This chapter discusses these three disorders from a neuropsychological viewpoint as well as by utilizing neuroimaging findings and a case report presentation.

Autism Spectrum Disorder

Psychologists in the schools are often called upon to identify and treat comorbid emotional and behavior problems in children with ASDs. A sizable minority of these children may also show intellectual disorders (IDs) while the majority have low average to above average cognitive skills. Few school clinicians receive extensive training in ASD and associated disorders (Aiello et al., 2017). They must rely on psychologists and other professionals to help formulate comprehensive treatment programs. At the present time, some school systems have autism specialists who are trained to administer the Autism Diagnostic Observation Schedule, Second Edition (ADOS-2; Lord & Rutter, 2012).

Neuropsychological evaluation of patterns of performance and aberrant behaviors can enhance diagnostic accuracy, which may be the single most important determinant of intervention success (Koegel et al., 2012). As children with ASD often have a broad array of problems and needs, careful examination and interdisciplinary coordination are required. Children with ASDs seldom show uniform patterns of performance on psychometric measures nor do children with ASDs plus ID—the so-called "flat profile" thought to be characteristic of the population with ID. Children with ASDs and IDs are just as complex as those with the higher-incidence disorders discussed throughout this book.

Characteristics and Comorbidities

Children with ASDs can be difficult to assess and treat, largely because behavioral interference with performance on standardized tests may limit the utility of these measures. It may be necessary to use behavioral observation and interviews to formulate diagnostic impressions. Knowing the characteristics and behavioral manifestations of these disorders is an important first step. Children with ASDs are characterized by impaired communication skills, poor sociability, and a limited range of interests and activities. Associated features include inattention, sensory–motor deficits, concrete thought, perseveration, affective blunting, poor insight, and sleep disturbance (Ozonoff et al., 2018).

Most children with ASDs display signs of neuropsychological deficits (Semrud-Clikeman, Walkowiak, Wilkinson & Butcher, 2010). Common neurological abnormalities in ASDs include abnormal gyri patterns, increased brain size (especially in the posterior regions), increased ventricular size, smaller corpus callosum, and cerebellar abnormalities (Eliez & Reiss, 2000). Studies of infants at high risk for ASDs have found differences in these regions prior to having a formal diagnosis (Hazlett et al., 2017). Interestingly, while the corpus callosum is smaller than expected in ASD, the enlarged occipital, temporal, and parietal areas are due to *excessive* white matter (Amaral, Schumann, & Nordahl, 2008).

The brains of children with ASDs tend to have microscopic abnormalities in both the cortex and subcortical structures, including the anterior cingulate, hippocampus, amygdala, and cerebellum (Amaral et al., 2008). The amygdala is of particular interest, given its relationship with "social intelligence" and the finding that children with ASDs do not use this region during mentalistic inferences (Baron-Cohen et al., 2000). The increased caudate volume observed in ASD, which is similar to that in obsessive–compulsive disorder (OCD) and Tourette syndrome, could account for the compulsive and ritualistic behavior observed in this population (Cody et al., 2002) as well as the difficulty modulating emotions (Semrud-Clikeman, Fine, et al., 2013). Differences in metabolism have been found in children with ASD, which lends support to the hypothesis that they may also have a disorder of energy production due to mitochondrial dysfunction (Frye, 2012) since mitochondria supply energy to the cell. Given the large number of brain areas associated with ASD, it is reasonable to speculate that the expression of autism can differ among children.

Unless they are "high-functioning," children with ASD often have low overall intelligence. Their speech and language may be impaired or delayed, characterized by intonation problems, difficult with supralinguistic language, pronoun reversal, meaningless echolalia, and pragmatic deficits affecting social reciprocity and conversation exchange (Ozonoff & Rogers, 2003). Frequently these children show delays in fine- and gross-motor, language, and cognitive flexibility skills. In contrast, their memory for rote material is often very good.

Children with ASD have been found to process facial features in a different manner compared to typically developing children. For example, they prefer to look at the mouth rather than the eyes (Joseph & Tanaka, 2003) and use the inferior temporal lobe to process faces, as if they were objects (Schultz et al., 2000). They also have poor eye contact, limited interest in or use of social cues, abnormal preoccupations and rituals, stereotypic or repetitive behavior patterns, and a need for environmental consistency (Klin & Volkmar, 2003).

Given the neurological problems in ASD, it is not surprising to find that these children have significant attention, memory, and executive function deficits (Semrud-Clikeman, Walkowiak, Wilkinson, & Minne, 2010). Additional deficits include perseveration and problems with cognitive flexibility or shifting cognitive sets (Hyseni et al., 2019). These difficulties with cognitive flexibility and executive functioning are likely to contribute to the social problems seen in ASD. A high number of autistic symptoms were found related to having significant neuropsychological problems. In an attempt to link executive function to social functioning or "mindblindness" deficits in ASD, researchers have used "theory-of-mind" tasks to assess children's understanding of the beliefs, thoughts, desires, and intentions of others (Scheeren et al., 2013). These researchers have found that children with ASDs may complete theory-of-mind tasks on neuropsychological measures adequately, but the real issue is the difficulty they have in applying these skills in everyday life.

Delays in most areas of academic functioning can be expected, and depending on the severity of these delays, a functional curriculum may be advised. Adaptive behavior is likely to be limited, especially in the areas of language and social activities, even in high-functioning individuals. Children with ASDs often have difficulty with language, particularly when the language skills involve higher-order abstract language (or supralinguistic language). Tests such as the Comprehensive Assessment of Spoken Language—Second Edition (CASL-2; Carrow-Woolfolk, 2017) help to evaluate the higher levels of language, which is particularly important for children with high functioning autism.

Difficulty with motor coordination, balance, gait, and implicit learning may be present in some children with ASDs due to possible cerebellar involvement. Careful monitoring of these behaviors, in conjunction with physical and/or occupational therapy, is good practice. For learning and behavior problems, strict operant conditioning procedures have been shown to be effective with children with ASDs (Foxx, 2008), but systematic monitoring is required to ensure efficacy. Stereotypic behaviors and/or self-injurious behaviors may require intensive behavioral and possibly psychotropic medication interventions.

You can use functional analysis to determine whether aberrant behaviors are driven by internal or external reinforcement (O'Reilly et al., 2010). However, the behaviors of children with autism were found to be self-reinforcing and not necessarily linked to external or internal reward systems. By identifying and operationalizing key problem behaviors, administering formal and informal cognitive measures, and systematically observing the behaviors during baseline and treatment conditions, psychologists in schools can help others monitor treatment response.

Asperger Syndrome

In previous editions of the DSM, Asperger syndrome (AS) was included as part of ASD but it is no longer a DSM diagnosis. It was not retained in the ICD-11 system but combined with childhood autism. The inclusion of AS with ASD continues to be a controversial decision. Children previously identified as having AS are now considered to have high-functioning autism (HFA). Children with HFA generally show extremely well-developed verbal skills with a sizable minority showing lower nonverbal reasoning skills (Semrud-Clikeman, Walkowiak, Wilkinson, & Christopher, 2010). These children also frequently show a pattern of stereotyped interests, difficulty when routines are changed, and problems with cognitive flexibility (Joseph & Tager-Flusberg, 2004). Although children with HFA are said to have language strengths, they are likely to present with idiosyncratic, agrammatical, and pedantic speech; preferences for rote, automatized verbal information; prosopagnosia; and marked difficulties with visual–perceptual–motor skills, prosody, and novel problem solving (Adolphs et al., 2001). Some have found differences between children diagnosed with AS versus HFA. One study found that children with AS were more likely to show fewer difficulties than children with HFA and to need fewer educational supports (de Giambattista et al., 2019). In contrast, children with AS showed more internalizing disorders (anxiety and depression) compared to those with HFA. This area of diagnosis continues to be controversial and is not resolved at this point in time. The astute clinician will be aware of possible differences within the spectrum of HFA as well as within ASD.

The differential neurocognitive and psychological deficits experienced by children with HFA may be identified through a comprehensive neuropsychological evaluation. Children with HFA are likely to display discordant/divergent language deficits; they have difficulty with understanding inference, implicit messages, metaphor, humor, and prosody. Despite being highly verbal, children with HFA are likely to miss the gist of social discourse, and to have significantly more academic and social problems during the middle childhood to adolescent years.

In addition to language issues, neuropsychological testing should allow for examination of frontal, right frontal, and right posterior brain functions, including the dorsal and ventral visual streams. This would include an examination of executive functions, working memory, attention, novel problem-solving and fluid reasoning skills, implicit receptive, and expressive language, receptive and expressive prosody, and visual–spatial as well as visual object memory.

Medical Issues

Many children with ASDs have concomitant medical disorders, particularly gastrointestinal difficulties and metabolic disturbances (Mayer et al., 2014). These medical problems often exacerbate emotional adjustment. It is hard for a child to be calm and manage frustration when his or her stomach hurts or when a child doesn't feel well. A thorough diagnostic workup that includes medical evaluations, as well as neuropsychological and educational assessment, can assist in developing the appropriate intervention program addressing medical, language, motor, adaptive, academic, and behavioral needs. The physician may suggest a trial of psychotropic medication. Careful neuropsychological and behavioral monitoring of medication response using multiple tools and informants is critical, especially if multiple medications are used for neurological and psychiatric symptoms (Murray et al., 2014).

ASD and ADHD

While many children with ASD show subclinical signs of ADHD, there is a sizable minority who qualify for both disorders (Grazdzinski et al., 2016). Some suggest that children who have a dual diagnosis of ADHD and ASD represent a separate subtype of ASD. More specifically, ADHD + ASD may be a different type of disorder than ASD without ADHD, with the former showing more severe symptoms and further compromise of neuropsychological skills (van der Meer et al., 2017). Therefore, when ADHD is more prominent in a child with ASD, the treatment of attention takes precedence. In contrast, when a child has ASD and less severe ADHD symptoms, the difficulty with social understanding is paramount.

Electroencephalogram (EEG) findings suggest that children with a combination disorder have more significant differences in electrical discharges while resting than either those with ADHD or ASD alone (Shephard et al., 2017). Severe forms of ADHD in children with ASD have been found to be related to more severe psychopathology compared to severe forms of ASD without ADHD (Mansour et al., 2017). Rommelse et al. (2018) investigated the overlap of ASD and ADHD. They suggested that a dual diagnosis should only be made for children with ASD when the ADHD causes significant distress in the child's life. Table 8.1 shows an overlap in the symptoms as well as symptoms that are unique to each disorder.

Nonverbal Learning Disorder

NVLDs generally include children who have visual–spatial deficits, problems with mathematics (particularly calculation), difficulty with attention, and problems with social

TABLE 8.1. Similarities and Differences in ASD and ADHD

ASD	ASD + ADHD	ADHD
Early signs		
Sometimes premature birth or delivery issues—but not necessarily	Sometimes premature birth/complicated delivery, etc.	Can have premature birth or delivery issues—but not necessarily
No significant sleep issues early on	Sleep problems	Frequently seen, particularly with restless sleep
May have self-regulation and self-soothing difficulties.	Difficulty with self-regulation and self-soothing	Some difficulty with self-regulation
Difficulty with eye contact and defensive to touch. May have difficulty bonding with parent.	Problems with social interactions in toddlerhood	More difficulty with impulsive behavior affecting social interactions than social issues
Later signs		
Reduced smiling	Friendship problems (ASD lack of interest; ADHD impulsive behaviors)	Good use of gestures and eye contact
Reduced joint attention/poor eye contact	Poor daily living skills	Motor restlessness
Atypical responses to sensory stimulation	Difficulties sharing toys and materials	Impatience and restlessness
Repetitive motor movements (rocking)	Difficulty with reciprocal conversation	Inattention to details/poor organization
Restricted interests	Voice volume is intense	Problems with sustained attention to nonpreferred activities
Lack of interest in other children/preference for playing alone/avoidance	Social disinhibition	Loses things or forgets
Excessive ordering of toys	Ordering of toys often seen; difficulty staying with one task—frequently impatient	Very short attention span playing with toys—quickly moving from one activity to another

relationships (Fine, Semrud-Clikesman et al., 2012). These children do have social problems but they are often seen as less severe than children with ASD or HFA. In addition, these children are often not identified until much older; they frequently respond well to social skills training; have very good reading skills but poor reading comprehension; and may have some difficulties with motor skills.

While the diagnosis of NVLD is controversial, clinicians often identify children with this disorder and it is hoped that revisions of DSM will recognize it as an actual disorder. Because NVLD is not recognized by DSM at this time, children do not generally qualify for services unless they have a learning disability in mathematics. However, a task force is recommending that NVLD be renamed Visual–Spatial Disorder (VSD) and included in the

DSM to more fully represent the difficulties experienced by these children. Two reviews of the NVLD literature have supported the existence of this diagnosis (Fine et al., 2013; Mammarella & Cornold, 2014). See Case Study 8.1 for an example of a child with NVLD.

Neuroimaging in ASD and NVLD

Neuroimaging and neuropsychological findings suggest that children with NVLD may be more similar to children with HFA than different (Fine, Musielak, et al., 2013). Initial findings report that children with NVLD or HFA show differences from neurotypical children in the area of the anterior cingulate—a structure important for error monitoring and changing of responses (Semrud-Clikeman, Fine, et al., 2013). Children with HFA show larger volumes in the amygdala region, which was not found in children with NVLD or neurotypical children. This finding suggests that children with HFA are more reactive, have more difficulty modulating their behavior, and adapting their behavior to new demands. In addition, the NVLD sample showed smaller volumes in the splenial area of the corpus callosum—an area important for visual spatial processing.

Case Study 8.1. Braydon's Baseball Blunder

Braydon was an 11-year-old boy who displayed a classic right-hemisphere pattern of performance on intellectual, neuropsychological, and psychosocial measures. He had fairly good verbal skills, scoring above average on the WISC-V Information and Vocabulary subtests, but his performance on the Comprehension subtest was poor, and his "SCAD" (Symbol Search, Coding, Arithmetic, and Digit Span) profile was also low. Braydon scored in the low average range on the Picture Completion and Picture Arrangement subtests, while his Block Design and Object Assembly skills were poor: Two configuration errors were noted on Block Design, and he failed to complete any of the abstract Object Assembly items. CHT results revealed poor fluid reasoning, spatial perception, and nonverbal memory, as well as inconsistent executive functions. Interestingly, Braydon had adequate visual memory for meaningful stimuli and faces, suggesting that his ventral stream was adequate. His mathematics skills were poor (due to computation and spatial errors), but his word reading was in the superior range, and his reading comprehension was average.

Behavior ratings, observation, and interview revealed that Braydon had social difficulties because he talked incessantly, often made off-task or irrelevant comments, had poor eye contact, and complained that others were whispering or yelling when talking with him. It did not help that he had very poor hygiene (due to self-neglect) and that his gross- and fine-motor skills were quite poor (because of poor visual–perceptual feedback to the motor system). Noting his social difficulties, his parents had encouraged him to join a Little League team. After all, baseball was Braydon's favorite sport, and he studied the statistics of his favorite players, such as batting averages and earned run averages. He tried to play baseball, but was quickly relegated to the bench for most games. When Braydon did play, he made several errors; his batting average was abysmal; and he often sat alone on the end of the bench. After a missed catch that resulted in a broken nose, Braydon quit the game, and his parents decided to seek a school evaluation. The teacher reported that Braydon was "fine—one of my best students," struggling only in math and writing class. She minimized any social problems, as he was "fine" during supplemental math instruction. However, the day before he was scheduled for a private evaluation, Braydon was suspended from school for hitting a "bully," and he was severely depressed upon presentation. Braydon is a child with all the features of NVLD: visual–spatial difficulties as well as social problems. Needless to say, we recommended intensive behavioral, social skills, and counseling support following our evaluation.

Margolis et al. (2019) studied the discrepancy between spatial IQ processing and verbal processing skills using functional magnetic resonance imaging (fMRI). They found that children with significant discrepancies that favored verbal comprehension over perceptual reasoning had less activation in the frontal lobe, basal ganglia, limbic (anterior cingulate), and temporal regions. These findings are not specific to NVLD or ASD but, as reviewed above, children with NVLD tend to show poorer perceptual reasoning skills compared to verbal skills. Further neuroimaging studies have found that the verbal IQ (VIQ)–Performance IQ (PIQ) discrepancy is related to significant thinning of the cortices with more thinning found in children with a greater discrepancy (VIQ > PIQ) (Margolis et al., 2013).

Two networks that support social processing are the default mode network (DMN) and the salience network (SN) (Laird et al., 2011; Menon, 2015a). The DMN includes the anterior cingulate, the precuneus (parietal lobe), and the parietal lobe. The SN includes the anterior insula and the prefrontal cortex. The DMN is activated when the child is processing social interactions and internally analyzing these interactions (Li et al., 2014). The SN has been implicated in the understanding of social norms as well as emotional processing (Xiang et al., 2013). These networks have been implicated in ASD with children showing less connectivity in the DMN region while other networks show higher connectivity when the child is asked to process social situations during fMRI (Hull et al., 2017). This finding is also true in the SN with increased and decreased connectivity found in these regions (Nielsen et al., 2016) when processing social interactions. These networks involve the anterior cingulate, which is a structure important for self-monitoring and in the social networks. Differences in this area have been found in ASD (Di Martino et al., 2009) and in NVLD (Semrud-Clikeman et al., 2013).

The two networks described above contribute to the central executive network which manages planning and problem-solving skills as well as making informed judgments based on information processed by the brain. Most importantly, this network manages working memory as well as the ability to make flexible judgments.

Margolis et al. (2019) compared children with ASD, NVLD, and controls using resting state MRI and looking at the SN and DMN areas. Children with ASD were found to show increased SN connectivity while those with NVLD showed reduced connectivity particularly in the anterior insula and anterior cingulate cortex areas. For the NVLD group, the left-hemispheric anterior insula and anterior cingulate were more compromised and strongly related to increased social problems. For the ASD group, the increase was found in the right hemisphere in the prefrontal cortex which is related to lower scores on language tasks. These findings underscore the hypothesis that there are differences between NVLD and ASD and that it is not simply a right–left hemisphere difference but rather that widespread networks are involved in social processing.

A meta-analysis of diffusion tensor imaging (DTI) studies evaluated white matter structures involved in ASD. It found microstructural differences in ASD in the development of white matter organization (Ameis & Catani, 2015). Differences in the connectivity between limbic regions were strongly related to complex socioemotional functioning and frontal and thalamic projection in children with ASD. These pathways were not found to be compromised in children without a diagnosis of ASD.

While some have speculated that HFA and NVLD may be due to right-hemispheric differences, this explanation is somewhat simplistic given the above findings. It is more likely that there is dysfunction in the cortical–limbic–reticular system with subsystems in the right-hemispheric centers that are important for processing novel stimuli also being involved. Using the model of Koziol and Budding (2009), the ability to cope with novel stimulation is likely problematic and anxiety producing for children with ASD or NVLD. Certainly an argument can be made that there needs to be overlap for some children who are diagnosed with ASD to also qualify for a diagnosis of NVLD. However, not all children with NVLD also show ASD.

Treatment

Interventions that have been found helpful for children with HFA and NVLD frequently include intensive cognitive-behavioral therapy, behavior management, and social skills instruction, instruction in theory of mind, and perspective taking. Research and clinical practice have now found that creative drama techniques can be quite helpful for children with HFA and NVLD (Guli et al., 2013; Minne & Semrud-Clikeman, 2012). These techniques utilize metacognitive instruction to improve self-monitoring and control as well as assisting the child in understanding his or her own reaction to situations. Teaching the processing of information from many perspectives also assists the child in developing new behaviors through the use of "game-like" activities.

Attention-Deficit/Hyperactivity Disorder

Characteristics

A plethora of research on the heterogeneous, disabling disorder of ADHD has been conducted in the last 30 years, but there is still considerable debate about its causes and treatment. The incidence of ADHD ranges from 4 to 7% worldwide (Spencer et al., 2007). It was originally thought that ADHD symptoms declined in adolescence and adulthood; however, more recent research found that it continues throughout adulthood in the majority of cases (Barkley, 2017). See In-Depth 8.1 for a look at attention and ADHD.

ADHD runs in families, with the heritability index estimated at 77% (Spencer et al., 2007). Most studies have utilized identical twins and fraternal twins to study this inheritability. When one identical twin has ADHD, there is a 75% chance the other twin also has ADHD. The remaining 25% seems to be due to nonshared environmental influences or measurement error (Boada et al., 2012). The genes that have been linked to ADHD include chromosomes 5, 6, 10, 12, and 16 (Willcutt et al., 2003). Even with our advanced knowledge of the genome, ADHD continues to be unexplained from a genetic point of view.

Risk Factors

Risk factors for the diagnosis of ADHD include problems during pregnancy such as toxemia, eclampsia, poor maternal health, maternal age, fetal postmaturity, fetal distress, and low birth weight (Mick et al., 2002). Moreover, maternal smoking and alcohol exposure during pregnancy as well as psychosocial adversity have been linked to ADHD (Huang et al., 2018; Wetherill et al., 2018). Factors of psychosocial adversity that are related to ADHD include severe marital discord, low social class, large family size, paternal criminality, maternal mental disorder, and foster care placement (Spencer et al., 2007). The hypothalamic–pituitary–adrenal (HPA) axis has been found to be affected by psychosocial adversity and results in these brain changes (Kazmierski et al., 2020). This axis affects the frontal lobes most directly, a brain area that has been linked to attentional difficulties. These factors can lead to permanent brain changes due to exposure to extreme environmental factors, thus resulting

IN-DEPTH 8.1. What Is Attention?

One of the first models of attention was published by Mirsky et al. (1999) involving the multiple brain areas. Focus/execute (striatum/superior temporal/inferior parietal), encode (hippocampus/amygdala), shift (prefrontal/anterior cingulate), and sustain/stability (reticular formation/thalamus) attention are the main elements. Posner (1994) further elaborated on this model and suggested that children with "real" ADHD have difficulty with what Posner and Raichle (1994) describe in their model as the anterior alerting/vigilance and executive/processing networks (i.e., frontal–subcortical circuits), but not the posterior orienting network (i.e., parietal function). In this model there is a posterior and anterior attentional system. The posterior system (Posner's first and second factor) develops early in the child's development and does not appear to be affected in children with ADHD (Huang-Pollock & Nigg, 2003). It has also been suggested that the cognitive load (complexity of the task) affects how well a child can focus his or her attention (Nigg, 2005b). As cognitive load increases, attention is stressed and more cognitive resources are required to complete the task.

The executive functions of working memory and set shifting have been linked to ADHD. Verbal working memory is often tested by a digit span task while tests of nonverbal working memory involve the recall of the location of a series of objects that had been placed in front of the person. Nonverbal working memory has been found to be particularly deficient in children with ADHD. *Set shifting* is the ability to be cognitively flexible when task demands suddenly change. Emerging research suggests that set shifting and cognitive flexibility may not be strongly associated with ADHD but be a related deficit (Barkely, 2006). Measures to evaluate these areas are discussed later.

Recent research has focused extensively on executive functioning as the main problem in ADHD. Executive functioning is lateralized to the frontal lobes (Koziol et al., 2012). The pathophysiology of ADHD is believed to arise from dysfunction of the dopaminergic and noradrenergic pathways that connect the prefrontal cortex and subcortical regions of the brain (Konrad et al., 2005; Semrud-Clikeman et al., 2006). Psychostimulant drugs block dopamine receptors and increase the availability of dopamine at the synapse. These medications have been found to be quite effective in improving performance on executive function measures (Mueller & Tomblin, 2012).

---

in altered brain activity as the brain is exposed to steroid hormones (Johnson et al., 2019). Maternal exposure to domestic violence also appears to negatively affect the HPA axis in the newborn, thereby setting up differences in how the brain develops (Fassaie & McAloon, 2020). Thus, during your interview, it is important to document what happened during the prenatal and postnatal environments as these experiences have been found to significantly affect brain development and place the child in a vulnerable position for the development of ADHD and likely other disorders.

How often have you evaluated a child, and the parent, after completing your questionnaires, then tells you, "I think I have ADHD"? Keep this comment in mind while working with the child. This disorder is frequently seen in the family, and you should be ready to provide accessible information about the disorder to parents. ADHD is variable in presentation and treatment course, but has three main presentations: predominantly inattentive (PI); predominantly hyperactive–impulsive (HI); and the combined type (C), both inattentive and hyperactive–impulsive.

Combined Presentation

ADHD:C is the most common form of ADHD and includes children who show significant symptoms of inattention, hyperactivity, and impulsivity. Longitudinal studies have found that ADHD:C continues throughout the lifespan and does not remit with adulthood (van Lieshout et al., 2016). This study also indicated that comorbid diagnoses, including oppositional defiant disorder and conduct disorder, decreased over time as did mood disorders. More severe symptoms were found in children with ADHD:C who had higher symptom severity at diagnosis, a family history of ADHD, and who had higher parental reported impairment. Medication was not found to improve symptom severity or overall functioning. Consistent with this finding, the dose of medication has been linked to problems with academic and social functioning, with higher doses related to poorer performance (Currie et al., 2014). Hale et al. (2011) found that higher dosages of methylphenidate improved behavior but decreased academic performance. Thus, it may be the level of medication that is most important for improving performance. As such, school personnel should be aware that optimal behavior control may not be consistent with academic improvement.

Further study of academic achievement in ADHD:C found that inattention negatively affects performance on measures of mathematics calculation, written expression, and visual–motor skills (Semrud-Clikeman, 2012). In this study children with ADHD:C and the predominantly inattentive presentation of ADHD (ADHD:PI), experienced difficulties with these types of academic tasks. Biederman et al. (2004) found that these difficulties are present independent of difficulties with executive functioning. Further studies have suggested that difficulty with inhibition and distractibility are independent of intellectual ability and cause children with both types of ADHD to experience problems in completing academic tasks (Penny et al., 2005; Passoulunghi et al., 2005).

Additional studies have implicated difficulties with fluid reasoning and problems with mathematics and written language (Horn & Blankson, 2012). *Fluid reasoning* is the ability to use different strategies to solve a problem as well as understanding abstract language (Woodcock et al., 2001). The neural network for fluid reasoning involves the association areas of the brain (parietal, temporal, and occipital lobes), areas implicated in the orienting aspect of attention. Findings of poorer fluid reasoning in ADHD:C and ADHD:PI suggest that the recruitment of this network is poorer in children with ADHD and thus negatively affects learning, particularly in mathematics and written language (Naidoo, 2006; Semrud-Clikeman, 2012).

Hyperactive–Impulsive Presentation

Children with ADHD: HI show significant problems with activity level but they do not reach the symptom level required for a diagnosis of inattention. Longitudinal studies have found a large majority of children diagnosed with ADHD:HI in preschool are re-diagnosed with ADHD:C at older ages (Lahey et al., 2007; Riley et al., 2008). Riley et al. (2008) found no difference between ADHD:C and ADHD:HI in preschool children on measures of externalizing behaviors, internalizing behaviors, social skills, or academic skills.

Studies have found that children with ADHD:HI have difficulty with processing of information, particularly with more complex tasks, as well as difficulty with accuracy on tasks (Tucha et al., 2006). Similar to children with ADHD:C, children with ADHD:HI show an increase in reaction time as well as consistency of response (Tucha et al., 2009). Attentional or impulsivity differences were not found between children with ADHD:C and those with ADHD:HI in this study. Attentional functions that were disrupted in both groups included vigilance, divided attention, flexibility, and focused attention.

The conclusion from these studies is that children with ADHD:HI and those with ADHD:C do not significantly differ from each other. It was also suggested that ADHD:HI may be an early variant of ADHD:C as most children identified as ADHD:HI are preschoolers (Riley et al., 2008).

Inattentive Presentation

ADHD:PI has symptoms of daydreaming, lethargy, staring, confusion, and passivity, Barkley (2014) suggests this type of ADHD is due to problems with focused or selective attention. In addition, children with ADHD:PI show slower processing speed compared to those with ADHD:C or those with reading disability (Weller et al., 2000). Compared to children with ADHD:C, children with ADHD:PI show fewer executive function difficulties, particularly with their ability to shift and inhibit responding, but they have more difficulty with working memory (Barkley, 2014; Semrud-Clikeman, Walkowiak, Wilkinson, & Butcher, 2010). Findings also suggest that girls with ADHD:PI show more internalizing difficulties (anxiety, depression) compared to boys. Both groups showed externalizing problems from teacher ratings (being off task, daydreaming) but not parent ratings (Becker et al., 2013).

Many hypothesize that ADHD:PI is a separate disorder rather than a subtype of ADHD (Barkley, 2006). Supportive evidence for this comes from neuroimaging. As discussed above, hyperactive–impulsive and combined types have been found to show a frontal–limbic circuit dysfunction. Fair et al. (2012) using resting-state fMRI (i.e., the child is not doing a task while in the MRI) found unique resting-state patterns in children with ADHD:PI compared to those with ADHD:C. Less connectivity was found in the cognitive control areas, including the dorsolateral prefrontal cortex and the cerebellum. In contrast, children with ADHD:C showed differences in the default network (described earlier).

DTI, as we've seen in earlier chapters, is a neuroimaging technique that allows for the visualization of white matter areas connecting gray matter regions. For this reason, it is an excellent tool to distinguish possible differences in connectivity throughout the brain. Emerging studies have suggested there are differences in structural connections (particularly in the right hemisphere) between ADHD:C and ADHD:PI (Hong et al., 2014). Moreover, findings of differences in connectivity between ADHD:C and ADHD:PI continue to support the hypothesis that these are two very separate disorders. Svatkova et al. (2014) found the ADHD:PI group showed more connectivity in the area connecting the anterior cingulate cortex, prefrontal cortex, and the thalamus. This supports the thinking that there are fronto–thalamic circuit deficits present in ADHD:PI. This difference was not found in the ADHD:C group. These circuits have been implicated in cognitive control, processing speed, and selective attention (Fair et al., 2012; Rossi et al., 2015). Taken together these findings support the hypothesis that ADHD:PI may be a separate disorder from ADHD:C and ADHD:HI. Neuroimaging demonstrates that the breakdown for ADHD:PI is the prefrontal–thalamic circuits rather than the prefrontal–limbic–precuneus circuits implicated in ADHD:C. Thus, there is strong evidence that these disorders really are separate and should be conceptualized as such.

Neuroimaging Findings

Neuroimaging studies have been done generally with ADHD:C males. As you can see from Table 8.2, there have been a number of neuroimaging studies, with most implicating the corpus callosum, the caudate, cingulate gyrus, and the frontal lobes. Additional findings include smaller total brain volume in some studies, smaller volume in the cerebellum, as well as differences in the right frontal lobe, caudate nucleus, anterior cingulate, and cerebellar vermis (Bledsoe et al., 2009; Castellanos et al., 1996; Castellanos & Tannock, 2002; Semrud-Clikeman et al., 2006; Semrud-Clikeman, Steingard, et al., 2000).

A feature-based study that evaluated the neuroimaging findings in ADHD:C to date found that the above structures were consistently compromised in these children (Xiao et al., 2016). Emerging evidence of the differences in the cerebellum, particularly in the vermis (the connection between the cerebellar lobes), has been found to be compromised in children with ADHD:C (Castellanos & Proal, 2012). In a study comparing boys with ADHD:C with and without a medication history, Bledsoe et al. (2009) found a smaller vermis in the boys without a history of stimulant medication. Boys with ADHD who had been on medication did not differ from the controls. Similarly, Semrud-Clikeman, Steingard, et al. (2006) found that treatment-naïve boys with ADHD:C showed a smaller anterior cingulate particularly in the right hemisphere. In contrast the ADHD:C boys with a history of stimulant medication did not show significant difference in this same structure compared to controls. Both ADHD

TABLE 8.2. Frontal-Subcortical Structures Implicated in ADHD

Source	Finding
Frontal lobe	
Casey et al. (1997)	Frontal volume/right frontal involvement
Castellanos et al. (1996)	
Filipek et al. (1997)	
Hynd et al. (1990)	Frontal–striatal network deficits found on fMRI as well as DTI
Semrud-Clikeman, Steingard, et al. (2000)	
Konrad & Eickhoff (2010)	
Rubia et al. (2009)	
Basal ganglia	
Semrud-Clikeman, Steingard, et al. (2000)	Smaller caudates in ADHD:C
Castellanos & Tannock (2002)	
Semrud-Clikeman et al. (2006)	
Max et al. (2002)	Ventral putamen
Frodl & Skokauskas (2012)	Stimulant medication found normalizing of subcortical networks
Nakao et al. (2011)	
Anterior cingulate (ACC)	
Svatkova et al. (2014)	More connectivity connecting ACC, prefrontal cortex, and thalamus in ADHD: PI compared to ADHD:C
Rossi et al. (2015)	
Semrud-Clikeman et al. (2006)	Treatment naïve boys showed smaller ACC compared to treated boy with ADHD:C
Frodl & Skokausakas (2012)	Adults with persistent ADHD show reduction in ACC
Banich et al. (2009)	Sustained attention networks involving the ACC and dorsolateral prefrontal cortex found deficient
Cerebellum	
Fair et al. (2012)	Unique resting state in ADHD:PI
Castellanos & Proal (2012)	Less connectivity between dorsolateral prefrontal cortex and cerebellum

groups showed smaller caudate volume compared to the controls. The caudate is responsible for inhibitory behaviors.

These findings suggest that medication affects brain structures, particularly those that are involved in attentional networks. Further studies are recommended to help us understand more fully the long-term effects of medication. A meta-analyses of imaging data has confirmed that stimulant medication may relate to normalization of subcortical structures and that many patients with ADHD may normalize the integrity of these networks with age and medication (Frodl & Skokauskas, 2011; Nakao et al., 2011). It should be noted that adults with persistent ADHD symptoms have continued to show reduction in the anterior cingulate, which is an important structure for self-monitoring (Frodl & Skokausakas, 2011).

Consistent findings of smaller caudate volumes implicate the dopaminergic system—a system that responds well to methylphenidate (Ritalin). These fronto–striatal network deficits have been repeatedly found using functional MRI as well as diffusion tensor imaging (Konrad & Eickoff, 2010; Rubia et al., 2009). Further studies have implicated the splenium of the corpus callosum (the region connecting the parietal lobes) and the cerebellum (Makris et al., 2003; Valera et al., 2007). The differences in these structures have led to a hypothesis that involves a cerebellar–prefrontal striatal network for attention and hyperactivity/impulsivity (Valera et al., 2005; Bledsoe et al., 2009).

Use of fMRI has found decreased functioning in the dorsolateral prefrontal cortex and the dorsal anterior cingulate for inhibitory control (Bush et al., 2008; Zang et al., 2005). For inhibition, activation is decreased in the right inferior prefrontal cortex, the precuneus of the parietal lobe, and the posterior cingulate cortex (Rubia et al., 2005).

Additional studies of attentional control have found neural dysfunction across a distributed network that includes the dorsolateral prefrontal cortex, anterior cingulate, posterior parietal cortex, and right inferior frontal cortex for sustained attention (Banich et al., 2009). Most researchers now view ADHD as a disrupted neural network. Studies using resting-state methodology require the child to merely rest with eyes closed while fMRI data are being collected. Findings from these studies suggest that ADHD is due to a default network disorder where stimuli is not regulated or competing behaviors (i.e., getting up from the desk, talking out of turn) are not suppressed. These networks have been further implicated in problems with inhibition and impulse control on an individual basis in children and adolescents with ADHD (Castellanos & Proal, 2012).

Comorbid Disorders

In addition to the hallmark symptoms of inattention and/or hyperactivity–impulsivity, children with ADHD frequently have comorbid LDs and behavior disorders. DuPaul et al. (2013) reviewed 17 studies examining ADHD and LD comorbidity and found a 45.1% positive rate. Further study has found approximately 47% of children with ADHD will also show mood disorders, 64% will show disruptive behavior disorders, with 27% showing no comorbid symptoms in their sample (Wilens et al., 2002). Conduct disorder (CD) and oppositional defiant disorder (ODD) are frequently comorbid with ADHD. It was found that ODD persists in a significant minority of children with ADHD over time in a longitudinal study of boys (Biederman et al., 2008). ODD was also found to be associated with major depression in these children and to increase the likelihood of a later diagnosis of CD. CD posed a large risk of later developing antisocial personality disorder as well as an increased risk for substance abuse, smoking, and bipolar disorder. Thus, the combination of CD and/or ODD with ADHD increases the possibility of later significant behavioral difficulties as well as mood disorders. Based on these findings, it is important to carefully evaluate children with ADHD for these frequently co-occurring disorders particularly in developing appropriate interventions.

ADHD:PI occurs more often with learning disabilities than the other two presentation types (Pennington, 2008). While children with the ADHD:HI subtype are more likely to receive comorbid diagnosis of ODD or CD; LDs are common in this population as well (Selenius et al., 2015). Of the LD subtypes discussed in earlier chapters, children with ADHD are more likely to have WLDs than other types of LDs (Semrud-Clikeman & Harder, 2011). These issues are likely related to a difficulty with the executive functions of planning, organization, and working memory, skills necessary for writing a cohesive narrative that are particularly at risk for children with ADHD. College students with ADHD have been found to show significant problems with written language, which negatively impacts their progress in many of their courses (Semrud-Clikeman & Harder, 2011).

Children with comorbid ADHD and LDs have been found to exhibit a pattern of deficits that is more pronounced than those found in either disorder alone (Willcutt et al., 2010). These children are also at higher risk for being retained at an almost 2 to 1 ratio compared to those children with a sole diagnosis, as well as having significant social impairment. ADHD and LD are comorbid at a higher rate than is expected based on their prevalence rates in the general population. Dyslexia and ADHD each occur in approximately 5% of the population, but 25–40% of children with ADHD or dyslexia also meet criteria for the other disorder (DuPaul et al., 2013).

A large sample found that family members of children with dyslexia or ADHD were more likely to meet criteria for either disorder at a rate of two to three times compared to those without a familial history (Willcutt et al., 2010). In this study, measures of response inhibition, processing speed, naming speed, phoneme awareness, verbal reasoning, and working memory were given to children with RDs, ADHD, RD + ADHD, and controls. While the clinical groups were impaired on all measures compared to controls, the RDs group was more impaired compared to the ADHD group. The comorbid group was the most impaired on measures of response inhibition and processing speed compared to the other groups. This finding was true for both the ADHD:PI and ADHD:C subtypes.

In order to avoid using categorical variables, and assuming attention issues are on a continuum, structural equation modeling was used to determine which cognitive constructs are able to predict dyslexic and ADHD symptoms (McGrath et al., 2011). Using this analysis, phoneme awareness, naming speed, and processing speed predicted reading scores while inhibition and processing speed predicted inattention and hyperactivity/impulsivity. Processing speed was the only shared cognitive risk factor that predicted all three symptom dimensions (single-word reading, inattention, and hyperactivity–impulsivity). Moreover, verbal working memory did not significantly predict any symptom dimension. Thus, deficits in processing speed are shared between ADHD and RD and may then be related to a genetic underpinning. This hypothesis was confirmed using a genetic analysis that is hierarchical in nature; namely, that once processing speed is accounted for there are no other genetic influences that are shared between the two disorders (Willcutt et al., 2010).

Neuropsychological Assessment

The most effective method for identifying ADHD continues to be the clinical interview (Davidson, 2008). Behavioral rating scales are also generally used with information gathered from the child or adolescent, parent, and teacher. In addition to the behavioral aspects of ADHD, a meta-analysis of ADHD has found deficits in attention, inhibition, interference, temporal relationships, planning, mental flexibility, maintaining/shifting cognitive set, and reaction time/processing speed (Mueller & Tomblin, 2012). The hyperactive–impulsive type has generally been found to involve less neuropsychological impairment than the inattentive or combined types (Pham & Riviere, 2015), with the combined type showing the greatest impairment (Barkely, 2006). Recent research has started to isolate neuropsychological weakness in the three presentations. Measures of executive function, working memory, and processing efficiency are associated with the inattentive and combined types, whereas inhibition measures help identify the hyperactive–impulsive type (Colbert & Bo, 2017).

Some clinicians may prefer to use behavioral approaches for diagnosis of ADHD, but we suggest that attention, working memory, and executive function measures should be used to supplement behavioral approaches. Notice that we say "supplement" rather than "substitute," as measures of executive function do not consistently discriminate between children with ADHD and those with other psychiatric disorders (Nigg, 2005a).

Executive functioning is generally measured through the use of the Wisconsin Card Sorting Test. In this test the child is asked to match four cards using a deck of cards. She is not told the rule but must discover it through trial and error. After a set number of correct trials, the correct answer changes without warning. Studies have found a small to moderate effect for set shifting.

A test frequently used to measure set shifting is Trails A and B (Reitan, 1958) or the Trail Making Test of the Delis–Kaplan Executive Function System (D-KEFS). Trails on the D-KEFS and the traditional trail making measure require the child to connect letters and numbers in sequential order and then to connect letters and numbers in alternating order as quickly as possible. The D-KEFS also provides a measure of motor speed to assist the psychologist in understanding whether the difficulty is in sequencing and automaticity of the task or if it is a motor control task. In addition, the inhibition measure on the NEPSY can also evaluate the child's ability to shift set as well as working memory and is useful for younger children (Korkman et al., 2007). On this measure, the child must connect numbers and letters in alternating order as quickly as possible.

Interference control is usually measured by the Stroop Test or the Color–Word subtest of the D-KEFS (Delis et al., 2001). The Stroop Test has three conditions. The first condition requires the child to name colors. In the second condition, the child reads the words of colors printed in black and white. The third condition (the interference condition) requires the child to read the color of the ink rather than the word. What makes this task difficult is that the word red is printed in green ink and the child must say green. To succeed on the task, a child must ignore the overlearned word red and say green, which is a competing response. Findings with children indicate small to large effects for this task and so it needs to be studied further. There are similar measures included in the D-KEFS with up-to-date norms (Delis et al., 2001).

While research does not support these measures solely as a diagnostic tool for ADHD, they can be useful in understanding the child's ability to retrieve information quickly and to keep information in mind while solving a problem (Gordon et al., 2006). Children with ADHD and learning disabilities may not have the same difficulty on the interference measure of the Stroop Test or Color–Word subtest of the D-KEFS because they do not read fluently. Similarly, on Trail Making, a child with ADHD and LD will often score poorly not due to attentional issues but because he or she does not know the letters automatically and needs to search through memory for the order of the letters.

Thus, the findings for the neuropsychological measures indicate that the strongest relation to ADHD is the CPT task for the commission variables and for the nonverbal working memory. Contrary to common belief, set shifting and cognitive flexibility only provide moderate relations as did the Stroop Test. Combining these measures with a good interview and behavioral rating scales seems to be the best practice for identifying children with ADHD.

Measures may become more specific and sensitive when we start to determine what true ADHD is and start to link subtype behavior and neuropsychological performance to frontal–subcortical circuits, as suggested in In-Depth 8.2.

There has been much research on ADHD, but several important questions remain, questions that we hope will be addressed in future neurophysiological, neuropharmacological, and neuropsychological research. These critical diagnostic and treatment questions include the following:

- Could the association between ADHD, particularly ADHD:PI, and depression and anxiety be related to the parietal attention network, or is this association related to the frontal executive problems found in both depression and ADHD? Can we differentiate between the inattention due to ADHD and depression, so the proper medication treatment is attempted? Given that anxiety is likely to be caused by too much orbital prefrontal activity, and the hyperactive–impulsive type of ADHD by too little, how do you make sure that a child's fidgety behavior isn't just nervousness?

- As the highest comorbidity rate for ADHD:C and ADHD:HI subtypes is with externalizing disorders, could both ADHD and externalizing disorders be related to underactive or hypoactive cortical functioning? Is the difference between them related to differences between cortical and subcortical causes of hypoactivity? How can you design instruction and interventions that maximize the cortical functioning level in these children, so they are available for learning?

- How do you differentiate among ADHD, OCD, and Tourette syndrome, as these disorders are also likely to show attention and executive deficits suggestive of frontal–subcortical circuit dysfunction? How do you discriminate between underactive (i.e., ADHD) and overactive (i.e., OCD) orbital frontal–subcortical circuits, especially when both these disorders occur comorbidly with Tourette syndrome? Could dysregulation (either an excess or an absence) of attention, impulse control, and motor activity be found in all of these disorders, suggesting a similar underlying pathophysiology?

Obviously, until these questions are addressed by systematic research, we are left with the available clinical tools and our clinical acumen to guide our practice. We present these questions in an attempt to guide your thinking about diagnostic and treatment issues. An advantage of the CHT approach is that you will quickly recognize it if you have gone down the wrong diagnostic path with a child. Through ongoing data collection and monitoring, you can assure treatment efficacy for the children you serve.

Treatment

Most studies confirm that the dopamine agonist methylphenidate (Ritalin) and other stimulants are highly effective in treating ADHD's associated executive and behavior deficits. However, a longitudinal study revealed substantial medication effects on behavioral but not academic outcomes, with little evidence that behavioral effects translated into academic gains (Molina et al., 2009). Why would a medication that is highly effective in reducing the problem behaviors associated with ADHD have little impact on academic achievement? We believe this happens because most medication management strategies typically rely on behavior observations and ratings in the classroom and home to determine treatment effects, and little attention is paid to the effects of medication on cognition. Although medication response can be systematically monitored through direct observation of the child or administration of rating scales, cognitive and behavior domains are often affected differentially by medications,

IN-DEPTH 8.2. ADHD as a Frontal–Subcortical Circuit Disorder

Although ADHD was once thought to be simply a behavior disorder, a growing body of evidence highlighted in Table 8.2 illustrates that ADHD is clearly a frontal–subcortical disorder. Consistent with findings of executive function deficits in ADHD, frontal–subcortical abnormalities found in children with ADHD include asymmetric/dysmorphic conditions (Hynd et al., 1990), abnormal electrical activity (Novak et al., 1995), and lowered cerebral blood flow (Ernst et al., 1994; Lou et al., 1984; Lou et al., 1989; Zametkin et al., 1993). In particular, the right frontal lobe, dorsolateral and orbital prefrontal cortex, or frontal cortical–subcortical systems may be differentially impaired (Voeller, 2001). As noted earlier, the right frontal lobe has been related to attention, whereas the orbital frontal cortex and striatum have been related to inhibition (Semrud-Clikeman, Steingard, et al., 2000; Starkstein & Kremer, 2001; Vaidya et al., 1998). Dopaminergic deficiencies may lead to frontal/striatal hypometabolism in children with ADHD (Rubia et al., 1999), which would account for the salutary effects of the dopamine agonist methylphenidate (Lou et al., 1989; Vaidya et al., 1998).

A comparison of dorsolateral–dorsal cingulate–striatal and orbital–ventral cingulate–striatal frontal–subcortical circuits suggests that the former may be related to the ADHD:PI type, whereas the ADHD:HI type could be related to the latter, with the ADHD:C type having both areas affected (Hale, Bertin, et al., 2004; Svaikova et al., 2016). However, as noted earlier, others suggest that ADHD:PI is related to parietal dysfunction and NVLDs, and indeed this may be the case for many children diagnosed with ADHD. However, we would argue that children with this type of attention problem will be unlikely to respond to medication, because their symptoms are actually secondary to parietal lobe dysfunction. This is consistent with research suggesting that children with the frontal type of ADHD respond to stimulant medication, but those with greater occipital–parietal involvement do not (Filipek et al., 1997). As stimulants have therapeutic effects because they are dopamine agonists (Swanson et al., 1998), it is not surprising that children with ADHD and IDs are less likely to respond to stimulant medication (DuPaul et al., 1994), possibly because their attention problems are associated with serotonin dysfunction and DE (e.g., Lahey et al., 1993).

---

even at the same dose. The best dose for behavior may have a limited or even a detrimental effect on cognitive functioning (Wilens & Kaminski, 2020).

Neuropsychological assessment and consultation may be necessary because many children respond to psychotropic medication in an idiosyncratic manner, especially when there are other diagnoses present in conjunction with ADHD. Given that children with ADHD respond differentially to medication, and that some doses may have a detrimental effect on learning (e.g., the "zombie" effect), the school psychologist must be ready to help monitor treatment response for physicians. We developed a multimethod double-blind placebo medication trial protocol designed to monitor methylphenidate dose–response relationships for children with ADHD (Hale et al., 2005). During the trials, neuropsychological, behavioral, and observational data are collected over a 4-week period of baseline, placebo, and low and high doses of methylphenidate. Following all data collection, the "blind" is broken, data are summarized, and the variables are rank-ordered across conditions from 1 (best performance) to 4 (lowest performance) to ensure that each measure has equal weight in determining response. The data are subjected to separate nonparametric analyses to determine statistical response. These results are provided to the physician in a summary report to help determine clinical response to medications.

An example of the type of report that can be generated for physicians to monitor dose response is provided by a hypothetical report on Doug. A medication trial for Doug showed a differential response for academics and behavioral control related to medication dose. After several unsuccessful attempts to treat his learning and behavior problems with different stimulant medications, school interventions, and behavior therapy, Doug was referred for the medication trial service. Doug's neuropsychological performance was better on 5 mg of methylphenidate, whereas his behavioral response was optimal on the 10 mg dose. Subsequent to the trial, Doug was successfully treated with a low medication dose and adjunctive behavior therapy to help control his out-of-seat, off-task, and calling-out behaviors. Figure 8.1 demonstrates these findings. Remember higher scores mean poorer performance.

Your skills in research design and measurement can be used to help physicians design similar trials to optimize psychotropic medication titration or monitor untoward effects for children with ADHD. This is the intervention part of CHT, where you hypothesize that medication will work, set up a data collection strategy, analyze the effects on and off medicine, and then help determine whether the treatment is effective. Although you may choose to use behavioral observations and/or ratings to help make this judgment, we feel it is critical to include some measure of cognitive or academic functioning as well, given the findings just presented.

Even if stimulant treatment is effective, it is not the cure-all that some hope it is. Medication just makes a child more available to learn from the environment (Silver, 1990). In addition to medication management to ameliorate attention and executive deficits, academic and behavioral strategies will be necessary for all children with ADHD, especially if a lower dose is chosen to optimize cognition. Learning strategies and metacognitive interventions are unlikely to be highly effective when children are unmedicated because of the executive deficits described earlier. However, as adjuncts to medication management, learning strategies can be highly effective in improving self-monitoring and awareness, mental flexibility, organizational strategies, inhibition, and persistence. Table 8.3 lists a number of interventions for children with ADHD and other executive function disorders.

Behavioral strategies, such as contingency management and behavioral contracting, are based largely on the operant conditioning techniques described in Chapter 4 (see In-Depth

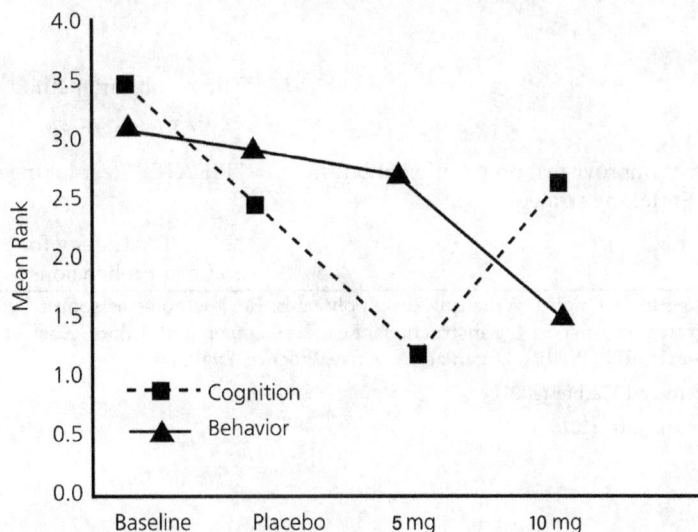

FIGURE 8.1. Medication trial results for Doug.

4.1). They have been shown to be highly useful as adjunctive therapies to medication, but again have limited effects without it. This is because medication may serve as an "establishing operation" necessary for a child with ADHD to respond to the discriminative stimulus. Without the beneficial effects of medication, the child is less likely to attend to a discriminative stimulus (e.g., teacher direction) or to inhibit a behavior (e.g., calling out an answer). Possibly this is because the medication also strengthens response to reinforcement and extinction interventions.

TABLE 8.3. Interventions for Metacognitive Processing and Executive Functions

Presenting problem	Goal of intervention	Intervention
Poor use of metacognitive strategies	Teach metacognitive strategy use	Think-alouds[a]
		Self-regulated strategy development[b, e]
		Mnemonics[c, d]
		Cognitive-behavior modification
		Child-generated strategies[b]
	Stimulate metacognitive strategy use with priming/prelearning activities	Anticipation guide[b]
		Semantic feature analysis: Concepts, vocabulary[c, d]
		Semantic maps: Advance organizers[c, d]
Poor use of academic strategies[f]	Improve note taking	
		Three-column method
		"AWARE" method[a]
	Improve test preparation and test-taking strategies	"PIRATES" test-taking strategy
		"PORPE" strategy for test preparation and comprehension[a]

Note. AWARE, *A*rrange to take notes, *W*rite quickly, *A*pply cues, *R*eview notes as soon as possible, *E*dit notes; PIRATES, *P*repare to succeed, *I*nspect the instructions, *R*ead, remember, and reduce; *A*nswer or abandon, *T*urn back; *E*stimate; *S*urvey; PORPE, Predict, Organize, Rehearse, Practice, Evaluate.

[a]Described in Goldstein and Mather (2001).
[b]Described in Mather and Jaffe (2016).
[c]Meltzer (2018).
[d]Meltzer (2010).
[e]Tamm et al. (2012).
[f]Dawson and Guare (2018).

ADHD Case Report

Case Report 8.1 illustrates an evaluation of a child with a previous diagnosis of ADHD with additional difficulties with mood.

Case Report 8.1. Summary of Neuropsychological Evaluation

Name: Kevin J

Reason for Evaluation

Kevin J is a 9-year, 5-month-old, Caucasian, right-handed male who has been recently diagnosed with attention-deficit/hyperactivity disorder (ADHD). He was referred by his primary care physician for an evaluation to assess his current neurobehavioral functioning and to assist with treatment and educational planning. Primary concerns were with Kevin's inattention and distractibility. Kevin is not prescribed medication at this time.

Background Information

Background information was gathered via parent interview, individual interview, developmental history questionnaire, school information form, and review of available records. For additional information, the interested reader is referred to Kevin's medical records.

Family History

Kevin lives with his mother, stepfather, an older brother, and a younger half-sister. Kevin's parents divorced when he was 5. He visits his father frequently and the families live in close proximity. Kevin's difficulties in school have also been somewhat stressful for the family. Family history includes mood disorders and ADHD.

Developmental and Medical History

Kevin was born weighing 8 pounds, 1 ounce following an uncomplicated full-term pregnancy and delivery. Kevin met early motor and language developmental milestones within normal limits. As an infant and toddler, he was interested in social contact. He was also adaptable and easy to please. The first developmental concerns appeared when Kevin was 2 years old when he appeared more easily distracted that his peers. Kevin was also noted to have tics beginning when he around 3 years of age, which included opening and closing his jaw and grimacing.

Medical history was generally normal. Adderall was prescribed when he was first identified with ADHD. He was tried on 5 mg, 10 mg, 15 mg, and 20 mg. The lower doses were not successful and the higher dose resulted in weight loss, an increase in tics, and staring-off behavior. Medication was discontinued. Kevin does not receive any specialized services outside of the school setting.

School History

Kevin attends 3rd grade at local parochial school. He does not have an Individualized Education Plan (IEP) nor does he receive any specialized services. He reportedly earns good grades. Kevin's teachers have reportedly indicated to his mother that Kevin has significant difficulty maintaining his attention in the classroom, which was a primary reason for pursuing this evaluation.

Kevin's teacher completed a school information form regarding Kevin's functioning in the classroom. She noted that Kevin's mother and all of his teachers have worked on helping him become more organized and engaged in learning but no formal supports have been put in place. She also indicated that he "bangs, rocks, shifts, and moves around most of the time." His teacher rated Kevin's overall reading skills as average, though she noted his reading fluency was slightly below grade level. She rated his mathematic skills as average. She rated his overall written language skills as average, though noted his letter formation and legibility were slightly below grade level.

Behaviorally, his teacher reported that Kevin tends to appear indifferent in terms of his motivation level. She reported that his behavior is not age appropriate, as he tends to act "very immature." For example, he plays with much younger children and does not play with children at his grade level. He tends to be uncooperative and will not speak to adults who ask a question about his behavior. Kevin also tends to be isolated from peers. He is easily distracted and has poor organizational skills. She additionally commented, "Kevin is extremely disorganized and very slow moving. It often takes up to 20 minutes for him to get ready for class after he gets to school. He loses books, papers, pencils, assignments, etc., on a daily basis."

His teacher also rated Kevin as having severe difficulty with his receptive language as he appears to not be listening or engaged when in class. Minor difficulties were noted with his expressive language. Fine- and gross-motor skills were reported to be poor for his age. She noted that Kevin is frequently tardy, which makes morning organization "even worse." She noted that he does not make eye contact during class or in conversation, does not engage in class discussions, and has "frequent meltdowns when he does not know what is going on." He becomes easily frustrated and cries often. His teacher reported that the school "has recommended testing and evaluation of Kevin's issues since kindergarten" and that they "await a diagnosis or best learning plan for Kevin."

His teacher also noted Kevin's strengths. She described him as an intelligent boy who wants to do well. He is honest when he chooses to answer adults. Kevin is kind to the younger students with whom he plays. She identified her primary concerns as relating to Kevin's behavior and learning difficulties. She also indicated that his organizational skills are problematic in that all attempts at helping him have been only temporarily successful. She emphasized that all of his teachers are interested in learning how to best teach Kevin so that he can be a happier and more successful child.

Previous Evaluations

This represents Kevin's first formal evaluation.

Current Functioning

Kevin's mother reported that Kevin has appeared easily distracted since the age of 2. Currently, he does not pay attention to detail or makes careless mistakes and has difficulty keeping focused what needs to be done. He frequently appears to not be listening when spoken to directly. He often fails to follow through when given directions or fails to finish activities, though his ability to do so depends on his motivation level. In addition, his mother reported that Kevin is easily distracted by noises or other stimuli and is forgetful in daily activities. She reported that Kevin sometimes "stares off" and does not always respond to his name. His mother reported observing this behavior 1–2 times per week, though his teacher has reported observing his staring behavior 1–2 times per day. Sometimes, Kevin needs to be touched in order to stop staring. His mother did not believe he appeared "checked out" or was experiencing seizure activity. Additionally, she noted that he is also nonresponsive when playing or engrossed in an activity. She initially thought that perhaps his hearing was a problem and that possibility was ruled out through audiology examination.

Kevin's mother reported that unless completely engrossed in an activity, Kevin has been highly active and moving about since he was an infant. He frequently fidgets with his hands or feet or squirms in his seat. He is always "on the go" or acts as if "driven by a motor." Kevin frequently blurts out answers before questions have been completed and interrupts or intrudes in on others' conversations or activities. His mother reported that Kevin's ADHD symptoms are problematic at home, although he is able to control himself better when motivated to earn rewards, such as video games or watching cartoons. He is able to get through tasks but is easily distracted and can only complete 2–3 steps at a time. Teachers have also noted that he is constantly rocking in his seat at school. Kevin's mother did not have any concerns about his fine-motor skills, although she noted he is clumsy and tends to bump into objects.

Mrs. Jones reported observing tics beginning when Kevin was about 3 years old. She reported that they typically occur when he is trying to stay focused. When asked to further describe these behaviors, she provided an example of Kevin pulling up his shirt (such as the collar or shoulder) and rubbing his cheek with his clothing. This behavior began when he was involved in a holiday program at school this year and was told he had to remain still on the stage. Kevin was able to stand still but then began engaging in this face-rubbing behavior. She reported that Kevin is compelled to rub his face any time he must stand or sit still. She noticed that he does not engage in this behavior when he wears a sweatshirt with a hood that he can wear. Kevin's mother did note behaviors that seemed more consistent with a tic due to their brief duration, including quickly opening his jaw and grimacing. He also takes breaths in the middle of words when speaking.

Mrs. Jones reported that Kevin's emotionality has decreased. Last year he cried 3–5 days out of the week for 15 minutes at a time. She was uncertain whether it was because he did not understand something, because he was being rigid, or because he missed information. Currently, Kevin becomes emotional half as often (approximately once per week) at home or at school. He has not demonstrated a loss of interest in previously enjoyed activities. He also does not present as irritable and, in fact, is less "cranky" now than he was in the past. His mother does not view him as having a depressed mood. Kevin has stated in the past that he wanted to kill himself, which his mother reported was "out of frustration." Last year he was "coming down really hard on himself about schoolwork." He would get upset when she asked him about his day and on one occasion said, "I just want to kill myself." He has never outlined a plan or made any attempts to hurt or kill himself. Mrs. Jones reported that she has never been concerned for his safety. In the past, Mrs. Jones reported that Kevin engaged in head banging; however, when questioned about this, she indicated that he repeatedly lifted and bumped his head against the surface in a noninjurious type of way. Her descriptions indicated it was more of a self-stimulating behavior. His head banging behavior has decreased, though if he is very tired, he engages in patting his head against his pillow repeatedly as a self-calming strategy. He has never hurt himself as a result of hitting his head against a surface.

Mrs. Jones reported that Kevin likes to be in control of his environment. He has emotional outbursts when he misses instructions and tends to withdraw and not speak when he is upset. His need for control over his environment is sometimes excessive, as he will ask many questions, such as "obsessing" over what he will eat for lunch. Kevin's mother noted that placing a calendar in his backpack with the daily menu for lunch has helped. In general, giving him information helps him to be less rigid.

Socially, Kevin tends to have closer friendships with younger children. His best friend, however, is 2 years older than him. Kevin is very affectionate toward his mother. He demonstrates empathy, such as saying to her, "I want to make sure you're okay." His mother reported that Kevin has been enrolled in karate and just earned his blue belt. She noted that he stands out in the class because of his attention issues. He has also been enrolled in swimming and gets along well with the other children in these activities. Kevin is able to converse about a variety of topics. He tends to become excited over typical interests, such as wanting a toy from a commercial for a week at a time and does not demonstrate any other narrow or restricted interests. He enjoys playing with Lego Blocks and is involved with a Lego Club at school. Kevin enjoys animals and reading books about animals. He also likes to read joke books. He has been reading the *Lord of the Rings* series with his mother. His mother reported that Kevin is able to remember intricate details from the story, even when it looks like he is not paying attention.

Academically, Kevin earns good grades, though teachers have consistently noted his lack of focus. They have also identified his hyperactivity as a significant problem. Mrs. Jones is worried that as he progresses in school, he will not receive as much support from teachers and his performance will decline. He has been offered a special mat to sit on in order to help his activity level, though there is not an occupational therapist at his school to oversee these types of interventions. Mrs. Jones also noted that, although he earns good grades, Kevin has trouble editing written work for grammar and capitalization.

Child Interview

Kevin reported that he is good at making friends, building with Lego blocks, swimming, and playing video games. He also stated that he does well in school and earns good grades. When asked what he has trouble with, Kevin responded, "nothing really." He reported feeling happy when he sees other people feeling happy. He also reported happiness related to playing with his friends and playing video games. Kevin reported sadness related to having to attend this evaluation. He also reported feeling sad when his classmates bully him. He stated that he usually "just tries to forget about it" which "does not go well." Kevin reported that his peers pick on him every day. He denied any physical bullying and stated that children often call him names. Kevin reported anger related to his brother's behavior. He stated that his brother "torments" him and punches him. When angry, Kevin said that he tries to attack his brother or walk away. He was not sure which strategy worked better. When asked about worry, Kevin denied any sources of anxiety. He denied worrying about what others think or worrying about his or his family's safety or future. He also denied worries related to school and could not think of an example of when he has felt nervous.

Kevin denied any thoughts or attempts of self-harm or suicidal ideation. He stated that he used to have thoughts of self-harm but did not want to talk about it. He was not able to say when the last time he had these thoughts. Kevin stated that he used to think about killing himself, "when I thought everyone was mean." He was unwilling to answer any follow-up questions. Kevin then became very tearful and stated, "I want to put it behind me."

Behavioral Observations

Kevin presented as a casually dressed and appropriately groomed boy who appeared his chronological age. He was tested over two appointments. At his first appointment, Kevin was extremely concerned about his performance and frequently made comments such as, "Did I get that one right?" and "I probably got that one wrong, didn't I?" Kevin completed many tasks at a slow pace and required frequent prompting from the examiner. He was agitated during a lengthy computerized attention task and said, "It's stupid" and "I want to break the screen." He interrupted the measure due to his frustration with the task. Mrs. Jones reported that Kevin was very frustrated following his first appointment and was unhappy about returning for a second appointment.

At his second appointment, Kevin waited in the hallway with the instruction to complete a self-report rating scale while the examiner interviewed his mother. Following interview, Kevin reported that he was not able to answer several of the questions and was upset because he viewed the questions as insulting. The examiner attempted to go through a couple of the questions with him. For example, he did not respond to the item, "I used to be happier." When asked about this item, he began crying and talking about how other children pick on him at school. Despite a few attempts from the examiner to engage him in answering self-report questions, Kevin became highly upset each time, expressed that he wanted to receive his mother's opinion about the questions, or stated that they were insulting. Kevin became frustrated and tearful on a few occasions following instructions with which he did not want to comply. He quickly became angered when encouraged to consider a guess and when he determined that he did not wish to comply with the directive, he remained insistent that he would not do so. At one point, this required he take a lengthy break with his mother to calm down and receive encouragement.

Kevin appeared much more upbeat when talking about his interest in video games. He initially talked extensively about his favorite video game with little regard for the examiner's level of interest or engagement in the conversation. At other times, he checked in with the examiner about her interests or opinions and was more reciprocal in his interactions. He used many gestures, both descriptively and to indicate his emotionality.

Kevin was observed to engage in some tic-like behaviors, such as raising his eyebrows. He was rather restless and was observed to engage in rubbing his face with his clothing when having to sit still in his chair. He also placed his shirt in his mouth on several occasions and fidgeted with a tissue. Kevin frequently interrupted the examiner's instructions.

Casual observation of Kevin's fine- and gross-motor skills did not reveal any notable concerns. His language contained age-appropriate grammar and syntax. His speech was within normal limits for rate, prosody, volume, and fluency. His overall mood was dour and he presented as easily frustrated and agitated. He became tearful on several occasions throughout the evaluation. Despite his emotionality and frustration with tasks, Kevin completed most measures presented to him. The evaluator at his first appointment noted that some measures might have underestimated his abilities due to his high level of anxiety and activity level (WISC-IV, TOVA). Those measures that he was able to complete at his second appointment are considered a valid estimate of his current neuropsychological functioning.

Neuropsychological Evaluation Methods and Instruments

Clinical Interview, Review of Records, Wechsler Intelligence Scale for Children, 4th Edition (WISC-IV),California Verbal Learning Test, Children's Version (CVLT-C),Test of Variables of Attention—Visual (TOVA),Wisconsin Card Sorting Test (WCST), Delis-Kaplan Executive Function System (DKEFS)—Color—Word Interference Test, Verbal Fluency Test, & Trail Making Test, Revised Children's Manifest Anxiety Scale, Second Edition (RCMAS-2), Beery-Buktenica Developmental Test of Visual-Motor Integration—6th Edition (VMI), Purdue Pegboard, Behavior Rating Inventory of Executive Function (BRIEF)—Parent form, Behavior Rating Inventory of Executive Function (BRIEF)—Teacher form

Behavior Assessment System for Children—2nd Edition (BASC-2)—Parent Rating Scale, Behavior Assessment System for Children—2nd Edition (BASC-2)—Teacher Rating Scale

Impressions

Kevin Jones is a 9-year, 5-month-old, Caucasian, right-handed male with a history of attention deficit/hyperactivity disorder (ADHD). He was referred to the clinic by his primary care physician for an evaluation to assess his current neurobehavioral functioning and to assist with treatment and educational planning. Kevin's mother identified her primary concerns as relating to Kevin's inattention and distractibility. Kevin is not prescribed medication at this time.

Kevin's neuropsychological evaluation indicated average verbal cognitive abilities and high average nonverbal cognitive abilities. Kevin's working memory, or ability to briefly hold information in mind, was also within the average range. In comparison, he demonstrated a relative weakness in his speed of mental processing, which was slightly below average. Kevin also demonstrated age-appropriate skills in other areas of functioning. These included his performance on a standardized measure of novel problem solving and ability to be flexible when rules change. Additionally, within the structured testing environment, he was able to quickly generate words belonging to a certain category or beginning with a certain letter (i.e., verbal fluency). Kevin's ability to quickly name words and colors was within the average range, though he had slightly more difficulty and low average performance when having to switch back and forth between response styles. Additionally, Kevin was able to demonstrate adequate performance on a measure of verbal learning and memory.

Kevin was previously assigned a diagnosis of AD/HD, combined type. Results of his current evaluation continue to support that diagnosis. He was highly impaired in his ability to maintain his attention, inhibit incorrect responding, and remain consistent over time. While parent rating scales of Kevin's attention were within normal limits, his mother reported that Kevin's inattention is highly problematic for him at home and interferes with his ability to complete tasks. Teachers have consistently identified inattention and hyperactivity as interfering with his academic progress. Current teacher rating scales were in the mild range for attention problems, though his primary classroom teacher identified his lack of focus as significantly problematic. Children with attention problems often struggle with executive functioning skills, which are cognitive skills used to problem solve and complete tasks in order to achieve a goal (e.g., initiating and organizing tasks, staying on task, inhibiting behaviors). Kevin's performance on clinical measures of executive functioning indicated mild difficulties with verbal inhibition and trouble with flexibility when having to switch back and forth between response styles during a sequencing task. His slowed processing speed combined with mild inhibition difficulties resulted in below average to impaired performance. In his daily life, executive functioning difficulties are seen in his tendency to interrupt or intrude on other's conversations, trouble inhibiting his behavioral responses, and tendency to become "stuck" or to perseverate when worried or upset. Overall, Mrs. Jones indicated that Kevin's tendency to be rigid has been highly problematic.

Kevin presents with a history of emotional outbursts and tendency to become tearful or withdrawn when faced with a conflict. While his mother reported that he has improved in his emotional reactivity, he continues to become tearful more often than his peers. His teacher also reported frequent meltdowns in the classroom and crying when he does not know what is going on. Parent ratings of Kevin's anxiety and depression were within normal limits, though his mother described Kevin's preference for control over his environment and frequent questioning, both of which are indicative of anxiety. Teachers noted clinically significant problems related to anxiety and depression, such as often worrying about things that cannot be changed, appearing sad, crying easily, being teased, having no friends, and being afraid to make mistakes. Based on Kevin's history of becoming easily agitated and ongoing emotional outbursts that interfere with his functioning at school and at home, he is described as having a mood disorder, not otherwise specified. Kevin presented with difficulties related to his motor skill functioning. His teacher noted that he has poor fine-motor skills that interfere with his legibility when writing and that his gross-motor skills are poor.

In summary, Kevin is a child who presents with many strengths. He is a compassionate and helpful child who aims to please others. He is both funny and engaging. He faces many challenges, primarily, difficulty regulating his attention and behavioral responses. Problems with self-regulation combined with his tendency to think in a rigid manner lead to quick escalation of his emotions. A broad set of recommendations aimed at providing accommodations in school, individual therapy, and follow-up with other medical specialists is outlined below. Recommendations are provided below to support Kevin in improving his functioning emotionally, behaviorally, and academically. Of additional note, Mrs. Jones's warm, caring support of Kevin and her positive relationship with his father have been important factors in supporting Kevin's development and emotional functioning.

Diagnoses

314.01	Attention-deficit/hyperactivity disorder, combined type (ADHD)
296.9	Mood disorder, not otherwise specified
307.20	Tic disorder, not otherwise specified

Recommendations

1. We recommend that Kevin receive individual cognitive behavior therapy (CBT). Therapy can help Kevin to better identify his emotions and when he is becoming frustrated, learn how to think in a more flexible manner, and learn various coping skills in order to better handle his emotional responses.

2. We recommend that within the private school setting, Kevin be provided with accommodations that are the equivalent of a 504 Plan. In other words, we recommend a contract that identifies accommodations for teachers to implement consistently across classrooms to address Kevin's difficulties with attention, executive functioning skills, and emotional regulation. Specific recommendations are provided below and can be incorporated into educational accommodation plans for Kevin. Additionally, he demonstrated a weakness in processing speed and should be considered for additional time to complete tests and shortened assignments.

3. Kevin's mood, ability to maintain his attention, and overall engagement in school has been and will continue to be negatively impacted by bullying. Encourage Kevin to discuss any teasing or bullying with a pre-designated individual (e.g., school counselor) to whom Kevin can go to review difficult social interactions or concerns. It is essential that Kevin trusts this individual and that this person truly respects him. This will help him to gain a better understanding of exactly what has happened in specific situations, as well as why a fellow student may have responded as he/she did and how Kevin might respond appropriately in the future.

Chapter 9

Neuropsychological Principles and Psychopathology

Most training programs provide a course or two on abnormal psychology and different types of psychiatric diagnoses. In these classes, students learn different theories of psychopathology, study differential diagnoses, and are taught to administer objective and projective measures of behavior and personality. Few programs outside of clinical psychology provide information about the American Psychiatric Association's *Diagnostic and Statistical Manual of Mental Disorders* (DSM) system or the World Health Organization's *International Classification of Diseases* (ICD). Even fewer programs provide classes in neuropsychology and they have little to no emphasis on the relationship between neuropsychology and psychopathology. Without a good background in typical and atypical child development, it becomes problematic to understand diagnoses of depression, anxiety, or other psychiatric conditions in schools. These behaviors are generally labeled as "sad" or as the child "acting out." If these children are academically underperforming, they are frequently labeled with "serious emotional disturbance," which merely indicates that the child is experiencing some type of emotional distress that is frequently unspecified. More troubling are those children who come to the attention of the child study team or school psychologist because of significant emotional distress but do not qualify for services due to adequate academic progress. As we discuss in the following sections, psychopathological disorders do exist in children, and recognizing the signs of such a disorder can lead to preventive early intervention, possibly limiting the impact of the condition.

All behavior can be viewed as typical or atypical, depending on the environment in which it is displayed, the frequency of its occurrence, and the severity of the difficulty. To view behavior in this way is to use a *transactional interpretive framework*—one that considers the interaction of biological and environmental factors in relation to brain development (Semrud-Clikeman & Ellison, 2009). When children interact with their environment, the behaviors they display in any given situation are invariably related to their previous experiences, the contingencies they have experienced, and the cognitive templates through which they perceive the world. These multiple realities that all children construct are what make them unique individuals. These multiple influences, coupled with changes in the developing brain, make the study of the neuropsychology of childhood psychopathology extremely difficult, though intriguing. At times these "different realities" are the child's attempt to adapt to a difficult situation or environment. When viewed in this way, it can be very helpful to understand where the child is coming from—behaviors are not necessarily abnormal—they may just be an attempt to adapt.

The school psychologist has an important role to play in identifying children who are experiencing significant emotional problems whether or not they have accompanying academic deficits. While many of these children need to be referred to a psychiatrist or a mental health professional for further evaluation and treatment, the majority of their day is still within the school, and teachers and health professionals will need to provide the needed support and guidance. School psychologists serve as the front line of mental health services for children and their families. Even children who have received mental health services in a hospital or residential setting were initially in a typical school setting, and are likely return to that school after treatment. With today's administrative climate in managed care clinical settings, there is an increased likelihood that you will be required to serve more children with significant mental health needs within the regular school setting. Hospital stays and residential care are quite expensive so they are most frequently short (generally even a matter of days) and the child is released with continuing difficulties. As we will discuss later, children who experience psychopathology have a greater tendency to have brain-based disorders. It is for this reason that neurologists and psychiatrists are required to have training in both neurology and psychiatry. Recognizing the interrelationship of brain and behavior also becomes essential for the school-based psychologist. Whether your training in personality and behavioral assessment and intervention was extensive or minimal, you must recognize the relationship among development, cognition, achievement, personality, and behavior if you are to gain a holistic understanding of a child. To begin, we briefly review the general system of evaluating children with significant emotional disturbance.

Neurological Underpinnings of Children's Mental Health

The taxonomies that are most commonly utilized for differential diagnosis are the *Diagnostic and Statistical Manual for Mental Disorders, Fifth Edition, Text Revision* (DSM-5-TR; American Psychiatric Association, 2022) or the *International Classification of Diseases, 11th Revision* (World Health Organization, 1993/2022). Within these systems, important information, including prevalence rates, etiological factors, associated characteristics, and diagnostic criteria for numerous disorders, is provided. Although a careful history and evaluation corroborated by medical, developmental, historical, and informant data may reveal classic signs and symptoms of specific disorders, the presence of neuropsychological symptoms, comorbid conditions, a rapid decline in academic performance or behavior, or poor response to intervention may indicate the need for a more comprehensive evaluation. When children are referred for an additional evaluation, the psychiatrist, neuropsychologist, or clinical psychologist often rely on observations from the teacher and the school psychologist about the presenting problem.

While the use of categorical models is helpful for understanding childhood disorders, the complex interplay of cognition, neuropsychology, behavior, and environment often requires a fine-grained understanding of diagnostic criteria for these disorders. Previously, behavior was given paramount importance without an appreciation of the interaction of behavior and brain systems. All behavior relies on the brain for modulation of what is perceived, how the perception is integrated with previous experience, and what action plan is selected from the variety of possibilities.

Although the famous case of Phineas Gage (the man who had the iron rod accident) demonstrated the first clear association between the frontal lobes and psychopathology in the mid-1800s, the relationship among brain, emotion, and behavior has only recently received much needed attention. In your training, you probably heard of the limbic system as the emotional area of the brain, but it is always unclear how this and other structures interact to produce the complexity of human behavior. Not only is neuroanatomy important in this study, but neurochemistry research has been instrumental as well. We know that stimulants (e.g., Ritalin, Adderall) may be the drugs of choice for ADHD and that selective serotonin reuptake inhibitors (SSRIs) are often used to treat depression. Researchers thus have evidence that the neurotransmitter dopamine is related to ADHD symptoms and serotonin is related to depression. We are only now beginning to understand how both of these neurotransmitters, and others, work together to produce the types of neuropsychological and behavioral patterns seen in these disorders. It is important to begin to understand the anomalous neural networks that are related to psychiatric difficulties and how these difficulties interact not only with brain development, but also with emotional development.

Subcortical Contributions to Psychopathology

This book largely examines cortical relationships and behavior, but this section necessarily begins with an exploration of subcortical structures associated with emotion and personality. Understanding the basis of psychiatric disorders helps with differential diagnosis and treatment strategies.

You will not be surprised to find that multiple structures and systems have been implicated in human emotions and behavior. The limbic system is made up of three networks that are important for us to understand. The network connecting the hippocampus to the corpus callosum has a role in memory (including the emotional part of memory) and in spatial orientation. The temporal lobe orbitofrontal network is involved with cognition. Finally, the default mode network (see Chapter 8) is important for autobiographical memory as well as introspection (Catani et al., 2013). This network has also been implicated in affective and social processing of information and environmental situations (Sethi et al., 2000).

The anterior portion of the limbic system includes the amygdala, anterior cingulate, and orbitofrontal cortex. This network is important for emotion, deciding upon how valuable the reward is for a behavior, and deciding whether to react to the stimulus (Rolls, 2015). The amygdala, with its "fight–flight–freeze" reputation, is the structure most likely to be associated with emotional valence (Isaacson, 2013)—from attraction (approach) to withdrawal (avoidance). It affects not only behavior, but endocrine and autonomic activity as well. The amygdala also helps identify emotionally laden information, and therefore has an important function for constructing long-term memories.

Developmentally the orbitofrontal region develops with age to override the amygdala (or more primitive responses to stimulation) and recruits the anterior cingulate to decide upon the best option that provides the most reward for the behavior. The more posterior network includes the hippocampus and the posterior cingulate and the thalamus and underlies the ability to recall information and situations from the past. This system in turn communicates with the anterior limbic system to process information emotionally and relate it back to past experiences and the consequences of previous behaviors. The hypothalamus is the subcortical structure essential for regulating drives such as eating and sexual behavior (Capote et al., 2001). The thalamic "relay station" can have a modulating effect on emotional processing; the striatum can affect executive and emotional regulation and motoric response to social or emotional stimuli; and the hippocampus may be involved in formulating emotional valence or memories.

Although cortical areas may be directly or indirectly related to emotional experiences, they also have a modulating influence. The prefrontal cortex allows individuals to think about the emotional consequences of their actions before they engage in a behavior, or mull over a behavior after they have completed it (Stuss & Benson, 2019). As a result, it is not surprising that the prefrontal–striatal–thalamic circuits have been strong candidates for many of the different psychopathological disorders, with the orbital (divided into the lateral and ventromedial sections) and dorsomedial prefrontal cortex seen as the prime culprits. Consistent with the activation hypothesis, orbital underactivation or dysfunction results in disinhibition, while overactivation results in inhibition or overcontrolled behavior. Later sections of this chapter will link this over- and underactivation to neuropsychopathological disorders.

This frontally based neural network may be one source of what has been termed *affective information processing* or *emotion regulation*—a dynamic process that allows for examination of intrinsic factors (self) in relation to extrinsic ones (others). This ability to regulate emotion is important not only for adaptive functioning, but also for cognitive flexibility. Flexible affective processing has been linked to positive mood and improved resilience (Grol & De Raedt, 2018). Damage to the orbital area has been associated with lability, irritability, poor judgment, antisocial behavior, distractibility, and socially inappropriate behavior (Reber & Tranel, 2019; Sethi et al., 2015). Damage to the dorsomedial prefrontal cortex is related to problems with planning and organization leading to a high output of effort with little payback in terms of project completion. Damage to the ventromedial portion of the orbitofrontal area causes difficulty with being able to select appropriate behaviors based on environmental input (Noonan et al., 2017). Figure 9.1 shows the demarcations of the frontal lobe.

While some have hypothesized that the orbital cortex is underactive in children with ADHD (Cubillo et al., 2012), more recent studies using neuroimaging have found that as the child with ADHD begins to prepare to respond, there is overactivity in the dorsolateral prefrontal cortex with the result that the child is less efficient in inhibiting a response (Fernandez-Ruiz et al., 2020). In OCD, the ventromedial prefrontal cortex with links to the ventral striatal area was found to be underactive, which is an important finding as this structure is helps to determine if an event is rewarding or not. In contrast, when OCD symptoms

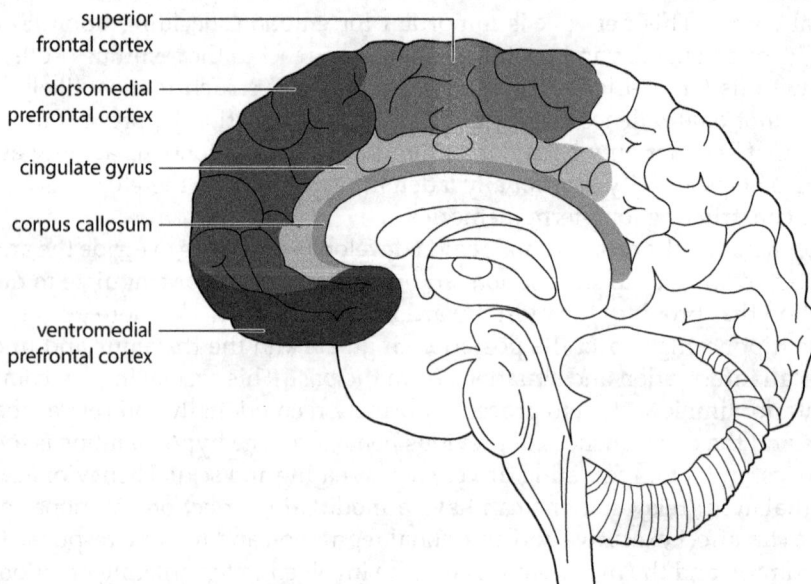

FIGURE 9.1. Demarcations of the frontal lobe.

were provoked, this study found that this same system was overactive, meaning that the symptoms were rewarding in reducing the anxiety (Norman et al., 2018). In the Norman et al. (2018) study, children with ADHD showed similar hypoactivation in the medial prefrontal cortex as well as the caudate during a reward condition. Thus, rewards must be stronger in order for the child to appreciate their worth. I am sure you have seen this in your practice with children who have ADHD; these children habituate to rewards and there must be a reward menu for effectiveness. These findings indicate that different disorders may show similar patterns of frontal lobe dysfunction but that the networks tied to the frontal lobes can vary depending on the diagnosis.

The orbital cortex has close connections with several subcortical structures, including the ventral anterior cingulate and ventral striatum (Palomero-Gallagher et al., 2009). These structures (as noted in Chapter 2) are related to online monitoring of environmental stimuli and self-control of behavior. The anterior cingulate has also been found to be important in regulating conflicting emotional information (Egner et al., 2008) and processing of emotional stimuli (Banks et al., 2007). Damage to the anterior cingulate has been found to be related to depression, particularly in the area of apathy, psychomotor slowing, and mood regulation (Riva-Posse et al., 2019). In addition, studies have found the anterior cingulate to be underactive in children diagnosed with anxiety disorders (Wheaton et al., 2014) and more active in those with depression (Eugene et al., 2010).

Oversimplifying the dorsolateral prefrontal cortex as the "executive function" area, and the orbital prefrontal cortex as the "emotion regulation" area, does not provide us with an accurate understanding of the complex relationship between these important areas and functions (Stuss & Benson, 2019). In addition, there may be left–right frontal differences that need elucidation. For instance, children with ADHD show right frontal–subcortical hypoactivity, while those with schizophrenia show underactivation in the left homologue frontal–subcortical areas (Rubia, Criuad, et al., 2019; Rubia, Smith, et al., 2019). While there have been studies about the effect of frontal lobe damage on executive functioning skills and reasoning, we are only now beginning to recognize how these frontal–subcortical relationships affect the social and emotional functioning of children (Szekely et al., 2017).

Although much of the emphasis on the neuropsychological causes of psychopathology has been on the frontal and temporal lobes, it is important to recognize that left- and right-hemisphere processes are probably also associated with emotion and behavior. A meta-analysis found that there is hemispheric specialization for positive and negative valence emotions (Fusar-Poli et al., 2009). It has been hypothesized that the left and right hemisphere are specialized to process positive and negative emotions respectively (Wyczesany et al., 2009). It has also been suggested that there is a left-hemispheric superiority for approach-related emotions (happiness, anger) with a right-hemispheric preference for avoidance-related emotions (fear) (Gable & Poole, 2014).

Could it be that novel, complex, and ambiguous situations cause individuals to experience negative emotions (i.e., right-hemisphere activation), while automatic, routinized, and familiar situations lead to positive emotions (i.e., left-hemisphere activation)? This possible link with our neuropsychological model discussed in Chapter 2 makes sense, given what we know about cognitive dissonance—we all like the things we know and tend to discount those ideas unfamiliar to us. Based on this left–right affect lateralization pattern, we might also suggest that if the left hemisphere is underactive or dysfunctional, then negative affect and avoidance behaviors may occur, and if the right is underactive, then positive affect and approach behaviors may occur. Consistent with this argument, crying, depressed behaviors, and catastrophic reactions have been associated with left-hemisphere lesions, while laughter, euphoria, or indifference are more likely associated with right-hemisphere lesions (Gainotti, 2019).

As we have seen in previous chapters, we are not surprised to find that cortical–subcortical structures act upon emotional information in complex and multifaceted ways. When it comes to cortical–subcortical relationships and psychopathology, the top-down or bottom-up question becomes a big one. The frontal–subcortical circuits can affect an individual's interest in the environment, with overarousal resulting in a tendency toward withdrawal (e.g., "Everything is too overwhelming; I need to avoid others") and underarousal associated with approach behaviors (e.g., "Everything is boring; I need to approach others").

Examining this propensity, Gray and McNaughton (2000) have argued that there are three interrelated systems: the behavioral activation system (BAS), which is sensitive to reward and escape from punishment; the behavioral inhibition system (BIS), which is sensitive to punishment and nonreward; and the fight–flight–freeze system (FFFS), which mediates reactions to all aversive stimuli resulting in panic and rage. Could psychological disorders be related to the interaction of these three systems? Individuals with externalizing disorders (e.g., conduct disorder) have cortical *underarousal,* while those with internalizing disorders (e.g., anxiety and depression) are likely to experience cortical *overarousal.* Individuals with internalizing disorders may be more vulnerable to heightened emotions or hypersensitivity to the environment (overarousal of the BAS system), which often causes an overreaction to stimulation (Alloy et al., 2015). Overactivation of the BIS system has been implicated in the inattention symptoms of ADHD as well as with anxiety and depression (Heym et al., 2015). Similarly, the BAS is involved in sensitivity to stimulation and is related to the impulsivity seen in ADHD:C presentation (Corr, 2008). Activation of the BAS system is also associated with aggression (Taubitz et al., 2015).

In the case of ADHD:C, the BAS works without BIS balance, while for anxiety, depression, and ADHD:PI, the BIS is overactive and limits the effects of the BAS (Mitchell & Nelson-Gray, 2006). This framework extends beyond the central nervous system to the autonomic nervous system as well, as children with internalizing disorders show high parasympathetic reactivity, and those with externalizing disorders show low reactivity in both the sympathetic and parasympathetic systems (Dornbach-Bender et al., 2020).

A New Way of Looking at Psychopathology

A new area of thought combines neuropsychological understanding and clinical understanding of psychopathology, or *neuropsychopathology* (Reddy, Koziol, et al., 2013). Neuropsychopathology combines our understanding of brain functioning with behavioral and emotional development. It is important to think about what function a behavior may serve. Within this framework there are four dimensions of volitional behavior that interact (Reddy, Koziol, et al., 2013):

1. Knowing when to start a behavior
2. Knowing when not to start a behavior
3. Knowing when to persist in a behavior
4. Knowing when to stop a behavior

When one or more of these dimensions is not effective, you generally see a breakdown in behavior and a resulting emotional reaction. For example, children with ADHD may have difficulty with starting and persisting in a behavior, often seen in the inability to complete tasks within a specified time. Other difficulties involve knowing when not to start (impulsivity) or to stop a behavior. Children who have ASD or OCD have difficulty stopping a behavior that either relieves anxiety or is soothing (i.e., self-stimulation, handwashing).

The Three-Axes Interpretation of Brain–Behavior Relationships

As was discussed in Chapter 2, there are many ways to look at how the brain is organized. The use of three axes to understand brain–behavior relationships translates into a better understanding of how psychopathology can arise as well as our understanding of the function that behavior and emotion play in the child or adolescent's behavior. To apply the tenets in Chapter 2 to psychopathology, it is necessary to review the interplay of brain structures that may be involved in the resulting behaviors.

The brain is a system that ties together cognition and behavior interactively for functional adaptation (Koziol et al., 2010). In this framework there are three axes: anterior–posterior, right–left, and superior–inferior. Novel learning and problem solving are generally within the right hemisphere, particularly in the frontal lobes, while routinized understanding and sequential thinking are the province of the left hemisphere. The frontal lobes are an important superstructure and basically rule over all aspects of behavior related to the self and to the environment. These systems develop motor programs that are important for successfully navigating the environment (Semrud-Clikeman, 2021).

Think about these systems as three dimensional by envisioning the vertical organization of the brain working from the cortex through the basal ganglia and into the cerebellum. As discussed in Chapter 2, the cortical–-basal ganglia system and cerebro–cerebellar systems modulate incoming and outgoing information by determining what information is or is not returned to the cortex for further processing. Feedback loops between the basal ganglia and the cortex and between the cortex and the cerebellum provide input that may either excite the brain by causing an act to be completed (direct pathway) or inhibit the action (indirect pathway). Another pathway bypasses the basal ganglia going directly from the subthalamic nucleus to the cortex and stops a behavior—or provides impulse control. Thus, difficulties in these circuits can result in problems executing a behavior or stopping it.

The main circuits that concern us in this chapter include frontal circuits that relay information to the cerebellum and back (Reddy, Weissman, et al., 2013). For our purposes the most important circuits are the dorsolateral circuit that is important for planning, organization, strategizing, monitoring, evaluating, and changing behavior. Similarly, the orbitofrontal circuit is important for internal or behavioral regulation functions. Included in these functions would be the ability to manage impulsivity for social judgment, and for problem solving. Finally, the medial circuit involves the anterior cingulate cortex (ACC) and nucleus accumbens, which regulate motivation, error monitoring, and decision making.

These systems can all be linked to executive functioning. When there are difficulties in these circuits, one sees maladaptive behavior that can interfere with the child's functioning—hence the term *neuropsychopathology*. Damage or dysfunction of the dorsolateral circuit relates to problems with the ability to change behaviors or to learn from doing incorrect things (Reddy, Koziol, et al., 2013). When hyperactive, this circuit could be related to ADHD, anxiety, and mania, and when hypoactive, it could be related to depression. The orbitofrontal circuit might also be involved in problems with impulse control seen in many childhood disorders (ASD, ODD, ADHD, and disruptive behavior disorder). The orbitofrontal circuit has been linked to a lack of emotional awareness or responsiveness when hypoactive and to anxiety and social phobia when hyperactive. The medial circuit would be related to OCD, anxiety, ADHD, and many other types of disorders. The medial circuit frequently works in conjunction with the dorsolateral circuit.

In conjunction with the frontal lobe systems, the basal ganglia is important for learning adaptive and maladaptive behaviors (Yin & Knowlton, 2006). Reddy, Weissman, et al. (2013) suggest that the basal ganglia bind elements of a movement program together so that a behavioral sequence is stored. If the program is effective, the basal ganglia releases dopamine that rewards the sequence and makes it more likely that the behavior will be repeated. If the sequence is not effective, dopamine is not released and the behavioral program is not rewarded, thus making it less likely to be repeated. This information in turn influences the amygdala to reward or not to reward (Blackford et al., 2010). Thus, aberrant behavioral programs are developed based on this reward or nonreward situation and can be tied ultimately to neuropsychopathology.

Similar to the reward circuits of the basal ganglia and amygdala, the cerebellum plays a significant role in affective and motivational behavior (Ito, 2008). In this loop the cerebellum modifies the input from the frontal lobes and basal ganglia and sends a refined and new message back to the cortex via the thalamus. As we noted, the three circuits relay to different parts of the cerebellum. In this chapter, our main interest is the lateral cerebellum where regulation of executive functioning, visual–spatial reasoning, linguistic and learning skills, and memory are managed. For the purposes of neuropsychopathology, the important role played by the lateral cerebellum is its regulation of the behavior rate, rhythm, and force allowing the child to manage the behavior. As stated by Reddy, Koziol, et al. (2013), the cortex decides what to do, the basal ganglia decides when to do it, and the cerebellum decides how to get things done efficiently. This system is very important for learning how to make appropriate anticipatory responses. In panic disorder and phobias, the anticipatory response is not related to the threat at hand and so is not modified in a useful manner by the cerebellum. Similarly, an important part to learning is automatization of the behavior—in other words, not having to think about what one is doing. When behaviors are not learned correctly, the incorrect behavior becomes automatic and leads to generalization that isn't adaptive (Koziol et al., 2012).

Thus, when a system is solely based on routine and relies heavily on automatic behavior, the child becomes inflexible and rigid. Similarly, if everything the child sees and perceives is novel without any automaticity, then all behavior is effortful. Rarely is this type of dichotomy seen in its purest form. Variations on this theme do occur. For example, children with ASD, anxiety, or OCD rely on automatic behavior and reject novelty, thus cutting themselves off from new experiences and new learning opportunities. Children with brain damage may find every new experience novel and be unable to apply previous learning to the situation. Both of these examples are very handicapping and make life quite difficult. Too much or too little higher-order control (frontal lobe systems) results in psychopathology.

Neuropsychopathology requires that you consider the interaction of brain systems, behavior, and the environment. Good neuropsychological assessment requires the ability to evaluate the child's response to novelty as well as his or her ability to automatize previously learned behavior. Too much or too little higher-level processing can lead to behaviors that are problematic for the child's adjustment to the environment. Similarly, if the relationship between cortical and subcortical functioning is not well regulated, difficulties likely will be present. For example, too much cortical control of automatic processes will disrupt novel problem solving while too little will result in impulsive behaviors and poor adaptation. The following sections will discuss various types of psychopathology from a neuropsychological perspective with suggestions for evaluation as well as treatment. One of the first aspects of any good neuropsychological assessment is a good interview of both the parents and the child or adolescent.

Assessment

An interview with the parents and child sets the stage for developing the assessment battery. A careful and comprehensive interview assists in determining what possible areas need to be evaluated and aids the practitioner in understanding the questions parents may have about their child's functioning. Interview techniques alone may not be effective for complex cases, and as we have discussed in earlier chapters, similar symptoms can result from very disparate neuropsychological disorders. As part of a team, you can become a key player in differential diagnosis and treatment of childhood disorders of psychopathology.

Your role in the assessment and treatment of child psychopathology requires a fine-grained examination of the interrelationship of neurological, cognitive, achievement, and behavioral characteristics. This analysis must be undertaken within an ecological and developmental framework, as the behavioral manifestations of neuropsychological impairment appear to change over time and situations (Semrud-Clikeman & Ellison, 2009). Gather the information necessary to confirm initial diagnostic impressions, rule out confounding or conflicting data, and monitor intervention efficacy. Although many children present with learning problems that may mask comorbid emotional and behavior disorders (Semrud-Clikeman, 2007), children with neuropsychological impairment are more likely to display overt signs of psychiatric disturbance (Benedek, 2012), and neuropsychological assessment is sensitive to both cerebral dysfunction and psychopathology (Dean & Noggle, 2013).

A child who presents with ADHD may have significant anxiety. The initial clinical impression of this child may be that he is fidgety, can't focus, is impulsive, and emotionally labile. At first glance, this looks like ADHD. After further discussion with his parent, it becomes clearer that he is experiencing significant worries and concerns to the extent that anxiety is significantly interfering with his performance. Solely treating ADHD in this child, or even starting to treat ADHD without acknowledging the anxiety component, will likely result in a poor outcome. Another child with a mathematics disorder may present with psychomotor slowing, poor abstract verbal comprehension, and both internalizing disorders such as depression and externalizing disorders such as CD. As is the case with cognitive and neuropsychological measures, your assessment strategy should be determined by the presenting problems and previous data acquired, because not all measures will be equally effective in addressing the wide array of childhood behavioral, social, and emotional problems (Merrell et al., 2022).

For a complex, multidimensional case, quantitative and qualitative analysis of neuropsychological patterns of performance can provide you with insight into the child's problems for subsequent treatment planning or modification (Bodin & Shay, 2012).

This insight is also critical for providing you with the necessary information for "manifestation determination," that is, determining whether the child's emotional or behavioral difficulties are related to his or her inappropriate behavior. This determination can affect subsequent disciplinary action (Hahn & Morgan, 2012).

Comorbidity and Child Psychopathology

As we have suggested throughout this book, the CHT model requires a comprehensive, yet flexible examination of brain–behavior relationships and their influence on a child's academic and behavioral functioning. This approach suggests that most children will not fit neatly into categories. When we think about the comorbidity of childhood psychopathological disorders, we need to think of an inherent tension between the "clumper" and "splitter" orientations (Fiorello et al., 2010). Clumpers tend to group children into large heterogeneous groups and adhere to a nomothetic or normative orientation. At the extreme end of the clumper continuum is the belief that all children are the same, learn the same way, and act the way they do for the same reasons. Although the number of groups in the clumper approach is fewer, these groups tend to be quite heterogeneous. The more clumping is done, the more heterogeneous the groups are.

Splitters, on the other hand, prefer to create smaller, more discrete groups by clumping only the most similar children together. Although doing this will reduce heterogeneity, it also increases the likelihood that the groups will be comorbid with each other (Sobanski et al., 2010). An extreme splitter will use idiographic analysis to evaluate the unique determinants of each child's cognition and behavior. No child is identical, so each child must be treated as a single-case study. Neither position serves any child well. It is important to recognize that categorical clumping or splitting is just a device for diagnosis—it doesn't necessarily provide the fine-grain analysis of what a child can do and what services are needed. The use of categories serves as a communication aid when talking about a child to another professional.

DSM-5-TR's (American Psychiatric Association, 2022) categorical approach is thought to be an atheoretical one, but it is really a "medical model" approach to differential diagnosis. In a *categorical approach*, a distinction is made between "normal" and "pathological" on the basis of category membership, not the degree that the two differ from each other (Scott & Schoenberg, 2011). Thus, this model is all or none—you either have sufficient symptoms for the diagnosis or you don't. Unfortunately, most of us do not fit neatly into a set category. It is even more complicated with children as one must take into account the stage of cognitive and emotional development as well as the child's reactions to his or her environment. A multimodal understanding of the child is more important than solely arriving at a diagnosis.

For instance, a child who meets only five of the DSM-5-TR (American Psychiatric Association, 2022) inattention criteria for ADHD does not qualify for a diagnosis while a child who meets six criteria for ADHD does. Qualitatively these children may appear quite similar. This discrepancy is one of the problems with a categorical approach for both practice and research, especially if services are only provided to children who meet the required number of criteria. A more important issue has to do with the reliability and validity of the categorical criteria. The *S* in DSM-5-TR stands for *Statistical*, but there is no statistical algorithm offered for assessment tools, so that you can be "sure" a child has a particular diagnosis. Low agreement has been found during trials of the DSM-5-TR criteria among professionals. To be fair, DSM-5-TR provides the latest information on disorders, and the criteria are often based on the results of empirical studies; however, these studies are often inconsistent in subject selection, methodology, data analysis, and interpretation, as we will see in our upcoming discussion of disorders.

Even if we assume that the diagnostic criteria are fairly reliable and valid, we must consider the thorny issue of whether a given child meets those criteria. Diagnostic uncertainty is a major limitation in developing and utilizing effective treatment strategies for children with psychopathology (Loberg et al., 2019), so it is not surprising that most of us want to use those left brains of ours to come up with a definitive decision about a child's diagnosis. We see our job as being one in which we answer that typical parent or teacher question: "So what is *it*? Did you find out what *the problem* is?" We often reluctantly fall for this ploy, saying definitively, "It's *X*," when we know that a host of diagnoses and factors are affecting the child's current status. After lengthy team discussions about a child, we are always amazed when the team looks at us in disbelief when we sheepishly say we should give a "provisional" diagnosis, as if this qualifier doesn't exist, or that we aren't doing a good job if we don't "know" the "truth." It's good practice to discuss characteristics, strengths, and needs rather than to just focus on labels; however, when a child shows a disorder and meets criteria, it is also important to provide that information to the parent, treating physician, and school. Thus, we need to recognize the limitations of our methods. Not only does a good clinician consider the reliability and validity of the various diagnostic criteria, he or she will also evaluate how the information was obtained and what other conditions may be present either comorbidly or instead of the presenting diagnosis. For example, we reviewed the reasons for referral to a university clinic and found that 80% of the children were referred for possible ADHD, but only 60% actually had that diagnosis when other possibilities were explored. An additional 20% showed ADHD plus another disorder.

Research has suggested that training in semistructured interview techniques results in fairly good reliability, but even if the data are reliable, you must consider whether the information is valid. Most agree that multimethod–multisource approaches lead to more accurate diagnoses and interventions (Allen & Becker, 2019). We see some parents who minimize a child's behavior problem, others who exaggerate it, and others who just don't see the problem, because they do not see it in their setting—all problems incurred during the use of informant ratings of behaviors. When one considers the low agreement rate between parent and teacher informants, particularly for internalizing disorder coupled with the high comorbidity rates between internalizing and externalizing disorders, complex, multifaceted approaches to assessment and intervention are required (Semrud-Clikeman, 2007).

Given these issues, it is extremely difficult to determine whether children really fall into one diagnostic category or another (i.e., have "pure" disorders). Indeed, comorbidity between disorders unfortunately appears to be the norm rather than the exception, with rates ranging from 19 to 75% (Hendren et al., 2019). Even this broad range of comorbidity rates is telling: If we can't decide what a disorder is, and accurately determine whether it is comorbid with other disorders, what good is a categorical system at all? For one thing, children with comorbid disorders are twice as likely to receive psychiatric services and comorbidity helps clinicians determine etiology, course, and treatment (Hendren et al., 2019). Meta-analyses found that comorbidity is not due to referral bias, rater expectancy effects, or use of multiple informants; nor is it the result of multiple or nonspecific symptoms (Costello & Angold, 2016).

Categories and their comorbidities serve a useful purpose. They give us a template to explore each child's unique characteristics and to determine how he or she differs from the category exemplar (a fictitious child who serves as conceptual anchor). As we've noted before, be careful, and don't make children try to "fit" into a category if they don't. You're always safer describing cognitive and behavioral functioning than justifying categorical labels.

Although categorical diagnoses and comorbidity appear to be verifiable phenomena, it is critical to use a developmental perspective when determining diagnoses. What might be acceptable at one age is likely not acceptable at another age. Some disorders also evolve over time and may look very different at age 3 compared to age 12. For example, children with high-functioning autism at age 3 show difficulty with peer relationships, joint attention, flexibility, and enjoyment of social activities. However, by age 10, many of these children have had many interventions and their social skills and their ability to manage novel situations has improved. That doesn't mean they don't continue to have autism, but rather that the disorder has modified based on good intervention, early identification, and improvement. Evaluating this child requires information as to how the child was at an early age as well as how he or she is functioning at the present time.

The variability in comorbidity rates we've described is related to the developmental manifestations of the overt symptoms displayed by children, which change according to their age and gender. For instance, depression symptoms are approximately equally distributed across genders until adolescence when girls report more symptoms (Semrud-Clikeman, 2007). Ongoing assessment and regular monitoring are critical for helping children with emotional or behavior disorders (Baron, 2016).

Understanding the relationship between symptom development and expression requires flexibility in thought and practice, as we have suggested in the CHT model (see Chapter 1). In CHT, we try to determine how much of a child's problem is related to the individual's temperament and constitution and what is related to—and shaped by—environmental contingencies in order to recognize the developmental continuum of psychopathology. The question we often face in clinical practice is not an "either–or" one, but a "how much" one. It is also important to recognize the neurological underpinnings of some of these disorders and to apply the information provided earlier in this chapter, as well as in Chapter 2, for your understanding of these disorders. Parents frequently welcome an explanation that provides a neurological foundation for what their child is experiencing. Laying this foundation provides guidance on interventions and for the ultimate understanding of the child's world.

In the following sections, we examine common childhood disorders that pose risks for both cognitive and psychosocial disturbance and offer intervention recommendations for each. As you review this material, you need to recognize that no particular pattern or sign on psychological or neuropsychological tests provides you with unequivocal evidence that a child has a particular neuropsychopathological disorder; it is rather the pattern of strengths and weaknesses that supports a diagnosis. The cursory examination that follows should serve to further your interest in and exploration of the neuropsychology of childhood psychopathology because this is a growing area that strengthens our understanding.

Selected Childhood Disorders

This section of the chapter briefly reviews the major disorders seen in childhood. We have selected common disorders that are most often seen, as it is not possible to review all disorders from a neuropsychological point of view within the confines of this volume. We cover internalizing and externalizing disorders, mood disorders, bipolar disorder, disruptive mood dysregulation disorder, conduct disorder, and oppositional defiant disorder.

Internalizing and Externalizing Disorders

As you read the heading to this section, you may be wondering why these disorders are in the same section. The fact is that for many children, it is not uncommon to find comorbidity among these apparently opposite conditions (Leech et al., 2006). Children with internalizing disorders such as depression or anxiety constitute a heterogeneous population that may have associated neuropsychological deficits. Similarly, children with externalizing disorders such as conduct disorder or disruptive behavior disorder also have neuropsychological deficits and may also evidence an internalizing disorder. Given the disorder, many children seem to show neuropsychological deficits because they are unable to maintain motivation or persistence on a task rather than having a true neuropsychological problem. One example is attention. Children with ADHD will have attentional problems but children with anxiety and/or depression will also experience attentional problems that may appear to be similar. A child who is resistant to testing or who feels threatened by having to perform may also display attentional problems indicative of ADHD, as you can see in Case Study 9.1.

While internalizing and externalizing disorders have been found to generally represent distinct factors in research, there is a fairly high incidence of these disorders being comorbid with each other. In a meta-analysis of the literature, CD and ODD coupled with ADHD often were accompanied by symptoms of depression but not anxiety (Hendren et al., 2018).

Children with anxiety show more ADHD symptoms compared to typically developing children (Llanes et al., 2020). When ADHD and anxiety overlap, it is very difficult to determine what part ADHD plays in the attentional symptoms and what part anxiety may play. At times clinical judgment is made as to which disorder to treat first and in what manner. For a child that shows significant anxiety on top of possible ADHD, cognitive-behavioral therapy (CBT) may be most appropriate and then a re-evaluation of progress to determine if medication is required at a later time.

Case Study 9.1. Steve's Best Friend

Steve was an 8-year-old boy referred for a psychological evaluation because the teacher felt he had "dyslexia." Described as a pleasant, compliant, and "sweet" boy, Steve was said to have no psychosocial problems, but he was failing most of his academic subjects. Except for word problems, math was said to be a relative strength for Steve, and he was only in the below-average range in this area during formal testing. His word attack skills were quite poor, and he couldn't do pseudoword decoding, but his reading fluency was fairly good on easy passages, and his reading comprehension was pretty good unless he had many word recognition errors. Surprisingly, he did quite well with writing, largely because he wrote creative and interesting prose. However, the passage he wrote received limited credit for vocabulary, grammar, capitalization, and punctuation. Cognitive testing revealed that Steve had significant strengths on the fluid, visual, and short-term/working memory subtests, but he did poorly on the crystallized, auditory processing, long-term memory, and processing speed measures. CHT results revealed poor auditory processing skills and both receptive and expressive language problems. His expressive language was notable for circumlocutions, poor fluency, and semantic paraphasias. Steve had limited crystallized knowledge, but only minor retrieval problems. A comparison of motor, visual, and visual–motor processing revealed that his problem was related to motor (left-hemisphere) rather than spatial processes, suggesting possible dyspraxic symptoms. The interview revealed similar fine-motor deficits, left–right confusion, and dressing dyspraxia. His Block Design performance, while in the average range, was notable for reversal, inversion, and rotation errors, but he performed all items quickly.

On the parent ratings, Steve was noted as having few problems, but clinical elevations were found on measures of anxiety, depression, withdrawal, and attention problems. The last of these appeared to be related to language or mood rather than to ADHD, given his strong working memory performance and executive functions. Additional personality testing suggested that Steve had poor self-esteem and a preference for solitary activities, such as watching television and playing with his "best friend"—his dog. He reported having many "friends," but he was not close to anyone outside his immediate family and spent little time with other children outside of school. Good relationships were noted with parents and the teacher. In addition, to academic interventions, we suggested that Steve receive individual counseling to address self-esteem and affect issues. The teacher was encouraged to help Steve work with a "study buddy" in the class, and to provide him with leadership opportunities in areas of his interest and success. We also recommended that Steve become involved in group activities, such as team sports and an environmental group he had expressed interest in.

Mood Disorders

Depression and anxiety in children often resemble each other and frequently are difficult to disentangle. For that reason, we will discuss anxiety and depression together. In addition, anxiety and depression often occur simultaneously in the same child or may occur with one disorder following the other (Costello et al., 2008; Garber & Weering, 2010). When both anxiety and depression co-occur, the prognosis is much more guarded with higher severity related to poorer outcome (Ezpeleta et al., 2006). Psychosocial treatments for anxiety and depression have not been found optimal for children with severe impairment (Nilesen et al., 2013). Nilsen et al. (2013) found that for anxiety, no demographic or clinic factors have been proven to moderate or predict outcomes. In contrast, baseline symptom severity and comorbid depression impact treatment response.

For much of the 20th century, children were not thought to have "adult" disorders such as major depression and anxiety. With the understanding that depression, anxiety, persistent depressive disorder (this is a low-grade form of sadness that is frequently coupled with irritability previously called dysthymia), withdrawal, and somatic complaints do occur in children, we have begun to explore the associated neuropsychological deficits in this population. These deficits can easily lead to misdiagnosis, with such children being seen as "slow" or "inattentive."

Children with anxiety disorders have been found to show frontal lobe volume reductions and fewer responses to tasks in the orbital frontal cortex. Children without anxiety disorders do not show a similar volume reduction, indicating an increased ability to cope with challenging life experiences and the presence of less negative affect (Grupe & Nitschke, 2013). It is also important to emphasize that the right–left hemisphere dichotomy is too simplistic for understanding these complex disorders. Neuroimaging findings have shown that worry and anxiety experiences activate the left prefrontal cortex while anxious arousal activates the right hemispheric region (Dolcos et al., 2016). Optimism has been found inversely related to anxiety as well as to orbital frontal cortical volume (more anxiety, less volume). Thus, resilience to anxiety increases the child's ability to emotionally regulate his or her feelings and involves a cognitive orientation toward positivity (D'Avanzato et al., 2013). These findings suggest that children with anxiety often use internally directed self-talk and possibly rumination, which interferes with efficient performance. This internal dialogue may in part account for their propensity to be self-focused and avoid social contact. Individuals with anxiety tend to be hypervigilant of their environment and exquisitely sensitive to people's emotions. Helping them narrow their concerns through cognitive-behavioral therapy has been found to be very helpful (Stark et al., 2011).

For depression, neuroimaging findings indicate that rumination is also present and is strongly correlated with the severity of depression (DeRaedt et al., 2015). This type of rumination can also be conceptualized as brooding. The default mode network (DMN; discussed in Chapter 8) has been implicated in depression particularly because it is the network involved in self-related processing (Fox et al., 2005). Functional abnormalities in the DMN have been found to be present during rumination (Hamilton et al., 2011). Findings support the role of rumination in depression, which is strongly linked to dysfunction in the DMN as well as in the dorsomedial prefrontal cortex (a subdivision of the orbital prefrontal cortex) (Zhou et al., 2020).

Thus, while anxiety and depression both involve the prefrontal cortex, the activity presents itself differently in this region. For anxiety, activation is widespread in the prefrontal cortex bilaterally, depending on the type of anxiety. For depression, the DMN is activated as well as the dorsomedial prefrontal cortex. These differences may well help in tailoring interventions to particular areas: for high anxiety, relaxation and improvement in self-talk; for depression, emphasis on rumination and corrective cognitive framing of tasks.

Depression Treatment

Studies have evaluated the efficacy of treatment for children with mood disorders. For those children with mood disorders, the best and most efficacious treatment involves parents as well as the child (Stark et al., 2012). Research has also found that parent involvement results in a significant improvement in the maintenance of treatment effects. This is particularly true for depression as many children who are depressed also have depressed parents. These families are frequently less communicative, support each other less, and are less cohesive, leading to stronger and more frequent interfamily conflict (Stark et al., 2012). These behaviors, as well as a genetic predisposition, frequently lead to depressed and anxious children, particularly as the modeling of appropriate problem-solving and coping skills is not present (Stark et al., 2012).

There is a very strong relationship found between parental depression and child psychopathology (Bifulco et al., 2002). Meeting with the parents about a child's needs and providing recommendations when a parent is already overwhelmed is not helpful and may actually be harmful. Referring the family for treatment in this case is likely more efficacious and successful in the long run.

Anxiety Treatment

CBT utilizes cognitive strategies (cognitive reframing and problem solving), relaxation techniques, emotional identification of feeling states, and exposure and reinforcement (Higa-McMillan et al., 2016). Exposure to the anxiety-producing situation and cognitive restructuring have been found to show the most efficacy for treatment while relaxation techniques have not shown as much efficacy (Whiteside et al., 2020). Treatment studies for anxiety disorders found improvement with CBT (Hedtke et al., 2009). Similar to studies of children with depression, family involvement in CBT led to stronger gain and improved outcome (Cooper et al., 2008). When anxiety and depression were comorbid, treatment efficacy was found to be more problematic, require significantly more sessions, and these children showed a greater chance of relapse (Melton et al., 2016).

Bipolar Disorder

Given the change in our understanding of depression in children, it is not surprising that researchers are discovering that pediatric mania is not as rare as once thought and accounts for 18% of all pediatric mental health hospitalizations (Connor et al., 2017). The diagnosis of bipolar disorder in children has been hotly debated with some finding an incidence of 1.8% (Duffy, 2020) while others finding no incidence of bipolar disorder (Vizard et al., 2018). Recent findings indicate bipolar disorder in adolescents is approximately 3% (Parru, Allison, & Bastiampallli, 2021). Children with bipolar disorder (BD) show elated mood, grandiosity, racing thoughts, hypersexuality, and decreased need for sleep (Van Meter et al., 2016). Pediatric BD has been found to be comorbid with several medical difficulties, including cardiovascular disease, obesity, and suicide (Elias et al., 2017).

This disease is highly heritable with a 10-fold greater risk of developing BD if there is a first-degree relative with BD (Duffy et al., 2014). Moreover, children of parents with BD, who do not respond to lithium (the current medication for BD), have a higher rate of ADHD, LDs, and difficulty with impulse control compared to those who do respond to lithium (Duffy et al., 2014). Finally, children of parents with BD have an earlier onset of BD and comorbid ADHD (Ramos et al., 2019). When your developmental history reveals that there is BD in a first- or second-degree relative, you need to consider BD as a possible diagnosis in your conceptualization.

Although individuals with BD have adequate intellectual skills, impaired performance skills can be seen during acute episodes, and attention, inhibition, verbal memory, verbal fluency, and executive function deficits are typical (Findling et al., 2018). In pediatric bipolar disorder, rapid cycling of mood is commonplace, suggesting extreme emotional lability, which can lead to explosive, aggressive outbursts and additional diagnoses of disruptive behavior disorder. These children also have a history of suicide attempts, hospitalizations, and psychotic symptoms (Axelson et al., 2006).

Comorbidity of child BD is common, especially with ADHD, CD, and anxiety. The most substantial overlap is between BD and ADHD (van Meter et al., 2011). This comorbidity may represent a distinct subtype that is different from other types of ADHD (Biederman et al.,

2013). A meta-analysis found 42% of children diagnosed with BD also show oppositional defiant disorder, 23% have comorbid anxiety disorder, and 27% qualified for a diagnosis of CD (van Meter et al., 2011). When ADHD and anxiety co-occur with BD, the outcome is generally worse, the symptoms more significant, and neurocognitive functioning is poorer (Frias et al., 2015).

Children with BD have higher verbal IQ than performance IQ as well as difficulty with executive functioning and processing speed (Mistry et al., 2019). Additional studies have found impairment on measures of attentional set-shifting and visual–spatial memory and in some instances in working memory and processing speed (Dickstein et al., 2004; Doyle et al., 2005). Memory skills have been found to be the most impaired in children with bipolar disorder and ADHD (McClure et al., 2005). These deficits have been found to continue even when the child has been adequately treated (Pavuluri et al., 2006). In contrast, children with ADHD have been found to improve on some but not all of these measures when treated with medication (Doyle, 2006; Gualitieri & Johnson, 2008).

Mattis et al. (2011) compared children with BD and those with BD and ADHD on numerous neuropsychological measures. They found difficulty with processing speed, with slower and more variable reaction time present in children in both groups. They concluded that these processing speed and motor issues were a specific endophenotype of BD independent of ADHD. Thus, it has been hypothesized that poor performance on repetitive motor tasks seen in children with ADHD is related to a core deficit in fronto–striatal circuitry. In contrast, the problems with sequential motor movements in children with BD are related more to problems with attentional set-shifting or frontal executive dysfunction (Dickstein et al., 2005).

One study compared children with BD and those with disruptive behavior disorder and negative mood (Connor & Doerfler, 2012). No differences were found between children with disruptive behavior disorder and depression and those with BD on measures of conduct problems, oppositionality, aggression, hostility, and psychopathology. The children with BD were found to experience higher rates of posttraumatic stress disorder, substance abuse, and suicidality. These findings suggest that it is difficult to distinguish between these two disorders and that children who present with these behaviors need to be carefully evaluated for posttraumatic disorder as well as suicidality.

Neurobiology of BD

DTI, which provides us with the ability to see connectivity in the brain, has found that children and adolescents with BD show less activation in the orbital prefrontal region,s particularly in the right hemisphere and the anterior corpus callosum (Kafantaris et al., 2009). Functional imaging found hyperactivation in the amygdala, and hypoactivation in the anterior cingulate cortex (Wegbreit et al., 2014). These findings suggest that the frontal–limbic connections are disrupted in BD, thus limiting the prefrontal lobes' ability to modulate behavior.

Treatment of BD

The empirically supported treatment for BD in children is psychopharmacology and psychosocial therapy (McClellan et al., 2007). Children with severe BD are most often prescribed two or more medications (Kowatch et al., 2013). Of concern is that approximately 38% of children and adolescents with a diagnosis of BD are not managed medically, thus leaving them vulnerable to continuing difficulty and significant problems with adjustment despite the fact that best practice indicates medication is most appropriate (Kowatch et al., 2013; McClellan et al., 2007). The most common medications are lithium, olanzapine (Zyprexa), divalprox, and risperidone for manic symptoms. Treatment of depressive symptoms is more problematic because antidepressants can precipitate a manic episode. Zyprexa and Prozac have been found to be effective in clinical trials for children and adolescents (Findling et al., 2018).

Psychotherapy is strongly recommended in conjunction with pharmacology, particularly when done with an accompanying family component (Fristad & McPherson, 2014). These interventions have been found to prevent relapse, improve social and emotional functioning, and improve adherence to medication. CBT has been found to be the most conducive to improvement in these areas.

Disruptive Mood Dysregulation Disorder

A relatively new diagnostic category, introduced in the 5th edition of the DSM, *disruptive mood dysregulation disorder* (DMDD), presents as persistent irritability and temper outbursts in children and was previously diagnosed, inaccurately, as BD (Baweja et al., 2016). There is a strong overlap with ADHD (81%) as well as with CD (13%) and ODD (96%) (Bruno et al., 2019). As this diagnosis is relatively new, there is not a great deal of information about its epidemiology and course (Bruno et al., 2019). This diagnosis is not appropriate for children under the age of 6 or adults over the age of 18. The core aspect of DMDD is irritability which is chronic, persistent, and occurs in more than one setting for most of the day every day. According to one large study, in addition to irritability, children with DMDD had disrupted relationships with others, particularly parents and siblings, and came from single-parent or poorer families (Copeland et al., 2013). Studies have also found that children with the highest number of externalizing behaviors and very poor executive functioning skills were more likely to develop significant impairment in later life (Matijasevich et al., 2015; Weissmann et al., 2016).

A large study found a prevalence of 0.8 to 3.3%, with a decrease in the diagnosis in later adolescence (Copeland et al., 2013). Emerging evidence using fMRI found decreased activation in the left amygdala, parietal cortex, and posterior cingulate, areas of the brain important for emotional regulation and reward awareness (Deveney et al., 2013). Other studies have also found abnormal amygdala activation, particularly related to the intensity of irritability and an increase in the intensity when viewing all facial emotions (Wiggins et al., 2016). These children differed from those with BD as there was amygdala overaction to fearful faces. Similarly, children with DMDD were found to show greater activation of the prefrontal regions and the anterior cingulate cortex, while those with BD showed reduced activation in the insula and increased superior frontal region activation (Rich et al., 2011).

Risk factors have not been well studied but the primary ones initially identified include early life trauma, recent divorce, and maternal depression (Bruno et al., 2019). Treatment has generally been achieved with medications, particularly psychostimulants and antidepressants (Tourian et al., 2015) as well as atypical antipsychotics, risperidone and aripiprazole (Owen et al., 2009). It has been strongly suggested that behavioral therapy (in particular, dialectical behavioral therapy) and parent training interventions need to be coupled with medication therapy for effective treatment of DMDD (Bruno et al., 2019). Findings from a study utilizing dialectical behavior therapy for pre-adolescent children found a 90.4% improvement for children with severe behavioral disorder (Perepletchikova et al., 2017). Parent management training utilizing the ADOPT program (affective dysregulation—optimizing prevention and treatment) has been found to help in improving parent and child interactions (Dopfner et al., 2019).

Comorbidity of Mood Disorders with ADHD

Approximately half of children diagnosed with ADHD continue to show ADHD in adulthood, particularly when they have associated mood disorders (Belanger et al., 2018). A diagnosis of ADHD:PI instead of anxiety or depression has been found to occur fairly frequently, while mood disorders with mood swings (BP and DMDD) can also show ADHD symptomatology, resulting in misdiagnosis. Anxiety disorder co-occurs with ADHD in about 30–40% of patients (Abramovich et al., 2015; Mitchison & Njardvik, 2019). These children tend to have more school refusal, poorer social skills, and more severe symptoms (Boylan et al., 2010). In addition, CBT can be successful with these children when paired with parent training (Sciberras et al., 2019). Medication is also problematic as stimulants can increase anxiety (Belanger et al., 2018).

ADHD is also comorbid with depression (Faraone et al., 2021). There is emerging evidence that these difficulties may increase as the child approaches adolescence and adulthood. Further studies have found approximately 22–50% incidence of comorbid depression with ADHD (Mitchison & Njardvik, 2019; Seymour & Miller, 2017). Girls with ADHD have been found to show internalizing symptoms more frequently compared to boys (Skogli et al., 2013).

Children with ADHD and depression often show irritability as part of their expression of sadness. This irritability is often associated with low frustration tolerance (Leibenluft & Stoddard, 2013). Signs of irritability are fairly frequent in children with ADHD compared to those without ADHD (Faraonoe et al., 2021). This irritability and frustration associated with both sadness and ADHD resulted in children quitting challenging tasks early and exhibiting poor emotional coping. These in turn can lead to feelings of sadness and hopelessness. The neurological networks associated with irritability and frustration include the amygdala, orbitofrontal cortex ,and the anterior cingulate, and these areas have been previously associated with ADHD (Seymour & Miller, 2017). Thus, the overlay of depression, irritability, and low frustration tolerance include the same networks involved with ADHD making children with ADHD perhaps, more susceptible to these emotional dyscontrol difficulties.

Children with ADHD plus mood disorders frequently have difficulty with working memory. When a child is anxious or sad it can be very difficult to attend to information that requires mental manipulation (Skirbekk et al., 2011). Studies have found that anxiety plus ADHD results in similar attentional difficulties as a sole diagnosis of ADHD (Jarrett et al., 2016). Moreover, children with a sole diagnosis of anxiety do not show more severe difficulty with symptoms than those children with ADHD plus anxiety.

Comorbidity of Mood Disorder with LDs

As described in Chapters 5–8, there are many causes and interventions for children with LDs. Research on the difficulties experienced by children with LDs is equivocal, with many authors not finding significant problems with social and adaptive functioning while others have found difficulty with these functions. Inconsistent study results may be related to the use of heterogeneous group designs, as differences between the LD groups and the control groups were often ones of severity. The poorest socioemotional adjustment is present in children with more than one type of LD (Willcutt et al., 2013). ADHD is also commonly comorbid with LDs and likely impacts the social and emotional development of the child.

One study sought to tease out why some children with LDs show social skills deficits and problems with emotional development and others do not. It hypothesized that the difference was due to social status (Meaden & Halle, 2004). Children with high social status were compared to those with low social status. Both groups were found to have adequate interpretation of facial expressions and emotions as well as a negative feeling about their need for resource room help but they did like the help. Children with lower social status were less attentive to facial details and interpreted the expression on those faces inaccurately. Those with higher social status indicated that they were no different from other children while those with lower social status felt different. Those with higher status were reported as behaving appropriately and attempting to control their behavior while those with lower status reported more aggressive behaviors, indicating that when they were mad they could not control their behavior. In addition, those with higher status indicated they liked to work and play with others while those with lower status said they preferred to play and work alone.

These findings begin to explain why the research on the adjustment of children with LDs has been equivocal. When group means are used without attention to mediating variables, differences are often not present due to statistical procedures. Many children with LDs may experience persistent maladaptive behavior patterns, but a large proportion of children with LDs experience no significant signs of psychopathology (Semrud-Clikeman, 2007).

A review of current research in dyslexia found that there is not a strong risk for elevated internalizing disorders, in general, for this group (Martinez & Semrud-Clikeman, 2004; Miller et al., 2005). When internalizing disorders such as anxiety or depression do exist, they are present similarly in boys and girls (Nelson & Gregg, 2012; Nelson & Harwood, 2011). Studies have found more depressive and anxious symptomatology in children and adolescents with dyslexia compared to the general child population but the symptoms were not necessarily sufficient to warrant a diagnosis (Daviss, 2008). Findings of lowered self-worth and feelings of not being accepted socially have been reported for adolescents with dyslexia (Undheim & Sund, 2008).

In a study comparing children with NVLD, neurotypicals, and those with RDs, it was found that children with NVLDs or RDs showed more anxiety and depressive symptoms (Mammarella et al., 2016). For the NVLD sample, significant anxiety and separation anxiety were found while the RD sample showed more depressive symptoms. It is important to note here that these children showed subclinical symptoms of depression and anxiety; in other words, they would not qualify for an official diagnosis but were, nevertheless, experiencing feelings of sadness, withdrawal, and worry—often centered around school performance.

The finding that students with LDs may feel additional stress is important. To date, the emphasis has been on finding whether anxiety and/or depression diagnoses are more common in children and adolescents with LDs. It has been suggested that a more appropriate approach may be to evaluate what mediating variables are involved in order for the student to develop this type of disorder (Nelson & Harwood, 2011). Identifying these variables can help put needed supports into place for these students in the K–12 and in higher education grades. Assessment needs to be multifactorial and include information from parents and teachers as well as self-reporting. Studies have found that adolescents with depressive and/or anxiety symptoms underreport the presence of these problems (Nelson & Harwood, 2011).

Comorbidity of Mood Disorder and ASD

Anxiety and ASD complicate our need to further understand what factors contribute to anxiety. Kerns and Kendall (2014) evaluated the symptoms of anxiety with ASD and found many similarities with a sole diagnosis of anxiety but also some striking differences. Differences were found in social discomfort, compulsive behavior not associated with symptom relief, and unusual phobias (Kerns et al., 2014). As we previously discussed in an earlier chapter, sensory dysfunction has been frequently found in children with ASD. There are two types of sensory difficulty: overresponsivity (experiencing stimuli as painful), and underresponsivity (repeated touching of objects), with both of these types co-occurring in children with ASD (Watts et al., 2016). Severity of anxiety has been found to be higher in children with more severe sensory dysfunction (Ulijarvic et al., 2016). Neuroimaging has found that children with ASD given sensory challenges during scanning show stronger activation in the amygdala and orbitofrontal cortices, thus suggesting that this overactivation triggers anxiety and sensory overload (Green et al., 2015). Children with ASD, unlike those without it, did not habituate to sensory input. thus continuing to show overresponsiveness to the environment.

The cortisol response to stress has also been found to be higher in children with ASD when interacting with peers, suggesting that stress is heightened in these situations (Corbett et al., 2016). Stress, in turn, increases emotional responses to incoming signals, and results in the prefrontal–anterior cingulate–amygdala network becoming unable to modulate emotional responses involving anxiety (Guistino & Maren, 2015). Also involved in this network is the insular region. The insula is critical to the child's ability to integrate introspective information with sensory information and thus regulate the emotional response to the environment (Bird et al., 2010). When this network is overstimulated, the child experiences significant emotional flooding and behaviors such as tantrums and avoidance are frequently seen (South & Rodgers, 2017). This network dysfunction also relates to more difficulty with social communication that impacts the child's peer relationships (Duvekot et al., 2018). Thus, as discussed above, anxiety coupled with ASD leads to a more severe presentation than ASD alone. Treatment is crucial for the child and it supports the combination of CBT with social skills interventions.

ASD can also co-occur with depression. The incidence of depression in ASD has been found to be approximately 20%, and was higher in children and adolescents with ASD without intellectual disability (Rai et al., 2018). In the general population, the incidence of depression is approximately 12% (Merikangas et al., 2010). Individuals with ASD plus depression may show an increase in obsessions and rituals, agitation, and self-injury (DeFilippis, 2018).

A longitudinal study of ASD and depression found that children with ASD showed more depressive symptoms at age 10 than children without ASD and these symptoms continue to be present through the age of 18 (Rai et al., 2013). For older adolescents, social communication deficits were found to be strongly associated with a comorbid diagnosis of depression. Moreover, bullying was frequently present and strongly related to more severe forms of depression in adolescents with ASD.

Children with ASD and depression diagnoses have a higher incidence of a family history of depression compared to those children with a sole diagnosis of ASD (DeFilippis, 2018). The most frequent strategy used by children and adolescents with ASD plus depression is avoidance of possibly stressful situations. Increased symptoms of depression have been found to be associated with poorer social functioning, thus, exacerbating the isolation already experienced by many individuals with ASD.

Treatment of depression in children and adolescents with ASD is generally based on research and treatment efficacy studies of children with a sole diagnosis of depression. Treatment includes psychotherapy and psychopharmacology (King et al., 2009). While there is an alarming lack of evidence for the use of SSRIs with children with ASD, the most commonly prescribed medication (33% of children) is an antidepressant (Thom et al., 2021). Due to the lack of evidence for the use of these medications, it's recommended to begin with low doses and titrate slowly while carefully monitoring the effects of the medication. Psychosocial interventions including CBT (both individual and group), mindfulness-based therapy, and social and vocational skills training have been effective with adults but have not been studied with children (Hiller et al., 2011; Pezzimenti et al., 2019; Spek et al., 2013).

CD and ODD

ODD is characterized by irritable mood, argumentativeness, acting-out behavior, defiance, and difficulty obeying authority (American Psychiatric Association, 2022). It is considered a form of disruptive behavior disorder. In contrast, CD is a more serious disorder with behaviors such as hurting others, setting fires, lying, breaking the law, truancy, and running away. It is not appropriate to make a dual diagnosis of ODD and CD. See Case Study 9.2 for an illustration of a child with these difficulties.

By definition, children with CD or ODD are likely to gain the attention of parents and teachers, but the neuropsychological characteristics of these disorders may go undetected because intervention efforts usually focus on the overt disruptive behaviors. Research has found that children diagnosed with either of these disorders do not necessarily go on to become delinquents or to be diagnosed with antisocial personality disorder in adulthood (Semrud-Clikeman, 2007). There is a strong overlap between these two disorders and ADHD—in fact approximately 80–90% of children with CD are thought to have comorbid ADHD (Hobson et al., 2011).

A majority of adolescents with conduct disorders show neuropsychological deficits in the areas of working memory, attention, and inhibitory control (Deters et al., 2020); approximately half have experienced traumatic brain injury with varying brain areas affected and types of deficits displayed across studies. Deficits in executive function suggest behavioral dyscontrol which is typical of children with both CD and ADHD. A mixed pattern of neuropsychological deficits has been found with verbal deficits found to be most common, and additional deficits present in attention, cognitive flexibility, and planning (Fairchild et al., 2019). These executive deficits could account for the fearless, disinhibited, stimulus-seeking characteristics of children with conduct disorder, which lead to aggressive and antisocial behavior.

Given the propensity for these adolescents to experience head trauma due to their risk-taking behaviors, the most common areas impacted are likely subcortical, prefrontal regions, and temporal-parietal injury (Teichner & Golden, 2000). These regions of injury are sensitive to premorbid factors such as previous head injuries, traumatic experiences, and timing of the injury, and they are more common in children who experience poverty. It has been suggested that rather than grouping adolescents on the basis of diagnosis or aggression, it would be more fruitful to examine the specific types of neuropsychological functioning within this group.

Studies have attempted to examine more carefully the type of executive function deficits seen with these children (Hobson et al., 2011). Given the high incidence of ADHD in this population, it is important to evaluate the contribution that ADHD has to these disorders. Functional neuroimaging with children with ODD or CD without ADHD and those children with ADHD has found dissociated underlying neurological differences between these groups. For the ADHD group, the lateral inferior prefrontal cortex has been found to be underactivated. In contrast, the ODD/CD group showed underactivation in the orbitofrontal cortex (particularly the ventromedial area), and the superior temporal lobe with the underlying limbic areas implicated (amygdala, hippocampus) (Rubia et al., 2008; Rubia, Smith, et al., 2009). In addition, smaller volume has been found in the amygdala, insula, and orbitofrontal cortex. Lower hypothalamic–pituitary–adrenal axis activation, as well as autonomic reactivity to stress, have been found (Fairchild et al., 2019). These findings further support our model, explained earlier in the chapter, of the three-dimension axes for understanding behavior.

Studies have found that children with ODD and CD without ADHD do not show significant problems with impulsivity, a finding that was not true for children with ADHD. These deficits have been considered "cool" executive function deficits—in other words, they happen when the child is not emotionally aroused. They are also associated with the lateral prefrontal cortex, which was discussed in the previous paragraph. In contrast, "hot" executive functioning tasks are those that are involved with reward and punishment. For these types of tasks, children with ODD and CD often show more problems than children with ADHD (Hobson et al., 2011). These tasks are related to increased risky decision making that is an inherent characteristic of children with ODD/CD. Children with ODD/CD were found to show more difficulty on the cool executive function tasks related to speed of inhibitory processes and response variability.

These are important findings because they begin to explain the behaviors that are frequently seen in children with ODD or CD but not necessarily in children with ADHD. Children with ODD or CD may not think through the consequences of their behavior because they relate to reward and punishment systems differently from neurotypical children. If the behavior is "worth" the risk, it is highly likely that they will engage in it. The differences in the amygdala circuits found in functional neuroimaging further supports this hypothesis— if these areas are underactivated, stimulating these areas through risky behavior becomes reinforcing in and of itself. These abnormalities in motivation control link directly to the behaviors frequently seen in children with ODD and CD. Helpful interventions may be those that include motivational approaches (directly teaching the advantages and disadvantages of specific antisocial behaviors). Moreover, teaching coping strategies for when the adolescent becomes impulsive would also be helpful. Some clinicians have suggested that channeling the risk-taking behaviors into more acceptable activities (i.e., skydiving, surfing, mountain climbing) may work for these children and adolescents. We have also found that enrolling in a martial arts class can assist the child or adolescent in developing self-control over impulses due to the emphasis in these classes on emotional control.

Not all adolescents with CD have neuropsychological deficits. The behavioral difficulties experienced by these adolescents are likely related to environmental factors and may include a history of abuse, substance abuse, chaotic family life, lack of parental monitoring, and the need for a peer group for support (i.e., gang activity). While this group may not have neuropsychological deficits at the onset of the problems, they are at higher risk for head injuries, which would complicate identifying the area of difficulty.

As with the other disorders explored in this chapter, there may be several subtypes of children with CD. For instance, many children with CD have problems with authority, school, and alcohol and drug abuse. Some children may show signs of a comorbid mood disorder, while others show antisocial behavior associated with thought disorder symptoms (Hofvander et al., 2018). Delinquents have been found to have persistent verbal deficits, particularly when the disorder is comorbid with ADHD and particularly with poorer short-term working memory skills independent of the ADHD. Verbal deficits interfere with abilities to solve problems, mediate verbal situations, and learn in school.

Consistent with our arguments that a hemispheric equilibrium is important in overall adjustment, children with large Verbal Comprehension–Perceptual reasoning splits, *in either direction*, have higher rates of delinquency than those whose verbal and visual spatial skills are comparable (Falk et al., 2017). Despite conflicting evidence regarding the relationship of brain dysfunction to CD, these children experience higher rates of learning deficits and suffer more brain injuries than other children (Narhi et al., 2010). Whether these conditions are

Case Study 9.2. Brain Functioning and Externalizing Disorders

Children with CD/ODD are a heterogeneous group who display a wide array of neuropsychological assets and deficits. Are there commonalities among these children that could explain their disruptive behavior? As we have suggested previously, the orbital prefrontal cortex, amygdala, and anterior cingulate play an important role in emotion regulation. Orbital frontal damage has been associated with impulsive aggression and individuals who display violent behavior show hypometabolism (Pliszka, 2016). However, unlike ADHD, externalizing disorder has been associated with serotonergic dysfunction (Chang et al., 2017). In addition to the frontal lobes, medial temporal lobe and limbic structures have been associated with anger and aggression. The right hemisphere has also been associated with conduct problems. Studies of antisocial and violent populations using fMRI have found decreased right-hemispheric functioning (Raine, 2001). Delinquents frequently show verbal, spatial, and global IQ deficits, which may be related to the difficulties seen in these adolescents (Raine et al., 2002).

It is possible that the type of delinquency seen may be related to differential hemispheric functioning. Those delinquents with right-hemispheric deficits may show difficulty due to their limited social information-processing skills and may be more likely to show undersocialized conduct problems (Frick & Matlasz, 2018). Children with right-hemisphere CD would lack insight into their own behavior or the behavior of others; these children may be the type that fail to show remorse for their actions. In contrast, those with left-hemisphere dysfunction may have socialized conduct problems. They understand the nature of their acts and abide by antisocial norms. The distinction between undersocialized and socialized delinquency could reflect child- and adolescent-onset subtype differences, as only children with the right-hemisphere subtype are likely to display neuropsychological deficits (Sijtsema & Ojanen, 2018). Generally, academic underachievement is most frequently recognized when these children reach early adolescence.

But do these findings apply to children with right, left, and/or frontal dysfunction? As we've mentioned, frontal factors likely play a primary or an additive role, with further research needed to clarify this issue. As for right–left differences, it is possible that children with CD and right-hemisphere dysfunction show early social problems and then begin to fail their academic subjects because of the complexity of the curriculum and unstructured instruction? It is possible that failure in school becomes associated with CD in the left-hemisphere dysfunction group in adolescence because the CD follows the continued failure and alienation that results from language-based learning challenges. Could this be an explanation for undersocialized versus socialized CD? This certainly warrants further investigation, as the diagnostic and treatment implications would be profound. Differentiating between the direct and indirect effects of brain dysfunction remains a critical task for the practitioner, especially when one considers the transactional and dynamic interplay among the brain, behavior, and environment (Semrud-Clikeman & Ellison, 2009).

the causes or the results of CD remains to be seen, but the brain–behavior correlates of CD and ODD are beginning to be recognized.

Neuropsychopathology

Future research will need to explore the complex interaction of neural networks that run anterior to posterior, right to left, and inferior to superior. The relation of these neural networks to different types of neuropsychopathology is just beginning to be explored. Although the search for brain–behavior relationships in these populations will undoubtedly continue, it is important to recognize that behavioral outcome is always a result of the complex interaction of neuropsychological and environmental determinants, as it is with all of the disorders we have discussed. Neuropsychological assessment can play an important role in helping determine whether neuropsychological assets or deficits exist in children with different types of neuropsychopathology.

The next step is to try to use these neuropsychological findings to predict what treatment is appropriate for each child. The effects of that treatment then need to be evaluated. For instance, if counseling is warranted, could the neuropsychological characteristics affect a child's response to the therapist, the therapist–child relationship, or the therapeutic strategies implemented? The research presented here suggests that children will respond variably to the same therapeutic techniques, strategies, and behaviors during individual or group counseling. Because children with neuropsychological deficits are likely to display a wide variety of neuropsychological and socioemotional issues, using the CHT model during counseling will allow adjustment of the treatment orientation and strategies to better meet each child's unique therapeutic needs as you can see in Case Study 9.3

As we have repeated throughout this book, for neuropsychological principles to be effectively applied in school settings, you must recognize that the assessment, interpretation, report writing, and feedback session are merely the beginnings of a successful intervention. It is up to you to work collaboratively with others to ensure that your understanding of neuropsychological principles is translated into effective interventions for the children you serve. CHT involves testing hypotheses not only about a child's neuropsychological strengths and weaknesses, but also about intervention. Even if your initial problem-solving intervention is less than optimal, you can recycle it as necessary until you achieve an intervention that successfully helps a child overcome his or her deficits. Despite all the promise of neuropsychological principles, it is up to you as a scientist–practitioner to reach the ultimate goal, making sure you meet the unique needs of the children you serve. The following case study offers an example of a child with suspected ADHD complicated by anxiety.

Case Study 9.3. Getting Terry's Behavior under Stimulus Control

Terry was an 8-year-old boy who was seen initially for a prereferral intervention consultation after repeated physical altercations with his peers. When Terry was observed in the classroom, momentary time sampling made it clear that he was frequently inattentive to task materials or the teacher (off-task behavior 55%, vs. 15% for a control peer) and that his motor activity was high (60%, vs. 10% for the control peer). He had nine (impulsive) call-outs during a 20-minute block of instruction, whereas the control peer had none. However, functional analysis (done through observation and teacher data collection) revealed that Terry only engaged in inappropriate peer interactions when the other children were either standing around their desks or lining up to go to lunch, recess, or other out-of-class events. Typically, Terry would become very animated and excited at these times. He'd start showing increased body movement and gestures, and would begin talking in a loud voice. Then he would often bump into someone, or another child would bump into him. The subsequent verbal exchange would inevitably lead to a shoving match, and one time a fight broke out. In the subsequent interview and follow-up consultation with the teacher, we decided to use differential reinforcement of incompatible behavior (DRI) whenever the children had to line up in the classroom. The other incidents could (we hoped) be reduced by the use of teacher proximity and interference. For the DRI program, we taught Terry to put his hands in his pockets whenever he stood up to get in line. When the teacher gave the direction for the class to rise, she would tap on his desk, and he would put his hands in his pockets on his way to the line. Verbal praise was used as a reinforcer.

After 1 week, we met again. The event-recording data produced by the teacher suggested that Terry had learned the operant behavior, but was using it inconsistently in the classroom. The teacher said she thought he was not sufficiently motivated by the praise, so we added 5 minutes of computer time at the end of each day for each time Terry complied with the DRI behavior. Two weeks later, the teacher stopped me (Hale) in the hall, and we went to her room to look at the data. Some days Terry earned 15–20 minutes of computer time, yet other days he earned no time. The teacher was upset because she felt that Terry's inconsistent performance was related to home problems or that he was being oppositional, but in reality his variable performance was what I had expected all along. The subsequent neuropsychological evaluation, including measures of attention, working memory, and executive functions, revealed the telltale signs of dorsolateral and orbital dysfunction associated with the combined type of ADHD. After the parents and teacher were helped to understand the condition, and various treatment options were offered, Terry underwent a double-blind placebo-controlled medication trial of methylphenidate. After the trial, the physician decided to choose the best dose to optimize cognition, and thereafter the DRI procedure worked without a problem. Apparently Terry's executive functions needed to be maximized for him to respond consistently to the behavioral treatment. Because the "brain boss" was now online, he could now easily recognize the discriminative stimuli (teacher direction and tap on desk), and the reinforcer (praise or computer time) was highly effective.

ADHD with Anxiety Case Report

Case Report 9.1 illustrates the frequent co-occurrence of ADHD and anxiety. It provides a window into understanding how to work with children with both disorders. Anxiety can mask ADHD as well as the opposite (ADHD can look like anxiety) Therefore it is important to carefully evaluate both possible disorders to arrive at the best treatment for the child.

Case Report 9.1. Summary of Neuropsychological Evaluation

Name: Matt J

Reason for Evaluation

Matt J is a 11-year, 1-month-old right-handed boy who was referred to the Pediatric Neuropsychology Clinic by Dr. Y due to concerns related to attention functioning, difficulty switching between tasks, and becoming easily fatigued. Matt also has a history of difficulties with reading, writing, and mathematics skills. In addition, Matt displays anxious behaviors related to his school performance and being tested (particularly timed tests), as well as other situations (e.g., being alone in a room, spiders).

Relevant History

Family History

Matt lives in a large East coast city with his parents and his 4-year-old sister. There is an immediate family history of depression, anxiety, and attention difficulties. Matt was born at full-term with no significant difficulties with pregnancy. Matt's Apgar scores were 1 at one minute and 9 at five minutes. Hospital course after delivery was unremarkable.

Developmentally, Matt met his milestones within normal limits. Matt was evaluated at age 7 by an OT and PT and diagnosed with hypermobility, weak grip strength, and poor overall coordination and received services for 6 months.

School History

Matt has been tested in the past and his ability measures have indicated above average to superior ability, but he has struggled with learning particularly in mathematics as well as difficulty with inattention. He was diagnosed with ADHD: inattentive type at the age of 8. He is not currently on any medications His teacher reported Matt frequently appears "overwhelmed" by the assignments but does not ask for help because he doesn't want to "bother" the teacher. Matt's mother reported that he has become increasingly anxious about his performance and can become upset when tasks are very hard. During these times, he will disengage from the task and shut down. He is also fearful about being left alone in a room and sleeping in his own bed. He frequently sleeps next to the parent's bed. He is also very afraid of spiders and will refuse to go into any room that has had a spider until it has been full checked. Matt is currently receiving CBT with partial success. Socially, Matt has many friends.

Behavioral Observations

Initially Matt did not want to separate from his mother and was slow to warm up to the examiner. After approximately 10 minutes, his mother left the session and Matt was fine after the testing was explained to him. Matt engaged in conversation readily with the examiner and displayed appropriate eye contact. His affect varied according to topic and was appropriate to the testing situation. Although he appeared to be putting forth his best effort, as the session progressed, Matt became increasingly distractible. He also appeared to have difficulty managing his impulsive responses. On some tests he needed frequent prompting to wait until the directions were completed before starting the task.

Impressions

Matt J is a 11-year, 1-month-old right-handed boy who was seen in the Pediatric Neuropsychology Clinic due to concerns regarding attention functioning, anxious behaviors, and problems with mathematics and writing. Matt's current neuropsychological evaluation revealed wide variation in his performance on different types of cognitive tasks. Matt demonstrated significant strengths in his ability to identify verbal concepts and reason with words (KABC-II Knowledge = 120), as well as his visual reasoning ability (KABC-II Simultaneous = 122). Matt's profile suggests that he excels on tasks that require visual and verbal reasoning, but performs relatively weaker on tests that require him to process information very rapidly or to hold and retain complex sequences of information in memory. Matt continues to show superior skills in several areas. There were no areas in which he demonstrated a deficit relative to others his age. Similar to his superior cognitive ability, Matt's executive functioning was in the superior range for his age. His visual spatial and visual motor skills were in the average range for his age. His social skills were also found to be a strength for him and he was reported by his teachers to be imaginative, thoughtful, and likeable. This is a wonderful quality that will likely serve him well personally and in future academic and professional settings.

Matt's reading skills are at or slightly above grade level. In contrast, Matt struggled with tests of mathematics. He scored in the significantly below average for his age on tests of his calculation abilities, his ability to rapidly solve arithmetic problems (math fluency), and his applied mathematics skills. Taken together, these results indicate that Matt qualifies for a diagnosis of a developmental learning disability in mathematics, which is a specific learning disorder in mathematics.

Significant concerns related to attention and executive functioning were also apparent on testing. Matt has previously diagnosed with Attention-Deficit/Hyperactivity Disorder, Predominately Inattentive Type. We feel that Matt continues to display characteristics and behaviors consistent with this diagnosis. He will become overwhelmed when there is a lot going on (as he is very observant and aware), or "hyperfocused" on certain things and miss important aspects of an activity. Matt struggled on a lengthy task of attention. He struggled to maintain vigilance and respond to the targets when required, showed significant impulsive errors, and his performance was variable across the computerized test of attention. Matt scored within the average range on tasks of visual scanning and graphomotor speed, as well as a test of number sequencing. However, during a letter-sequencing task, Matt performed in the impaired range for his age. At one point in the task, he seemed to "space out" and had difficulty determining the next letter in the sequence. Similarly, when required to switch between two different sequences (i.e., numbers and letters), he again scored in the impaired range. Matt also had difficulty with a task requiring him to inhibit his responses. In line with these test results, Matt's mother and teacher both indicated clinically significant concerns regarding aspects of executive functioning, including Matt's ability to initiate tasks, hold information in mind while using it, and use successful planning and organizational strategies.

Regarding social–emotional functioning, results of neuropsychological testing indicate that *Matt's emotional health and academic performance are significantly impacted by anxiety*. Matt rated himself as having clinically significant symptoms of anxiety (e.g., he reported that he often worries, is afraid of a lot of things, is bothered by little things, gets nervous, is bothered by thoughts about death, and worries when he goes to bed at night). His responses also indicated that Matt may feel he has little control over what happens to him (e.g., feeling that he is often blamed for problems, that people get mad at him even when he does nothing wrong, or that things go wrong for him even when he tries hard). Matt also reported a highly negative attitude toward school, which may be the result of feeling that he is not able to achieve success and heightened levels of anxiety about his performance or about failing. Matt's anxiety is best described with the diagnosis **Unspecified Anxiety Disorder**. It should be noted that many individuals with significant anxiety also have problems with attention and concentration. However, based in Matt's history and test results, we feel that Matt's anxiety does not fully explain the difficulties that he has with attention. Importantly, Matt's difficulties with attention seem to have an onset prior to his symptoms of anxiety. According to parent report, Matt's anxiety has worsened in the past 1-2 years, a time frame subsequent to his original diagnosis of ADHD.

Recommendations

Emotional Functioning

1. It is recommended that Matt continue to work with a therapist trained in cognitive-behavioral therapy (CBT) to develop and practice strategies to manage his anxiety.
2. Matt may respond best when warned in advance of any expected changes in his daily schedule, and suggestions for appropriate behavior (including use of coping strategies) should be reviewed frequently with him, particularly prior to potentially problematic situations.
3. It is recommended that Matt's parents contact his school and share this report with them for a possible referral to a child study team for consideration for mathematics learning disability support as well as ADHD support.

Chapter 10

Neuropsychology of Chronic Medical Disorders

Is Medicine Relevant for the Practice of School Neuropsychology?

The school psychology field has a long history of leaders decrying the medical model in favor of ecological approaches for serving children (see Gutkin, 2012). We agree that a strict medical model approach in psychology has many limitations in addressing the systems-level changes we have advocated in this book. But to say this translates into a disavowal of the medical model and modern medical advances is a mistake. We know of a few school psychologists who avoid taking a thorough medical and developmental history from parents because they are only concerned with the child's "current" functioning due to perceived environmental causes for their behavior (i.e., behavioral orientation). This is a significant problem because a thorough medical history is worth its weight in gold in understanding a child's current functioning, which in turn can lead to appropriate assessment and intervention strategies. In fact, medical professionals, such as pediatricians, psychiatrists, and even neurologists, will base much of their diagnoses on a thorough history, not only of the symptoms presented, but what their patient experienced prior to the presenting problem for the day's visit.

In today's climate of brief medical care and quick school reintegration for children with medical conditions, physicians are counting more and more on teachers, psychologists, and allied professionals to do the work that was once done in hospitals or rehabilitation settings. In the recent past, it was not uncommon to hear school psychologists say things like "It's a medical problem, it isn't my responsibility," and "I don't know that, the physician will take care of it," but times have changed dramatically. The nature–nurture question, as you will recall from your Introductory Psychology course, led to the conclusion that both are important to consider. That conclusion remains relevant today, even with "environmental" problems such as posttraumatic stress disorder (PTSD) that lead to brain function changes that can affect attention memory, and emotion regulation (De Bellis et al., 2010; Wilson et al., 2011). As noted earlier, the environment can make brains better or worse, so plasticity is a double-edged sword worth your constant clinical consideration, and early intervention efforts. That is because some of the things we typically do for children with disabilities in schools actually work against brain development and instead potentially lead to lifelong disability (Hale et al., 2018). In fact, when we teach to a child's strengths, or provide classroom accommodations to "get around" the disability, neuroscience has taught us that while we may get these students through an assignment or test, we may be perpetuating their weaknesses, leading to potentially hardwired, lifelong disabilities (e.g., Koziol et al., 2013).

Of interest here is ADHD, one of the common childhood disorders, which you read about in Chapter 8. You may feel you have a good understanding of what true ADHD is, but what if the attention problems are not ADHD but rather problems associated with a medical condition? How do you know if a child's attention problem is due to a sleep disturbance, since sleep apnea can cause significant attention problems (Sedky et al., 2013). Maybe the attention problem is caused by a child's absence seizures (Vega et al., 2010) or the medications she is taking for her asthma (Saricoban et al., 2011), or the enduring effects of a concussion (called postconcussive syndrome, which we discuss later in the chapter) he experienced during a hockey game last month (Bigler, 2008). Case Study 10.2 highlights how we can easily be led astray using behavioral criteria alone to diagnose ADHD, especially the inattentive presentation, instead of understanding the relationship between what we observe and brain functioning.

Prevalence rates of school-age children with chronic medical disorders have skyrocketed in recent decades, with over 15 to 18% of children living with these conditions that affect their school functioning on a daily basis (Crump et al., 2013). There is a great need for practitioners to be aware of the neuropsychological effects of chronic medical conditions (Phelps et al., 2013). Unfortunately, few training programs offer graduate students sufficient education about these conditions, leading some to advocate advanced training in what has been termed *pediatric school psychology* (Barraclough & Machek, 2010; Shaw et al., 2011).

As the medical field has advanced, more children are surviving life-threatening conditions, and returning to school after illnesses once thought to be permanently disabling. Therefore, administrators, teachers, psychologists, allied professionals, and parents alike must increase their understanding of these conditions and adjust their efforts to meet the needs of affected children. School psychologists have become increasingly aware of the need to address the psychological, academic, behavioral, and adaptive challenges of children with chronic medical conditions. These can stem from many different causes, such as genetic mutation or traumatic injury. Interdisciplinary efforts are needed to help other school-based professionals and parents understand conditions and facilitate optimal communication and service delivery outcomes for affected children (Conroy & Logan, 2014; Sulkowski et al., 2011).

This chapter addresses how a school neuropsychological approach can optimize service delivery for these children to maximize adjustment to both the medical condition and classroom environment upon reintegration into school settings. Although an entire book could be written on this topic, we provide an overview of the most common conditions that are likely to affect learning and behavioral adjustment of children in classrooms, as listed on Table 10.1.

Neurodevelopmental Insults Affecting Neuropsychological Functioning

Prematurity, Low Birthweight, Neonatal Trauma

Children are surviving at ever younger gestational ages leading and many have extremely low birthweight or preterm histories that often lead to cognitive and emotional/behavioral consequences well beyond the child's medical stabilization. In addition to the medical complications associated with prematurity and low birthweight, these children are born with immature nervous systems that can lead to cerebral palsy, asthma, low intellectual and adaptive functioning, and executive, memory, and motor impairments (Taylor et al., 2006). Frequent attention, executive, working memory, visual–perceptual, social, internalizing, and learning problems are noted because of reduced white matter function and hippocampal volume (Anderson & Doyle, 2003; Skranes et al., 2007; Spittle et al., 2009). It should not be surprising that many of these children have learning and behavior problems, with about 40%

TABLE 10.1. Pediatric Medical Condition Symptoms and Associated Learning and Behavior Problems

Medical condition	Possible neuropsychological symptoms	Possible learning and behavior problems
Prematurity/low birthweight	• Inattention • Poor self-regulation • Social awareness, processing, and empathy • Poor motor skills	• ADHD:PI • Internalizing/tics • Separation anxiety • Low intelligence • Adjustment/adaptive • Graphomotor • Learning problems
Neonatal stroke	• Attention • Visual–spatial skills • Verbal and spatial memory • Problem solving, fluid reasoning, and cognitive flexibility • Processing speed	• Psychosocial adjustment • ADHD • Inattention • Apathy • Academic fluency • Math calculation and word problems
Cerebral palsy	• Seizure disorder • Learning and memory • Expressive language • Fine- and gross-motor skills, body posture • Divided and sustained attention • Working memory, set-shifting, and inhibitory control	• Psychosocial and socioemotional • Internalizing and externalizing psychopathology • Low global intellectual functioning • Reading comprehension • Handwriting and written expression • Math computation and word problems • Graphomotor
Neoplasms/brain tumors	• Hydrocephalus • Arousal and basic attention • Learning and memory • Frontal–subcortical and executive functions • Working memory, processing speed, response inhibition, sustained attention • Sequential and visual–spatial processing • Expressive language	• Cerebellar cognitive affective syndrome • ADHD • Other psychopathologies, depending on lesion location • Psychosocial adjustment • Word reading and reading comprehension • Oral and written expression • Math computation and word problems
Cancer and leukemia	• Working memory • Speed of information processing • Fine-motor skills • Poor inhibition	• Attention • Mathematics • Handwriting • Reading (comprehension)
Viral/bacterial encephalitis	• Attention and memory • Specific executive deficits, including problem solving, organization, and cognitive flexibility	• Attention and disinhibition • Aggression • Depression • Intellectual decline • Oral and written expression • Math computation and word problems
HIV/AIDS	• Verbal/visual perceptual • Executive functions such as mental flexibility, working memory, attention control, and processing speed	• Socioemotional, behavioral, and psychosomatic • ADHD • Conduct disorder • Anxiety and depressive symptoms • Intellectual and adaptive behavior decline • Reading, math, and/or writing learning disability *(continued)*

TABLE 10.1. (continued)

Lyme disease	• Persistent headache, confusion, and neuritis • Attention • Auditory and visual sequential processing • Fine-motor control • Planning, memory retrieval, mental flexibility, and processing speed	• Internalizing disorders (e.g., autism, or schizophrenia symptoms) • Externalizing disorders (less common) • Depressive symptoms • Oral and written expression • Academic fluency
Fetal alcohol spectrum disorder	• Growth retardation • White matter hypoplasia • Neurodevelopmental delays • Low arousal, increased activity, and slow habituation • Attention control, response inhibition, working memory • Planning and problem solving • Learning and memory, verbal retrieval • Visual–spatial • Psychomotor skills, reaction time, decision speed, fluency	• Poor social skills • ADHD • Emotionally dysregulation and irritability • Early-onset bipolar disorder • Depression/anxiety • Oppositional defiant/conduct disorder • Intellectual, academic (reading, writing, math), and adaptive disability common • Academic fluency • Graphomotor
Lead exposure	• Attention and sensory memory • Working memory (visual < auditory) • Verbal, visual, and fine motor	• Externalizing problems (e.g., ADHD and antisocial behavior) • Intellectual and achievement deficits • Graphomotor
Epilepsy	• Attention • Memory • Language (varies depending on type) • Fine motor (mostly for frontal) • Psychomotor speed (variable) • Planning, organization, mental flexibility, working memory, response inhibition	• ADHD (ADHD:PI more common) • Poor functional and psychosocial adaptation • Social skills • Lower educational and occupational attainment • Mood and anxiety disorders • Oral expression and memory encoding and/or retrieval • Reading, math, and/or writing disability
Concussion/mild traumatic brain injury	• Attention, concentration, and processing speed • Reaction time • Verbal memory • Hemispheric integration and bimanual control	• ADHD • Mood disorders • Oppositional/conduct disorder • Mood symptoms • Psychosocial adjustment • Academic fluency • Oral and written expression
Traumatic brain injury	• Diffuse axonal injury • Edema, intercranial pressure, and secondary injury • Frontal–subcortical circuit functioning • Fluid reasoning and most executive functions • Impulse control, self-regulation, empathy • Processing speed	• Socioemotional, and social competence • Secondary ADHD • Emotional lability, mood swings • Depression/anxiety • Oppositional/conduct disorder • Academic fluency • Oral and written expression • Math computation and word problems • Graphomotor

of these children exhibiting psychosocial concerns (Jantzie et al., 2008). Of the neuropsychiatric disorders identified, ADHD:PI is the most common, likely due to the reduction in white matter, including corpus callosum thinning observed in many of these children (Indredavik et al., 2005). Thus, these children are likely to have internalizing problems such as anxiety, depression, autism, and tic disorders (Indredavik et al., 2010) and if diagnosed with "comorbid" ADHD, they are less likely to respond to stimulant medications as a result (Hale et al., 2011).

Although these birth history complications are significant, birth traumas such as lack of oxygen (anoxia) or neonatal stroke (cerebral vascular accidents or infarcts) can lead to widespread diffuse cortical dysfunction. Even though forceps delivery is no longer used, there are complications with its replacement (vacuum assist), which can also lead to brain trauma (Elvander & Cnittigius, 2015). This is because the bony plates of our skull (i.e., meninges) are not fused at birth, which can lead to brain tissue damage during a traumatic birth. In the case of a stroke, there may be impairment on verbal and spatial memory, visual–spatial skills, problem solving, and cognitive flexibility measures (Max, 2004). Selective attention, sustained attention, attention orientation, and processing speed concerns are common and may suggest ADHD and math disability (Max, 2004) A commonly recognized manifestation is cerebral palsy, which has many possible causes, including intracranial hemorrhage, genetic abnormalities, birth trauma/anoxia, low birthweight, maternal infections, or prematurity (Bottcher et al., 2009). Cerebral palsy can also be caused by traumatic brain injury (accidental or abuse-related, e.g., shaken baby syndrome) or brain infection (Straub & Obrzut, 2009). Thus, if a child is diagnosed with cerebral palsy, brain damage has occurred. Upon noting this diagnosis, the astute school neuropsychology practitioner must subsequently delve into the medical records, including neuroimaging, to see the potential impact of the brain damage that is occurent on the child's present academic and behavioral functioning.

Cerebral palsy causes more than motor impairments or medical problems, with approximately 80% of affected children also showing significant cognitive, academic, and/or behavioral problems (Odding et al., 2006). It can lead to deficits in attention, set-shifting, working memory, inhibitory control, language, and academic deficits, especially in math and written language (Bottcher et al., 2009; Jenks et al., 2009). ADHD and internalizing and externalizing symptoms have been found in this population, so careful analysis of psychosocial functioning is required (Sipal et al., 2009). While some children with prematurity, low birthweight, neonatal stroke, or cerebral palsy may have only motor impairments, the likelihood of multiple academic and psychosocial impairments is likely.

Neoplasms/Brain Tumors

How do you know if a child has a brain tumor? Many people might think there are telltale signs, such as severe headache or seizures, or that the medical doctor will pick it up during a regular physical exam, but this often not the case. Tumors can grow for some time before overt symptoms appear, and valuable treatment time can be lost, which can lead to a poorer response to treatment and poorer overall prognosis. School psychologists are like the battlefield medics who must triage their children, keeping in the back of their mind that the problem presented may be a symptom of a much more serious condition. Being on the "front line" of medical care means careful attention to history and changes in the child's status to see if further evaluation and/or referral is necessary. That can't be done when operating from a strict behavioral orientation, which attributes all problems to the environment. The lesson here is that it is essential that school-based practitioners and outpatient neuropsychologists catch the "red flags," hopefully before there are clear signs of a tumor, so treatment can begin, as suggested in Case Study 10.1.

Case Study 10.1. A Mistaken Diagnosis

Ethan was referred for evaluation due to a significant deterioration in cognitive, academic, and behavioral functioning. His parents requested the neuropsychological evaluation after the school psychologist decided the boy only needed a reading and math CBM at his 3-year re-evaluation, and no further testing was needed even though the boy's grades had dropped dramatically from the B to C range to the C to D range. The school psychologist decided it was his lack of motivation, noncompliant behavior, and parent–child conflict that was causing the deterioration, and recommended a behavior plan.

In conducting the CHT evaluation, a significant drop in his academic and cognitive scores (up to 30 points in some cases) and increased behavioral problems (clinical range aggression, conduct, and executive problems) were found. In addition, CHT evaluation showed some focal signs (deterioration of receptive language and right-hand sensory perception and motor control). Prior to the scheduled feedback session, Ethan had a grand mal seizure and a neurology consult was obtained. Neuroimaging revealed a brain tumor (grade II glioma) in the left posterior region, and following surgery and treatment he made a good recovery. Precious time had been lost since the school psychologist concluded Ethan had a "behavior problem." The persistence of his parents in obtaining help for him coupled with prompt medical treatment saved this child and prevented further brain damage.

Childhood Cancer

Pediatric cancers are the most common cause of death in children ages 5 to 16. One out of 8 children with cancer do not survive (Stone et al., 2017). Of the children who do survive, around 60% suffer from late effects from the treatment (Ward et al., 2014). Cancer is a genetic disease caused by DNA changes and altered gene expression and results in uncontrolled cell growth (Vogelstein & Kinzler, 2015). These cells expand and develop vascular support to feed them and allow the cells to spread. Infectious agents can also increase the likelihood of cancer with about 15–20% of cancers associated with viruses (Fernandez & Esteller, 2010). Obesity is another risk factor for adults and children. Recent research has linked an increased risk for obesity in adults who were treated for cancer in childhood (Wilson et al., 2015). Chemotherapy has increased the survival from childhood cancer to an 80% 5-year survival rate and now approaching a 90% cure rate (Lam et al., 2019). As a result, those who undergo medical treatment for cancer may have lingering effects of chemotherapy and/or radiation, which is sometimes reported as "chemo brain" or "chemo fog." Symptoms include attention, concentration, memory, retrieval, confusion, fatigue, and slow processing speed.

Medulloblastomas, astrocytomas, gliomas, medulloblastomas, and ependymomas are not very common in children, but they do occur, with an incidence of about 4 cases per 100,000 children (McKean-Cowdin et al., 2013). The effects, as noted in Case Study 10.1, can be significant, not only due to the tumor's direct effects on brain tissue, but also as a result of radiation and chemotherapy, which can lead to considerable executive dysfunction (Mulhern & Butler, 2004). Of particular note are posterior tumors around the cerebellum, which can lead to a blockage of the cerebral aqueduct (i.e., aqueductal stenosis) and obstructive hydrocephalus. This occurs because there is a very small path between the third and fourth ventricles of the brain. If damage occurs to the cerebellar vermis, then attention, executive, automaticity, and psychosocial problems may result in a condition called *cerebellar cognitive affective syndrome* (CCAS; Levisohn et al., 2000). There are many risk factors for pediatric cancer, including exposure to diagnostic X-rays, genetic syndromes, and high birthweight (Tikellis et al., 2018).

Specific cognitive functions often show difficulty and increase over time, including attention, spatial–holistic processing, working memory, and processing speed deficits (Briere et al., 2008). White matter (e.g., roads and highways) degradation is often the likely cause, which can lead to problems with new learning, abstract thinking, sustained attention, response inhibition (Stone et al., 2017), and lower social competence (Ross et al., 2003). These effects often do not show up until later in life for the younger child and as such the child is said to "grow into the deficit." For example, a child of 3 is not yet expected to show significant executive functioning in the area of working memory, planning, and organization. As the child matures, he or she will be expected to develop these skills. These children with late effects of treatment will now encounter difficulty not seen previously.

Leukemia

Childhood acute lymphoblastic leukemia (ALL) is a cancer where the bone marrow makes too many lymphocytes (white blood cell type) (*www.cancer.gov/types/leukemia/patient/child-all-treatment-pdq*). It can also affect other white, as well as red, blood cells and platelets. This cancer of the blood and bone marrow will quickly worsen if not treated. Similar to other cancers, risk factors include being exposed to X-rays prior to birth, being exposed to radiation, past treatment with chemotherapies, and certain genetic conditions (e.g., Down syndrome, neurofibromatosis type 1, Fanconi anemia). The initial signs of leukemia include fever, easy bruising or bleeding, dark-red spots under the skin caused by bleeding, bone and joint pain, lumps in the neck, underarm, stomach or groin, weakness, and loss of appetite. It is diagnosed through blood counts, bone marrow biopsy, and a lumbar puncture, so catching these symptoms early could be important for further medical care. There are three risk groups in childhood ALL that affect treatment:

1. Standard risk (low): ages 1 to 10 with a white blood cell count that is moderately elevated
2. High risk: ages 10 and older or who have a very high white blood cell count
3. Very high risk: children younger than 1 who have a slow response to initial treatment and who show continuing signs of leukemia after 1 month of treatment

Approximately 4,000 cases of childhood ALL are diagnosed every year in the United States. It is the most common cancer in children and adolescents, with a cure rate at approximately 80% (Dores et al., 2012). In contrast, adult recovery from ALL is much poorer with cure rates less than 40% (Katz et al., 2015). A sizable number of minority of children do not have access to good medical care and thus do not have good outcomes. In the past, males were more likely to have poor ALL survival rates, but this is no longer the case with improvements in treatment (McKean-Cowdin et al., 2013).

Treatment for ALL is directed by the phenotype, genotype, and risk factors. Children with a mature B-cell ALL are treated with short-term intensive chemotherapy. (A mature B cell is a specific type of white blood cell that is necessary to fight off infections; Pui, Sandlund, et al., 2004). This type of ALL is also called Burkitt ALL and is fairly rare.

For patients with T-cell ALL, the thymus is enlarged. This type of ALL is more common and treated with remission-induction therapy, which eradicates almost 99% of the leukemia cells. It includes the use of a glucocorticoid (prednisone, prednisolone, or dexamethasone), vincristine, and one other agent. Those children in the high-risk category often receive four or more drugs and the remission rate is approximately 98% for these children (Pui & Evans, 2006). Children in remission are then treated with a high dose of methotrexate with additional medications and more than one regimen may be used in those children in the high- and very high-risk categories to ensure complete recovery physically (Schrappe et al., 2000). Bone marrow transplantation can be used with some children who are in the very high-risk category or who do not respond well to treatment (Sanders et al., 2005).

Similar to other childhood cancers, there are late effects from the treatment. Generally, these include problems with memory, attention, processing speed, planning, and working memory (Hearps et al., 2017). Deficits are also frequently seen on measures of intelligence with lower scores for the Full Scale IQ, Verbal IQ, and less difficulty, although still significant on the PIQ (Iyer et al., 2015). This study also found that Digit Span forward and backward, information processing speed, fine-motor functioning, and verbal memory were significantly affected. No significant difficulty was found in this review on measures of visual–motor integration or on the ability to plan, organize, and sequence information. Because this was a retrospective study, it is not possible to conclude long-term effects of treatment from these results. Similarly, van der Plas et al. (2018) found difficulties with working memory and response inhibition, particularly with the WISC-IV Working Memory and Processing Speed Indices and the Delis–Kaplan Trails Making Test. These findings suggest that developing an IEP or interventions requires attention to continuing problems with working memory, processing speed, and memory, as well as mild difficulties with attention. It is important that psychologists provide this information to teachers as the child may look like they have recovered from their disease, but still have difficulties with attention and executive function. Thus, executive deficits can affect many academic functions, especially reading comprehension, written expression, and applied math problems (as discussed in Chapters 5, 6, and 7).

Infectious Diseases and Neurotoxins

Infectious Diseases

Common infectious diseases that have meaningful neuropsychological, academic, and behavioral implications include encephalitis (e.g., meningitis), perinatally acquired HIV/AIDS, and Lyme disease. You might be surprised to learn that there are about 16 cases of encephalitis per 100,000 children, with rates even higher in developing countries (Starza-Smith et al., 2007). There are many infectious causes of this brain inflammation condition, including viral (69%) and bacterial (20%) causes (Ebaugh, 2007). Encephalitis typically leads to fever, headache, and focal neurological signs from the infection, but hypoxic-ischemic, inflammatory, metabolic, or seizure-related damage can occur secondary to the infection (Carter et al., 2003). In one study, over 90% of infected children demonstrated "considerable" cognitive deficits, most of which were executive impairments (Starza-Smith et al., 2007). Of these deficits, planning, goal setting, organizational skills, visual problem solving, psychomotor speed, and academic difficulties are most common (Anderson, Anderson, et al., 2004; Koomen et al., 2004). Viral encephalitis can lead to problems with attention, inhibition, aggression, and/or depression (Kneen & Solomon, 2008), whereas bacterial encephalitis is associated with learning, organization, problem solving, cognitive flexibility, and language deficits (Grimwood et al., 2000).

We turn to two key examples of viral and bacterial infection: HIV and Lyme disease. Children exposed to human immunodeficiency virus (HIV) and acquired immune deficiency syndrome (AIDS) have considerable neuropsychological, academic, and behavioral problems, even if the child does not have full-blown AIDS (Hochhauser et al., 2008). HIV-related progressive viral encephalitis has been associated with intellectual and developmental deficits and cerebral atrophy (Wood et al., 2009). These children experience deficits in verbal–visual perceptual skills, mental flexibility, working memory, attentional control, and processing speed, often leading to SLD, emotional, and behavior problems, with a large proportion of patients (between one-third and two-thirds) experiencing significant psychosocial disturbance (Hazra et al., 2010; Wood et al., 2009). This likelihood is decreased with successful antiviral treatment regimens, but the symptoms persist in poor responders to treatment. In addition, while survival is common now, there can be psychosocial concerns leading to poor overall adjustment to living with this chronic medical condition, so mental health support is needed. As with other medical disorders, treatment compliance can be a struggle for some individuals living with AIDS (Havens et al., 2016), and cognitive-behavioral therapy approaches have been shown to be useful in addressing this concern (Havens et al., 2016).

If the family likes to go hiking in the woods, then Lyme disease is a significant concern, especially in areas that have deer populations. It is a common tick-borne bacterial disease of particular interest given its frequency in children, with approximately 20,000 cases reported annually in the United States alone (McAuliffe et al., 2008). In addition to a "bulls-eye" rash, symptoms include persistent fever, headache, joint pain, nausea, vomiting, confusion, lability, and neuritis. A secondary inflammatory response or neurotoxin release can cause additional neurological impairment (McAuliffe et al., 2008). Although long-term effects are controversial, reports of associated neuropsychological deficits are common, particularly when encephalitis is present (Cairns & Godwin, 2005). Poorer performance on attention, auditory and visual sequential processing, memory retrieval, processing speed, fine-motor control, and spatial planning/mental flexibility measures have been noted (Cameron, 2010). Internalizing disorders, such as depressive symptoms of anhedonia and lethargy, can be expected, but some children have autism- or schizophrenia-like reactions (Marzillier, 2009). Meta-analyses suggest these symptoms can persist well beyond the initial exposure and subsequent antibiotic treatment (Cairns & Godwin, 2005).

Neurotoxins

Toxins are all around us, many of which cannot be easily recognized by our senses. Concern over exposure to teratogens (any agent that can cause brain damage) has led to many changes in prenatal and postnatal care of children. Neurotoxins can result in frontal–subcortical circuit dysfunction at any time during brain maturation, not just prenatally. Prenatal exposure is especially problematic because teratogenic substances ingested by the mother can cross the blood–brain barrier, exposing the fetus. Alcohol and lead exposure are common causes of neurotoxin disability, but there are many agents that can lead to disability. If exposure to a teratogen is reported or suspected, it is a good strategy to research the potential effects online to review articles and textbooks on the cognitive and other effects of exposure.

Alcohol Exposure

Fetal alcohol spectrum disorder (FASD) is caused by the mother's alcohol intake during pregnancy. Considering alcohol intake is especially important for women who may be having unprotected sexual intercourse and have irregular periods. A mother interviewed by one of the authors (J. B. H.) reported that she drank heavily until she found out she was pregnant, then she "stopped immediately." But she had been pregnant for almost 2 months before she was tested. (She thought she had just missed her period.) The fetus had been exposed to alcohol for nearly 2 months during a crucial gestational period. FASD occurs in approximately 1 out of every 1,000 births, and this number balloons with fetal alcohol effects (FAE; exposure not great enough to lead to facial dysmorphic features), making this a true spectrum disorder. School-age population prevalence rates may be as high as 2–5% of children (Lange et al., 2017). Alcohol exposure in utero often leads to prenatal and/or postnatal growth retardation, intellectual and academic disability, neurodevelopmental delays, and neuropsychiatric disorders, even when facial dysmorphic features (found in severe cases) are not present (Mattson et al., 2011).

Frontal–subcortical circuit impairment typical in FASD leads to poor attention control, response inhibition, working memory, decision speed, reaction time, psychomotor skills, planning, problem solving, fluency, and set-shifting (Mattson et al., 2011) that lead to poorer social skills and greater behavioral impairment (Schonfeld et al., 2006). Given that the hippocampus appears to be particularly vulnerable, learning and memory are often impaired in FASD (Mattson et al., 2011). Reduced cingulate volume in addition to global white matter

Case Study 10.2. Inattention and School Performance

Zane was an 8-year, 2-month-old boy who had a long history of language and attention problems. A psychoeducational evaluation revealed poor DAS-II Verbal Ability scores only, reading and math achievement deficits relative to DAS-II Nonverbal Ability and Spatial Ability scores (also diagnostic subtests) were within normal limits as were speech and language delays on the Comprehensive Evaluation of Language Fundamentals—Fifth Edition (CELF-5). Graphomotor skills on the VMI were also poor. The teacher reported inattentive, distractible, and daydreaming behavior in the classroom, and difficulty following oral directions and completing tasks. Zane was diagnosed with ADHD:PI, specific learning disability, developmental coordination disorder, and a language disorder. Despite some improvement with the speech, language, and occupational therapy interventions, classroom progress was slow and stimulant medication treatment was unsuccessful.

Zane was subsequently referred for a comprehensive school neuropsychology evaluation. First, his profile was reviewed and the types of problems we would expect to see if he had ADHD were not present. (Other than Digits Forward, his working memory and processing speed were adequate.) He was not hyperactive or impulsive, but he was in the clinical range for the BASC-2 Inattention subscale. The teacher interview was conducted and Zane was observed in his classroom. The functional analysis revealed Zane had more difficulty with on-task behavior when there was whole- or small-group instruction, especially when it was verbal in nature. In contrast, he was mostly on-task and engaged during individual instruction or seat work. The observation also showed some strange facial expressions that might be tics. Next, this evaluation found results fairly similar to the earlier evaluation, but no sign of executive problems consistent with ADHD. A more fine-grained analysis of his processing weaknesses during hypothesis testing was conducted. Phonological processing was fairly good, but auditory–sequential and language skills appeared weak, and he struggled with long-term memory storage. The problem seemed more related to integration than to specific processes, especially for language functions, with peculiar oromotor difficulties inconsistently found during oral expression. He had a lot of saliva and drooling on occasion, and the facial twitching made a diagnosis of tic disorder or a possible seizure disorder as hypotheses. A parent report about sleep patterns indicated that Zane had difficulty sleeping with some unusual facial expressions when he was "restless," but he didn't show any other signs of a tic disorder.

A referral for an EEG evaluation was made and Zane was diagnosed with benign rolandic epilepsy, which fit well with the symptoms observed. Clearly, Zane did not have the type of ADHD that would respond to stimulant medication. Although most cases of benign rolandic epilepsy resolve by adulthood, the lingering effects of cognitive, academic, and/or behavioral deficits may persist, so luckily his neurologist treated him with levetiracetam—a seizure medication. This combined with other interventions already in place started to turn Zane around, and improvements were made in all areas of functioning.

hypoplasia appear to add to the disruptive, inattentive, and emotionally dysregulated behavioral profiles seen in this population (Bjorkquist et al., 2010). In their FASD review, O'Connor and Paley (2009) reported that irritability, inattention, slow habituation, low arousal, emotional activity, and hyperactivity were often present, but reported no consistent finding regarding internalizing or externalizing disorders, with mood, anxiety, ADHD, ODD, and CD problems. An additional difficulty these children face is the failure to consider different approaches to a problem as a result of poor cognitive flexibility and difficulty with shifting or switching mental sets.

Functional connectivity (i.e., white matter functioning) has also been found to be deficient in children with FASD. Global efficiency was found to be compromised in children with FASD with controls that suggested decreased network connectivity particularly for integrative cognitive functioning (Wozniak et al., 2011, 2013). Children with FASD were also found to show thinner cortical thickness in the frontal, temporal, and parietal regions. Disruption in white matter is also associated with cognitive dysfunction particularly the inability to learn from experience, poor perceptual organization, limited processing speed, and visual–motor coordination deficits (Spottiswoode et al., 2011; Wozniak et al., 2009). These are important findings because functional connectivity is a measure of distributed brain function that allows the brain to communicate with itself. It also involves the default mode network (described in Chapters 8 and 9), which is important for memory consolidation and planning (Raichle & Snyder, 2007). For children, this network is often not connected front to back and right to left. As typical children mature, these connections are strengthened and by adulthood the system is well distributed throughout the brain (Fair et al., 2008). These networks are disrupted in children with FASD resulting in significant difficulty with executive functioning, learning, and problem solving.

Lead Exposure

The older standard of 10 pg/dl previously set by the Centers for Disease Control and Prevention yielded an incidence of only 1% of children with unacceptable levels of lead in their blood. By contrast, the newer levels of 5 pg/dl yield an incidence rate of 2.6% or 535,000 children under the age of 5 having blood levels at unacceptable ranges. Some researchers have concluded that any lead exposure is detrimental (Castro et al., 2019). High lead levels clearly lead to deficits in learning and behavior as well as difficulty with global intelligence, sustained attention, response inhibition, verbal, visual–motor, short-term memory, and fine-motor skills deficits (Ris et al., 2004). Even low-level lead exposure can lead to deficits in intelligence, achievement, attention, and working memory, and externalizing ADHD and antisocial behavior (Bellinger, 2008), but findings are controversial.

Neuropsychology of Epilepsy

Epilepsy represents a diverse neurological condition associated with several underlying causes, with different cognitive, academic, adaptive, and psychosocial characteristics. Even "benign" epilepsies (e.g., benign rolandic epilepsy, childhood absence epilepsy) are known to be associated with neuropsychological deficits (e.g., attention problems, memory impairment, language deficits) as well as psychosocial problems (Lee et al., 2000). For an example, see Case Study 10.2, earlier in the chapter. There are many characteristics associated with epilepsy, including frequency and duration of epileptic seizures. The outcomes and quality of life for the child can vary, depending on multiple drug therapy, overall adaptive functioning, psychosocial functioning, and parental adjustment (Sillanpaa et al., 2004). This suggests that neuropsychological evaluations must address cognitive, adaptive, academic, behavioral, and personality factors.

Types of Epilepsy

The International League Against Epilepsy (ILAE) classifies seizure into two types: *focal* and *generalized* seizures with known or unknown onset (Fisher et al., 2017). Focal seizures originate within one hemisphere and within that hemisphere can be localized or distributed. Focal seizures are further characterized by the level of awareness present during the seizure as well as motor symptoms such as automatisms (i.e., smacking the lips), clonic (jerking of limbs), tonic (stiffening of limbs), spasms, jerking, or loss of muscle tone (atonic). Nonmotor seizures will show autonomic symptoms (drooling, gastrointestinal sensations, goosebumps etc.), stopping in the middle of an activity, and cognitive (deficits in talking, thinking, hallucinations), emotional (fear, anxiety, anger, etc.) or sensory dysfunction (smelling items not present, seeing things, hearing things, etc.). The new classification of a *focal aware seizure* corresponds to the previous term *simple partial seizure,* while a *focal-impaired awareness seizure* is synonymous with the older term *complex partial seizure.*

Generalized seizures begin in the brain and quickly spread throughout brain networks. Generalized seizures involve many brain networks from the beginning of the seizure, while focal seizures can extend into generalized seizures. There is impaired awareness from the beginning of a generalized seizure. The main division for generalized seizures is *motor* or *nonmotor* seizures.

Motor seizures include the *generalized tonic–clonic seizure,* which was classified as a grand mal seizure in the past and *myoclonic*. Myoclonic seizures occur prior to the tonic–clonic seizures with awareness lost prior to the tonic–clonic seizure's beginning. Myoclonic seizures are generally briefer and often occur in children with genetic disorders (Berth & Kossof, 2019). With myocolonic seizures, the child loses muscle tone, particularly in the leg, and will fall backward onto the buttocks or forward. In contrast, tonic–clonic seizures cause the child to fall backward on his/her back. Generalized clonic seizures begin and end with sustained bilateral jerking of limbs as well as jerking of the head and neck. These seizures are less common than tonic–clonic seizures and generally occur with infants (Fisher et al., 2017). Generalized tonic seizures are characterized by bilateral limb stiffness as well as neck stiffening. Frequently during this type of seizure, the child shows abnormal posture. *Epileptic spasms* (previously called "infantile spasms") occur in infancy. These seizures present as a sudden flexion, extension, or extension–flexion of the chest and back.

Absence seizures would be classified as nonmotor seizures, and these were classified previously as petit mal seizures. These are seizures where there is no motor movement as the child stops an activity without awareness. Absence seizures can happen frequently, even several times a minute and for brief durations. As a result, absence seizures can appear to be brief lapses of attention and mislabeled as inattentiveness, as the child appears to be staring blankly ahead. The major difference between an ADHD-like inattentiveness and absence seizure is that the child is not aware of the environment during an absence seizure. If you snap your fingers in front of a child with an absence seizure, there will be no response. Although rare, some absence seizures can present with changes in tone and these are seen as atypical absence seizures. A myoclonic type of absence seizure is characterized by rhythmic three per second movements with the upper limbs gradually moving upward. Impairment of consciousness may not be present in these seizures. These seizures can also present as jerks of the eyelids and/or an upward movement of the eyes. They can be present when the child closes his or her eyes or if light is suddenly present.

A final type of classification is whether the onset of the seizure activity is known or unknown. When seizures occur with an unknown onset, they can be motor or nonmotor. These are most often seen with tonic–clonic seizures where it is unknown when the child experienced the first seizure. As is the case with other medical conditions, it is worth your effort to do research on the particular seizure disorder and try to understand the location(s) of the seizure activity from the neurological report. This can provide you with information on the impact the seizures have on learning and behavior. For instance, even "benign rolandic epilepsy" (sometimes called Childhood Epilepsy with Centrotemporal Spikes) can impair memory and phonological processing, which can affect both reading and spelling (Northcott et al., 2005).

Comorbidity of ADHD

ADHD is about five times more common in children with epilepsy, with the predominately inattentive presentation being much more common than the combined presentation (Hermann et al., 2007). This is the opposite pattern found in typical ADHD samples. Interestingly, symptoms of ADHD are seen in a vast majority of children *before* the onset of their seizures (Hermann et al., 2007). Children with ADHD and epilepsy show executive deficits in motor/psychomotor speed and response inhibition, mental flexibility, and working memory leading to poorer school performance (Hoie et al., 2006). Unilateral frontal lobe epilepsy appears to affect selective attention tasks (e.g., mediating executive functions and motor planning) but not global intellectual functioning or verbal/nonverbal memory (Riva et al., 2005), while the profile is the opposite with temporal lobe epilepsy (Culhane-Sjelburne et al., 2002). Early age of seizure onset, greater frequency of seizure activity, and poor response to anti-seizure medications are significant predictors of executive deficits (Hoie, Mykletun, et al., 2006).

Children with epilepsy may also have mood disorders, such as those found in temporal lobe personality disorder, which was examined in previous chapters, but few with these mental health issues receive proper treatment (Caplan et al., 2005). Approximately 12% of children with motor focal seizures can have either depression or anxiety, while 13% with absence epilepsy have depression or anxiety (Ott et al., 2001). Girls with epilepsy are more likely to report depression than boys. If the frequency of seizures is high, more severe affective problems may be evident, especially in children with intellectual disabilities (Mula, 2018). Finally, children with epilepsy may also experience social skills difficulties and self-esteem issues because of their condition (Hamiwka et al., 2011), especially if seizures are not controlled and regularly lead to loss of school time or social time with peers. Education of teachers and peers is crucial to head off misinformation about, or maltreatment of, a child with epilepsy. Children with epilepsy are more likely to be bullied than other children (Hamiwka & Wirrell, 2009), so it is crucial that educators be aware of this potential and hopefully head off the behavior before it emerges.

The neuropsychological approach must not only examine the child, but the family as well, given the impact this chronic medical condition has on all family members. Again, epilepsy severity, medical requirements, child and family restrictions, family coping skills, and available financial and psychosocial resources all contribute to family impact (Camfield et al., 2001). Depression and other psychiatric problems are often evident in family members that are poorly adjusted, suggesting that psychological support is needed not only for the child with epilepsy, but potentially for other family members as well (Ferro & Speechley, 2009).

Acquired Brain Injuries Affecting Neuropsychological Functioning

We feel that acquired brain injuries have been generally neglected in school psychology (and even medical) practice, despite their disturbingly high prevalence. As a result, we pay considerable attention here to the neuropsychological issues and services for this medical condition.

Concussion/Mild Traumatic Brain Injury

In the past, concussions were not seen as significant events in a child or adolescent's life. We now know that they can have an effect on the child and the child's development. Frequently, school personnel see these children or adolescents once they have recovered sufficiently to return to school. It is, therefore, important to discuss concussions from a neuropsychological point of view with an eye toward assessment and intervention. Children as young as 3 years participate in sports and the effect of concussion at this young age is currently unknown. Approximately 20% of children and adolescents who are admitted to a hospital have a TBI or concussion. There are many who are not seen in the emergency department and the incidence may be higher (Thurman, 2014).

There is a popular myth still around today that "all children fall and hit their heads," so recovery is complete and inconsequential, but, in reality, there is no such thing as a *good* head injury (Hale, Metro, et al., 2010). Concussions occur when there is a blow to the head which disrupts normal brain cellular activity, a process which is termed a *neurometabolic cascade* (McCrea, 2013). This cascade results in clinical symptoms of headache, dizziness, confusion, concentration problems, nausea, and problems with light sensitivity. In addition, problems with irritability and mood can be seen. Cognitively, the child experiences problems with memory, attention, reaction time, and processing speed and may either sleep too little or too much. It has been found that high school football players received an average of 652 hits to the head in excess of 15g of force (Broglio et al., 2011). Breedlove et al. (2012) found that subconcussive hits had a substantial impact on cognitive functioning and brain physiology was altered by the repeated exposure to these blows. Thus, repeated blows to the brain, whether a concussion was experienced or not, can alter the neurophysiology of the brain and thus change neuropsychological functioning (Prins & Giza, 2011).

An object (e.g., thrown baseball, rock, or even a hard punch) striking the head is a *coup injury*. When a moving child's head hits a stationary object, that is a *coup-contre coup* or *acceleration–deceleration injury*, for example, hitting one's head on the ground after falling off a bike, there may be subtle or even significant brain damage associated with it. While the brain is plastic and can recover quickly without apparent long-term effect, do not assume that mild traumatic brain injury occurs without *any* consequence. Otherwise, this may lead you to dismiss subtle signs and symptoms of dysfunction (DeMatteo et al., 2010). These subtle, persistent signs of brain injury may lead to a diagnosis of postconcussive syndrome (PCS). PCS can lead to behavioral dysfunction or even psychopathology (Gerring et al., 2009) if left unrecognized or untreated. PCS has been recognized in athletes who engage in contact sports, with some, like football players, who experience repeated concussions showing more significant neuropsychological and psychiatric problems (Broshek et al., 2014) that likely have a neurophysiological basis (Breedlove et al., 2012). Those with PCS are more likely to experience retrograde amnesia, difficulty concentrating, disorientation, insomnia, loss of balance, and sensitivity to light or noise (Kerr et al., 2018), thus coordination between medical and educational professionals becomes crucial in the recovery process (Ellis et al., 2016).

Educators need to be aware of the signs and symptoms of a concussion and take them seriously. Key signals include problems with paying attention (particularly if this was not a problem previously), problems learning or remembering new material, inappropriate or impulsive behavior, greater irritability, problems with organization, fatigue in class, and headaches (Master et al., 2012).

While much of the research on concussions has been conducted with older adolescents or adults, there is a burgeoning amount of information about concussions at younger ages. Working with younger children with concussions can be challenging due to the rapidly changing brain and the child's developmental stage. Support for parents and school personnel is crucial, particularly ensuring that all involved are properly educated about concussion. Gather information about the injury characteristics and history variables to determine what measures are best suited for the particular child. For instance, as we've mentioned, a child with significant ADHD is at higher risk for head injury than a child without it (Semrud-Clikeman, 2001). Age has also been seen to play a role in recovery with younger athletes/children taking significantly longer to recover than collegiate athletes (Ganesalingam et al., 2011).

Many of the concussion symptoms improve after the first 7 days but approximately 10% of patients with concussions will require more than 7 days for recovery while an additional 5% will take more than 45 days (McCrea et al., 2013). Along with improved cognitive functioning, fMRI has found that recovery in connectivity improves by 7 weeks (McCrea et al., 2010). Repeated injury will extend physiological recovery by at least 15 days and likely longer (McCrea et al., 2013). Higher risk is found for concussions that occur at younger ages, and recurrent concussions, including a history of multiple concussions particularly within 10 days of the initial concussion (Giza et al., 2013). Case Study 10.3 illustrates a case of a concussion.

Neuropsychological Assessment of Concussion

Experts in the field have strongly suggested that patients be assessed using concussion scales and neuropsychological testing (Echemendia et al., 2013; Gosselin et al., 2010) to examine the initial impact of concussion and return to play guidelines. Neuropsychological testing consists of measurement of memory performance, reaction time, processing speed, and attention. We also recommend that balance and sensory organization be assessed to test physiological functioning (Giza et al., 2013).

An integrated recovery model has been proposed that links concussions to acute, postacute, and full recovery (McCrea, 2013). In this model the acute symptoms are functionally impairing and there is neurocognitive as well as physiological dysfunction present (balance, light sensitivity, etc.). During the postacute phase, there is generally full clinical recovery but persistent physiological dysfunction. This phase occurs within 7 days of the original injury and frequently the patient returns to play and is at higher risk for a repeat concussion. Full recovery is only present when both cognitive and physiological symptoms resolve. Adolescent girls show the most pronounced effects when cognitive exertion is required (Broshek et al., 2012). Thus, girls may show more vulnerability to these effects compared to boys, particularly in adolescence (Gioia, 2013).

These are important findings because school is the child's work. Cognitive exertion is required for new learning and practice to take place. Concussions can be accompanied by problems with headaches, light and noise sensitivity, fatigue, and blurred vision—and these all interfere with learning. The worsening of symptoms with any type of cognitive task makes learning very difficult. Cognitive rest is frequently prescribed to avoid excessive demands on the neurometabolism of the brain. However, it would be important to not fill this idle time with television and video game activities, at least initially following injury. Cognitive rest is very important for the child's recovery and school personnel need to be cognizant of this need. It is important for the clinician to stress with teachers and other school personnel that pushing the child is counterproductive (Majerske et al., 2008).

Case Study 10.3. A Case of Repeated Concussions

Tommy was a 15-year, 10-month-old young man with a love for ice hockey, having played the game competitively since he was a small child. Over the years, he had repeated concussions (9 in total), none of which were aggressively treated. Several of them happened within a very short time frame before "return to play" rules were instituted. One concussion came just days after an initial serious concussion because Tommy didn't want to miss a playoff game.

His poor work performance, deteriorating school grades, and limited social skills were readily reported by both school and parent reports during the school neuropsychological evaluation. However, the school had attributed these problems to his drinking habits and marijuana smoking, which began during his early teenage years. The evaluation revealed poor visual–spatial skills, novel problem solving, and considerable executive deficits, with processing speed very low. Not surprisingly, he had the most difficulty with oral and written expression, and comprehension problems, with academic fluency impaired across all domains. Tommy also complained that he couldn't "keep up" with what the teacher or his peers were saying, so he "checked out" when others were talking. All these symptoms are suggestive of the white matter dysfunction expected from repeated traumatic brain injury. For interventions, we suggested slower rate of oral presentation, identifying key words, tape recording, or supplemental notes or notetaking. We suggested task analysis of complex tasks. For increasing processing speed, we suggested repeated readings and overlearning to build automaticity, and other compensatory activities to help Tommy overcome his executive deficits. These interventions proved successful and enabled Tommy's good progress.

Concussion and ADHD

ADHD symptoms may exist in a large number of children with concussions (Schrieff et al., 2011; Yeates et al., 2005). The externalizing diagnoses following this type of traumatic brain injury may be due to cortical hypoarousal (Hale, Reddy, et al., 2009), representing a loss of function (e.g., cortical control of impulsive behavior). Other children may experience cortical overactivity which would suggest a release of function problem, such as anxiety and obsessive–compulsive symptoms due to orbital dysfunction (Grados et al., 2008) that are not due to posttraumatic stress disorder (Mather et al., 2003).

Emotional Issues Following Concussion

Children and adolescents who suffer concussions frequently experience psychological symptoms including irritability, sadness, and anxiety. These issues can be exacerbated by preexisting difficulties in these areas (Semrud-Clikeman, LaFavor, et al., 2017). Psychological factors play a prominent role in concussions. These factors include the new feeling of vulnerability and a "shaken sense of self." (Broshek, 2013). It is not uncommon for feelings of depression to be present within the first 2 weeks to 1 month following a concussion when the symptoms are at their highest level (Kontos et al., 2012).

An interesting study of athletes with concussion and depression using fMRI found reduced activation in the dorsolateral prefrontal cortex and striatum as well as in the medial frontal and temporal regions (Chen et al., 2008). Depression severity was significantly related to reduced gray matter volume in these regions, leading to the conclusion that the depressed mood following a concussion may be a related, underlying disturbance in the limbic–frontal connections.

In addition to depression, anxiety is frequently seen in concussion patients (Ponsford et al., 2012). This type of anxiety generally occurs within 1 month of the injury and, for most, will subside within 3 months. An exception to this finding is for patients who had preinjury physical or psychiatric problems whose anxiety problems continued following recovery from the head injury. Anxiety management is very important for recovery from a concussion, particularly for patients with a previous history of anxiety.

In an attempt to isolate cognitive and affective factors following traumatic brain injury, Clarke et al. (2012) evaluated three groups: adults with concussion, those with spinal injury but no traumatic brain injury, and controls. Depression, anxiety, and neurotic symptoms were the best predictors of postconcussive affective symptoms compared to neuropsychological testing. In contrast, neuropsychological testing was a better predictor for cognitive difficulties found in these patients. The presence of both cognitive and affective difficulties appears to exacerbate the difficulties the patient experiences and likely makes the concussion that much more severe, strongly suggesting that we cannot separate affective and cognitive skills when talking about the recovery of the patient; both areas of functioning need to be addressed. It may also be that anxiety contributes to patients feeling that their symptoms are more severe and that they will not have a full recovery. Treating this anxiety will likely assist with improvement in cognition.

Do not ignore the child's feelings of isolation and loss of activity. These feelings improve, along with cognitive functioning, with mild to moderate exercise, particularly for children who show a slower recovery (Gagnon et al., 2009). This finding was replicated with adolescents who were also slow to recover. Increasing exercise gradually and under supervision of a trainer resulted not only in symptom-free recovery for 80% of the patients but also to full return to work and school for all of the participants in the study (Leddy et al., 2012). Thus, exercise enhances recovery through increased neurotrophic factors that play a key role in neuronal plasticity. Brain-derived neurotrophic factor (BDNF) is important for long-term potentiation functions of the hippocampus, which is a key mechanism for learning and memory (Griesbach, Hovda, & Gomez-Pinilla, 2009). Postinjury exercise can assist in regulation of the postconcussion neuroendocrine dysfunction frequently seen with the neurometabolic cascade.

For patients with anxiety and depression, cognitive-behavioral therapy assists in restructuring cognitions and fears about recovery. It can also provide support to help the child or adolescent face many of the challenges that can be present initially during recovery. Strategies such as breathing exercises, relaxation, and reattribution of feelings can all be of assistance to the child or adolescent as recovery continues.

Return to School

Once a trained medical provider has cleared the student to come back to the classroom following a concussion, the school needs to begin preparing for the student's return to classes. This process requires coordination and communication among family members, medical providers, allied health care providers, educators, and athletics personnel (Hale et al., 2011). It will be important for the school to regularly monitor the symptoms and to communicate regularly with the family. Too often, school personnel tend to attribute psychological changes to a child's adjustment after injury, when there could be a biological basis for such changes. One obstacle to proper monitoring is the lack of training in concussion management for school personnel. This is an area in which the school psychologist and school counselor can provide much needed assistance. Materials are available from the Centers for Disease Control and Prevention that can assist schools with understanding concussions. The need for policies and programs for managing concussions is significant. A recent study asking parents about the types of program provided to their children upon return to school found that only 24% were aware of a written plan for concussion management (Sady et al., 2011).

Serving children with acquired brain injuries is complex. The school neuropsychologist must consider the interrelationship of premorbid functioning, injury type and severity, adaptation to injury and life skills, and family functioning. The variability in traumatic brain injury presentation, developmental considerations at time of the injury, and changes following rehabilitation require careful interdisciplinary coordination of medical, neuropsychological, and school-based services (Hale et al., 2010), as you can see in In-Depth 10.1

IN-DEPTH 10.1. Providing School Neuropsychology Services to Children with Traumatic Brain Injury

School personnel need to be aware of the signs and symptoms of all forms of TBI, like concussion, and take them seriously. Key signals to look for include problems with paying attention and processing speed, difficulty with learning or remembering new material, inappropriate or impulsive behavior, greater irritability, disorganization, fatigue in class, and headaches (Master et al., 2012; McLeod & Gioia, 2010).

Younger children with concussions pose a particular challenge because of the child's developmental stage. For instance, executive deficits experienced in small children may not completely surface until these skills are needed in later years of schooling. It is important to gather information about the injury characteristics and history in order to determine what measures are best suited to help assess and treat the particular child, and how premorbid functioning is affecting current status (Hale, Metro, et al., 2010). For instance, a child with significant ADHD is at higher risk for head injury than a child without ADHD (Semrud-Clikeman, 2001), so attention problems may have predated the injury. Age not only affects the manifestation of the injury, but it has also been shown to play a role in recovery, with younger athletes/children taking significantly longer to recover (Gioia et al., 2009).

What's the best way to avoid excessive cognitive exertion and worsening of symptoms? Frequently, in initial recovery, the child should not watch TV, work on a computer, use a cell phone, read, play video games, or listen to loud music. Many will not attend school. This is a particularly difficult time for parents and children alike as boredom sets in and it is hard to prioritize rest while still allowing some activity (Sady et al., 2011). However, this rest is crucial for the child's recovery and it is important for parents and school personnel to recognize this need (Majerske et al., 2008). The fine line between too much cognitive exertion and not enough needs to be monitored by parents and teachers.

Clearly, the presence of both cognitive and affective difficulties appears to exacerbate the problems the child experiences and likely makes the TBI that much more severe. It is difficult to separate affective and cognitive skills when talking about the recovery of the child; both areas of functioning need to be addressed. Improving processing speed and hemispheric integration is key along with targeting complex problem solving, written expression, academic fluency, and social skills for improvement.

Chapter 11

Common Genetic Disorders in Childhood

As you work in the schools, you will see children with various genetic disorders. Generally, these children have a different look to their face, hair, ears, eyes, and sometimes hands. While some genetic disorders are not as common as ADHD or learning disabilities, they do occur, and you will likely have at least one or more of these children on your case load. There are over 600 neurodegenerative genetic diseases, with approximately 50 of these seen frequently in pediatric neuropsychology and neurology clinics. The first section of this chapter offers a brief review of basic genetics. It can act as a framework for understanding these disorders.

The Basics of Genetics

Genes are basically molecules of DNA. There are approximately 3 billion base pairs of DNA divided into 23 pairs of chromosomes, including one pair of sex chromosomes (McMahon et al., 2017). Deoxyribonucleic acid (DNA) replicates itself allowing for the transmission and expression of genetic traits. The DNA molecule is a double helix with two long, thin strands twisted around each other. The strands are made up of phosphates and sugars (nucleotides). There are four *nucleotides* (also referred to as *bases*) contained in these strands: adenine (A), thymine (T), guanine (G), and cytosine (C). One of the four is attached to each sugar. The strands are held together by hydrogen bonds, and adenine forms a base pair with thymine and cytosine forms a base pair with guanine. If there is an adenine on one side of the helix, there will always be a thymine on the other side. Conversely if there is a cytosine on one side of the helix, there will always be a guarnine on the other side. There can be 1,000 base pairs for one gene or on a really big gene, there can be 10,000 base pairs! DNA also regulates ribonucleic acid (RNA) synthesis, which is important for the formation of amino acids that build proteins to establish the metabolic functioning for the cells of the body. Genes appear in sequential order on the chromosomes.

With one exception, every cell in the body has 23 pairs of chromosomes for a total of 46. Each chromosome has a long arm (called the q arm) and a short arm (p). The one exception is the cells of the egg and sperm, which include only one sex chromosome each. When an egg is fertilized by a sperm, the resulting zygote inherits one set of chromosomes from the sperm and one set from the egg to create 23 new pairs. Most women have XX sex chromosomes, most men have XY. The X chromosome is bigger than the Y and is thought to be responsible for most traits. The Y chromosome is primarily responsible for male gender determination. The 22 pairs of nonsex chromosomes are called *autosomes*. They are similar in shape and their genes are arranged in sequence at specific sites on the chromosome. When the genes inherited from both parents are identical, they are called *homozygous* and when dissimilar, they are called *heterozygous*.

A gene that is expressed (shows a trait) on only one chromosome of a pair is considered to be a *dominant* trait. A gene that must be on both chromosomes to be expressed is considered a *recessive* trait. A child can have the following modes of genetic transmission: an autosomal (nonsex) dominant trait, an autosomal (nonsex) recessive trait, and an X-linked trait. There are also incidences of chromosomal abnormalities that spark a genetic disorder.

Chromosomal abnormalities can be either structural or numerical (Nussbaum et al., 2015). Numerical abnormalities are alternations in the chromosome number sequence. Duplication of one of the 46 chromosomes is called *aneuploidy*, an extra chromosome is *trisomy*, and a missing chromosome is *monosomy*. All monosomies are lethal except for Turner syndrome, which results from missing one X chromosome (Descartes, 2017).

Autosomal Dominant Disorders

Autosomal dominant disorders are caused by a dominant gene on a nonsex chromosome. Each person with an autosomal dominant disorder has a 50% chance of having children with the disorder. People who do not inherit the affected gene are genetically normal and have normal children that are genetically normal. Males and females can be equally affected with this type of disorder. This type of disorder is generally expressed in every generation, so if a child has it, one or both parents typically have the disorder. It is important to recognize this, since the parent(s) may also show the disorder, which could affect their understanding or efforts to help the child with the disorder.

Neurofibromatosis

Neurofibromatosis (NF), Noonan syndrome (discussed below), and other disorders are known as *RASopathies*. RASopathies are caused by a gene mutation related to a protein pathway. The affected protein pathway involves several brain circuits involved in the prefrontal cortex and basal ganglia that regulate attention and executive functioning (Pierpont et al., 2015). These disorders are frequently associated with cognitive impairment. There are two types of neurofibromatosis: NF1 and NF2.

NF1 is the most common form of neurofibromatosis and has an incidence of approximately 1 in 300 (Serdaroglu et al., 2019). Approximately 50% of these children do not have a family history of NF. Diagnostic criteria include neurofibromas (a tumor in the peripheral nervous system), café au lait macules (they look like birthmarks), freckling, lisch nodules (seen as yellow glints in the iris of the eye), optic gliomas, and a first-degree relative with NF1. Very often NF1 is accompanied by short stature, a tendency to develop malignancies, large skull size, learning disabilities, and epilepsy. Both verbal and nonverbal learning disabilities are frequently seen in NF1, as well as attention deficit hyperactivity disorder, hypotonia, and receptive and expressive language problems (Thiele & Korf, 2017). In addition, these children frequently have difficulty with sleep and an increased incidence of autism. Treatment generally includes being closely followed by a physician to monitor the possible increase in neurofibromas particularly in the optic nerve and the spinal cord. Neurofibromas that occur on the peripheral nerves are generally not removed unless there is irritation or malignancy. Symptomatic tumors are generally treated with chemotherapy.

A defining criterion for the second type of neurofibromatosis, *NF2*, is the occurrence of vestibular schawnnomas (tumors on the vestibular nerve in the ear). These present as tinnitus and/or hearing loss as well as problems with balance. While these schawnnomas can occur along any cranial nerve, the fifth nerve (trigeminal: jaw) is the most common after the eighth (vestibular: auditory). Prevalence is approximately 1 in 60,000 live births. This disorder has been mapped to chromosome 22. Management is generally through surgery.

Noonan Syndrome

Noonan syndrome (NS) is one of the more common RASopathies. It occurs in approximately 1 in 1,000 to 1 in 2,500 live births. Children with this disorder show distinctive facial features, short stature, congenital heart disease, skeletal difficulties, and other areas of deficits. Most children with NS show motor delays, cognitive impairment, language deficits, and learning disabilities (Pierpont et al., 2013). Many children with NS are diagnosed with ADHD and attentional problems, as well and have difficulty with working memory, self-monitoring, and social skills (Pierpont et al., 2015). Moreover, the working memory deficits seen in children with NS require significant support in the school as the child will forget the steps required to complete a task or the directions provided or have difficulty with academic functioning, especially in the areas of reading comprehension, applied math problems, and/or written expression. Children with NS show significant problems with insight into their behavior, thus making it difficult for them to learn from past mistakes, and they are unaware of how their behavior affects others. Neurobiologically, children with NS show reduced activity in the connections between the frontal lobe and the basal ganglia, which are structures important for inhibition and impulse control, and they are related to problems with working memory (Shilyansky et al., 2010).

Tuberous Sclerosis

Tuberous sclerosis (TS) affects multiple organ systems and is one of the most common single gene disorders in children with an estimated incidence of 1 in 5,800 live births (Thiele & Korf, 2017). There are several criteria for a diagnosis, but in each case, difficulties are found on the skin and/or brain; either skin or brain criteria are sufficient for diagnosis. Generally, children with TS show tumors in the brain (on a brain scan, these look similar to the eyes you see on a potato), fibromas which are reddish around the fingernails (ungual fibromas), leathery like skin in the lower back, retinal hamartoma (which looks like cream-colored lesions in the eye), nodules around the nose called *astrocytomas*, and more minor features (skin lesions, pits in the teeth, and others). Epilepsy is common in TS with 80–90% of patients having seizures, with onset generally in childhood. Infantile spasms often occur with TS and are associated with poorer developmental outcome. Treatment includes close management by the physician. Learning disabilities are frequently seen and can be severe (Ferguson et al., 2002). In addition, autism can occur with TS in as many as 9% of children with autism also showing TS. Behavioral difficulties are frequently seen in TS and pose the most difficulty for management. Treatment of these difficulties includes therapy as well as parent training. As a practitioner, consider what you've learned about the brain in Chapter 2, because it is important to consider the location and size of the tumors to understand how they might affect neuropsychological, academic, and psychosocial functioning.

Sturge–Weber Syndrome

Sturge–Weber syndrome (SWS) is characterized by a facial angioma (port wine stain) and has an incidence of 1 in 20,000 to 50,000 cases. This angioma is often accompanied by angiomas of the ophthalmic and jaw nerves. Glaucoma can often occur with SWS and seizures are frequently seen, with 20% having tonic–clonic seizures and 40% showing partial and generalized seizures (Thiele & Korf, 2017). The clinical course includes intellectual disability stroke-like episodes, seizures (Thomas-Sohl et al., 2004), and frequent migraines. Treatment generally includes management of seizures and headaches with 50% of children having seizures that can be controlled with antiepileptic drugs. The children who do not respond to these medications are often considered for epilepsy surgery. Treatment of the wine stain includes laser therapy, which is most effective when begun early in life. The treatment team for SWS should include a physician, psychologist, and social worker. School neuropsychologists are an important part of this team to help with adjustment in school and to assist school personnel if stroke-like episodes occur during the school day.

Huntington's Chorea

Huntington's chorea is an autosomal dominant disorder on chromosome 4. It is most commonly found in people of northern European descent, particularly from the United Kingdom (Snowden, 2017). It is detected through genetic screening, and the average age of onset occurs from 30 to 50 years but it has been seen in children as young as 5. Approximately 5–13% first manifest symptoms in childhood or adolescence but these signs are generally subtle and often diagnosed as ADHD. Difficulties are often seen in executive functions, memory, and psychomotor slowing. Further along in the disorder there are significant personality changes that include depression and paranoia, as well as symptoms of chorea, which includes facial grimaces, dysfluent speech, ataxia, and eventually profound dementia. Neuropathology has found gross atrophy of the caudate, basal ganglia, and frontal lobes.

Williams Syndrome

Some consider Williams syndrome (WS) to be an autosomal dominant disorder, while others feel it is not clear (Brawn & Porter, 2018), however, Williams syndrome is a rare disorder that is caused by a microdeletion on chromosome 7 on the q arm. The prevalence is approximately 1 in 7,500 live births (Brawn & Porter, 2018). Physical features include small stature, dysmorphic facial features, attention deficits, hypersociability, as well as heightened anxiety, fears, and phobias (Meyer-Lindenberg et al., 2006). These children have been described as looking "elfin-like" and frequently have congenital heart disease and endocrine deficits (Kimura et al., 2019). Young children with WS usually show developmental delay with mild to moderate impairment in intellectual functioning, including learning disabilities (Porter & Coltheart, 2005). The intellectual impairment ranges from severe to average (Mervis & John, 2010). Strengths are found in verbal and literal nonverbal reasoning, speech, and short-term memory for verbal information. Another strength is that the child with WS can recognize emotions from facial expressions (Ibemon et al., 2018). Weaknesses are generally present in tasks such as block design, abstract language, and pragmatics. Adaptive functioning is another area that is compromised in children with WS, particularly in personal and daily living skills as well as motor skill. Socialization appears to be strong because of good explicit verbal communication skills (Brawn & Porter, 2018). However, difficulties with adaptive functioning continue into adulthood for the majority of children with WS, and because implicit language is sometimes poor, there can be higher-order academic and social concerns. Concerns about treatment for children with WS are that school professionals lack experience with this disorder, and it is easy to misdiagnose because the cognitive profile for WS might look like NVLD (discussed in Chapter 8) to the average school psychologist. Less than 11% of teachers working with children with genetic disorders have any information about these disorders (Reilly et al., 2015). Even more concerning is that a survey of school professionals found that the majority did not feel these children required specialist support (Van Herwegen et al., 2019). Thus, it is incredibly important for neuropsychologists in the schools to research and provide information about the disorder to both parents and educators, recognizing the child's strengths and weaknesses, with the goal of developing the most appropriate school-based interventions. Such interventions need to include implicit language therapy to develop abstract language skills. Although these children are often mistakenly thought to have well-developed language skills, for the most part, their language is generally superficial and socially driven by left-hemisphere explicit language skills that may be average or higher. Support for motor skill development, particularly fine-motor skills and visuo–constructive skills, are important interventions particularly for developing mathematics skills, map reading, and graphing. Attentional skills also need to be dealt with in the IEP with recommendations similar to those developed for children with ADHD (Shalev et al., 2019). For those children with intellectual disability, appropriate daily living skills need to be addressed.

Autosomal Recessive Disorders

With autosomal recessive disorder, males and females are affected similarly. When two carriers have a child, there is a 25% chance the child will show the disorder, 25% will be carriers, and 50% will have a normal karyotype (how chromosomes appear in the cell). Table 11.1 shows this incidence pattern.

TABLE 11.1. Autosomal Recessive Disorder Inheritance

When both parents have a recessive gene, neither parent shows the disease

1. Males and females affected equally
2. When 2 carriers produce children, 25% of the children are affected
3. 25% of their children will be carriers
4. 50% of their children will be genetically normal

Phenylketonuria

Phenylketonuria (PKU) is caused by a deficiency in the phenylalanine hydroxylase enzyme that allows for conversion of this enzyme into tyrosine (a precursor of dopamine). Phenylalanine is toxic and when it builds up in the system, it causes significant intellectual disability as well as microcephaly, seizures, tremors, and spatisticity (Gallagher et al., 2017). Mandatory testing for PKU was established in the 1960s, since damage from this disorder can be prevented through diet, but testing may not be uniform in developing countries and this disorder is sometimes misdiagnosed as cerebral palsy. With the large number of immigrant families we see in our daily practices, there is a chance that one or more of your students has PKU. Because the artificial sweetener aspartame contains phenylalanine, diet soda made with the sweetener contains a statement warning people with this disorder to not drink the soda. Many children who do not have controlled PKU will show neurodevelopmental, psychiatric, and behavioral problems. Neuropsychological deficits include problems with visual–spatial reasoning, mathematics, and some aspects of executive functioning (Canton, Le Gall, et al., 2019). MRIs have found dysmyelination in the periventricular white matter that may be reversible with the appropriate diet (Gallagher et al., 2017). Children with white matter abnormalities that extended to subcortical/frontal regions showed more severe deficits in cognition and executive functioning (Anderson, Wood, et al., 2004). In terms of neuropsychiatric and behavioral issues, depression and anxiety are the most common for children with PKU (Gentile et al., 2010). Although diet is the main treatment, it is difficult to adhere to because it is quite restrictive and involves low-protein foods and vegetables and fruits. Treatment with diet after the age of 3 is too late. Less than half of children and adults with PKU keep their phenylalnine at the recommended levels (Brown & Lichter-Konecki, 2016).

X-Linked Disorders

X-linked disorders involve mutations or other changes on the X sex chromosome. Since males do not have two X chromosomes (one from each parent), the likelihood of X-linked disorders is greater in males than females. See Table 11.2 for an overview of the inheritance pattern for X-linked disorders.

Fragile X Syndrome

Fragile X syndrome affects males and results in intellectual disability, while females experience less cognitive disability. It is inherited from the mother and is caused by an expansion of the CGG DNA sequence on the X chromosome. It has been well described as a single-gene cause of intellectual disability (Kover et al., 2013). The incidence is approximately 1 in 400 children for affected males. Longitudinal studies have found that the IQ score of these boys declined as the child developed, showing a slowing of intellectual development occurring in late childhood and adolescence. Difficulty is seen on tasks measuring frontal lobe functioning, in particular executive function and working memory (Langfranchi et al., 2009). Increased autistic symptoms are also frequently seen in children with fragile X (Loesch et al., 2007). Girls may show learning disabilities and some social emotional deficits, particularly with anxiety and mood disorders. The incidence of seizures in fragile X is approximately 15% in males and 5% in females. Speech and language therapy, occupational therapy, and educational support through an IEP are crucial for these children. For children with autistic symptoms, social and emotional support are important (Garber et al., 2008).

TABLE 11.2. The Inheritance Pattern for X-Linked Disorders

	X-Linked Dominant Disorders	
Affected father	Affected mother	Carrier mother
Transmit only to daughter	Transmit to all children	50% of children—boys and girls equally
	X-Linked Nondominant Disorders	
Boys affected	50% of daughters are carriers	50% of daughters are carriers
	100% of sons affected	

Turner Syndrome

Turner syndrome is a relatively common genetic abnormality that occurs exclusively in girls and is the result of the complete or partial loss of a sex chromosome (Baker & Reiss, 2015). It is associated with short stature, webbed neck, and a low hairline. In this syndrome, IQ is generally spared but difficulty is generally seen in mathematics and visual–spatial reasoning (Hong et al., 2009). Deficits are seen in calculation rather than in understanding numerosity. In addition, children with Turner syndrome have difficulty with visual–perception but not with tactile spatial skills (Baker et al., 2020). Studies have found that the difficulties seen in mathematics performance are related to difficulties with visual tracking, visual-motor coordination and figure-ground processing (Baker et al., 2020). Moreover, these skills continue to be an area of difficulty throughout development. Girls with Turner syndrome have also been found to show NVLD (Semrud-Clikeman & Trauner, 2017). Communication skills are generally intact except for the ability to sequence verbal information and to understand and use implicit language. Consistent with their NVLD profile, girls with Turner syndrome also frequently show attentional difficulty, but this is not the same as in children with ADHD (see Chapter 8). Neuroimaging studies have found reduction in the gray matter volume in the parietal and occipital regions (Zhao et al., 2019). DTI has also found difficulties with white matter integrity (Semrud-Clikeman & Trauner, 2017). Brain development has also been shown to have a different trajectory in girls with Turner syndrome. Over time (from ages 2 to 9), the left parietal white matter volume and the thickness of the right parietal lobe were smaller by the age of 8 or 9.

X-Linked Adrenoleukodystrophy

There are three phenotypes of this disorder, with the childhood-onset cerebral form the most common (35%). It occurs primarily in males, and symptoms generally begin in boys ages 4–8. Early symptoms include ADHD and hyperactivity (Lund et al., 2018). This is a progressive disease and motor difficulties, deteriorating academic performance, and difficulty with handwriting and behaviors are early indications. The disease can progress quickly, often leading to total disability within 6 months to 2 years. Feeding often becomes difficult as motor control decreases significantly during this period. Adrenal insufficiency is also seen and can be fatal. This disorder involves the deficient production or action of glucocorticoids which are required for adequate functioning of the immune system and the hypothalamic–pituitary axis. Most patients with adrenoleukodystrophy (ALD) will die within a decade after diagnosis unless they are treated with a bone-marrow transplant. Bone-marrow transplant is the only known effective treatment for cerebral ALD, and it needs to be performed at an early stage of the disease. Those boys with a pronounced case of cerebral ALD generally do not do well after transplant (van der Knaap et al., 2019). Early identification of ALD is important, with school-based practitioners being key in this identification, particularly when boys show decline in their performance.

Metachromatic Leukodystrophy

One of the more prevalent inherited white matter disorders, metachromatic leukodystrophy (MLD), is an autosomal recessive disorder (Vanderver & Wolf, 2017). Presentation of MLD depends on the age of the child. The most common form of MLD is the late infantile form in which some children will present by the age of 30 months after normal development. Initially symptoms may be slow to develop with walking difficulties and speech sound deficits noticed first. With development of further symptoms, a specialist is contacted and the definitive diagnosis is made. As the disease progresses the child can become blind, deaf, and paralyzed, and death becomes likely. The juvenile form of MLD first shows between ages 4 and 16 years. The first signs of the disorder may be behavioral problems and increasing difficulty with schoolwork. Progression is slower than for the infantile form. Adult-onset MLD appears in the teen years and later with symptoms including cognitive and behavioral difficulties. Motor difficulties, speech articulation problems, and worsening behavioral problems present with worsening presentation over time. Seizures may occur. Progression is slower than with the early type of MLD. MRI findings show periventricular and deep white matter demyelination. Similar to cerebral ALD, bone-marrow transplant is the sole treatment available and is most effective when done early (Thibert et al., 2016). Gene therapy and enzyme replacement therapies have shown promise (Gieselmann, 2008).

Structural Abnormalities in Genetic Disorders

Prader–Willi Syndrome

Prader–Willi syndrome is the result of an abnormal imprinting of the paternal copy of chromosome 15 on the q arm (the long arm of the chromosome). The incidence of Prader–Willi is 1 per 10,000 to 30,000 (Cassidy et al., 2011). At infancy, the child shows hypotonia and failure to thrive as well as dysmorphic eye opening and small hands and small feet. (Paciorkowski et al., 2017). However, Prader–Willi is often not diagnosed until an older age. When diagnosed at an early age, growth hormone is the general treatment. Children with Prader–Willi are frequently morbidly obese due to an inability to stop eating. Developmental milestones are generally significantly delayed, with sitting not occurring until 12 months of age and walking not until after 2 years of age (Paciorkowski et al., 2017). Most children with Prader–Willi show mild intellectual disability, with approximately 40% showing below average to average ability. Temper tantrums are very common as well as stubbornness and compulsive behaviors. At older ages, these children may show obsessive–compulsive behavior as well as significant mood disorders. Approximately 1 in 5 show autistic-like symptoms and would qualify for a diagnosis of ASD (Descheemaeker et al., 2006). In our experience with one such child, there were explosive outbursts and uncontrollable rage, but behavioral intervention helped the child overcome those challenges.

Angelman Syndrome

Angelman syndrome is characterized by inappropriate laughter, developmental disability, and difficulty walking (Pelc et al., 2008). The syndrome is due to the loss of expression of the maternal copy of a gene on chromosome 15. Neuropsychological features include intellectual disability as well as a total lack of language with accompanying hyperactivity and aggression (Paciorkowski et al., 2017). Children with Angelman syndrome often show ataxic gait, jerky arm movements, and sleep disturbances. Eighty to 90% of children with Angelman syndrome have intractable epilepsy with multiple seizure types, and these seizures continue into adulthood. There are no known treatments for the syndrome. Some children with Angelman can use communication devices but most remain nonverbal (Clayton-Smith & Laan, 2003).

22q11.2 Deletion Syndrome

Once called velocardiofacial syndrome, DiGeorge syndrome, and Shprintzen syndrome because it was thought these were all different conditions, 22q11.2 deletion syndrome is a relatively common genetic syndrome with an estimated prevalence of 1 in 2,000 (Beaton et al., 2010). It occurs as the result of a deletion on the long arm of chromosome 22. Heart disease, hypercalcemia, cleft palate, short stature, and facial dysmorphology are common in children with 22q11.2 deletion syndrome, along with autism, intellectual disability, and ADHD. Significant difficulties are seen in visual–spatial skills, executive functioning, and mathematics (Semrud-Clikeman & Trauner, 2017). In adulthood there evidence of a higher incidence of schizophrenia, affective bipolar disorder, and schizophreniform disorder (Niklasson et al., 2001). Support through an IEP throughout grades K–12 is crucial for these children with continued support provided throughout adulthood, particularly for psychiatric issues.

Mucopolysaccharidoses

A group of rare disorders, mucopolysaccharidoses (MPS), are caused by a difficulty in lysosomal enzyme storage. There are three types of MPS: MPS I, II, and III. All but one of these disorders are an autosomal recessive disease. The exception is MPS II, which is an X-linked disorder that affects males. Lysosomes are important in the processing of enzymes, and when disrupted, will lead to an accumulation of lysosomes in organs, which degrade cellular functioning resulting in tissue and organ damage (Shapiro et al., 2017). Frequent deficits are found in skeletal and joint abnormalities, cardiac disease, vision and/or hearing difficulties as well as aggressive and hyperactive behaviors, global developmental delay, and a decline in language and cognitive abilities (Wegrzyn et al., 2015).

MPS I

Children with MPS I have coarse facial features, large livers, corneal clouding, and cardiac valve abnormalities. There are three types of MPS I: Hurler, Hurler–Scheie, and Scheie. Hurler syndrome is the most severe form of MPS I. Children with Hurler syndrome show cognitive impairment, rapid disease progression, and early death. The other two subtypes of MPS I show milder or no cognitive impairment and slower disease progression (Beck et al., 2014). Most children with Hurler syndrome are treated with hematopoietic stem-cell transplants (bone-marrow transplants), which can halt the cognitive decline and central nervous system damage, but will not correct damage that has already occurred. If not treated, children with Hurler generally show intelligence that is more than two standard deviations below the average by the age of 2 (Beck et al., 2014). Hurler patients that receive treatment frequently show attentional difficulties after treatment. Adolescents with MPS I frequently present with depression and social withdrawal and require therapy and an IEP for support (Shapiro et al., 2017).

MPS II

MPS II, or Hunter syndrome, is also caused by a malfunction of an enzyme and is generally identified around the ages of 2 to 4 years of age. It is a rare X-linked lysosomal disorder and impacts all organ systems (Eisengart et al., 2020). A large tongue, tonsils, liver or spleen, and joint stiffness are frequently seen. Some children with Hunter syndrome have progressive neurological impairments while others do not. Those with progressive neurological disorders have neurocognitive decline as well as significant behavioral symptoms; death occurs in the second decade of life without treatment. Those without neurological symptoms generally have average ability but do have difficulty with attention, executive functioning, and visual–motor skills. These children frequently require an IEP to provide educational support as well as social-emotional assistance.

MPS III

Also called Sanfilippo syndrome, MPS III is characterized by severe neurological deficits without the somatic features seen in the other MPS types. These children show normal development until the age of 3 and then show rapid decline, but they do not have restricted behaviors or deficits in communicative skills prior to the age of 3. Autistic-like behavioral problems generally occur around the age of 4 (Shapiro et al., 2016). By the age of 6, these children are generally functioning at approximately a 2-year-old level. Speech and language difficulties are generally the first symptoms seen prior to the cognitive decline, which includes the development of severe behavioral problems, including hyperactivity, poor attention, sleep disturbances, and extreme difficulty with emotional control (Heron et al., 2011). There is no known effective treatment for these children at this time. Given their severe cognitive deficits, an IEP is an absolute must for these children.

Genetic Disorders Case Report

There are many more genetic disorders that are beyond the scope of this chapter. The disorders we've described provide you with a picture of how difficult these children find school and the importance of IEPs and related services to support them. Continued support is frequently needed for these children once they attain adulthood since many of them are now surviving disorders that would have proven fatal in the past. The neuropsychologist and school psychologist are generally charged with providing leadership in determining appropriate educational interventions and, as a result, you need to be fully informed about how these genetic disorders present. As we've noted, school personnel may never have seen children with these disorders, so it is important for you to provide the information that will assist teachers and other personnel about how best to approach the education of these children (see Chapter 10 for a discussion of this important role of the school psychologist). Case Report 11.1 is offered as a guide to appropriate support that can be provided for these children.

Case Report 11.1. Summary of Neuropsychological Evaluation

Reason for Re-Evaluation

Amy S is a 6-year, 10-month-old left-handed White female with mucopolysaccharidosis type I, Hurler syndrome (MPS IH), who was diagnosed in utero due to family history. She underwent a 6/6 unrelated umbilical cord blood transplant (UCBT) in 2019 when she was 8 months old. Amy did not experience any posttransplant complications and is fully engrafted. She is now 6 years posttransplant. Specific concerns were expressed regarding continued attention difficulties.

Relevant History

Developmental and Medical History

Amy was born at 38 weeks, 16 days gestation, following an uncomplicated pregnancy. A prenatal screen for Hurler syndrome was performed, given that Amy's sister is also diagnosed with MPS IH.

Amy's medical records have indicated that her features are mild, with regard to her Hurler syndrome diagnosis. An MRI (magnetic resonance imaging) of Amy's brain, conducted at age 3, indicated findings consistent with Hurler syndrome. A laparoscopic gastrostomy tube (G-tube) was placed due to "failure to thrive in preparation for bone-marrow transplant." As is consistent with her Hurler syndrome, Amy has experienced a number of medical complications, including visual problems (corneal clouding, hyperopia, astigmatism, monocular estropia, and strabismic amblyopia) that require a prescription for her to wear eyeglasses full time, and orthopedic problems (joint stiffening at the elbows, hips, knees, digits; mild kyphosis; carpal tunnel). Her brain imaging was also consistent with Hurler syndrome, including "multiple prominent bilateral perivascular spaces in the region of the basal ganglia as well as in the peri-atrial white matter." According to radiologic report, brain imaging has remained consistent over the years, and her myelination pattern is unremarkable. This past year Amy was referred for an electroretinogram (ERG). Results revealed abnormality, indicating dysfunction of the photoreceptors in both eyes.

Family History

Amy currently resides with her biological parents and her brother (age 10 and previously diagnosed with Hurler syndrome). They have two pet dogs.

School History

Amy recently completed kindergarten. Ms. Smith reported that Amy did well in school and has not needed any additional support. The school has not expressed any concern with Amy's attention. Some concern in attention is reported in the home setting. Amy's mother reported Amy is "mostly happy."

Behavioral Observations

Amy was accompanied to the appointment by her mother. Amy engaged in appropriate eye contact with the neuropsychologist upon being greeted. Rapport was established quickly and maintained throughout testing. Most conversations were initiated by Amy as she demonstrated good spontaneous and reciprocal conversation. Her speech was unremarkable from rate tone and prosody. Amy displayed minor articulation errors, but they did not interfere with the intelligibility of her speech. No atypical motor movements or mannerisms were observed during testing. Amy wore her corrective eyeglasses during testing. She demonstrated mild inattention and hyperactivity (e.g., easily distracted by sounds and objects around her, fidgeting in her chair). Despite this behavior, she was easily redirected to the task at hand and responded well to limit setting, praise, and positive reinforcement. She was very verbal and appropriately commented on her performance.

Child Interview

Amy shared that she enjoys singing, painting, and playing with a hula hoop and with her Barbie's. She reported having a "bunch of besties" with whom she likes to play gymnastics. When asked to name some things that make her happy, Amy's response was snuggling with her dogs and playing "tickle monster" with her father.

Results and Impressions

It is important to know that Amy's medical condition, Hurler syndrome, places her at a greater risk for neurocognitive problems as a result of the condition itself and the treatments she has received (e.g., chemotherapy, transplant). Results from the current evaluation indicate that Amy continues to maintain an average to above average developmental trajectory in relation to her cognitive abilities. Her above average verbal comprehension skills (accessing and applying acquired word knowledge) were particularly encouraging as children with Hurler syndrome are susceptible to language delays and slowing in their language development. Amy's processing speed (speed and accuracy of visual identification, decision making, and decision implementation) was a relative weakness for her, which may be a result of some mild inattention and executive functioning deficits.

Amy is at a greater risk for attention difficulties and executive functioning deficits as a result of the chemotherapy she received to prepare for her bone-marrow transplant. Amy was administered a computerized sustained attention test and made a significant number of errors on the sustained attention portion of this measure. Amy demonstrated average impulse control; however, she consistently and frequently missed responding to the stimuli on the screen. On parent and teacher behavior rating scales, it was reported that Amy often has a short attention span, is easily distracted, and has trouble concentrating. She did not fall in the clinically significant range on a structured behavioral rating scale for attention or hyperactivity concerns. While Amy does not currently qualify for a diagnosis of Attention-Deficit/Hyperactivity Disorder (ADHD), her attentional symptoms should be monitored going forward and addressed in the future should her attention difficulties worsen or impact her functioning. On measures of executive functioning Amy showed difficulty with organization of materials (orderliness of work, play, and storage spaces), working memory (holding an appropriate amount of information in mind for further processing), and planning/organizing (managing current and future-oriented task demands). Executive functioning affects the way a person thinks and approaches problems.

Amy's visual motor skills were found to be in the low average range for her ability, with difficulty noted in attention to detail. On a measure that evaluated her ability to solve geometric puzzles, Amy scored in the above average range, indicating she has no difficulty in visual perception.

Amy's memory was also evaluated as memory skills can be affected by her past treatment. No significant memory difficulties were found.

Adaptive behaviors are those skills that require the child to function independently in their environment. There were no significant areas of concern and Amy's scores are commensurate with past assessments indicating she continues to make progress in her independent functioning.

Emotionally, Amy is reported to be a happy young girl and that is the child we saw in our clinic. She is not reported to show significant signs of difficulty in an area and continues to make good progress in her development.

Moving forward, it will be important to continue monitoring Amy's progress over time as research has shown that she is at risk for a slowing in her developmental progress, associated with her medical condition, prolonged hospitalization, and/or effects of treatment. Therefore, proactive implementation of therapies in addition to continued monitoring of her progress via follow-up neuropsychological evaluations are critical.

Diagnoses

E76.01   Mucopolysaccharidosis Type IH (Hurler Syndrome)
Z92.21   Status Post Chemotherapy
Z94.81   Status Post Transplant

Recommendations

1. Children with Hurler syndrome are at increased risk of losing skills without the support of ongoing therapy. We, therefore, recommend that Amy restart occupational therapy (OT). The evidence is that children with Hurler syndrome benefit greatly from intensive intervention. Amy will likely need the therapy services on an ongoing basis, even if she progresses within age-level expectations, to ensure that she does not lose ground during the next year.

2. Amy's parents will no doubt continue nurturing interactions with her, which are just the types of interactions that facilitate child development. As we previously recommended, activities that are helpful include reading books with visually stimulating pictures together, doing artwork, copying letters and symbols, modeling problem-solving skills. We strongly encourage Amy's family to continue to cultivate a multisensory learning environment for Amy to promote her cognitive, language, and physical development.

3. Amy is entering first grade in the Fall, and we strongly encourage her parents to contact their school district to discuss Amy's condition. Accommodations and supports will be needed for her med-

ical condition and related issues (e.g., attention difficulties) to ensure she benefits from the academic instructions at school. Physical therapy (PT), occupational therapy (OT), as well as speech and language therapy, may be beneficial for Amy as she continues to develop.

4. Since Amy displays mild attention and behavioral regulation issues, some behavioral strategies for children with attention-deficit hyperactivity disorder may be helpful. It is recommended that Amy's parents consult resources to become familiar with behavioral strategies related to individuals with attention difficulties for both the home and academic settings. Some helpful resources can be found at:

- National Resource Center on ADHD (*https://chadd.org/about/about-nrc*)
- Understood (*www.understood.org/en*)
- *Taking Charge of ADHD: The Complete, Authoritative Guide for Parents (Fourth Edition)* by Russell A. Barkley, 2020. Guilford Press, New York.

5. It will be important for Amy's neurocognitive development that she be evaluated on a regular basis as recommended by her medical team. Yearly follow-up is recommended at this point in her care.

References

Aaron, P. G. (2003). *Poor reading performance: Is it dyslexia or ADHD?* Paper presented at the 54th Annual Conference of the International Dyslexia Association, San Diego, CA.

Abbott, R. D., Berninger, V. W., & Fayol, M. (2010). Longitudinal relationships of levels of language in writing and between writing and reading in grades 1 to 7. *Journal of Educational Psychology, 102*(2), 281.

Abramovich, A., Dar, R., Mittleman, A., & Wilhelm, S. (2015). Comorbidity between attention deficit/hyperactivity disorder and obsessive–compulsive disorder across the lifespan: A systematic and critical review. *Harvard Review of Psychiatry, 23,* 245–262.

Achenbach, T. M., & Rescorla, L. A. (2001). *Manual for the ASEBA school-age forms & profiles.* University of Vermont Research Center for Children, Youth, & Families.

Ackerman, J. (2008). *Sex sleep eat drink dream: A day in the life of your body.* Houghton Mifflin Harcourt.

ADA Amendments Act of 2008. Pub.L. 110-325.

Adams, W., & Sheslow, D. (2021). *WRAML 3: Wide Range Assessment of Memory and Learning.* Wide Range.

Adolphs, R., Sears, L. L., & Piven, J. (2001). Abnormal processing of social information from faces in autism. *Journal of Cognitive Neuroscience, 13*(2), 232–240.

Adolphs, R., Tranel, D., Damasio, H., & Damasio, A. R. (1995). Fear and the human amygdala. *Journal of Neuroscience, 15*(9), 5879–5891.

Agate, F. T., & Garcia-Barrera, M. (2020). Assessment issues within neuropsychological settings. In M. Selborn & J. A. Suhr (Eds.), *The Cambridge handbook of clinical assessment and diagnosis* (pp. 472–484). Cambridge University Press.

Aiello, R., Ruble, L., & Esler, A. (2017). A national study of school psychologists' use of evidence-based assessment in autism spectrum disorder. *Journal of Applied School Psychology, 33,* 67–88.

Alamiri, B., Nelson, C., Fitzmaurice, G. M., Murphy, J. M., & Gilman, S. E. (2018). Neurological soft signs and cognitive performance in early childhood. *Developmental Psychology, 54*(11), 2043.

Albritton, K., & Truscott, S. (2014). Professional development to increase problem-solving skills in a response to intervention framework. *Contemporary School Psychology, 18,* 44–58.

Alexander, M. P., & Annett, M. (1996). Crossed aphasia and related anomalies of cerebral organization: Case reports and a genetic hypothesis. *Brain and Language, 55*(2), 213–239.

Allen, D. N., & Becker, M. L. (2019). Clinical interviewing. In G. Goldstein, D. N. Allen, & J. DeLuca (Eds.), *Handbook of psychological assessment* (4th ed., pp. 307–336). Academic Press.

Allen, S. J., & Graden, J. L. (2002). Best practices in collaborative problem solving for intervention design. In A. Thomas & J. Grimes (Eds.), *Best practices in school psychology IV* (Vol. 1, pp. 565–582). National Association of School Psychologists.

Alloway, T. P., & Passolunghi, M. C. (2011). The relationship between working memory, IQ, and mathematical skills in children. *Learning and Individual Differences, 21,* 133–137.

Alloy, I. B., Nusslock, R., & Boland, E. M. (2015). The development and course of bipolar spectrum disorders: An integrated reward and circadian rhythm dysregulation model. *Annual Review of Clinical Psychology, 11*, 213–250.

Alquraini, T., & Gut, D. (2012). Critical components of successful inclusion of students with severe disabilities: Literature review. *International Journal of Special Education, 27*(1), 42–59.

Altemeier, L. E., Abbott, R. D., & Berninger, V. W. (2008). Executive functions for reading and writing in typical literacy development and dyslexia. *Journal of Clinical and Experimental Neuropsychology, 30*(5), 588–606.

Amalric, M., Wang, L., Pica, P., Figueira, S., Sigman, M., & Dehaene, S. (2017). The language of geometry: Fast comprehension of geometrical primitives and rules in human adults and preschoolers. *PLOS Computational Biology, 13*(1), e1005273.

Amaral, D. G., Schumann, C. M., & Nordahl, C. W. (2008). Neuroanatomy of autism. *Trends in Neurosciences, 31*, 137–145.

Ameis, S. H., & Catani, M. (2015). Altered white matter connectivity as a neural substrate for social impairment in Autism Spectrum Disorder. *Cortex, 62*, 158–181.

American Educational Research Association, American Psychological Association, & National Council on Measurement in Education. (2014). *Standards for educational and psychological testing.* Authors.

American Psychiatric Association. (2022). *Diagnostic and statistical manual of mental disorders* (5th ed., text rev.). Author.

Americans with Disabilities Act (ADA). 42 U.S.C. § 12101 et seq. (1990).

Amitay, S., Ben-Yehudah, G., Banai, K., & Ahissar, M. (2002). Disabled readers suffer from visual and auditory impairments but not from a specific magnocellular deficit. *Brain, 125*, 2272–2285.

Anderson, P., & Doyle, L. W. (2003). Neurobehavioral outcomes of school-age children born extremely low birth weight or very preterm in the 1990s. *Journal of the American Medical Association, 289*(24), 3264–3272.

Anderson, P. J., Wood, S. J., Francis, D. E., Coleman, L., Warwick, L., Casanelia, S., et al. (2004). Neuropsychological functioning in children with early-treated phenylketonuria: Impact of white matter abnormalities. *Developmental Medicine and Child Neurology, 46*, 230–238.

Anderson, V., Anderson, P., Grimwood, K., & Nolan, T. (2004). Cognitive and executive function 12 years after childhood bacterial meningitis: Effect of acute neurologic complications and age of onset. *Journal of Pediatric Psychology, 29*, 67–81.

Anderson, V., Spencer-Smith, M., & Wood, A. (2011). Do children really recover better? Neurobehavioural plasticity after early brain insult. *Brain, 134*(8), 2197–2221.

Andersson, U. (2008). Mathematical competencies in children with different types of learning difficulties. *Journal of Educational Psychology, 100*, 48–66.

Ansari, D., & Dhital, B. (2006). Age-related changes in the activation of the intraparietal sulcus during nonsymbolic magnitude processing: An event-related functional magnetic resonance imaging study. *Journal of Cognitive Neuroscience, 18*, 1820–1828.

Ardila, A. (2008). Cultural values underlying psychometric cognitive testing. *Neuropsychology Review, 15*, 185–195.

Ardila, A. (2020). Cross-cultural neuropsychology: History and prospects. *RUDN Journal of Psychology and Pedagogics, 17*, 64–88.

Arns, M., & Vollebregt, M. A. (2019). Time to wake up: Appreciating the role of sleep in attention-deficit/hyperactivity disorder. *Journal of the American Academy of Child and Adolescent Psychiatry, 58*(4), 398–400.

Arnsten, A. F., & Rubia, K. (2012). Neurobiological circuits regulating attention, cognitive control, motivation, and emotion: disruptions in neurodevelopmental psychiatric disorders. *Journal of the American Academy of Child & Adolescent Psychiatry, 51*(4), 356–367.

Arsalidou, M., & Taylor, M. J. (2011). Is 2 + 2 = 4? Meta-analyses of brain areas needed for numbers and calculations. *NeuroImage, 54*, 2382–2393.

Ashkenazi, S., Black, J. M., Abrams, D. A., Hoeft, F., & Menon, V. (2013). Neurobiological underpinnings of math and reading learning disabilities. *Journal of Learning Disabilities, 46*, 549–569.

Ashkenazi, S., & Henik, A. (2010). Attentional networks in developmental dyscalculia. *Behavioral and Brain Function, 6*, 1–12.

Ashkenazi, S., Rosenberg-Lee, M., Tenison, C., & Menon, V. (2012). Weak task-related modulation and stimulus representations during arithmetic problem solving in children with developmental dyscalculia. *Developmental Cognitive Neuroscience, 2*(Suppl. 1), S152–S166.

Atkinson, T. M., Konold, T. R., & Glutting, J. J. (2008). Patterns of memory: A normative taxonomy of the Wide Range Assessment of Memory and Learning–Second Edition (WRAML-2). *Journal of the International Neuropsychological Society, 14*(5), 869–877.

Axelson, D., Birmaher, B., Strober, M., Gill, M. K., Valeri, S., Chiappetta, L., et al. (2006). Phenomenology of children and adolescents with bipolar spectrum disorders. *Archives of General Psychiatry, 63*, 1139–1148.

Aylward, E. H., Richards, T. L., Berninger, V. W., Nagy, W. E., Field, K. M., Grimme, A. C., et al. (2003). Instructional treatment associated with changes in brain activation in children with dyslexia. *Neurology, 61*, 212–219.

Ayres, R. R., & Cooley, E. J. (1986). Sequential versus simultaneous processing on the K-ABC: Validity in predicting learning success. *Journal of Psychoeducational Assessment, 4*(3), 211–220.

Babiloni, C., Vecchio, F., Bultrini, A., Luca Romani, G., & Rossini, P. M. (2006). Pre- and poststimulus alpha rhythms are related to conscious visual perception: a high-resolution EEG study. *Cerebral Cortex, 16*(12), 1690–1700.

Bachevalier, J., & Loveland, K. A. (2006). The orbitofrontal–amygdala circuit and self-regulation of social–emotional behavior in autism. *Neuroscience & Biobehavioral Reviews, 30*(1), 97–117.

Backenson, E. M., Holland, S. C., Kubas, H. A., Fitzer, K. R., Wilcox, G., Carmichael, J. A., et al. (2015). Psychosocial and adaptive deficits associated with learning disability subtypes. *Journal of Learning Disabilities, 48*(5), 511–522.

Baker, J. M., Klabunde, M., Booil, J., Green, T., & Reiss, A. L. (2020). On the relationship between mathematics and visuospatial processing in Turner syndrome. *Journal of Psychiatric Research, 121*, 135–142.

Baker, J. M., & Reiss, A. L. (2015). A meta-analysis of math performance in Turner syndrome. *Developmental Medicine and Child Neurology, 58*, 123–130.

Baker, L., & Cantwell, D. P. (1987). A prospective psychiatric follow-up of children with speech/language disorders. *Journal of the American Academy of Child and Adolescent Psychiatry, 26*, 546–553.

Balaban, N., Friedmann, N., & Ziv, M. (2016). Theory of mind impairment after right-hemisphere damage. *Aphasiology, 30*(12), 1399–1423.

Baldo, J. V., Shimamura, A. P., Delis, D. C., Kramer, J., & Kaplan, E. (2001). Verbal and design fluency in patients with frontal lobe lesions. *Journal of the International Neuropsychological Society, 7*, 586–596.

Balu, R., Zhu, P., Doolittle, F., Schiller, E., Jenkins, J., & Gersten, R. (2015). *Evaluation of response to intervention practices for elementary school reading* (NCEE 2016-4000). National Center for Education Evaluation and Regional Assistance.

Bandura, A. (1978). Self-efficacy: Toward a unifying theory of behavioral change. *Advances in Behaviour Research and Therapy, 1*(4), 139–161.

Banich, M. T., Burgess, G. C., Depue, B. E., Ruzic, L., Bidwell, L. C., & Hitt-Laustsen, S. (2009). The neural basis of sustained and transient attentional control in young adults with ADHD. *NeuroImage, 53*, 3095–3104.

Banks, S. J., Eddy, K. T., Angstadt, M., Nathan, P. J., & Phan, K. L. (2007). Amygdala-frontal connectivity during emotion regulation. *Social Cognitive and Affective Neuroscience, 2*, 303–312.

Bao, A. M., Meynen, G., & Swaab, D. F. (2008). The stress system in depression and neurodegeneration: focus on the human hypothalamus. *Brain Research Reviews, 57*(2), 531–553.

Barbey, A. K., Koenigs, M., & Grafman, J. (2013). Dorsolateral prefrontal contributions to human working memory. *Cortex, 49*(5), 1195–1205.

Barkely, R. A. (2006). The inattentive type of ADHD as a distinct disorder: What remains to be done. *Clinical Psychology, 8*, 489–493.

Barkley, R. A. (2014). Sluggish cognitive tempo (concentration deficit disorder?): Current status, future directions, and a plea to change the name. *Journal of Abnormal Psychology, 42*, 117–125.

Barkley, R. A. (Ed.). (2015). *Attention-deficit/hyperactivity disorder* (4th ed.). Guilford Press.

Barkley, R. A. (2017). *When an adult you love has ADHD*. American Psychological Association.

Barkley, R. A. (2020). *Taking charge of ADHD: The complete, authoritative guide for parents* (4th ed.). Guilford Press.

Baron, I. S. (2000). Clinical implications and practical applications of child neuropsychological evaluations. In K. O. Yeates, H. D. Ris, & H. G. Taylor (Eds.), *Pediatric neuropsychology: Research, theory, and practice* (pp. 439–454). Guilford Press.

Baron, I. S. (2016). *Neuropsychological evaluation of the child: Domains, methods, and case studies*. Oxford University Press.

Baron, I. S. (2018). *Neuropsychological evaluation of the child: Domains, methods, & case studies*. Oxford University Press.

Baron-Cohen, S., Tager-Flusberg, H., & Cohen, D. J. (2000). *Understanding other minds: Perspectives from developmental cognitive neuroscience* (2nd ed). Oxford University Press.

Barraclough, C., & Machek, G. (2010). School Psychologists' role concerning children with chronic illnesses in schools. *Journal of Applied School Psychology, 26*, 132–148.

Barth, A. E., Stuebing, K. K., Anthony, J. L, Denton, C. A., Mathes, P. G., Fletcher, J. M., & Francis, D. J. (2008). Agreement among response to intervention criteria for identifying responder status. *Learning and Individual Differences, 18*, 296–307.

Bates, P., & Silberman, W. (2007). *Modelling risk management in inclusive settings*. National Development Team.

Batsche, G. M., Curtis, M. J., Dorman, C., Castillo, J. M., & Porter, L. J. (2007). The Florida problem-solving/response to intervention model: Implementing a statewide initiative. In S. R. Jimerson, M. K. Burns, & A. M. VanDerHeyen (Eds.), *Handbook of response to intervention: The science and practice of assessment and intervention* (pp. 378–395). Springer Science + Business Media.

Bauman, M. L., & Kemper, T. L. (2005). Neuroanatomic observations of the brain in autism: a review and future directions. *International Journal of Developmental Neuroscience, 23*(2–3), 183–187.

Baweja, R., Mayes, S. D., Hameed, U., & Waxmonsky, J. G. (2016). Disruptive mood dysregulation disorder: Current insights. *Neuropsychiatric Disorder Treatment, 12,* 2115–2124.

Beach, K. D. (2012). *Early response-to-intervention measures and criteria as predictors of reading disability in 3rd grade.* University of California, Riverside.

Beaton, E. A., Stoddard, J., Lai, S., Lackey, J., Shi, J., Ross, J. L., & Simon, T. J. (2010). Atypical functional brain activation during a multiple object tracking task in girls with Turner syndrome: neurocorrelates of reduced spatiotemporal resolution. *American Journal on Intellectual and Developmental Disabilities, 115*(2), 140–156.

Beauregard, M., Chertkow, H., Bub, D., Murtha, S., Dixon, R., & Evans, A. (1997). The neural substrate for concrete, abstract, and emotional word lexica: A positron emission tomography study. *Journal of Cognitive Neuroscience, 9,* 441–461.

Beck, M., Arn, P., Giugliani, R., Muenzer, J., Muenzer, J., Okuyama, T., et al. (2014). The natural history of MPS I: global perspectives from the MPS I Registry. *Genetic Medicine, 16,* 759–765.

Becker, S. P., McBurnett, K., Hinshaw, S. P., & Pfiffner, L. J. (2013). Negative social preference in relation to internalizing symptoms among children with ADHD predominantly inattentive type: Girls fare worse than boys. *Journal of Clinical Child & Adolescent Psychology, 42*(6), 784–795.

Bednarz, H., & Kana, R. (2019). A-24 Metacognition and behavioral regulation associated with distinct connectivity patterns in autism spectrum disorder. *Archives of Clinical Neuropsychology, 34*(6), 883–883.

Beeman, M. (1993). Semantic processing in the right hemisphere may contribute to drawing inferences from discourse. *Brain and Language, 44,* 80–120.

Beeman, M. J., & Chiarello, C. (Eds.). (2013). *Right hemisphere language comprehension: Perspectives from cognitive neuroscience.* Psychology Press.

Beery K. E., & Beery N. A. (2010). *Administration, scoring, and teaching manual for the Beery-VMI* (6th ed.). Pearson.

Beers, S. F., Berninger, V. W., Mickail, K., & Abbott, R. (2018). Online writing processes in translation cognition into language transcribing written language by stylus and keyboard in upper elementary and middle school students with persisting dysgraphia or dyslexia. *Learning Disabilities, 23,* doi:10.18666/LDMJ-2018-V23-I2-9008.

Belanger, S. A., Andrews, D., Gray, C., & Korczak, D. (2018). ADHD in children and youth: Part 1—Etiology, diagnosis, and comorbidity. *Paediatrics & Child Health, 23,* 447–453.

Belger, A., & Banich, M. T. (1998). Costs and benefits of integrating information between the two hemispheres: A computational perspective. *Neuropsychology, 12,* 380–398.

Bellinger, D. C. (2008). Neurological and behavioral consequences of childhood lead exposure. *PLOS Medicine, 5*(5), 115.

Bellocchi, S., Muneaux, M., Bastien-Toniazzo, M., & Ducrot, S. (2013). I can read it in your eyes: What eye movements tell us about visuo-attentional processes in developmental dyslexia. *Research in Developmental Disabilities, 34,* 452–460.

Bender, W. N. (2012). *Differentiating instruction for students with learning disabilities: New best practices for general and special educators.* Corwin Press.

Benedek, E. P. (2012). Review of practical child and adolescent psychiatry and primary care. *Bulletin of the Menninger Clinic, 76,* 94–96.

Benson, N. F., Maki, K. E., Floyd, R. G., Eckert, T. L., Kranzler, J. H., & Fefer, S. A. (2020). A national survey of school psychologists' practices in identifying specific learning disabilities. *School Psychology, 35*(2), 146.

Benton, A., & Tranel, D. (1993). Visuoperceptual, visuospatial, and visuoconstructive disorders. In K. M. Heilman & E. Valenstein (Eds.), *Clinical neuropsychology* (3rd ed., pp. 165–213). Oxford University Press.

Ben-Yehudah, G., Sackett, E., Malchi-Ginzberg, L., & Ahissar, M. (2001). Impaired temporal contrast sensitivity in dyslexics is specific to retain-and-compare paradigms. *Brain, 124,* 1381–1395.

Berch, D. B. (2017). Why learning common fractions is uncommonly difficult: Unique challenges faced by students with mathematical disabilities. *Journal of Learning Disabilities, 50*(6), 651–654.

Berlucchi, G. (2012). Frontal callosal disconnection syndromes. *Cortex, 48*(1), 36–45.

Berninger, V. W. (2007a). *Process assessment of the learner, second edition: Diagnostics for math (PAL-II Math).* Pearson.

Berninger, V. W. (2007b). *Process assessment of the learner, second edition: Diagnostics for reading and writing (PAL-II Reading and Writing).* Pearson.

Berninger, V. W. (2008). Evidence-based written language instruction during early and middle childhood. In R. D. Morris & N. Mather (Eds.), *Evidence-based interventions for students with learning and behavioral challenges* (pp. 215–235). Erlbaum.

Berninger, V. W. (2009). Highlights of a programmatic, interdisciplinary research on writing. *Learning Disabilities Research and Practice, 24,* 69–80.

Berninger, V. W., Abbott, R. D., Billingsley, F., & Nagy, F. W. (2001). Processes underlying timing and fluency of reading: Efficiency, automaticity, coordination, and morphological awareness. In M. Wolf (Ed.), *Dyslexia, fluency, and the brain* (pp. 383–414). York Press.

Berninger, V. W., Abbott, R., & Garcia, N. (2009). Comparison of pen and keyboard transcription modes in children with and without learning disabilities. *Learning Disability Quarterly, 32,* 123–141.

Berninger, V. W., Abbott, R. D., Jones, J., Wolf, B. J., Gould, L., Anderson-Youngstrom, M., et al. (2006). Early development of language by hand: Composing, reading, listening, and speaking connections; three letter-writing modes; and fast mapping in spelling. *Developmental Neuropsychology, 29*(1), 61–92.

Berninger, V. W., Abbott, R. D., Nagy, W. E., & Carlisle, J. (2010). Growth in phonological, orthographic, and morphological awareness in grades 1 to 6. *Journal of Psycholinguistic Research, 39,* 141–163.

Berninger, V. W., & Dunn, M. (2012). Brain and behavioral response to intervention for specific reading, writing, and math disabilities: What works for whom? In B. Wong & D. L. Butler (Eds.), *Learning about learning disabilities* (4th ed., pp. 59–88). Elsevier Academic Press.

Berninger, V. W., Lee, T.-L., Abbott, R. D., & Breznitz, Z. (2013). Teaching children with dyslexia to spell in a reading-writers' workshop. *Annals of Dyslexia, 63,* 1–24.

Berninger, V. W., & Niedo, J. (2012). Individualizing instruction for students with oral and written language difficulties. In J. T. Mascolo, V. C. Alfonso, & D. P. Flanagan (Eds.), *Essentials of planning, selecting and tailoring intervention: Addressing the needs of unique learners* (pp. 231–264). Wiley.

Berninger, V. W., Nielsen, K. H., Abbott, R. D., Wijsman, E., & Raskind, W. (2008a). Gender differences in severity of writing and reading disabilities. *Journal of School Psychology, 46,* 151–172.

Berninger, V. W., Nielsen, K. H., Abbott, R. D., Wijsman, E., & Raskind, W. (2008b). Writing problems in developmental dyslexia: Under-recognized and under-treated. *Journal of School Psychology, 46,* 1–21.

Berninger, V. W., & O'Malley May, M. (2011). Evidence-based diagnosis and treatment for specific learning disabilities involving impairments in written and/or oral language. *Journal of Learning Disabilities, 44*(2), 167–183.

Berninger, V. W., Raskind, W., Richards, T., Abbott, R. D., & Stock, P. (2008). A multidisciplinary approach to understanding developmental dyslexia within working-memory architecture. *Developmental Neuropsychology, 33,* 707–744.

Berninger, V. W., & Richards, T. L. (2012). The writing brain: Coordinating sensory/motor, language, and cognitive systems in working memory. In V. W. Berninger (Ed.), *Past, present, and future contributions of cognitive writing research to cognitive psychology* (pp. 537–563). Psychology Press.

Berninger, V. W., Richards, T. L., & Abbott, R. D. (2015). Differential diagnosis of dysgraphia, dyslexia, and OWL LD: Behavioral and neuroimaging evidence. *Reading and Writing, 28,* 1119–1153.

Berninger, V. W., Richards, T. L., & Abbott, R. D. (2017). Brain and behavioral assessment of executive functions for self-regulating levels of language in reading brain. *Journal of Natural Science, 3,* 1–14.

Berninger, V. W., Swanson, H. L., & Griffin, W. (2015). Understanding developmental and learning disabilities within functional-systems frameworks: Building on the contributions of J. P. Das. In T. C. Papadopoulos, R. K. Parrila, & J. R. Kirby (Eds.), *Cognition, intelligence, and achievement: A tribute to J. P. Das* (pp. 397–418). Elsevier Academic Press.

Berninger, V. W., Vaughan, K., Abbott, R. D., Begay, K., Coleman, K. B., Curtin, G., et al. (2002). Teaching spelling and composition alone and together: Implications for the simple view of writing. *Journal of Educational Psychology, 94*(2), 291.

Berninger, V. W., Winn, W., Stock, P., Abbott, R. D., Eschen, K., Lin, C., et al. (2008). Tier 3 specialized writing instruction for students with dyslexia. *Reading and Writing, 21,* 95–129.

Bernstein, J. H. (2000). Developmental neuropsychological assessment. In K. O. Yeates, M. D. Ris, & H. G. Taylor (Eds.), *Pediatric neuropsychology: Research, theory, and practice* (pp. 405–438). Guilford Press.

Bernstein, S. E. (2009). Phonology, decoding, and lexical compensation in vowel spelling errors made by children with dyslexia. *Reading and Writing, 22,* 307–331.

Berth, S. H., & Kossoff, E. H. (2019). Adolescent-onset absence epilepsy years after resolution of childhood epilepsy with myoclonic-atonic seizures. *Epilepsy & Behavior Reports, 12,* 1–5.

Best, J. R., Miller, P. H., & Naglieri, J. A. (2011). Relations between Executive Function and Academic Achievement from Ages 5 to 17 in a Large, Representative National Sample. *Learning and Individual Differences, 21*(4), 327–336.

Biederman, J., Faraone, S .V., Petty, C., Martelon, M., Woodworth, K. Y., & Wozniak, J. (2013). Further evidence that pediatric-onset bipolar disorder comorbid with ADHD represents a distinct subtype: Results from a large controlled family study. *Journal of Psychiatric Research, 47,* 15–22.

Biederman, J., Monuteaux, M. C., Doyle, A. E., Seidman, L., Wilens, T. & Ferrero, F. (2004). Impact of executive function deficits and attention-deficit hyperactivity disorder (ADHD) on academic outcomes in children. *Journal of Consulting and Clinical Psychology, 72,* 757–766.

Biederman, J., Petty, C. R., Dolan, C., Hughes, S., Mick, E., Monuteaux, M. C., & Faraone, S. V. (2008). The long-term longitudinal course of oppositional defiant disorder and conduct disorder in ADHD boys: Findings from a controlled 10-year prospective longitudinal follow-up study. *Psychological Medicine, 38,* 1027–1036.

Bifulco, A. T., Moran, P. M., Ball, C., Jacobs, D., Baines, R., Bunn, A., & Cavagin, J. (2002). Child adversity, parental vulnerability and disorder: Examination of inter-generational transmission of risk. *Journal of Child Psychology & Psychiatry & Allied Disciplines, 43,* 1075–1086.

Bigler, E. D. (2008). Neuropsychology and clinical neuroscience of persistent post-concussive syndrome. *Journal of the International Neuropsychological Society, 14,* 1–22.

Binder, J. R., Desai, R. H., Graves, W. W., & Conant, L. L. (2009). Where is the semantic system? A critical review and meta-analysis of 120 functional neuroimaging studies. *Cerebral Cortex, 19,* 2767–2796.

Binder, J. R., Medler, D. A., Westbury, C. F., Liebenthal, E., & Buchanan, L. (2006). Tuning of the human left fusiform gyrus to sublexical orthographic structure. *NeuroImage, 33,* 739–748.

Binet, A., & Simon, T. (1905). Methodes nouvelles pour le diagnostic du niveau intellectuel anormaux. *L'Année Psychologique, 11,* 191–244.

Bird, G., Silani, G., Brindley, R., White, S., Frith, U., & Singer, R. (2010). Empathic brain responses in insula are modulated by levels of alexithymia but not autism. *Brain, 133,* 1515–1525.

Bjorkquist, O. A., Fryer, S. L., Reiss, A. L., Mattson, S. N., & Riley, E. P. (2010). Cingulate gyrus morphology in children and adolescents with fetal spectrum disorders. *Psychiatry Research, 181*(2),101–107.

Blackford, J. U., Buckholtz, J. W., Avery, S. N., & Zald, D. H. (2010). A unique role for the human amygdala in novelty detection. *NeuroImage, 50,* 1188–1193.

Blair, K. P., Rosenberg-Lee, M., Tsang, J. M., Schwartz, D. L., & Menon, V. (2011). Beyond natural numbers: Representation of negative numbers in the parietal cortex. *Frontiers in Human Neuroscience, 6,* 7.

Bledsoe, J., Semrud-Clikeman, M., & Pliszka, S. R. (2009). An MRI study of the cerebellar vermis in chronically-treated and treatment-naive children with ADHD-Combined type. *Biological Psychiatry, 64,* 620–624.

Blum, C., & Bakken, J. P. (2010), Labeling of students with disabilities: Unwanted and not needed. In F. E. Obiakor, J. P. Bakken, & A. F. Rotatori (Eds.), *Current issues and trends in special education: Identification, assessment and instruction* (pp. 115–125). Emerald Group.

Blum, D., & Holling, H. (2017). Spearman's law of diminishing returns: A meta-analysis. *Intelligence, 65,* 60–66.

Boada, R., Willcutt, E., & Pennington, B. F. (2012). Understanding the comorbidity between dyslexia and attention-deficit/hyperactivity disorder. *Topics in Language Disorders, 32,* 264–284.

Bodin, D., & Shay, N. (2012). Cognitive screening and neuropsychological assessment. In M. W. Kirkwood & K. O. Yeates (Eds.), *Mild traumatic brain injury in children and adolescents: From basic science to clinical management* (pp. 264–278). Guilford Press.

Boll, T. J. (1993). *Children's Category Test.* Psychological Corporation.

Bolton, S., & Hattie, D. S. (2017). Cognitive and brain development: Executive function, Piaget, and the prefrontal cortex. *Archives of Psychology, 1*(3), 1–36.

Bookheimer, S. Y., Zeffiro, T. A., Blaxton, T., Gaillard, W., & Theodore, W. (1995). Regional cerebral blood flow during object naming and word reading. *Human Brain Mapping, 3,* 93–106.

Booth, J. L., & Newton, K. J. (2012). Fractions: Could they really be the gatekeeper's doorman? *Contemporary Educational Psychology, 37,* 247–253.

Bornstein, M. H., Putnick, D. L., & Esposito, G. (2017). Continuity and stability in development. *Child Development Perspectives, 11*(2), 113–119.

Bottcher, L., Flachs, E. M., & Uldall, P. (2009). Attentional and executive impairments in children with spastic cerebral palsy. *Developmental Medicine & Child Neurology, 52,* 42–47.

Bowers, P. G., & Wolf, M. (1993). *A double-deficit hypothesis for developmental reading disorders.* ERIC Number: ED355495.

Bowman, D. B., Markham, P. M., & Roberts, R. D. (2001). Expanding the frontier of human cognitive abilities: So much more than (plain) *g! Learning and Individual Differences, 13,* 127–158.

Boylan, K., Georgiades, K., & Szatmari, P. (2010). The longitudinal association between oppositional and depressive symptoms across childhood. *Journal of the American Academy of Child and Adolescent Psychiatry, 49,* 152–161.

Boyle, C., Scriven, B., Durning, S., & Downes, C. (2011). Facilitating the learning of all students: The "professional positive" of inclusive practice in Australian primary schools. *Support for Learning, 26*(2), 72–78.

Bracken, B. A. (1988). Ten psychometric reasons why similar tests produce dissimilar results. *Journal of School Psychology, 26,* 155–166.

Braden, J. P., & Kratochwill, T. R. (1997). Treatment utility of assessment: Myths and realities. *School Psychology Review, 26,* 475–485.

Brawn, G., & Porter, M. (2018). Adaptive functioning in Williams Syndrome: A systematic review. *International Journal of Disability, Development and Education, 65,* 123–147.

Braze, D., Mencl, W. E., Tabor, W., Pugh, K., Constable, R. T., Fulbright, R. K., et al. (2011). Unification of sentence processing via ear and eye: An fMRI study. *Cortex, 47*, 416–431.

Breaux, R. P., Brown, H. R., & Harvey, E. A. (2017). Mediators and moderators of the relation between parental ADHD symptomatology and the early development of child ADHD and ODD symptoms. *Journal of Abnormal Child Psychology, 45*, 443–456.

Breedlove, E. L., Robinson, M., Talavage, T. M., Morigaki, K. E., Yoruk, U., O'Keefe, K., et al. (2012). Biomechanical correlates of symptomatic and asymptomatic neurophysiological impairment in high school football. *Journal of Biomechanics, 45*, 1265–1272.

Breznitz, Z. (2001). The determinants of reading fluency: A comparison of dyslexic and average readers. In M. Wolf (Ed.), *Dyslexia, fluency, and the brain* (pp. 245–276). York Press.

Brière, M.-E., Scott, J. G., McNall-Knapp, R. Y., & Adams, R. L. (2008). Cognitive outcome in pediatric brain tumor survivors: Delayed attention deficit at long-term follow-up. *Pediatric Blood & Cancer, 50*, 337–340.

Brodmann, K. (1909). *Vergleichende lokalisationslehre der grosshirnrinde in ihren prinzipien dargestellt auf Grund des zellenbaues.* J. A. Barth.

Brody, N. (1997). Intelligence, schooling, and society. *American Psychologist, 52*, 1046–1050.

Broglio, S. P., Eckner, J. T., Martini, D., Sosnoff, J. J., Kutcher, J. S., & Randolph, C. (2011). Cumulative head impact burden in high school football. *Journal of Neurotrauma, 28*, 2069–2078.

Brooks, A. D., Berninger, V. W., & Abbott, R. D. (2011). Letter naming and letter writing reversals in children with dyslexia: Momentary inefficiency in the phonological and orthographic loops of working memory. *Developmental Neuropsychology, 36*, 847–868.

Brooks, B. L., & Iverson, G. L. (2012). Improving accuracy when identifying cognitive impairment in pediatric neuropsychological assessments. In E. M. S Sherman & B. L. Brooks (Eds.), *Pediatric forensics neuropsychology* (pp. 66–88). Oxford University Press.

Broshek, D. K. (2013). *Psychological factors associated with concussion.* Paper presented at the 2013 International Sports Concussion Symposium, Minneapolis.

Broshek, D. K., Samples, H., Beard, J., & Goodkin, H. P. (2014). Current practices of the child neurologist in managing sports concussion. *Journal of Child Neurology, 29*(1), 17–22.

Brown, C. S., & Lichter-Konecki, U. (2016). Phenylketonuria (PKU): A problem solved? *Molecular Genetics and Metabolism, 6*, 8–12.

Brown-Chidsey, R., & Andren, K. J. (2012). Intelligence tests in the context of emerging assessment practices: Problem-solving applications. In D. P. Flanagan & P. L. Harrison (Eds.), *Contemporary intellectual assessment* (pp. 839–851). Guilford Press.

Brumback, R. A., & Weinberg, W. A. (1990). Pediatric behavioral neurology: An update on the neurologic aspects of depression, hyperactivity, and learning disabilities. *Pediatric Neurology, 8*, 677–703.

Bruno, A., Celebre, L., Torre, G., Pandolfo, G., Mento, C., Cedro, C. et al (2019). Focus on disruptive mood dysregulation disorder: A review of the literature. *Psychiatry Research, 279*, 323–330.

Bruya, B. (2010). Introduction: Toward a theory of attention that includes effortless attention. In B. Bruya (Ed.), *Effortless attention: A new perspective in the cognitive science of attention and actions* (pp. 1–28). MIT Press.

Bryan, K. L., & Hale, J. B. (2001). Differential effects of left and right hemisphere accidents on language competency. *Journal of the International Neuropsychological Society, 7*, 655–664.

Bryden, M. P. (1988). Does laterality make any difference?: Thoughts on the relation between cerebral asymmetry and reading. In D. L. Molfese & S. J. Segalowitz (Eds.), *Brain lateralization in children: Developmental implications* (pp. 509–525). Guilford Press.

Buckner, R. L., Andrews-Hanna, J. R., & Schacter, D. L. (2008). The brain's default network: Anatomy, function, and relevance to disease. *Annals of the New York Academy of Sciences, 1124*, 1–38.

Burgess, P. W., & Stuss, D. T. (2017). Fifty years of prefrontal cortex research: Impact on assessment. *Journal of the International Neuropsychological Society, 23*(9–10), 755–767.

Burianova, H., McIntosh, A. R., & Grady, C. L. (2010). A common functional brain network for autobiographical, episodic, and semantic memory retrieval. *Neuroimage, 49*(1), 865–874.

Burns, M., & Gerstenberger, S. L. (2014). Implications of the new Centers for Disease Control and Prevention blood lead reference value. *American Journal of Public Health, 104*, 1131–1149.

Burns, M. K., & Gibbons, K. (2013). *Implementing response-to-intervention in elementary and secondary schools.* Routledge.

Burns, M. K., Peters, R., & Noell, G. H. (2008). Using performance feedback to enhance implementation fidelity of the problem-solving team process. *Journal of School Psychology, 46*(5), 537–550.

Burton, L. (Ed.). (2012). *Learning mathematics: From hierarchies to networks.* Routledge.

Bush, G., Luu, P., & Posner, M. I. (2000). Cognitive and emotional influences in anterior cingulate cortex. *Trends in Cognitive Science, 4*, 215–222.

Bush, G., Spencer, T. J., Holmes, J., Shin, L. M., Valera, E., & Seidman, L. (2008). Functional magnetic resonance imaging of methylphenidate and placebo in attention-deficit hyperactivity disorder during the multi-source interference task. *Archives of General Psychiatry, 65*, 102–114.

Butterworth, B., Varma, S., & Laurillard, D. (2011). Dyscalculia: From brain to education. *Science, 332*, 1049–1053.

Caemmerer, J. M., Maddocks, D. L., Keith, T. Z., & Reynolds, M. R. (2018). Effects of cognitive abilities on child and youth academic achievement: Evidence from the WISC-V and WIAT-III. *Intelligence, 68*, 6–20.

Caggiano, P., & Jehkonen, M. (2018). The "Neglected" personal neglect. *Neuropsychology Review, 28*, 417–435.

Cairns, V., & Godwin, J. (2005). Post-Lyme borreliosis Syndrome: A meta-analysis of reported symptoms. *International Journal of Epidemiology, 34*, 1340–1345.

Caldani, S., Gerard, C. L., Peyre, H., & Bucci, M. P. (2020). Visual attentional training improves reading capabilities in children with dyslexia: An eye tracker study during a reading task. *Brain Sciences, 10*(8), 558.

Cameron, D. J. (2010). Proof that chronic Lyme Disease exists. *Interdisciplinary Perspectives on Infectious Diseases.* Available at https://doi.org/10.1155/2010/876450.

Camfield, C., Breau, L., & Camfield, P. (2001). Impact of pediatric epilepsy on the family: A new scale for clinical and research use. *Epilepsia, 42*(1), 104–112.

Canivez, G. L., & Gaboury, A. R. (2016). Construct validity and diagnostic utility of the Cognitive Assessment System for ADHD. *Journal of Attention Disorders, 20*(6), 519–529.

Canivez, G. L., McGill, R. J., Dombrowski, S. C., Watkins, M. W. Pritchard, A. E., & Jacobson, L. A. (2020). Construct validity of the WISC-V in clinical cases: Exploratory and confirmatory factor analyses of the 10 primary subtests. *Assessment, 27*(2), 274–296.

Canivez, G. L., Watkins, M. W., & Dombrowski, S. C. (2017). Structural validity of the Wechsler Intelligence Scale for Children–Fifth Edition: Confirmatory factor analyses with the 16 primary and secondary subtests. *Psychological Assessment, 29*(4), 458.

Canton, M., Le Gall, D., Feillet, F., Bonnemains, C., & Roy, A. (2019). Neuropsychological profile of children with early and continuously treated phenylketonuria: systematic review and future approaches. *Journal of the International Neuropsychological Society, 25*(6), 624–643.

Capano, L., Minden, D., Chen, S. X., Schachar, R. J., &

Ickowicz, A. (2008). Mathematical learning disorder in school-age children with Attention-Deficit Hyperactivity Disorder. *The Canadian Journal of Psychiatry, 53*, 392–398.

Caplan, R., Siddarth, P., Gurbani, S., Hanson, R., Sankar, R., & Shields, W. D. (2005). Depression and anxiety disorders in pediatric epilepsy. *Epilepsia, 46*(5), 720–730.

Capote, A., Flaherty, L., & Lichter, D. G. (2001). Addictions and subcortical circuits. In D. Lichter & J. L. Cummings (Eds.), *Frontal–subcortical circuits in psychiatric and neurological disorders* (pp. 231–257). Guilford Press.

Cappa, S. F., & Perani, D. (2003). The neural correlates of noun and verb processing. *Journal of Neurolinguistics, 16*(2–3), 183–189.

Carey, E., Hill, F., Devine, A., & Szucs, D. (2016). The chicken or the egg? The direction of the relationship between mathematics anxiety and mathematics performance. *Frontiers of Psychology, 6*, 1987.

Carlson, A. G., Rowe, E., & Curby, T. W. (2013). Disentangling fine motor skills' relations to academic achievement: The relative contributions of visual–spatial integration and visual-motor coordination. *The Journal of Genetic Psychology, 174*(5), 514–533.

Carmichael, J. A., Fraccaro, R. L., Miller, D. C., & Maricle, D. E. (2014). Academic achievement and memory differences among specific learning disabilities subtypes. *Learning Disabilities: A Multidisciplinary Journal, 20*(1), 8–17.

Carmichael, J. A., Kubas, H. A., Carlson, H. L., Fitzer, K. R., Wilcox, G., & Lemay, J. F. (2015). Reconsidering "inattention" in attention-deficit hyperactivity disorder: implications for neuropsychological assessment and intervention. *Applied Neuropsychology: Child, 4*(2), 97–105.

Carota, F., Kriegeskorte, N., Nili, H., & Pulvermüller, F. (2017). Representational similarity mapping of distributional semantics in left inferior frontal, middle temporal, and motor cortex. *Cerebral Cortex, 27*(1), 294–309.

Carroll, J. B. (1993). *Human cognitive abilities: A survey of factor-analytic studies.* Cambridge University Press.

Carrow-Woolfolk, E. (1999). *Comprehensive assessment of spoken language.* American Guidance Service.

Carrow-Woolfolk, E. (2011). *Oral and Written Language Scales, Second edition.* Pearson.

Carrow-Woolfolk E. (2017). *Comprehensive Assessment of Spoken Language, Second Edition* (CASL-2) [Manual]. Western Psychological Services.

Carter, C. S., & Sellman, E. (2013). A view of dyslexia in context: Implications for understanding differences in essay writing experience amongst higher education students identified as dyslexic. *Dyslexia, 19*, 149–164.

Carter, J. A., Neville, B., & Newton, C. (2003). Neurocognitive impairment following acquired central nervous system infections in childhood: A systematic review. *Brain Research Reviews, 43,* 57–69.

Casaletto, K. B., & Heaton, R. K. (2017). Neuropsychological assessment: Past and future. *Journal of the International Neuropsychological Society, 23*(9–10), 778–790.

Casanova, M., El-Baz, A. S., Giedd, J. N., Rumsey, J. M., & Switala, A. E. (2010). Increased white matter gyral depth in dyslexia: Implications for corticocortical connectivity. *Journal of Autism and Developmental Disorders, 40,* 21–29.

Casey, B. J., Tottenham, N., Liston, C., & Durston, S. (2005). Imaging the developing brain: what have we learned about cognitive development? *Trends in Cognitive Sciences, 9*(3), 104–110.

Casey, B. J., Trainor, R., Giedd, J., Vauss, J., Vaituzis, C. K., Hamburger, S., et al. (1997). The role of the anterior cingulate gyrus in automatic and controlled processes: A developmental neuroanatomical study. *Developmental Psychobiology, 30,* 61–69.

Cassidy, S. B., Schwartz, S., Miller, J. L., & Driscoll, D. J. (2011). Prader–Willi Syndrome. *Genetics in Medicine, 14,* 10–26.

Castellanos, F. X., Giedd, J. N., Marsh, W. L., Hamburger, S. D., Vaituzis, A. C., Dickstein, D. P., et al. (1996). Quantitative brain magnetic resonance imaging in attention-deficit hyperactivity disorder. *Archives of General Psychiatry, 53,* 607–616.

Castellanos, F. X., & Proal, E. (2012). Large-scale brain systems in ADHD: Beyond the prefrontal–striatal model. *Trends in Cognitive Science, 16,* 17–26.

Castellanos, F. X., & Tannock, R. (2002). Neuroscience of attention-deficit/hyperactivity disorders: The search for endophenotypes. *Neuroscience, 3,* 617–628.

Castles, A., & Coltheart, M. (2004). Is there a causal link from phonological awareness to success in learning to read? *Cognition, 91,* 77–111.

Castles, A., Rastle, K., & Nation, K. (2018). Ending the reading wars: Reading acquisition from novice to expert. *Psychological Science in the Public Interest, 19*(1), 5–51.

Castro, I. E., Larsen, D. A., Hruska, B., Parsons, P. J., Palmer, C. D., & Gump, B. B. (2019). Variabilities in the spatial density of properties contributes to background lead (Pb) exposure in children. *Environmental Research, 170,* 463–471.

Catani, M., Dell'Acqua, F., & Thiebaut de Schotten, M. (2013). A revised limbic system model for memory, emotion, and behaviour. *Neuroscience and Behavioral Reviews, 37,* 1724–1737.

Centers for Disease Control. (2010). Childhood lead poisoning. Retrieved May 19, 2010, from *www.cdc.gov/lead/default.html*.

Chamberlin, J. M., Gagne, C. L., Spalding, T. L., & Loo, K. (2019). Detecting spelling errors in compound and pseudocompound words. *Journal of Experimental Psychology: Learning, Memory and Cognition, 46,* 580–602.

Chang, C., Gou, S., Huang, W.-S., Shiue, C.-Y., & Yeh, C.-B. (2017). Abnormal serotonin transporter available in the brains of adults with conduct disorder. *Journal of Formosan Medical Association, 116,* 469–475.

Chang, S., & Yu, N. (2016). Comparison of motor praxis and performance in children with varying levels of developmental coordination disorder. *Human Movement Science, 48,* 7–14.

Chapleau, N., & Beaupré-Boivin, K. (2019). Interventions to support the development of spelling knowledge and strategies for children with dyslexia. *Education, 9*(1), 1–8.

Chen, J.-K., Johnston, K. M., Petrides, M., & Ptito, A. (2008). Neural substrates of symptoms of depression following concussion in male athletes with persisting postconcussion symptoms. *JAMA Psychiatry, 65,* 81–89.

Chen, J.-Q., & Gardner, H. (2018). Assessment from the perspective of Multiple-Intelligences Theory: Principles, practices, and values. In D. P. Flanagan & E. M. McDonough (Eds.), *Contemporary intellectual assessment: Theories, tests, and issues* (4th ed., pp. 164–173). Guilford Press.

Chiron, C., Jambaque, I., Nabbout, R., Lounes, R., Syrota, A., & Dulac, O. (1997). The right brain hemisphere is dominant in human infants. *Brain, 120,* 1057–1065.

Chong, S. L., & Siegel, L. S. (2008). Stability of computational deficits in math learning disability from second through fifth grades. *Developmental Neuropsychology, 33,* 300–317.

Chu-Shor, C. J., Caviness, V. S., & Cash, S. S. (2012). Neural networks in the developing human brain. In M. T. Bianchi, V. S. Caviness, & S. S. Cash (Eds.), *Network approaches to diseases of the brain* (pp. 21–31). Bentham Books.

Cicchetti, D. V., & Rourke, B. P. (Eds.). (2004). *Methodological and biostatistical foundations of clinical neuropsychology and medical and health disciplines.* CRC Press.

Cioni, G., D'Acunto, G., & Guzzetta, A. (2011). Perinatal brain damage in children: neuroplasticity, early intervention, and molecular mechanisms of recovery. *Progress in Brain Research, 189,* 139–154.

Clarke, L. A., Genat, R. C., & Anderson, J. F. I. (2012). Long-term cognitive complaint and post-concussive symptoms following mild traumatic brain injury: The role of cognitive and affective factors. *Brain Injury, 26,* 298–307.

Clayton-Smith, J., & Laan, J. (2003). Angelman syndrome: A review of the clinical and genetic aspects. *Journal of Medical Genetics, 40,* 87–95.

Clements, A. M., Rimrodt, S. L., Abel, J. R., Blankner, J. G., Mostofsky, S. H., Pekar, J. J., et al. (2006). Sex differences in cerebral lateraltiy of language and visuospatial processing. *Brain and Language, 98,* 150–158.

Clements, S., Christner, R. W., McLaughlin, A. L., & Bolton, J. B. (2011). Assessing student skills using process-oriented approaches. In T. M. Lionetti, E. P. Snyder, & R. W. Christner (Eds.), *A practical guide to building professional competencies in school psychology* (pp. 101–119). Springer Science + Business Media.

Cloutman, L., Gingis, L., Newhart, M., Davis, C., Heidler-Gary, J., Crinion, J., & Hillis, A. E. (2009). A neural network critical for spelling. *Annals of Neurology, 66,* 249–253.

Cody, H., Pelphrey, K., & Piven, J. (2002). Structural and functional magnetic resonance imaging of autism. *International Journal of Developmental Neuroscience, 20,* 421–438.

Cohen, J. D., Botvinick, M., & Carter, C. S. (2000). Anterior cingulate and prefrontal cortex: Who's in control? *Nature Neuroscience, 3,* 421–424.

Cohen, M. (1997). *Children's Memory Scale.* Psychological Corporation.

Colbert, A. M., & Bo, J. (2017). Evaluating relationships among clinical working memory assessment and inattentive and hyperactive/impulsive behaviors in a community sample of children. *Research in Developmental Disabilities, 66,* 34–43.

Cole, W. R., Mostofsky, S. H., Larson, J. C., Denckla, M. B., & Mahone, E. M. (2008). Age-related changes in motor subtle signs among girls and boys with ADHD. *Neurology, 71,* 1514–1520.

Compton, D. L., Fuchs, L. S., Fuchs, D., Lambert, W., & Hamlett, C. L. (2011). The cognitive and academic profiles of reading and mathematics learning disabilities. *Journal of Learning Disabilities, 45,* 79–95.

Conant, L. L., Liebenthal, E. Desai, A., & Binder, J. R. (2013). fMRI of phonemic perception and its relationship to reading development in elementary- to middle-school-age children. *Neuroimage, 89,* 192–202.

Connelly, V., Campbell, S., MacLean, M., & Barnes, J. (2006). Contribution of lower order skills to the written composition of college students with and without dyslexia. *Developmental Neuropsychology, 29,* 175–196.

Conners, C. K., Sitarenios, G., & Ayearst, L. E. (2018). *Conners' continuous performance test.* Multi-Health Systems.

Connor, D. F., & Doerfler, L. A. (2012). Characteristics of children with juvenile bipolar disorder or disruptive behavior disorders and negative mood: Can they be distinguished in the clinical setting? *Annals of Clinical Psychiatry, 24,* 261–270.

Connor, D. F., Ford, J. D., Pearson, G. S., Scranton, V. L., & Dusad, A. (2017). Early-onset bipolar disorder: Characteristics and outcomes in the clinic. *Journal of Child and Adolescent Psychopharmacology, 27,* 875–883.

Conroy, C., & Logan, D. E. (2014). Pediatric multidisciplinary and interdisciplinary teams and interventions. In M. C. Roberts, B. S. Aylward, & Y. P. Wu (Eds.), *Clinical practice of pediatric psychology* (pp. 93–108). The Guilford Press.

Constable, R. T., Pugh, K., Berroya, E., Mencl, W. E., Westerveld, M., Ni, W., & Shankweiler, D. P. (2004). Sentence complexity and input modality effects in sentence comprehension: A fMRI study. *NeuroImage, 22,* 11–21.

Cooper, P. J., Gallop, C., Willets, L., & Creswell, C. (2008). Treatment response in child anxiety is differentially related to the form of maternal anxiety disorder. *Behavioral and Cognitive Psychotherapy, 36,* 41–48.

Copeland, W. E., Angold, A., Costello, E. J., & Egger, H. (2013). Prevalence, comorbidity and correlates of DSM-5 proposed disruptive mood dysregulation disorder. *American Journal of Psychiatry, 170,* 173–179.

Corbett, B. A., Constantine, L. J., Hendren, R., Rocke, D., & Ozonoff, S. (2009). Examining executive functioning in children with autism spectrum disorder, attention deficit hyperactivity disorder and typical development. *Psychiatry Research, 166*(2–3), 210–222.

Corbett, B. A., Muscatello, R. A., & Blain, S. D. (2016). Impact of sensory sensitivity on physiological stress response and novel peer interaction in children with and without autism spectrum disorder. *Frontiers of Neuroscience, 10,* 278.

Cormier, D. C., McGrew, K. S., Bulut, O., & Funamoto, A. (2017). Revisiting the relations between the WJ-IV measures of Cattell-Horn-Carroll (CHC) cognitive abilities and reading achievement during the school-age years. *Journal of Psychoeducational Assessment, 35*(8), 731–754.

Corr, P. J. (2008). *The reinforcement sensitivity theory of personality.* Cambridge University Press.

Costello, E. J., & Angold, A. (2016). *Developmental epidemiology.* Wiley.

Costello, E. J., Mustillo, S., Erkanli, A., Keeler, G., & Angold, A. (2008). Prevalence and development of psychiatric disorders in childhood and adolescence. *Archives of General Psychiatry, 60,* 837–844.

Council of the Great City Schools. (2017). *Annual report.* Retrieved from *www.dgcs.org.*

Coutinho, M. J., & Oswald, D. P. (2000). Disproportionate representation in special education: A synthesis and recommendations. *Journal of Child and Family Studies, 9,* 135–156.

Cragg, L., & Gilmore, C. (2014). Skills underlying mathematics: The role of executive function in the development of mathematics proficiency. *Trends in Neuroscience and Education, 3*(2), 63–68.

Crepaldi, D., Berlingeri, M., Paulesu, E., & Luzzatti, C. (2011). A place for nouns and a place for verbs? A critical review of neurocognitive data on grammatical-class effects. *Brain and Language, 116*(1), 33–49.

Crockett, J. B., & Kauffman, J. M. (2013). *The least restrictive environment: Its origins and interpretations in special education.* Routledge.

Crone, D. A., Hawken, L. S., & Horner, R. H. (2015). *Building positive behavior support systems in schools* (2nd ed.). Guilford Press.

Crump, C., Rivera, D., London, R., Landau, M., Erlandson, B., & Rodriguez, E. (2013). *Annals of Epidemiology, 23,* 179–184.

Cubillo, A., Halari, R., Smith, A., Taylor, E., & Rubia, K. (2012). A review of fronto–striatal and fronto-cortical brain abnormalities in children and adults with attention deficit hyperactivity disorder (ADHD) and new evidence for dysfunction in adults with ADHD during motivation and attention. *Cortex, 48,* 194–215.

Culhane-Shelburne, K., Chapieski, L., Hiscock, M., & Glaze, D. (2002). Executive functions in children with frontal and temporal lobe epilepsy. *Journal of the International Neuropsychological Society, 8,* 623–632.

Cummings, K. D., Dewey, E. N., Latimer, R. J., & Good III, R. H. (2011). Pathways to word reading and decoding: The roles of automaticity and accuracy. *School Psychology Review, 40*(2), 284–295.

Currie, J., Stabile, M., & Jones, L. (2014). Do stimulant medications improve educational and behavioral outcomes for children with ADHD? *Journal of Health Economics, 37,* 58–69.

Cutler, L., & Graham, S. (2008). Primary grade writing instruction: A national survey. *Journal of Educational Psychology, 100*(4), 907.

Cutting, L. E., Clements, A. M., Courtney, S., Rimrodt, S. L., Schafer, J. G. B., Biesesi, J., & Pugh, K. (2006). Differential components of sentence comprehension: Beyond single word reading and memory. *NeuroImage, 29,* 429–438.

Cutting, L. E., Eason, S. H., Young, K. M., & Alberstadt, A. L. (2009). Reading comprehension: Cognition and neuroimaging. In K. Pugh & P. McCardle (Eds.), *How children learn to read: Current issues and new directions in the integration of cognition, neurobiology, and genetics of reading and dyslexia research and practice* (pp. 195–213). Psychology Press.

Cutting, L. E., Materek, A., Cole, C. A. S., Levine, T.

M., & Mahone, E. M. (2009). Effects of fluency, oral language, and executive function on reading comprehension performance. *Annals of Dyslexia, 59,* 34–54.

Damasio, H., Grabowski, T. J., Tranel, D., Hichwa, R. D., & Damasio, A. R. (1996). The neural basis of lexical retrieval. *Nature, 380,* 499–505.

D'Amato, R. C., & Hartlage, L. C. (2008). *Essentials of neuropsychological assessment: Treatment planning for rehabilitation.* Springer.

D'Amato, R. C., Rothlisberg, B. A., & Rhodes, R. L. (1997). Utilizing a neuropsychological paradigm for understanding common educational and psychological tests. In C. R. Reynolds & E. Fletcher-Janzen (Eds.), *Handbook of clinical child neuropsychology* (pp. 270–295). Plenum Press.

Daniele, A., Giustolisi, L., Silveri, M. C., Colosimo, C., & Gainotti, G. (1994). Evidence for a possible neuroanatomical basis for lexical processing of nouns and verbs. *Neuropsychologia, 32,* 1325–1341.

Daroczy, G., Wolska, M., Meurers, W. D., & Nuerk, H. C. (2015). Word problems: A review of linguistic and numerical factors contributing to their difficulty. *Frontiers in Psychology, 6,* 348.

Das, J. P., Carlson, J., Davidson, M. B., & Longe, K. (1997). *PREP: PASS remedial program.* Hogrefe.

Das, J. P., Kar, R., & Parrila, R. K. (1996). *Cognitive planning: The psychological basis of intelligent behavior.* Sage.

Das, J. P., Naglieri, J. A., & Kirby, J. R. (1994). *Assessment of cognitive processes: The PASS theory of intelligence.* Allyn & Bacon.

Das, J. P., & Varnhagen, C. K. (1986). Neuropsychological functioning and cognitive processing. In J. E. Obrzut & G. W. Hynd (Eds.), *Child neuropsychology: Vol. 1. Theory and research* (pp. 117–140). Academic Press.

Daselaar, S. M., Veltman, D. J., Rombouts, S. A., Raaijmakers, R. B., & Jeroen, G. W. (2002). Medial temporal lobe activity during semantic classification using a flexible fMRI design. *Behavioral Brain Research, 136,* 399–404.

D'Avanzato, C., Joormann, J., Siemer, M., & Gotlib, I. H. (2013). Emotion regulation in depression and anxiety: Examining diagnostic specificity and stability of strategy use. *Cognitive Therapy and Research, 37*(5), 968–980.

Davidson, M. A. (2008). ADHD in adults: A review of the literature. *Journal of Attention Disorders, 11,* 628–641.

Davidson, R. J. (1995). Cerebral asymmetry, emotion, and affective style. In R. J. Davidson & K. Hugdahl (Eds.), *Brain asymmetry* (pp. 361–387). MIT Press.

Davidson, R. J. (1998). Affective style and affective disorders: Perspectives from affective neuroscience. *Cognition and Emotion, 12,* 307–330.

Davis, A. S. (Ed.). (2010). *Handbook of pediatric neuropsychology*. Springer.

Davis, A. S., & Dean, R. S. (2010). Assessing sensory-motor deficits in pediatric traumatic brain injury. *Applied Neuropsychology, 17*(2), 104–109.

Davis, J. M., & Broitman, J. (2011). *Nonverbal learning disabilities in children: Bridging the gap between science and practice*. Springer.

Davis, N., Cannistraci, C. J., Rogers, B. P., Gatenby, J. C., Fuchs, L. S., Anderson, A. W., & Gore, J. C. (2009). Aberrant functional activation in school age children at-risk for mathematical disability: A functional imaging study of simple arithmetic skills. *Neuropsychologia, 47*, 2470–2479.

Daviss, W. B. (2008). A review of co-morbid depression in pediatric ADHD: Etiologies, phenomenology, and treatment. *Journal of Child and Adolescent Psychopharmacology, 18*, 565–571.

Dawson, P., & Guare, R. (2018). *Executive skills in children and adolescents* (3rd ed.). Guilford Press.

Dealberto, M. J. (2011). Prevalence of autism according to maternal immigrant status and ethnic origin. *Acta Psychiatrica Scandinavica, 123*(5), 339–348.

Dean, R. S., & Noggle, C. A. (2013). Neuropsychological assessment within the psychiatric setting. In C. A. Noggle & R. S. Dean (Eds.), *The neuropsychology of psychopathology* (pp. 459–471). Springer.

Dean, R. S., Woodcock, R. W., Decker, S. L., & Schrank, F. A. (2003). A cognitive neuropsychology assessment system. In F. A. Schrank & D. P. Flanagan (Eds.), *WJ III clinical use and interpretation* (pp. 345–376). Academic Press.

DeBellis, M. D., Hooper, S. R., Woolley, D. P., & Shenk, C. E. (2010). Demographic, maltreatment, and neurobiological correlates of PTSD symptoms in children and adolescents. *Journal of Pediatric Psychology, 35*, 570–577.

de Chambrier, A.-F., & Zesiger, P. (2018). Is a fact retrieval deficit the main characteristic of children with mathematical learning disabilities? *Acta Psychologica, 190*, 95–102.

Decker, S. L., Englund, J. A., Carboni, J. A., & Brooks, J. H. (2011). Cognitive and developmental influences in visual–motor integration skills in young children. *Psychological Assessment, 23*(4), 1010.

Decker, S. L., Hale, J. B., & Flanagan, D. P. (2013). Professional practice issues in the assessment of cognitive functioning for educational applications. *Psychology in the Schools, 50*(3), 300–313.

Decker, S. L., Hill, S. K., & Dean. R. S. (2007). Evidence of construct similarity in executive functions and fluid reasoning abilities. *International Journal of Neuroscience, 117*(6), 735–748.

Decker, S. L., Schneider, W. J., & Hale, J. B. (2012). Estimating base rates of impairment in neuropsychological test batteries: A comparison of quantitative models. *Archives of Clinical Neuropsychology, 27*(1), 69–84.

DeFilippis, M. (2018). Depression in children and adolescents with autism spectrum disorder. *Children, 5*, 112–121.

de Giambattista, C., Ventura, P., Trerotoli, P., Margari, M., Palumbi, R., & Margari, L. (2019). Subtyping the autism spectrum disorder: Comparison of children with high functioning autism and Asperger syndrome. *Journal of Autism and Developmental Disorders, 49*(1), 138–150.

Dehaene, S., Cohen, L., Morais, J., & Kolinsky, R. (2015). Illiterate to literate: Behavioural and cerebral changes induced by reading acquisition. *Nature Reviews Neuroscience, 16*(4), 234–244.

Dehaene-Lambertz, G., Monzalvo, K., & Dehaene, S. (2018). The emergence of the visual word form: Longitudinal evolution of category-specific ventral visual areas during reading acquisition. *PLOS Biology, 16*(3), e2004103.

de Hevia, M. D., & Spelke, E. S. (2009). Spontaneous mapping of number and space in adults and young children. *Cognition, 111*, 198–207.

Dehn, M. J. (2008). *Working memory and academic learning: Assessment and intervention*. Wiley.

Dehn, M. J. (2010). *Long-term memory problems in children and adolescents: Assessment, intervention, and effective instruction*. Wiley.

Dehn, M. J. (2013). *Essentials of processing assessment* (2nd ed.). Wiley.

Delis, D. C., Kaplan, E., & Kramer, J. H. (2001). *Delis–Kaplan Executive Function System*. Psychological Corporation.

Delis, D. C., Kramer, J. H., Kaplan, E., & Holdnack, J. (2004). Reliability and validity of the Delis-Kaplan Executive Function System: An update. *Journal of the International Neuropsychological Society, 10*(2), 301–303.

Delis, D. C., Kramer, J. H., Kaplan, E., & Ober, B. A. (1994). *CVLT-C: California Verbal Learning Test—Children's Version*. Psychological Corporation.

Delis, D. C., Robertson, L., & Efron, R. (1986). Hemispheric specialization of memory for visual hierarchical stimuli. *Neuropsychologia, 24*, 205–214.

DeMatteo, C., Hanna, S., Mahoney, W., Hollenberg, R., Scott, L., Law, M., et al. (2010). "My child doesn't have a brain injury, he only has a concussion": Understanding how clinicians use the word "concussion" in pediatric hospitals. *Pediatrics, 125*, 327–334.

DeMatteo F. J. (2021). *Delivering psychoeducational results to parents*. Routledge.

Demonet, J-F., Taylor, M. J, & Chaix, Y. (2004). Developmental dyslexia. *Lancet, 363*, 1451–1460.

Dennis, M. (2000). Developmental plasticity in children: The role of biological risk, development, time, and reserve. *Journal of Communication Disorders, 33*(4), 321–332.

Dennis, M. (2010). Language disorders in children with central nervous system injury. *Journal of*

Clinical and Experimental Neuropsychology, 32(4), 417–432.

Deno, S. L. (1990). Individual differences and individual difference: The essential difference of special education. *Journal of Special Education, 24,* 160–173.

DeRaedt, R., Vanderhasselt, M. C., & Baeken, C. (2015). Neurostimulation as an intervention for treatment resistant depression: From research on mechanisms towards targeted neurocognitive strategies. *Clinical Psychology Review, 41,* 61–69.

Descartes, M., Korf, B. R., & Mikhail, F. M. (2017). Chromosomes and chromosomal abnormalities. In K. W. Swaiman (Ed.), *Swaiman's pediatric neurology* (pp. 268–276). Elsevier.

Descheemaeker, M. J., Govers, V., Vermeulen, P., & Fryns, J. P. (2006). Pervasive developmental disorders in Prader–Willi syndrome: The Leuven experience in 59 subjects and controls. *American Journal of Medical Genetics A, 140,* 136–142.

De Smedt, B., Taylor, J., Archibald, L., & Ansari, D. (2010). How is phonological processing related to individual differences in children's arithmetic skills? *Developmental Science, 13,* 508–520.

Deters, R. K., Naaijen, J., Rosa, M., Aggensteiner, P. M., Banaschewski, T., Saam, M. C., et al. (2020). Executive functioning and emotional recognition in youth with oppositional defiant disorder and/or conduct disorder. *The World Journal of Biological Psychiatry, 21,* 539–551.

Deveney, C. M., Connolly, M. E., Haring, C. T., Bones, B. L., Reynolds, R. C., Kim P, et al. (2013). Neural mechanisms of frustration in chronically irritable children. *American Journal of Psychiatry, 170,* 1186–1194.

Devine, A., Hill, F., Carey, E., & Dzucs, D. (2018). Cognitive and emotional math problems largely dissociate: Prevalence of developmental dyscalculia and mathematics anxiety. *Journal of Educational Psychology, 110,* 431–444.

Dickstein, D. P., Garvey, M., Pradella, A. G., Greenstein, D., Sharp, W. S., & Castellanos, F. X. (2005). Neurologic examination abnormalities in children with bipolar disorder or attention-deficit/hyperactivity disorder. *Biological Psychiatry, 58,* 517–524.

Dickstein, D. P., Treland, J. E., Snow, J., McClure, E. B., Mehta, M. S., & Towbin, K. W. (2004). Neuropsychological performance in pediatric bipolar disorder. *Biological Psychiatry, 55,* 32–39.

DiMartino, A., Ross, K., Uddin, L. Q., Sklar, A. B., Castellanos, F. X., & Milham, M. P. (2009). Functional brain correlates of social and nonsocial processes in autism spectrum disorders: An activation likelihood estimation meta-analysis. *Biological Psychiatry, 65,* 63–74.

Dirks, E., Spyer, G., Van Lieshout, E. C. D. M., & De Sonneville, L. (2008). Prevalence of combined reading and arithmetic disabilities. *Journal of Learning Disabilities, 41,* 460–473.

Dolcos, S., Hu, Y., Iordan, A. D., Moore, M., & Dolcos, F. (2016). Optimism and the brain: Trait optimism medicates the protective role of the orbitofrontal cortex gray matter volume against anxiety. *Social Cognitive and Affective Neuroscience, 11,* 263–271.

Dombrowski, S. C., Canivez, G. L., Watkins, M. W., & Beaujean, A. A. (2015). Exploratory bifactor analysis of the Wechsler Intelligence Scale for Children—Fifth Edition with the 16 primary and secondary subtests. *Intelligence, 53,* 194–201.

Dopfner, M., Katzmann, J., Hanisch, C., Fegert, J. M., Kölch, M., Ritschel, A., et al. (2019). Affective dysregulation in childhood—optimizing prevention and treatment: Protocol of three randomized controlled trials in the ADOPT study. *BMC Psychiatry, 19,* 264–284.

Dores, G. M., Devesa, S. S., Curtis, R. E., Linet, M. S., & Morton, L. M. (2012). Acute leukemia incidence and patient survival among children and adults in the United States. *Blood, 119,* 34–43.

Dornbach-Bender, A., Ruggero, C. J., Smith, P., Schuler, K., Bennett, C. B., Neumann, C. S., & Callahan, J. L. (2020). Association of behavior activation system sensitivity to lower level facets of positive affect in daily life. *Personality and Individual Differences, 153,* 1–8.

Dowker, A., Sarkar, A., & Looi, C. Y. (2016). Mathematics anxiety: What have we learned in 60 years? *Frontiers in Psychology, 7,* 508.

Doyle, A. E. (2006). Executive functions in attention-deficit/hyperactivity disorder. *Journal of Clinical Psychiatry, 67,* 21–26.

Doyle, A. E., Wilens, T., Kwon, A., Seidman, L. J., Faraone, S .V., & Fried, R. (2005). Neuropsychological functioning in youth with bipolar disorder. *Biological Psychiatry, 58,* 540–548.

Dreary, I. J., Lawn, M., & Bartholomew, D. J. (2008). A conversation between Charles Spearman, Godfrey Thomson, and Edward L. Thorndike: The international examinations inquiry meetings 1931–1938. *History of Psychology, 11*(2), 122–142.

Drevets, W. C., & Raichle, M. E. (1995). Positron emission tomographic imaging studies of human emotional disorders. In M. S. Gazzaniga (Ed.), *The cognitive neurosciences* (pp. 1153–1164). MIT Press.

Ducrot, S., & Grainger, J. (2007). Deployment of spatial attention to words in central and peripheral vision. *Perception and Psychophysics, 64,* 1130–1144.

Duffy, A., Carlson, G., Dubicka, B., & Hillegers, M. H. J. (2020). Pre-pubertal bipolar disorder: Origins and current status of the controversy. *International Journal of Bipolar Disorder, 8,* 18.

Duffy, A., Horrocks, J., Doucette S., Keown-Stoneman, C., McCloskey, S., & Grof, P. (2014). The developmental trajectory of bipolar disorder. *British Journal of Psychiatry, 204,* 122–128.

Dumont, R., Willis, J. O., & Elliott, C. D. (2008). *Essentials of DAS-II assessment.* Wiley.

Dumonthell, I., & Klingberg, R. (2012). Brain activity during a visuospatial working memory task predicts arithmetical performance 2 years later. *Cerebral Cortex, 22,* 1078–1085.

Dunn, L. M., & Dunn, L. M. (1997). *Peabody Picture Vocabulary Test–II.* American Guidance Service.

DuPaul, G. J., Barkley, R. A., & McMurray, M. B. (1994). Response of children with ADHD to methylphenidate: interaction with internalizing symptoms. *Journal of the American Academy of Child & Adolescent Psychiatry, 33*(6), 894–903.

DuPaul, G., Gormley, M. J., & Laracy, S. D. (2013). Comorbidity of LD and ADHD: Implications of DSM 5 for assessment and treatment. *Journal of Learning Disabilities, 46,* 43–51.

Duvekot, J., van der Ende, J., Verhulst, F. C., & Greaves-Lord, K. (2018). Examining bidirectional effects between the autism spectrum disorder (ASD) core symptom domains and anxiety in children with ASD. *The Journal of Child Psychology and Psychiatry, 59,* 277–284.

Dymock, S., & Nicholson, T. (2017). To what extent does children's spelling improve as a result of learning words with the look, say, cover, write, check, fix strategy compared with phonological spelling strategies? *Australian Journal of Learning Difficulties, 22*(2), 171–187.

Ebaugh, F. G. (2007). Neuropsychiatric sequelae of acute epidemic encephalitis in children. *Journal of Attention Disorders, 11,* 336–338.

Echemendia, R. J., Iverson, G. L., McCrea, M. A., Macciocchi, S. A., Gioia, G. A., Putukian, M., & Comper, P. (2013). Advances in neuropsychological assessment of sport-related concussion. *British Journal of Sports Medicine, 47,* 294–298.

Egner, T., Etkin, A., Gale, S., & Hirsch, J. (2008). Dissociable neural systems resolve conflict from emotional versus nonemotional distracters. *Cerebral Cortex, 18,* 1475–1484.

Ehri, L. C., Nunes, S. R., Willows, D. M., Schuster, B. V., Yaghoub-Zadeh, Z., & Shanahan, T. (2001). Phonemic awareness instruction helps children learn to read: Evidence from the National Reading Panel's meta-analysis. *Reading Research Quarterly, 36*(3), 250–287.

Eisengart, J. B., King, K. E., Shapiro, E. G., Whitley, C. B., & Muenzer, J. (2020). The nature and impact of neurobehavioral symptoms in neuronopathic Hunter syndrome. *Molecular Genetics and Metabolism Reports, 22,* 100549.

Elias, L. R., Miskowiak, K. W., Vale, A. M., Köhler, C. A., Kjærstad, H. L., Stubbs, B., et al. (2017). Cognitive impairment in euthymic pediatric bipolar disorder: A systematic review and meta-analysis. *Journal of the American Academy of Child and Adolescent Psychiatry, 56,* 286–296.

Eliez, S., & Reiss, A. L. (2000). Annotation: MRI neuroimaging of childhood psychiatric disorders: A selective review. *Journal of Child Psychology and Psychiatry, 41,* 679–694.

Elliott, C. D. (2007). *Differential ability scales—Second edition (DAS-II).* Pearson.

Elliott, C. D. (2008). Identifying a learning disability: Not just product, but process. In E. Fletcher-Janzen & C. R. Reynolds (Eds.), *Neuropsychological perspectives on learning disabilities in the era of RTI: Recommendations for diagnosis and intervention* (pp. 210–218). Wiley.

Elliott, C. D. (2023). *Differential Ability Scales (2nd ed., DAS–II): Normative update school-age manual.* NCS Pearson.

Elliott, C. D., Hale, J. B., Fiorello, C. A., Dorvil, C., & Moldovan, J. (2010). Differential abilities scales–second edition prediction of reading performance: Global scales are not enough. *Psychology in the Schools, 47,* 698–720.

Ellis, M. J., Leddy, J., & Willer, B. (2016). Multidisciplinary management of athletes with post-concussion syndrome: an evolving pathophysiological approach. *Frontiers in Neurology, 7,* 136.

Elvander, C., & Cnattingius, S. (2015). Outcome of attempted vaginal delivery after a previous vacuum extraction: A population-based study. *Obstetrics & Gynaecology Scandinavia, 95,* 362–367.

Epstein, H. T. (2001). An outline of the role of the brain in human cognitive development. *Brain and Cognition, 45,* 44–51.

Erchul, W. P., & Martens, B. K. (2010). *School consultation: Conceptual and empirical bases of practice* (3rd ed.). Springer.

Ernst, M., Liebenauer, L. L., King, A. C., Fitzgerald, G. A., Cohen, R. M., & Zametkin, A. J. (1994). Reduced brain metabolism in hyperactive girls. *Journal of the American Academy of Child & Adolescent Psychiatry, 33*(6), 858–868.

Etscheidt, S., & Curran, C. M. (2010). Reauthorization of the Individuals with Disabilities Education Improvement Act (IDEA, 2004): The peer-reviewed research requirement. *Journal of Disability Policy Studies, 21*(1), 29–39.

Eugene, G., Joormann, J., Cooney, R. E., Atlas, L. Y., & Gotlib, I. H. (2010). Neural correlates of inhibitory deficits in depression. *Psychiatry Research: Neuroimaging, 181,* 30–35.

Evans, J. J., Floyd, R. G., McGrew, K. S., & Leforgee, M. H. (2002). The relations between measures of Cattell-Horn-Carroll (CHC) cognitive abilities and reading achievement during childhood and adolescence. *School Psychology Review, 31*(2), 246–262.

Evans, M. A., Shedden, J. M., Hevenor, S. J., & Hahn, M. C. (2000). The effect of variability of unattended information on global and local processing: Evidence for lateralization at early stages of processing. *Neuropsychologia, 38,* 225–239.

Ezpeleta, L., Domonech, J. M., & Angold, A. (2006). A comparison of pure and comorbid CD/ODD and depression. *Journal of Child Psychology & Psychiatry & Allied Disciplines, 47,* 704–712.

Fair, D. A., Cohen, A. L., Dosenbach, N. U., Church, J. A., Miezen, M. A., Barcch, D. M. et al. (2008). The maturing architecture of the brain's default network. *Proceedings of the National Academy of Sciences USA, 105,* 4028–4032.

Fair, D. A., Nigg, J. T., Iyerm S., Bathulam D., Millsm K. L., Dosenbach, N. U., et al. (2012). Distinct neural signatures detected for ADHD subtypes after controlling for micro-movements in resting state functional connectivity MRI data. *Frontiers in Systems Neuroscience, 6,* 80–95.

Fairchild, G., Hawes, D. J., Frick, P. J., Copeland, W. E., Odgers, C. L., Franke, B., et al. (2019). Conduct disorder. *Nature Reviews, 5,* 43–50.

Falk, A. E., Lee, S. S., & Chorpita, B. F. (2017). Differential association of youth attention-deficit/hyperactivity disorder and anxiety with delinquency and aggression. *Journal of Clinical Child and Adolescent Psychology, 46,* 653–660.

Faraone, S. V., Banaschewski, R., Coghill, D., Zhen, Yi, Biederman, J., Bellgrove, M. A., et al. (2021). The World Federation of ADHD international consensus statement: 208 Evidence-based conclusions about the disorder. *Neuroscience & Behavioral Reviews, 128,* 789–818.

Farris, E. A., Odegard, T. N., Richards, T. L., Aylward, E. H., Thomson, J., & Berninger, V. W. (2011). Functional connectivity between the left and right inferior frontal lobes in a small sample of children with and without reading difficulties. *Neurocase, 17,* 425–439.

Fassaie, S., & McAloon, J. (2020). Maternal distress, HPA activity, and antenatal interventions: A systematic review. *Psychoneuroendocrinology, 112,* 104477.

Fayol, M., Alamargot, D., & Berninger, V. W. (2012). *Translation of thought to written text while composing: Advancing theory, knowledge, research methods, tools, and applications.* Psychology Press.

Feder, K. P., & Majnemer, A. (2007). Handwriting development, competency, and intervention. *Developmental Medical & Child Neurology, 49,* 312–317.

Feifer, S. G. (2011). The neuropsychology of written language disorders. In A. Davis (Ed.), *Handbook of pediatric neuropsychology* (pp. 689–697). Springer.

Feifer, S. G. (2015). *Feifer Assessment of Reading (FAR).* PAR.

Feifer, S. G. (2016). *Feifer Assessment of Mathematics (FAM).* PAR.

Feifer, S. G. (2020). *Feifer Assessment of Writing.* PAR.

Feifer, S. G., & DeFina, P. D. (2002). *The neuropsychology of written language disorders: Diagnosis and intervention.* School Neuropsychology Press.

Feifer, S. G., Nader, R. G., Flanagan, D., Fitzer, K. R., & Hicks, K. (2014). Identifying specific reading disability subtypes for effective educational remediation. *Learning Disabilities: A Multidisciplinary Journal, 20*(1), 18–30.

Feigenson, L., Dehaene, S., & Spelke, E. (2004). Core systems of number. *Trends in Cognitive Science, 8,* 307–314.

Fenwick, M. E., Kubas, H. A., Witzke, J. W., Fitzer, K. R., Miller, D. C., Maricle, D. E., et al. (2016). Neuropsychological profiles of written expression learning disabilities determined by concordance–discordance model criteria. *Applied Neuropsychology: Child, 5*(2), 83–96.

Ferguson, A. P., McKinlay, I. A., & Hunt, A. (2002). Care of adolescents with severe learning disabilities. *Developmental Medicine and Child Neurology, 44,* 256–262.

Fernandez, A. F., & Esteller, M. (2010). Viral epigenomes in human tumorigenesis. *Oncogene, 29,* 1405–1420.

Fernandez-Ruiz, J., Schwerdtfeger, R. M. H., Alahyane, N., Brien, D. C., Coe, B. C. & Munoz, D. P. (2020). Dorsolateral prefrontal cortex hyperactivity during inhibitory control in children with ADHD in the antisaccade task. *Brain Imaging and Behavior, 14*(6), 2450–2463.

Ferro, M. A., & Speechley, K. N. (2009). Depressive symptoms among mothers of children with epilepsy: A review of prevalence, associated factors, and impact on children. *Epilepsia, 50*(11), 2344–2354.

Ferstl, E. C., Neumann, J., Bogler, C., & von Cramon, Y. (2007). The extended language network: A meta-analysis of neuroimaging studies on text comprehension. *Human Brain Mapping, 29,* 581–593.

Figueras, B., Edwards, L., & Langhorn, D. (2008). Executive function and language in deaf children. *Journal of Deaf Studies in Deaf Education, 13,* 362–377.

Filipek, P. A., Semrud-Clikeman, M., Steingard, R. J., Renshaw, P. F., Kennedy, D. N., & Biederman, J. (1997). Volumetric MRI analysis comparing attention-deficit/hyperactivity disorder and normal controls. *Neurology, 48,* 589–601.

Finch, H., Davis, A., & Dean, R. S. (2010). Factor Invariance Assessment of the Dean–Woodcock Sensory–Motor Battery for Patients With ADHD Versus Nonclinical Subjects. *Educational and Psychological Measurement, 70*(1), 161–173.

Findling, R. L., Stepanova, K., Youngstrom, E. A., & Young, A. S. (2018). Progress in diagnosis and treatment of bipolar disorder among children and adolescents: An international perspective. *Evidence Based Mental Health, 21,* 177–181.

Fine, E. M., Delis, D. C., & Holdnack, J. (2011). Normative adjustments to the D-KEFS trail making test:

Corrections for education and vocabulary level. *The Clinical Neuropsychologist, 25*(8), 1331–1344.

Fine, J. G., Musielak, K., & Semrud-Clikeman, M. (2013). Functional magnetic resonance findings in children with Asperger disorder, nonverbal learning disabilities, and controls. *Child Neuropsychology, 19*(2), 190–223.

Fine, J. G., Semrud-Clikeman, M., & Bledsoe, J. (2012). Nonverbal learning disability. In A. Davis (Ed.), *Handbook of pediatric neuropsychology* (pp. 721–734). Springer.

Fine, J. G., Semrud-Clikeman, M., & Bledsoe, J. (2013). A critical review of the literature on NLD as a developmental disorder, *Child Neuropsychology, 19*, 190–223.

Finn, S. E., Fischer, C. T., & Handler, L. (Eds.). (2012). *Collaborative/therapeutic assessment: A casebook and guide.* Wiley.

Fiorello, C. A., Flanagan, D. P., & Hale, J. B. (2014). The utility of the pattern of strengths and weaknesses approach. *Learning Disabilities, 20*(1), 57–61.

Fiorello, C. A., Hale, J. B., Decker, S. L., & Coleman, S. (2010). Neuropsychology and school psychology. In E. Garcoa-Vazquez, T. D. Crespi, & C. Riccio (Eds.), *Handbook of education, training, and supervision of school psychologists in school and community* (pp. 213–232). Routledge.

Fiorello, C. A., Hale, J. B., Holdnack, J. A., Kavanagh, J. A., Terrell, J., & Long, L. (2007). Interpreting intelligence test results for children with disabilities: Is global intelligence relevant? *Applied Neuropsychology, 14*(1), 2–12.

Fiorello, C. A., Hale, J. B., McGrath, M., Ryan, K., & Quinn, S. (2001). IQ interpretation for children with flat and variable test profiles. *Learning and Individual Differences, 13*(2), 115–125.

Fiorello, C. A., Hale, J. B., & Snyder, L. E. (2006). Cognitive hypothesis testing and response to intervention for children with reading problems. *Psychology in the Schools, 43*, 835–853.

Fiorello, C. A., Hale, J. B., Snyder, L. E., Forrest, E., & Teodori, A. (2008). Validating individual differences through examination of converging psychometric and neuropsychological models of cognitive functioning. In S. K. Thurman & C. A. Fiorello (Eds.), *Applied cognitive research in K–3 classrooms* (pp. 232–254). Routledge.

Fiorello, C. A., Hale, J. B., & Wycoff, K. L. (2012). Cognitive Hypothesis Testing (CHT): Linking test results to the real world. In D. P. Flanagan & P. L. Harrison (Eds.), *Contemporary intellectual assessment: Theories, tests, and issues* (3rd ed., pp. 484–496). Guilford Press.

Fiorello, C. A., & Jenkins, T. K. (2018). Best practices in Intellectual Disability identification. *Communiqué, 46*(5), 1, 18–20.

Fiorello, C. A., Liebman, R. B., & Levine-Dawson, S. (1999, April). *Inclusion: What works? What doesn't?* Paper presented at the annual meeting of the National Association of School Psychologists, Las Vegas, NV.

Fiorello, C. A., & Wycoff, K. L. (2018). Cognitive hypothesis testing: Linking test results to the real world. In D. P. Flanagan & E. M. McDonough (Eds.), *Contemporary intellectual assessment: Theories, tests, and issues* (4th ed., pp. 715–730). Guilford Press.

Fischer, K. W., & Daley, S. G. (2007). Connecting cognitive science and neuroscience to education. In L. Meltzer (Ed.), *Executive function in education: From theory to practice* (pp. 237–160). Guilford Press.

Fisher, G. L., Jenkins, S. J., Bancroft, M. J., & Kraft, L. M. (1988). The effects of K-ABC-based remedial teaching strategies on word recognition skills. *Journal of Learning Disabilities, 21*, 307–312.

Fisher, R. S., Cross, J. H., D'Souza, C. D., French, J. A., Haut, S. R., Higurashi, N., et al. (2017). Instruction manual for the ILAE 2017 operational classification of seizure types. *Epilepsia, 58*, 531–542.

Flanagan, D. P., & Alfonso, V. C. (2017). *Essentials of WISC-V assessment.* Wiley.

Flanagan, D. P., Alfonso, V. C., & Dixon, S. G. (2014). Academic achievement batteries. In S. G. Little & A. Akin-Little (Eds.), *Academic assessment and intervention* (pp. 33–78). Routledge.

Flanagan, D. P., Alfonso, V. C., Mascolo, J. T., & Hale, J. B. (2011). The Wechsler Intelligence Scale for Children, Fourth Edition, in neuropsychological practice. In A. S. Davis (Ed.), *Handbook of pediatric neuropsychology* (pp. 397–414). Springer.

Flanagan, D. P., Alfonso, V. C., & Ortiz, S. O. (2012). The cross-battery assessment approach: An overview, historical perspective, and current directions. In D. P. Flanagan & P. L. Harrison (Eds.), *Contemporary intellectual assessment: Theories, tests, and issues* (3rd ed., pp. 459–483). Guilford Press.

Flanagan, D. P., Alfonso, V. C., & Ortiz, S. O. (2025). *Essentials of cross-battery assessment* (4th ed.). Wiley.

Flanagan, D. P., Fiorello, C. A., & Ortiz, S. O. (2010). Enhancing practice through application of Cattell–Horn–Carroll theory and research: A "third method" approach to specific learning disability identification. *Psychology in the Schools, 47*, 739–760.

Flanagan, D. P., & McDonough, E. M. (Eds.). (2018). *Contemporary intellectual assessment: Theories, tests, and issues* (4th ed.). Guilford Press.

Flanagan, D. P., Ortiz, S. O., & Alfonso, V. C. (2013). *Essentials of cross-battery assessment* (3rd ed.). Wiley.

Flanagan, R. (Ed.). (2024). *Clinical guide to effective*

psychological assessment and report writing: Integrating research into practice. Springer.

Flapper, B. C., Houwen, S., & Schoemaker, M. M. (2006). Fine motor skills and effects of methylphenidate in children with attention-deficit/hyperactivity disorder and developmental coordination disorder. *Developmental Medicine and Child Neurology, 48*(3), 165–169.

Fletcher, J. M. (2012). Classification and identification of learning disabilities. In B. Y. L. Wong & D. L. Butler (Eds.), *Learning about learning disabilities* (pp. 1–25). Elsevier.

Fletcher, J. M., Coulter, W. A., Reschly, D. J., & Vaughn, S. (2004). Alternative approaches to the definition and identification of learning disabilities: Some questions and answers. *Annals of Dyslexia, 54*(2), 304–331.

Fletcher, J. M., Levin, H. S., Landry, S. H., Almli, C. R., & Finger, S. (1984). Behavioral consequences of cerebral insult in infancy. *Early Brain Damage, 1,* 189–213.

Fletcher-Janzen, E. (2005). The school neuropsychological examination. In R. C. D'Amato, E. Fletcher-Janzen, & C. R. Reynolds (Eds.), *Handbook of school neuropsychology* (pp. 172–212). Wiley.

Fletcher-Janzen, E., & Reynolds, C. R. (Eds.). (2010). *Neuropsychological perspectives on learning disabilities in the era of RTI: Recommendations for diagnosis and intervention.* Wiley.

Floyd, R. G., McGrew, K. S., & Evans, J. J. (2008). The relative contributions of the Cattell–Horn–Carroll cognitive abilities in explaining writing achievement during childhood and adolescence. *Psychology in the Schools, 45*(2), 132–144.

Follmer, D. J., Sperling, R. A., & Suen, H. K. (2017). The role of MTurk in education research: Advantages, issues, and future directions. *Educational Researcher, 46*(6), 329–334.

Foorman, B. R., Herrera, S., Petscher, Y., Mitchell, A., & Truckenmiller, A. (2015). The structure of oral language and reading and their relation to comprehension in Kindergarten through Grade 2. *Reading and Writing, 28,* 655–681.

Forrest, B. (2007). Diagnosing and treating right hemisphere disorders. In S. J. Hunter & J. Donders (Eds.), *Pediatric neuropsychological intervention* (pp. 175–192). Cambridge University Press.

Fox, M. D., Snyder, A. Z., Vincent, J. L., Corbetta, M., Van Essen, D. C., & Raichle, M. E. (2005). The human brain is intrinsically organized into dynamic, anticorrelated functional networks. *Proceedings of the National Academy of Sciences USA, 102,* 9673–9678.

Foxx, R. M. (2008). Applied behavior analysis treatment of autism: The state of the art. *Child and Adolescent Psychiatric Clinics of North America, 17,* 821–834.

Franceschini, S., Gori, S., Ruffino, M., Pedrolli, K., & Facoetti, A. (2012). A causal link between visual spatial attention and reading acquistion. *Current Biology, 22,* 814–819.

Francis, D. J., Fletcher, J. M., & Rourke, B. P. (1988). Discriminant validity of lateral sensorimotor tests in children. *Journal of Clinical and Experimental Neuropsychology, 10*(6), 779–799.

Franzen, M. D. (2013). *Reliability and validity in neuropsychological assessment.* Springer Science + Business Media.

Frías, Á., Palma, C., & Farriols, N. (2015). Comorbidity in pediatric bipolar disorder: prevalence, clinical impact, etiology and treatment. *Journal of Affective Disorders, 174,* 378–389.

Frick, P. J., Barry, C. T., & Kamphaus, R. W. (2010). *Clinical assessment of child and adolescent personality and behavior.* Springer.

Frick, P. J., & Matlasz, T. (2018). Clinical classification of aggression in children. In T. Malti & K. H. Rubin (Eds.) *Handbook of child and adolescent aggression* (pp. 20–40). Guilford Press.

Friederici, A. D. (2018). The neural basis for human syntax: Broca's area and beyond. *Current Opinion in Behavioral Sciences, 21,* 88–92.

Friedman, G. N., Johnson, L., & Williams, Z. M. (2018). Long-term visual memory and its role in learning suppression. *Frontiers in Psychology, 9,* 1896.

Frijters, J. C., Lovett, M. W., Steinbach, K. A., Wolf, M., Sevcik, R. A., & Morris, R. D. (2011). Neurocognitive predictors of reading outcomes for children with reading disabilities. *Journal of Learning Disabilities, 44*(2), 150–166.

Fristad, M. A., & MacPherson, H. A. (2014). Evidence-based psychosocial treatments for child and adolescent bipolar spectrum disorders. *Journal of Clinical and Child Adolescent Psychology, 43,* 339–355.

Frodl, T., & Skokauskas, N. (2012). Meta-analysis of structural MRI studies in children and adults with attention deficit hyperactivity disorder indicates treatment effects. *Acta Psychiatrica Scandinavica, 125*(2), 114–126.

Frye, R. E. (2012). Biomarkers of abnormal energy metabolism in children with autism spectrum disorder. *North American Journal of Medicine and Science, 5,* 141–148.

Frye, R. E., Liederman, J., Hasan, K. M., Lincoln, A. J., Malmberg, B., McLean, J., III., & Papanicolaou, A. C. (2011). Diffusion tensor quantification of the relations between microstructural and macrostructural indices of white matter and reading. *Human Brain Mapping, 32,* 1220–1235.

Fuchs, D., & Fuchs, L. S. (2006). Introduction to response to intervention: What, why, and how valid is it? *Reading Research Quarterly, 41,* 93–99.

Fuchs, D., Fuchs, L. S., & Compton, D. L. (2012). Smart RTI: A next-generation approach to multilevel prevention. *Exceptional Children, 78*(3), 263–279.

Fuchs, D., Hale, J. B., & Kearns, D. (2011). Cognitive and neuropsychological assessment data that inform educational intervention: An introduction to the special issue and critical analysis. *Journal of Learning Disabilities, 44,* 99–104.

Fuchs, D., McMaster, K. L., & Kearns, D. M. (2017). Evidence-based interventions for reading disabilities in children and adolescents. In L. Theodore (Ed.), *Handbook of evidence-based interventions for children and adolescents* (pp. 85–98). Springer.

Fuchs, L. S. (2003). Assessing intervention responsiveness: Conceptual and technical issues. *Learning Disabilities Research & Practice, 18,* 172–186.

Fuchs, L. S., Geary, D. C., Compton, D. L., Fuchs, D., Hamlett, C. L., & Bryant, J. D. (2010). The contributions of numerosity and domain-general abilities to school readiness. *Child Development, 81,* 1520–1533.

Fuchs, L. S., Powell, S. R., Seethaler, P. M., Cirino, P., Fletcher, J. M., Fuchs, D., & Hamlett, C. L. (2010). The effects of strategic counting instruction with and without deliberate practice, on number combination skill among students with mathematics difficulties. *Learning and Individual Differences, 20,* 89–100.

Fuchs, L. S., Powell, S. R., Seethaler, P. M., Cirino, P., Fletcher, J. M., Fuchs, D., et al. (2008). Remediating number combination and word problem deficits among students with mathematics difficulties: A randomized control trial. *Journal of Educational Psychology, 101,* 561–576.

Fuentes, P., Barrós-Loscertales, A., Bustamante, J. C., Rosell, P., Costumero, V., & Ávila, C. (2012). Individual differences in the Behavioral Inhibition System are associated with orbitofrontal cortex and precuneus gray matter volume. *Cognitive, Affective, & Behavioral Neuroscience, 12,* 491–498.

Fusar-Poli, P., Placentino, A., Carletti, F., Landi, P., Allen, P., Surguladze, S., et al. (2009). Functional atlas of emotional faces processing: A voxel-based meta-analysis of 105 functional magnetic imaging studies. *Journal of Psychiatry and Neuroscience, 34,* 418–432.

Gable, P. A., Mechin, N. C., Hicks, J. A., & Adams, D. L. (2015). Supervisory control system and frontal asymmetry: Neurophysiological traits of emotion-based impulsivity. *Social Cognitive and Affective Neuroscience, 10*(10), 1310–1315.

Gable, P. A., & Poole, B. D. (2014). Influence of trait behavioral inhibition and behavioral approach motivation systems on the LPP and frontal asymmetry to anger pictures. *Social Cognitive and Affective Neuroscience, 9,* 182–190.

Gagnon, I., Galli, C., Friedman, D., Grilli, L., &

Iverson, G. L. (2009). Active rehabilitation for children who are slow to recover following sport-related concussion. *Brain Injury, 23,* 956–964.

Gainotti, G. (2019). Some psychopathological implications of hemispheric asymmetries for emotions. In G. Gainotti (Ed.), *Emotions and the right side of the brain* (pp. 81–91). Springer.

Galaburda, A. M., LoTurco, J., Ramus, F., Fitch, R. H., & Rosen, G. D. (2006). From genes to behavior in developmental dyslexia. *Nature Neuroscience, 9,* 1213–1217.

Galaburda, A. M., Sherman, G. P., Rosen, G. D., Aboitiz, F., & Geschwind, N. (1985). Developmental dyslexia: Four consecutive patients with cortical anomalies. *Annals of Neurology, 18,* 222–233.

Gallagher, R. C., Enns, G. M., Cowan, T. M., Mendelsohn, B., & Packman, S. (2017). Aminoacidemias and organize acidemias. In K. Swaiman, S. Ashwayl, D. M. Ferriero, N. F. Schor, R. S. Finkel, A. L. Gropan, P. L. Pearl, & M. I. Shevell (Eds.), *Swaiman's Pediatric Neurology* (6th ed., pp. 286–297). Elsevier.

Galuschka, K., Gorgen, R., Kalmar, J., Haberstroh, S., Schmalz, X., & Schulte-Korne, G. (2020). Effectiveness of spelling interventions for learners with dyslexia: A meta-analysis and systematic review. *Educational Psychologist, 55,* 1–20.

Galuschka, K., Ise, E., Krick, K., & Schulte-Körne, G. (2014). Effectiveness of treatment approaches for children and adolescents with reading disabilities: A meta-analysis of randomized controlled trials. *PLOS One, 9*(2), e89900.

Ganesalingam, K., Yeates, K. O., Taylor, H. G., Walz, N. C., Stancin, T., & Wade, S. (2011). Executive functions and social competence in young children 6 months following traumatic brain injury. *Neuropsychology, 25,* 466–476.

Garber, J., & Weering, V. R. (2010). Comorbidity of anxiety and depression in youth: Implications for treatment and prevention. *Clinical Psychology and Science Practice, 17,* 293–306.

Garber, K. B., Visootsak, J., & Warren, S. T. (2008). Fragile X syndrome. *European Journal of Human Genetics, 16,* 666–672.

Garcia, N., Abbott, R. D., & Berninger, V. W. (2010). Predicting poor, average, and superior spellers in grades 1 to 6 from phonological, orthographic, and morphological, spelling or reading composites. *Written Language and Literacy, 13,* 61–99.

Gartland, D., & Strosnider, R. (2020). The use of response to intervention to inform special education eligibility decisions for students with specific learning disabilities. *Learning Disability Quarterly, 43*(4), 195–200.

Gazzaniga, M. S. (2013). Shifting gears: Seeking new approaches for mind/brain mechanisms. *Annual Review of Psychology, 64,* 1–20.

Gazzaniga, M. S., Ivry, R. B., & Mangun, G. R. (2008). *Cognitive neuroscience: The biology of the mind* (3rd ed.). Norton.

Gazzaniga, M. S., Ivry, R. B., & Mangun, G. R. (2013). *Cognitive neuroscience: The biology of the mind* (4th ed.). Norton.

Gazzaniga, M. S., & Miller, M. B. (2009). The left hemisphere does not miss the right hemisphere. In S. Laureys & G. Tononi (Eds.), *The neurology of consciousness: Cognitive neuroscience and neuropathology* (pp. 261–270). Elsevier.

Geary, D. C. (2004). Mathematics and learning disabilities. *Journal of Learning Disabilities, 37,* 4–15.

Geary, D. C. (2011a). Cognitive predictors of achievement growth in mathematics: A 5-year longitudinal study. *Developmental Psychology, 47*(6), 1539–1552.

Geary, D. C. (2011b). Consequences, characteristics, and causes of mathematical learning disabilities and persistent low achievement in mathematics. *Journal of Developmental and Behavioral Pediatrics, 32,* 250–263.

Geary, D. C. (2013). Learning disabilities in mathematics: Recent advances. In H. L. Swanson, K. Harris, & S. Graham (Eds.), *Handbook of learning disabilities* (pp. 239–256). Guilford Press.

Geary, D. C., Hamson, C. O., & Hoard, M. K. (2000). Numerical and arithmetical cognition: A longitudinal study of process and concept deficits in children with learning disability. *Journal of Experimental Child Psychology, 77,* 236–263.

Geary, D. C., Hoard, M. K., Byrd-Craven, J., Nugent, L., & Numtee, C. (2007). Cognitive mechanisms underlying achievement deficits in children with mathematical learning disability. *Child Development, 78,* 1343–1359.

Geary, D. C., Hoard, M. K., Nugent, L., & Bailey, D. H. (2012). Mathematical cognition deficits in children with learning disabilities and persistent low achievement: A five-year prospective study. *Journal of Educational Psychology, 104,* 206–223.

Gehring, W. J., & Knight, R. T. (2000). Prefrontal–cingulate interactions in action monitoring. *Nature Neuroscience, 3,* 516–520.

Gentile, J. K., Hoedt, A. E. T., & Bosch, A. M. (2010). Psychosocial aspects of PKU: Hidden disabilities. *Molecular Genetic Metabolism, 99,* S64–S67.

George, M. S., Ketter, T. T., & Post, R. M. (1994). Prefrontal cortex dysfunction in clinical depression. *Depression, 2,* 59–72.

Georgiou, N., Delfabbro, P., & Balzan, R. (2020). COVID-19-related conspiracy beliefs and their relationship with perceived stress and pre-existing conspiracy beliefs. *Personality and Individual Differences, 166,* 110201.

Gerring, J. P., Grados, M. A., Slomine, B., Christensen, J. R., Salorio, C. F., Cole, W. R., et al. (2009). Disruptive behaviour disorders and disruptive symptoms after severe pediatric traumatic brain injury. *Brain Injury, 23,* 944–955.

Geschwind, N. (1983). Biological associations of left-handedness. *Annals of Dyslexia, 33,* 29–40.

Geschwind, N., & Galaburda, A. M. (1985). Cerebral lateralization: Biological mechanisms, associations, and pathology: I. A hypothesis and a program for research. *Archives of Neurology, 42,* 521–552.

Giedd, J. N., & Rapoport, J. L. (2010). Structural MRI of pediatric brain development: what have we learned and where are we going? *Neuron, 67*(5), 728–734.

Giedd, J. N., Rosenthal, M. A., Rose, A. B., Blumenthal, J. D., Molloy, E., Dopp, R. R., et al. (2004). Brain development in healthy children and adolescents: Magnetic resonance imaging studies. In M. S. Keshavan, J. L. Kennedy, & R. M. Murray (Eds.), *Neurodevelopment and schizophrenia* (pp. 35–44). Cambridge University Press.

Giedd, J. N., Schmitt, J. E., & Neale, M. C. (2007). Structural brain magnetic resonance imaging of pediatric twins. *Human Brain Mapping, 28*(6), 474–481.

Gieselmann, V. (2008). Metachromatic leukodystrophy: Genetics, pathogenesis and therapeutic options. *Acta Paediatrica, Supplement, 97,* 15–21.

Gilchrist, A., Green, J., Cox, A., Burton, D., Rutter, M., & LeConteur, A. (2001). Development and current functioning of adolescents with Asperger syndrome: A comparative study. *Journal of Child Psychology and Psychiatry, 42,* 227–240.

Gioia, G. A. (2013). *Special considerations in managing concussion in children and adolescents.* Paper presented at the 2013 International Sports Concussion Symposium, Minneapolis, MN.

Gioia, G. A., Isquith, P. K., Guy, S. C., & Kenworthy, L. (2015). *Behavior Rating Inventory of Executive Function.* (2nd ed.). Psychological Assessment Resources.

Gioia, G. A., Schneider, J. C., Vaughn, C. G., & Isquith, P. K. (2009). Which symptom assessments and approaches are uniquely appropriate for paediatric concussion? *British Journal of Sports Medicine, 43,* 13–22.

Giza, C. C., Kutcher, J. S., Ashwal, S., Barth, J. T., Gesthius, T. S. D., Gioia, G. A., et al. (2013). Summary of evidence-based guideline update: Evaluation and management of concussion in sports. *Neurology, 80,* 2250–2257.

Glezer, L. S., Jiang, X., & Riesenhuber, M. (2009). Evidence for highly selective neuronal tuning to whole words in the "Visual Word Form Area." *Neuron, 62,* 192–204.

Glosser, G. (1993). Discourse production patterns in neurologically impaired and aged populations.

In H. H. Brownell & Y. Joanette (Eds.), *Narrative discourse in neurologically impaired and normal aging adults* (pp. 191–212). Singular.

Glossner, G., & Koppell, S. (1987). Emotional–behavioral patterns in children with learning disabilities: Lateralized hemispheric differences. *Journal of Learning Disabilities, 20*, 365–368.

Glutting, J. J., Watkins, M. W., Konold, T. R., & McDermott, P. A. (2006). Distinctions without a difference: The utility of observed versus latent factors from the WISC-IV in estimating reading and math achievement on the WIAT-II. *Journal of Special Education, 40*, 103–114.

Goodglass, H., & Kaplan, E. (1987). *The assessment of aphasia and related disorders* (2nd ed.). Lea & Febiger.

Gogtay, N., Giedd, J. N., Lusk, L., Hayashi, K. M., Greenstein, D., Vaituzis, A. C., et al. (2004). Dynamic mapping of human cortical development during childhood through early adulthood. *Proceedings of the National Academy of Sciences USA, 101*(21), 8174–8179.

Goldberg, E., & Costa, L. D. (1981). Hemispheric differences in the acquisition and use of descriptive systems. *Brain and Language, 14*, 144–173.

Goldberg, E., Harner, R., Lovell, M., Podell, K., & Riggio, S. (1994). Cognitive bias, functional cortical geometry, and the frontal lobes: Laterality, sex, and handedness. *Journal of Cognitive Neuroscience, 6*, 276–296.

Golden, C. J. (2004). The adult Luria-Nebraska Neuropsychological Battery. In G. Goldstein, S. R. Beers, & M. Hersen (Eds.), *Comprehensive handbook of psychological assessment: Intellectual and neuropsychological assessment* (vol. 1, pp. 133–146). Wiley.

Golden, C. J., Espe-Pfeifer, P., & Wachsler-Felder, J. (2000). *Neuropsychological interpretation of objective psychological tests.* Kluwer Academic.

Golden, C., Freshwater, S. M., & Golden, Z. (2002). *Stroop Color and Word Test* [Database record]. APA PsycTests.

Golden, C. J., Freshwater, S. M., & Vayalakkara, J. (2000). The Luria Nebraska Neuropsychological Battery. In G. Growth-Marnat (Ed.), *Neuropsychological assessment in clinical practice: A guide to test interpretation and integration* (pp. 263–289). Wiley.

Golden, C. J., Purisch, A., & Hammeke, T. (1985). *Manual for the Luria–Nebraska Neuropsychological Battery.* Western Psychological Services.

Goldstein, G., Allen, D. N., Thaler, N. S., Luther, J. F., Panchalingam, K., & Pettegrew, J. W. (2014). Developmental aspects and neurobiological correlates of working and associative memory. *Neuropsychology, 28*(4), 496.

Goldstein, S., & Mather, N. (2001). *Learning disabilities and challenging behaviors: A guide to intervention and classroom management.* Brookes.

Goldstein, S., Naglieri, J. A., & DeVries, M. (Eds.). (2011). *Learning and attention disorders in adolescence and adulthood: Assessment and treatment.* Wiley.

Goldstein, S., & Reynolds, C. R. (Eds.). (2010). *Handbook of neurodevelopmental and genetic disorders in children* (2nd ed.). Guilford Press.

Golestani, N., Molko, N., Dehaene, S., LeBihan, D., & Pallier, C. (2007). Brain structure predicts the learning of foreign speech sounds. *Cerebral Cortex, 17*, 575–583.

Good, R. H., III, Vollmer, M., Creek, R. J., Katz, L., & Chowdhri, S. (1993). Treatment utility of the Kaufman Assessment Battery for Children: Effects of matching instruction and student processing strength. *School Psychology Review, 22*, 8–26.

Gonzalez-Escamilla, G., Chirumamilla, V. C., Meyer, B., Bonertz, T., von Grotthus, S., Vogt, J., et al. (2018). Excitability regulation in the dorsomedial prefrontal cortex during sustained instructed fear responses: a TMS-EEG study. *Scientific Reports, 8*(1), 14506.

Gordon, M., Barkley, R. A., & Lovett, B. J. (2006). Tests and observational measures. In R. A. Barkley (Ed.), *Attention-deficit/hyperactivity disorder: A handbook for diagnosis and treatment* (3rd ed., pp. 369–388). Guilford Press.

Gorno-Tempini, M. L., & Price, C. J. (2001). Identification of famous faces and buildings: A functional neuroimaging study of semantically unique items. *Brain, 124*(10), 2087–2097.

Gosselin, N., Singh, S. R., Chen, J. K., Bottari, C., Johnston, K., & Ptito, A. (2010). Brain function after sport concussion or mild traumatic brain injury: Insights from event-related potentials and functional magnetic resonance imaging. *The Physician and Sportsmedicine, 38*, 27–37.

Goto, Y., & Grace, A. A. (2005). Dopaminergic modulation of limbic and cortical drive of nucleus accumbens in goal-directed behavior. *Nature Neuroscience, 8*(6), 805–812.

Gottfredson, L. S. (1997). Why *g* matters: The complexity of everyday life. *Intelligence, 24*, 79–132.

Gottfredson, L. S. (2005). Suppressing intelligence research: Hurting those we intend to help. In R. H. Wright & N. A. Cummings (Eds.), *Destructive trends in mental health* (pp. 155–186). Routledge.

Gottfredson, L. S. (2008). Of what value is intelligence? In A. Prifitera, D. H. Saklofske, & L. G. Weiss (Eds.), *WISC-IV clinical assessment and intervention* (2nd ed., pp. 545–563). Elsevier Science.

Gottfredson, L. S. (2010). Lessons in academic freedom as lived experience. *Personality and Individual Differences, 49*(4), 272–280.

Goulardins, J. B., Rigoli, D., Licari, M., Piek, J. P., Hasue, R. H., Oosterlaan, J., & Oliveira, J. A. (2015). Attention deficit hyperactivity disorder and developmental coordination disorder: Two separate disorders or do they share a common etiology. *Behavioural Brain Research, 292,* 484–492.

Gourovitch, M. L., Kirkby, B. S., Goldberg, T. E., Weinberger, D. R., Gold, J. M., Esposito, G., et al. (2000). A comparison of rCBF patterns during letter and semantic fluency. *Neuropsychology, 14,* 353–360.

Grados, M. A., Vasa, R. A., Riddle, M. A., Slomine, B. S., Salorio, C., Christensen, J., et al. (2008). New onset obsessive–compulsive symptoms in children and adolescents with severe traumatic brain injury. *Depression and Anxiety, 25,* 398–407.

Graesser, A. C., McNamara, D. S., Louwerse, M. M., & Cai, Z. (2004). Coh-Metrix: analysis of text on cohesion and language. *Behavioral Research Methods, 36,* 193–202.

Graham, S., Harris, K. R., & Adkins, M. (2018). The impact of supplemental handwriting and spelling instruction with first grade students who do not acquire transcription skills as rapidly as peers: A randomized control trial. *Reading and Writing, 31,* 1273–1294.

Graham, S., Harris, K. R., & Hebert, M. (2011). It is more than just the message: Presentation effects in scoring writing. *Focus on Exceptional Children, 44,* 1–10.

Graham, S., & Santangelo, T. (2014). Does spelling instruction make students better spellers, readers, and writers? A meta-analytic review. *Reading and Writing, 27,* 1703–1743.

Granet, D. B., Gomi, C. F., Ventura, R., & Miller-Scholte, A. (2005). The relationship between convergence insufficiency and ADHD. *Strabismus, 13*(4), 163–168.

Graves, S. L., Jr., & Nichols, K. (2016). Intellectual assessment of ethnic minority children. In S. L. Graves, Jr., & J. J. Blake (Eds.), *Psychoeducational assessment and intervention for ethnic minority children: Evidence-based approaches* (pp. 61–76). American Psychological Association.

Graves, S. L., Smith, L. V., & Nichols, K. D. (2021). Is WISC V a fair test for Black children? *Contemporary School Psychology, 25*(2), 157–169.

Gray, J. A., & McNaughton, N. (2000). *The neuropsychology of anxiety: An enquiry into the functions of the septo–hippocampal system.* Clarendon Press/ Oxford University Press.

Green, C. T., Bunge, S. A., Chiongbian, V. B., Barrow, M., & Ferrer, E. (2017). Fluid reasoning predicts future mathematical performance among children and adolescents. *Journal of Experimental Child Psychology, 157,* 125–143.

Green, S. A., Hernandez, L., Tottenham, N., Krasileva, K., Bookheimer, S. Y., & Dapretto, M. (2015). Neurobiology of sensory overresponsivity in youth with autism spectrum disorder. *JAMA Psychiatry, 72,* 778–786.

Gregg, N. G., Coleman, C., Davis, M., & Chalk, J. C. (2007). Timed essay writing: Implications for high-stakes test. *Journal of Learning Disabilities, 40,* 306–318.

Gregory, G. H., & Chapman, C. (2012). *Differentiated instructional strategies: One size doesn't fit all.* Corwin Press.

Gresham, F. M. (2016). Social skills assessment and intervention for children and youth. *Cambridge Journal of Education, 46,* 319–332.

Gresham, F. M., & Witt, J. C. (1997). Utility of intelligence tests for treatment planning, classification, and placement decisions: Recent empirical findings and future directions. *School Psychology Quarterly, 12,* 249–267.

Gresham, G. (2017). Following the trail of mathematics anxiety from preservice to inservice. In T. A. Olson & L. Venenciano (Eds.), *Proceedings of the 44th Annual Meeting of the Research Council on Mathematics Learning: Engage, Explore, and Energize Mathematics Learning* (pp. 49–56). Research Council on Mathematics Learning.

Greven, C. U., Kovas, Y., Willcutt, E. G., Petrill, S. A., & Plomin, R. (2014). Evidence for shared genetic risk between ADHD symptoms and reduced mathematics ability. *Journal of Child Psychology and Psychiatry, 55,* 39–48.

Griesbach, G. S., Hovda, D. A., & Gomez-Pinilla, F. (2009). Exercise-induced improvement in cognitive performance after traumatic brain injury in rats is dependent on BDNF activation. *Brain Research, 1288,* 105–115.

Grigorenko, E. L. (2007). Rethinking disorders of spoken and written language: Generating workable hypotheses. *Journal of Developmental and Behavioral Pediatrics, 28,* 478–486.

Grigorenko, E. L., Compton, D. L., Fuchs, L. S., Wagner, R. K., Willcutt, E. G., & Fletcher, J. M. (2020). Understanding, educating, and supporting children with specific learning disabilities: 50 years of science and practice. *American Psychologist, 75*(1), 37.

Grimwood, K., Anderson, P., Anderson, V., Tan, L., & Nolan, T. (2000). Twelve-year outcomes Following bacterial meningitis: Further evidence for persisting effects. *Archives of Disease in Childhood, 83,* 111–116.

Grol, M., & De Raedt, R. (2018). The effect of positive mood on flexible processing of affective information. *Emotion, 18,* 819–833.

Groth-Marnat, G. (2009). The five assessment issues you meet when you go to heaven. *Journal of Personality Assessment, 91*(4), 303–310.

Grupe, D. W., & Nitschke, J. B. (2013). Uncertainty and anticipation in anxiety: An integrated neurobiological and psychological perspective. *Nature Reviews Neuroscience, 14,* 488–501.

Grzadzinski, R., Dick, C., Lord, C., & Bishop, S. (2016). Parent-reported and clinician-observed autism spectrum disorder (ASD) symptoms in children with attention deficit hyperactivity disorder (ADHD): Implications for practice under DSM 5. *Molecular Autism, 7, https://doi.org/10.1186/s13229-016-0072-1.*

Gualitieri, C. T., & Johnson, L. G. (2008). Medications do not necessarily normalize cognition in ADHD patients. *Journal of Attention Disorders, 11,* 459–469.

Giustino, T. F., & Maren, S. (2015). The role of the medial prefrontal cortex in the conditioning and extinction of fear. *Frontiers in Behavioral Neuroscience, 9,* 298.

Guilford, J. P. (1967). *The nature of human intelligence.* McGraw-Hill.

Guilmette, T. J., Sweet, J. J., Hebben, N., Koltai, D., Mahone, E. M., . . . Spiegler, B. J. (2020). American Academy of Clinical Neuropsychology consensus conference statement on uniform labeling of performance test scores. *The Clinical Neuropsychologist, 34*(3), 437–453.

Guli, L. A., Semrud-Clikeman, M., Lerner, M., & Britton, M. (2013). Use of creative drama as intervention for children with social competence deficits. *The Arts in Psychotherapy, 40,* 37–44.

Gustafson, S., Ferreira, J., & Ronnberg, J. (2007). Phonological or orthographic training for children with phonological or orthographic deficits. *Dyslexia: An International Journal of Research and Practice, 13,* 211–228.

Gutkin, T. (2012). Ecological psychology: Replacing the medical model paradigm for school-based psychological and psychoeducational services. *Journal of Educational and Psychological Consultation, 22,* 1–20.

Habib, R., Nyberg, L., & Tulving, E. (2003). Hemispheric asymmetries of memory: The HERA model revisited. *Trends in Cognitive Sciences, 7*(6), 241–245.

Haddad, F. A., Garcia, Y. E., Naglieri, J. A., Grimditch, M., McAndrews, A., & Eubanks, J. (2003). Planning facilitation and reading comprehension: Instructional relevance of the pass theory. *Journal of Psychoeducational Assessment, 21*(3), 282–289.

Hahn, L. G., & Morgan, J. E. (2012). Neuropsychological contributions to independent education evaluations: Forensic perspectives. In E. M. S. Sherman & B. L. Brooks (Eds.), *Pediatric forensic neuropsychology* (pp. 288–317). Oxford University Press.

Hain, L. A., & Hale, J. B. (2010). Nonverbal learning

disabilities or Asperger's syndrome: Clarification through cognitive hypothesis testing. In N. Mather & L. Jaffe (Eds.), *Comprehensive evaluations: Case reports for psychologists, diagnosticians, and special educators* (pp. 372–387). Wiley.

Hain, L. A., Hale, J. B., & Kendorski, J. G. (2009). Comorbidity of psychopathology in cognitive and academic SLD subtypes. In S. G. Feifer & G. Rattan (Eds.), *Emotional disorders: A neuropsychological, psychopharmacological, and educational perspective* (pp. 199–234). School Neuropsychology Press.

Hajovsky, D. B., Villeneuve, E. F., Schneider, W. J., & Caemmerer, J. M. (2020). An alternative approach to cognitive and achievement relations research: An introduction to quantile regression. *Journal of Pediatric Neuropsychology, 6,* 83–95.

Hale, J. B. (2006). Implementing IDEA with a three-tier model that includes response to intervention and cognitive assessment methods. *School Psychology Forum: Research and Practice, 1,* 16–27.

Hale, J., Alfonso, V., Berninger, V., Bracken, B., Christo, C., Clark, E., et al. (2010). Critical issues in response-to-intervention, comprehensive evaluation, and specific learning disabilities identification and intervention: An expert white paper consensus. *Learning Disability Quarterly, 33*(3), 223–236.

Hale, J. B., Bertin, M., & Brown, L. (2004). *Modeling frontal–subcortical circuits for ADHD subtype identification.* Unpublished manuscript.

Hale, J. B., Betts, E. C., Morley, J., & Chambers, C. (2010, March). *SLD third method approaches for combining RTI and comprehensive evaluation.* In Mini Skills Workshop presented at the Annual Convention of the National Association of School Psychologists, Chicago.

Hale, J. B., Chen, S. A., Tan, S. C., Poon, K., Fitzer, K. R., & Boyd, L. A. (2016). Reconciling individual differences with collective needs: The juxtaposition of sociopolitical and neuroscience perspectives on remediation and compensation of student skill deficits. *Trends in Neuroscience and Education, 5*(2), 41–51.

Hale, J. B., & Fiorello, C. A. (2001). Beyond the academic rhetoric of *g*: Intelligence testing guidelines for practitioners. *The School Psychologist, 55*(4), 113–139.

Hale, J. B., & Fiorello, C. A. (2002). Cross-battery cognitive assessment approaches to test interpretation: Are you a clumper or a splitter? *Communiqué, 31*(1), 37–40.

Hale, J. B., & Fiorello, C. A. (2004). *School neuropsychology: A practitioner's handbook.* Guilford Press.

Hale, J. B., Fiorello, C. A., & Brown, L. L. (2005). Determining medication treatment effects using teacher ratings and classroom observations of children with ADHD: Does neuropsychological impairment matter? *Educational and Child Psychology, 22,* 39–61.

Hale, J. B., Fiorello, C. A., Dumont, R., Willis, J. O., Rackley, C., & Elliott, C. D. (2008). Differential Ability Scales—Second Edition (neuro)psychological predictors of math performance for typical children and children with math disabilities. *Psychology in the Schools, 45,* 838–858.

Hale, J. B., Fiorello, C. A., Kavanagh, J. A., Hoeppner, J. B., & Gaither, R. A. (2001). WISC-III predictors of academic achievement for children with learning disabilities: Are global and factor scores comparable? *School Psychology Quarterly, 16,* 31–55.

Hale, J. B., Fiorello, C. A., Kavanagh, J. A., Holdnack, J. A., & Aloe, A. M. (2007). Is the demise of IQ interpretation justified? A response to special issue authors. *Applied Neuropsychology, 14,* 37–51.

Hale, J. B., Fiorello, C. A., Miller, J. A., Wenrich, K., Teodori, A., & Henzel, J. N. (2008). WISC-IV interpretation for specific learning disabilities identification and intervention: A cognitive hypothesis testing approach. In A. Prifitera, D. H. Saklofske, & L. G. Weiss (Eds.), *WISC-IV clinical assessment and intervention* (2nd ed., pp. 109–171). Elsevier Academic Press.

Hale, J. B., Fiorello, C. A., & Thompson, R. (2010). Integrating neuropsychological principles with response to intervention for comprehensive school-based practice. In E. R. Arzubi & E. Mambrino (Eds.), *A guide to neuropsychological testing for health care professionals* (pp. 229–261). Springer.

Hale, J. B., & Fitzer, K. R. (2015). Evaluating orbital-ventral medial system regulation of personal attention: A critical need for neuropsychological assessment and intervention. *Applied Neuropsychology Child, 4*(2), 106–115.

Hale, J. B., Flanagan, D. P., & Naglieri, J. A. (2008). Alternative research-based methods for IDEA (2004) identification of children with specific learning disabilities. *Communiqué, 36*(8), 1–17.

Hale, J. B., Hain, L. A., Murphy, R., Cancelliere, G., Bindus, D. L., & Kubas, H. A. (2013). The enigma of learning disabilities: Examination via a neuropsychological framework. In C. A. Noggle & R. S. Dean (Eds.), *The neuropsychology of psychopathology* (pp. 75–96). Springer.

Hale, J. B., Hoeppner, J. B., & Fiorello, C. A. (2002). Analyzing Digit Span components for assessment of attention processes. *Journal of Psychoeducational Assessment, 20,* 128–143.

Hale, J. B., Kaufman, A., Naglieri, J. A., & Kavale, K. A. (2006). Implementation of IDEA: Integrating response to intervention and cognitive assessment methods. *Psychology in the Schools, 43,* 753–770.

Hale, J. B., Metro, N., Glass-Kendorski, J., Hain, L., Whitaker, J., & Moldovan, J. (2010). Facilitating school reintegration for children with traumatic brain injury. In A. S. Davis (Ed.), *Handbook of pediatric neuropsychology* (pp. 1155–1168). Springer.

Hale, J. B., Reddy, L. A., Decker, S. L., Thompson, R., Henzel, J., Teodori, A., et al. (2009). Development and validation of an attention-deficit/hyperactivity disorder (ADHD) executive function and behavior rating screening battery. *Journal of Clinical and Experimental Neuropsychology, 31*(8), 897–912.

Hale, J. B., Reddy, L. A., Semrud-Clikeman, M., Hain, L. A., Whitaker, J., Morley, J., et al. (2011). Executive impairment determines medication response: Implications for academic achievement. *Journal of Learning Disabilities, 44,* 196–212.

Hale, J. B., Reddy, L. A., & Weissman, A. S. (2018). Recognizing frontal-subcortical circuit dimensions in child and adolescent neuropsychopathology. In J. N. Butcher & P. C. Kendall (Eds.), *APA handbook of psychopathology: Child and adolescent psychopathology* (pp. 97–122). American Psychological Association.

Hale, J. B., Reddy, L. A., Wilcox, G., McLaughlin, A., Hain, L., Stern, A., et al. (2009). Assessment and intervention for children with ADHD and other frontal–striatal circuit disorders. In D. C. Miller (Ed.), *Best practices in school neuropsychology: Guidelines for effective practice, assessment and evidence-based interventions* (pp. 225–279). Wiley.

Hale, J. B., Wilcox, G., & Reddy, L. A. (2016). Neuropsychological assessment. In J. C. Norcross, G. R. VandenBos, D. K. Freedheim, & R. Krishnamurthy (Eds.), *APA handbook of clinical psychology: Applications and methods* (pp. 139–165). American Psychological Association.

Hale, J. B., Wycoff, K. L., & Fiorello, C. A. (2010). RTI and cognitive hypothesis testing for specific learning disabilities identification and intervention: The best of both worlds. In D. P. Flanagan & V. C. Alfonso (Eds.), *Essentials of specific learning disability identification* (pp. 173–202). Wiley.

Hale, J. B., Yim, M., Schneider, A. N., Wilcox, G., Henzel, J. N., & Dixon, S. G. (2012). Cognitive and neuropsychological assessment of attention-deficit/hyperactivity disorder: Redefining a disruptive behavior disorder. In D. P. Flanagan & P. L. Harrison (Eds.), *Contemporary intellectual assessment: Theories, tests, and issues* (3rd ed., pp. 687–707). Guilford Press.

Hamilton, J. P., Farmer, D. J., Chang, C., Thomason, M. E., Dennis, E., & Gotlib, L. H. (2011). Default-mode and task-positive network activity in major depressive disorder: Implications for adaptive and maladaptive rumination. *Biological Psychiatry, 70,* 327–333.

Hamiwka, L. D., Hamiwka, L. A., Sherman, E. M., & Wirrell, E. (2011). Social skills in children with epilepsy: How do they compare to healthy and chronic disease controls? *Epilepsy & Behavior, 21*(3), 238–241.

Hamiwka, L. D., & Wirrell, E. C. (2009). Comorbidities in pediatric epilepsy: Beyond "just treating the seizures." *Journal of Child Neurology, 24*(6), 734–742.

Hammill, D. D., & Larsen, S. C. (1974). The relationship of selected auditory perceptual skills and reading ability. *Journal of Learning Disabilities, 7*(7), 429–436.

Harn, B. A., Damico, D. P., & Stoolmiller, M. (2017). Examining the variation of fidelity across an intervention: Implications for measuring and evaluating student learning. *Preventing School Failure: Alternative Education for Children and Youth, 61*, 289–302.

Harris, M. J. (1991). Controversy and cumulation: Meta-analysis and research on interpersonal expectancy effects. *Personality and Social Psychology Bulletin, 17*, 316–322.

Harry, B., & Klinger, J. (2007). Improving instruction for students with learning needs. *Educational Leadership, 64*(5), 16–21.

Hart, S. A., Petrill, S. A., & Thompson, L. S. (2010). A factorial analysis of timed and untimed measures of mathematics and reading abilities in school aged twins. *Learning and Individual Differences, 20*, 61–134.

Haslinger, B., Erhard, P., Weilke, F., Ceballos-Baumann, A. O., Bartenstein, P., Grafin von Einsiedel, H., et al. (2002). The role of lateral premoto–cerebellar–parietal circuits in motor sequence control: A parametric fMRI study. *Cognitive Brain Research, 13*, 159–168.

Hassabis, D., & Maguire, E. A. (2007). Deconstructing episodic memory with constuction. *Trends in Cognitive Science, 11*, 299–306.

Hasson, U., Nusbaum, H. C., & Small, S. L. (2007). Brain networks subserving the extraction of sentence information and its encoding to memory. *Cerebral Cortex, 17*, 2899–2913.

Havens, J. F., Mellins, C. A., & Ryan, S. (2016). Mental health treatment of children and families affected by HIV/AIDS. In L. A. Wicks (Ed.), *Psychotherapy and AIDS* (pp. 101–114). Taylor & Francis.

Hawelka, S., Gagl, B., & Wimmer, H. (2010). A dual-route perspective on eye movements of dyslexic readers. *Cognition, 115*, 367–379.

Hawes, Z., Moss, J., Caswell, B., Seo, J., & Ansari, D. (2019). Relations between numerical, spatial, and executive function skills and mathematics achievement: A latent-variable approach. *Cognitive Psychology, 109*, 68–90.

Hay, D. B. (2007). Using concept maps to measure deep, surface, and non-learning outcomes. *Studies in Higher Education, 32*, 39–57.

Hayes, S. A., & Watson, S. L. (2013). The impact of parenting stress: A meta-analysis of studies comparing the experience of parenting stress in parents of children with and without autism spectrum disorder. *Journal of Autism and Developmental Disorders, 43*, 629–642.

Haywood, H. C., & Lidz, C. S. (2006). *Dynamic assessment in practice: Clinical and educational applications.* Cambridge University Press.

Hazlett, H. H., Gu, H., Munsell, B. C., Kim, S. H., Styner, M., Wolff, J. J., et al. (2017). Early brain development in infants at high risk for autism spectrum disorder. *Nature, 542*, 348–351.

Hazra, R, Siberry, G. K., & Mofenson, L. M. (2010). Growing up with HIV: children, adolescents, and young adults with perinatally acquired HIV infection. *Annual Review of Medicine, 61*, 169–185.

Hearps, S., Seal, M., Anderson, V., McCarthy, M., Connellan, M., Downie, P., & De Luca, C. (2017). The relationship between cognitive and neuro-imaging outcomes in children treated for acute lymphoblastic leukemia with chemotherapy only: A systematic review. *Pediatric Blood & Cancer, 64*, 225–233.

Heaton, R. K. (2004). *Revised comprehensive norms for an expanded Halstead–Reitan Battery: Demographically adjusted neuropsychological norms for African American and Caucasian adults, professional manual.* Psychological Assessment Resources.

Heaton, R. K., Chellune, G. J., Talley, J. L., Kay, G. G., & Curtis, G. (1993). *Wisconsin Card Sorting Test (WCST) manual revised and expanded.* Psychological Assessment Resources.

Hebben, N., & Milberg, W. (2009). *Essentials of neuropsychological assessment.* John Wiley & Sons.

Hecaen, H. (1976). Acquired aphasia in children and the ontogenesis of hemispheric functional specialization. *Brain and Language, 3*, 114–134.

Hedtke, K. A., Kendall, P. C., & Tiwari, S. (2009). Safety-seeking and coping behavior during exposure tasks with anxious youths. *Journal of Clinical Child Adolescence, 38*, 1–15.

Heilman, K. M., & Rothi, L. J. G., 2003. Apraxia. In K. M. Heilman & E. Valenstein (Eds.), *Clinical Neuropsychology* (pp. 215–235). Oxford University Press.

Helland, T. (2006). Dyslexia at a behavioural and a cognitive level. *Dyslexia: An International Journal of Research and Practice, 13*, 25–41.

Helland, T., Tjus, T., Hovden, M., Ofte, S., & Heimann, M. (2011). Effects of bottom-up and top-down intervention principles in emergent literacy in children at risk of developmental dyslexia: A longitudinal study. *Journal of Learning Disabilities, 44*(2), 105–122.

Heller, W. (1993). Neuropsychological mechanisms of individual differences in emotion, personality, and arousal. *Neuropsychology, 7*, 476–489.

Heller, W., Nitschke, J. B., & Miller, G. A. (1998). Lateralization in emotion and emotional disorders. *Current Directions in Psychological Science, 7,* 26–32.

Hendren, R. L., Haft, S. L., Black, J. M., White, N. C., & Hoeft, F. (2018). Recognizing psychiatric comorbidity with reading disorders. *Frontiers in Psychiatry, 9,* 101–109.

Hendricks, E. L., & Fuchs, D. (2020). Are individual differences in response to intervention influenced by the methods and measures used to define response? Implications for identifying children with learning disabilities. *Journal of Learning Disabilities, 53*(6), 428–443.

Henson, R., Shallice, T., & Dolan, R. (2000). Neuroimaging evidence for dissociable forms of repetition priming. *Science, 287,* 1269–1272.

Herbster, A. N., Mintun, M. A, Nebes, R. D., & Becker, J. T. (1997). Regional cerebral blood flow during word and nonword reading. *Human Brain Mapping, 5,* 84–92.

Hermann, B., Jones, J., Dabbs, K., Allen, C. A., Sheth, R., Fine, J., et al. (2007). The frequency, complications and aetiology of ADHD in new onset paediatric epilepsy. *Brain: A Journal of Neurology, 130*(Pt 12), 3135–3148.

Herrnstein, R. J., & Murray, C. (1994). *The bell curve: Intelligence and class structure in American life.* Free Press.

Heron, Y., Mikaeloff, R., Froissart, G., Caridade, I., Maire, I., Caillaud, C., et al. (2011). Incidence and natural history of musopolysaccaharidosis type III in France and comparison with United Kingdom and Greece. *American Journal of Medical Genetics A, 115A,* 58–68.

Hess, J. A., Matson, J. L., & Dixon, D. R. (2010). Psychiatric symptom endorsements in children and adolescents diagnosed with autism spectrum disorders: a comparison to typically developing children and adolescents. *Journal of Developmental and Physical Disabilities, 22,* 485–496.

Hessler, G. L., & Sosnowsky, W. P. (1979). A review of aptitude-treatment interaction studies with the handicapped. *Psychology in the Schools, 16*(3), 388–394.

Heumann, J. E., & Hehir, I. (1994). *Intent/scope of LRE requirement.* 21 IDELR §1152 (Office of Special Education Programs Memorandum No. 95-9).

Heym, N., Kantini, E., Checkley, H. L. R., & Cassaday, H. J. (2015). Gray's revised reinforcement sensitivity theory in relation to attention-deficit/hyperactivity and Tourette-like behaviors in the general population. *Personality and Individual Differences, 78,* 24–28.

Hickok, G., Pickell, H., Klima, E., & Bellugi, U. (2009). Neural dissociation in the production of lexical versus classifier signs in ASL: Distinct patterns of hemispheric asymmetry. *Neuropsychologia, 47*(2), 382–387.

Higa-McMillan, C. K., Francis, S. E., Rith-Najarian, L., & Chorpita, B. F. (2016). Evidence base update: 50 years of research on treatment for child and adolescent anxiety. *Journal of Clinical Child & Adolescent Psychology, 45,* 91–113.

Hildebrand, D. K., & Ledbetter, M. F. (2001). Assessing children's intelligence and memory: The Wechsler Intelligence Scale for Children—Third Edition and The Children's Memory Scale. In J. J. W. Andrews, D. H. Saklofske, & H. L. Janzen (Eds.), *Handbook of psychoeducational assessment: Ability, achievement, and behavior in children* (pp. 13–32). Academic Press.

Hill, F., Mammarella, I. C., Devine, A., Caviola, S., Paaolunghi, M. C., & Dzucs, D. (2016). Math anxiety in primary and secondary school students: Gender differences, developmental changes and anxiety specificity. *Learning and Individual Differences, 48,* 45–53.

Hiller, A. J., Fish, T., Siegl, J. H., & Beverdorf, D. Q. (2011). Social and vocational skills training reduces self-reported anxiety and depression among young adults on the autism spectrum. *Journal of Developmental and Physical Disabilities, 23,* 267–276.

Hillis, A. E., Kane, A., Tuffiash, E., Beauchamp, N. J., Barker, P. B., Jacobs, M. A., et al. (2002). Neural substrates of the cognitive processes underlying spelling: Evidence from MR diffusion and perfusion imaging. *Aphasiology, 16,* 425–438.

Hobson, C. W., Scott, S., & Rubia, K. (2011). Investigation of cool and hot executive function in ODD/CD independently of ADHD. *Journal of Child Psychology and Psychiatry, 52,* 1035–1043.

Hochhauser, C. J., Gaur, S., Marone, R., & Lewis, M. (2008). The impact of environmental risk factors on HIV-associated cognitive decline in children. *AIDS Care, 20,* 692–699.

Hoeft, F., Meyler, A., Hernandez, A., Juel, C., Taylor-Hill, H., Martindale, J. L., et al. (2007). Functional and morphometric brain dissociation between dyslexia and reading ability. *Proceedings of the National Academy of Sciences USA, 104,* 4234–4239.

Hoeft, F., Torgesen, J. K., Wagner, R. K., & Rashotte, C. A. (2011). The relations between phonological processing abilities and emerging individual differences in mathematical computation skills: A longitudinal study from second to fifth grades. *Journal of Experimental Child Psychology, 79,* 192–227.

Hofvander, B., Anckarsater, H., Wallinius, M., & Billstedt, E. (2018). Mental health in young adults in prison: The importance of childhood onset conduct disorder. *British Journal of Psychiatry, 3,* 78–84.

Hoie, B., Mykletun, A., Waaler, P. E., Skeidsvoll, H., & Sommerfelt, K. (2006). Executive functions and seizure-related factors in children with epilepsy in western Norway. *Developmental Medicine and Child Neurology, 48*(6), 519–525.

Hoien, T., Lundberg, I., Stanovich, K. E., & Bjaalid, I-K. (1995). Components of phonological awareness. *Reading and Writing, 7,* 171–188.

Hong, D. S., Scaletta Kent, J., & Kesler, S. (2009). Cognitive profile of Turner syndrome. *Developmental Disabilities Research Review, 15,* 270–278.

Hong, S. B., Zalesky, A., Fornito, A., Park, S., Yang, Y. H., Park, M. H., et al. (2014): Connectomic disturbances in attention-deficit/hyperactivity disorder: A whole-brain tractography analysis. *Biological Psychiatry, 76,* 656–663.

Horn, J. L, & Blankson, A. N. (2012). Foundations for better understanding of cognitive abilities. In D. P. Flanagan & P. L. Harrison (Eds.), *Contemporary intellectual assessment* (3rd ed., pp. 73–98). Guilford Press.

Horn, J. L., & Cattell, R. B. (1967). Age differences in fluid and crystallized intelligence. *Acta Psychologica, 26,* 107–129.

Horowitz-Kraus, T., Vannest, J. J., Gozdas, E., & Holland, S. K. (2014). Greater utilization of neural-circuits related to executive functions is associated with better reading: A longitudinal fMRI study using the verb generation task. *Frontiers in Human Neuroscience, 8,* 447.

Horowitz-Kraus, T., Vannest, J. J., Kadis, D., Cicchino, N., Wang, Y. Y., & Holland, S. K. (2014). Reading acceleration training changes brain circuitry in children with reading difficulties. *Brain and Behavior, 4*(6), 886–902.

Horská, A., & Barker, P. B. (2010). Imaging of brain tumors: MR spectroscopy and metabolic imaging. *Neuroimaging Clinics, 20*(3), 293–310.

Horton, A. M., Jr., Soper, H. V., & Reynolds, C. R. (2010). Executive functions in children with traumatic brain injury. *Applied Neuropsychology, 17*(2), 99–103.

Hosp, M. K., Hosp, J. L., & Howell, K. W. (2016). *The ABCs of CBM* (2nd ed.). Guilford Press.

Howard, D., Patterson, K., Wise, R., Brown, W. D., Friston, K., Weiller, C., et al. (1992). The cortical localization of the lexicons. Positron emission tomography evidence. *Brain, 115,* 1769–1782.

Huang, L., Wan, U., Zhang, L., Zheng, Z., Zhu, T., Qu, Y., & Mu, D. (2018). Maternal smoking and attention-deficit/hyperactivity disorder in offspring: A meta-analysis. *Pediatrics, 141,* 1–11.

Huang-Pollock, C. L., & Nigg, J. T. (2003). Searching for the attention deficit in attention deficit hyperactivity disorder. *Clinical Psychology Review, 23,* 801–830.

Hübner, R., & Volberg, G. (2005). The integration of object levels and their content: A theory of global/local processing and related hemispheric differences. *Journal of Experimental Psychology: Human Perception and Performance, 31*(3), 520.

Hudson, R. F., Pullen, P. C., Lane, H. B., & Torgesen, J. K. (2008). The complex nature of reading fluency: A multidimensional view. *Reading and Writing Quarterly: Overcoming Learning Difficulties, 25,* 4–32.

Hughes, T., Tansy, M., & Fallon, C. (2017). Evidence-based interventions for children and adolescents with emotional and behavioral disorders. In L. A. Theodore (Ed.), *Handbook of evidence-based interventions for children and adolescents* (pp. 205–216). Springer.

Hull, J. V., Dokovna, L. B., Jacokes, Z. J., Torgerson, C. M., Irimia, A., & van Horn, J. D. (2017). Resting-state functional connectivity in autism spectrum disorders: A review. *Frontiers of Psychiatry, 7,* 205.

Hung, Y. H., Frost, S. J., & Pugh, K. R. (2018). Domain generality and specificity of statistical learning and its relation with reading ability. In T. Lachmann & T. Weis (Eds.), *Literacy studies: Vol. 16. Reading and dyslexia* (pp. 33–55). Springer International.

Huslander, J., Talcott, J. B., Witton, C., DeFries, J. C., Pennington, B. F., Wadsworth, S., et al. (2004). Sensory processing, reading, IQ, and attention. *Journal of Experimental Child Psychology, 88,* 274–295.

Hutton, J. S., Dudley, J., Horowitz-Kraus, T., DeWitt, T., & Holland, S. K. (2020). Associations between home literacy environment, brain white matter integrity and cognitive abilities in preschool-age children. *Acta Paediatrica, 109,* 1376–1386.

Hynd, G. W., & Obzrut, J. E. (1981). School neuropsychology. *Journal of School Psychology, 19,* 45–50.

Hynd, G. W., & Semrud-Clikeman, M. (1989). Dyslexia and brain morphology. *Psychological Bulletin, 106,* 447–482.

Hynd, G. W., Semrud-Clikeman, M., Lorys, A. R., Novey, E. S., & Eliopulos, D. (1990). Brain morphology in developmental dyslexia and attention deficit disorder/hyperactivity. *Archives of Neurology, 47*(8), 919–926.

Hynes, C. A., Baird, A. A., & Grafton, S. T. (2006). Differential role of the orbital frontal lobe in emotional versus cognitive perspective-taking. *Neuropsychologia, 44*(3), 374–383.

Hyseni, F., Blanken, L. M., Muetzel, R., Verhulst, F. C., Tiemeier, H., & White, T. (2019). Autistic traits and neuropsychological performance in 6- to 10-year-old children: A population-based study. *Child Neuropsychology, 25,* 352–369.

Ibemon, L., Touchet, C., & Pochon, R. (2018). Emotion recognition as a real strength in Williams syndrome: Evidence from a dynamic nonverbal task. *Frontiers in Psychology, 9,* 463.

Indredavik, M. S., Skranes, J. S., Vik, T., Heyerdahl, S., Romundstad, P., Myhr, G. E., et al. (2005). Low-birth-weight adolescents: psychiatric symptoms and cerebral MRI abnormalities. *Pediatric Neurology, 33,* 259–266.

Indredavik, M. S., Vik, T., Evensen, K. A., Skranes, J., Taraldsen, G., & Brubakk, A. M. (2010). Perinatal risk and psychiatric outcome in adolescents born preterm with very low birth weight or term small for gestational age. *Journal of Developmental and Behavioral Pediatrics, 31,* 286–294.

Insel, T. R. (2014). The NIMH research domain criteria (RDoC) project: Precision medicine for psychiatry. *American Journal of Psychiatry, 171*(4), 395–397.

Isaacson, R. (2013). *The limbic system.* Springer Science + Business Media.

Iseman, J. S., & Naglieri, J. A. (2011). A cognitive strategy instruction to improve math calculation for children with ADHD and LD: a randomized controlled study. *Journal of Learning Disabilities, 44*(2), 184–195.

Ishai, A., Schmidt, C. F., & Boesiger, P. (2005). Face perception is mediated by a distributed cortical network. *Brain Research Bulletin, 67*(1–2), 87–93.

Ito, M. (2008). Control of mental activities by internal models in the cerebellum. *Nature Reviews Neuroscience, 9,* 304–313.

Iyer, N. S., Balsamo, L. M., Bracken, M. B., & Kadan-Lottick, N. S. (2015). Chemotherapy-only treatment effects on long-term neurocognitive functioning in children ALL survivors: A review and meta-analysis. *Blood, 126,* 346–354.

Jackson, J. H. (1958). *Selected writings of John Hughlings Jackson.* Basic Books. (Original work published 1868)

Jacoby, N., & Fedorenko, E. (2020). Discourse-level comprehension engages medial frontal theory of mind brain regions even for expository texts. *Language, Cognition and Neuroscience, 35*(6), 780–796.

Jagger-Rickels, A. C., Kibby, M. Y., & Constance, J. M. (2018). Global gray matter morphometry differences between children with reading disability, ADHD, and comorbid reading disability/ADHD. *Brain and Language, 185,* 54–66.

James, K. H., & Gathier, I. (2006). Letter processing automatically recruits a sensory-motor brain network. *Neuropsychologia, 44,* 2937–2949.

Jang, J., Dixon, D. R., Tarbox, J., & Granpeesheh, D. (2011). Symptom severity and challenging behavior in children with ASD. *Research in Autism Spectrum Disorders, 5*(3), 1028–1032.

Jantzie, L. L., Todd, K. G., & Cheung, P. (2008). Neonatal ischemic stroke: A hypoxic–ischemic injury to the developing brain. *Future Neurology, 3,* 99–102.

Jarrett, M. A., Wolff, J. C., Davis III, T. E., Cowart, M. J., & Ollendick, T. H. (2016). Characteristics of children with ADHD and comorbid anxiety. *Journal of Attention Disorders, 20,* 626–644.

Jenks, K. M., de Moor, J., & van Lieshout, E. C. D. M. (2009). Arithmetic difficulties in children with cerebral palsy are related to executive function and working memory. *Journal of Child Psychology and Psychiatry, 50,* 824–833.

Jensen, A. R. (1998). *The g factor: The science of mental ability.* Praeger.

Jobard, G., Crivello, F., & Tzourio-Mazoyer, N. (2003). Evaluation of the dual route theory of reading: A metanalysis of 35 neuroimaging studies. *NeuroImage, 20,* 693–712.

Johnson, A. E., Perry, N. B., Hostinar, C. E., & Gunnar, M. R. (2019). Cognitive–affective strategies and cortisol stress reactivity in children and adolescents: Normatic development and effects of early life stress. *Developmental Psychobiology, 61,* 999–1013.

Jones, D., & Christensen, C. A. (1999). Relationship between automaticity in handwriting and students' ability to generate written text. *Journal of Educational Psychology, 91*(1), 44.

Jordan, N. C., Kaplan, D., Locuniak, M. N., & Ramineni, C. (2007). Predicting first-grade math achievement from developmental number sense trajectories. *Learning Disabilities Research & Practice, 22*(1), 36–46.

Jordan, N. C., Kaplan, D., Ramineni, C., & Locuniak, M. N. (2009). Early math matters: Kindergarten number competence and later mathematics outcomes. *Developmental Psychology, 45,* 850–867.

Jorge, R. E., Robinson, R. G., Moser, D., Tateno, A., Crespo-Facorro, B., & Arndt, S. (2004). Major depression following traumatic brain injury. *Archives of General Psychiatry, 61*(1), 42–50.

Joseph, R. M., & Tager-Flusberg, H. (2004). The relationship of theory of mind and executive functions to symptom type and severity in children with autism. *Development and Psychopathology, 16,* 137–155.

Joseph, R. M., & Tanaka, J. (2003). Holistic and part-based face recognition in children with autism. *Journal of Child Psychology and Psychiatry, 44,* 529–542.

Kadosh, R. C., Kadosh, K. C., Linden, D. E., Gevers, W., Berger, A., & Henik, A. (2007). The brain locus of interaction between number and size: A combined functional magnetic resonance imaging and event-related potential study. *Journal of Cognitive Neuroscience, 19*(6), 957–970.

Kafantaris, V., Kingsley, P., Ardekani, B., Saito, E., Lencz, T., Lim, K., & Szeszko, P. (2009). Lower orbital frontal white matter integrity in adolescents with bipolar I disorder. *Journal of the American Academy of Child and Adolescent Psychiatry, 48,* 79–86.

Kaminski, R. A., & Good, R. H. (1998). Assessing

early literacy skills in a problem solving model: Dynamic indicators of basic early literacy skills. In M. R. Shinn (Ed.), *Advanced applications of curriculum-based measurement* (pp. 113–142). Guilford Press.

Kamphaus, R. W., Benson, J., Hutchinson, S., & Platt, L. O. (1994). Identification of factor models for the WISC-III. *Educational and Psychological Measurement, 54*(1), 174–186.

Kaplan, R. M. (1990). Behavior as the central outcome in health care. *American Psychologist, 45*(11), 1211.

Kapur, S., Rose, R., Liddle, P. F., Zipursky, R. B., Brown, G. M., Stuss, D., et al. (1994). The role of the left prefrontal cortex in verbal processing: Semantic processing or willed action. *NeuroReport, 5,* 2193–2196.

Karavasilis, E., Christidi, F., Velonakis, G., Giavri, Z., Kelekis, N. L., Efstathopoulos, E. P., et al. (2019). Ipsilateral and contralateral cerebro–cerebellar white matter connections: A diffusion tensor imaging study in healthy adults. *Journal of Neuroradiology, 46*(1), 52–60.

Karlsdottir, R., & Stefansson, T. (2002). Problems in developing functional handwriting. *Perceptual and Motor Skills, 94,* 623–662.

Katusic, S. K., Colligan, R. C., Weaver, A. L., & Barbaresi, W. J. (2009). The forgotten learning disability: Epidemiology of written-language disorder in a population-based birth cohort (1976–1982), Rochester, Minnesota. *Pediatrics, 123,* 1306–1313.

Katz, A. J., Chia, V. M., Schoonen, W. M., & Kelsh, M. A. (2015). Acute lymphoblastic, leukemia: An assessment of international incidence, survival, and disease burden. *Cancer Causes & Control, 26,* 1627–1642.

Kaufman, A. S. (1994). *Intelligent testing with the WISC-III.* Wiley.

Kaufman, A. S. (2009). *IQ testing 101.* Springer.

Kaufman, A. S. (2018). Foreword. In D. P. Flanagan & E. M. McDonough (Eds.), *Contemporary intellectual assessment: Theories, tests, and issues* (4th ed., pp. ix–xii). Guilford Press.

Kaufman, A. S., & Kaufman, N. L. (1983). *Kaufman Assessment Battery for Children: Interpretive manual.* American Guidance Service.

Kaufman, A. S., Lichtenberger, E. O., Fletcher-Janzen, E., & Kaufman, N. L. (2005). *Essentials of KABC-II assessment.* Wiley.

Kaufman, A. S., Raiford, S. E., & Coalson, D. L. (2015). *Intelligent testing with the WISC-V.* Wiley.

Kaufman, J. C., Kaufman, S. B., & Lichtenberger, E. O. (2011). Finding creative potential on intelligence tests via divergent production. *Canadian Journal of School Psychology, 26*(2), 83–106.

Kaufmann, L., Mazzocco, M. M., Dowker, A., von Aster, M., Göbel, S. M., Grabner, R. H., et al. (2013). Dyscalculia from a developmental and differential perspective. *Frontiers in Psychology, 4,* 516.

Kaufmann, L., Wood, G., Rubinsten, O., & Henik, A. (2011). Meta-analyses of developmental fMRI studies investigating typical and atypical trajectories of number processing and calculation. *Developmental Neuropsychology, 36*(6), 763–787.

Kavale, K. A., & Forness, S. R. (1999). Effectiveness of special education. In C. R. Reynolds & T. B. Gutkin (Eds.), *The handbook of school psychology* (3rd ed., pp. 984–1024). Wiley.

Kazmierski, K. F. M., Beam, C. R., & Margolin, G. (2020). Family aggression and attachment avoidance influence neuroendocrine reactivity in young adult couples. *Journal of Family Psychology, 34*(6), 664–675.

Keen, D. V., Reid, F. D., & Arnone, D. (2010). Autism, ethnicity and maternal immigration. *The British Journal of Psychiatry, 196*(4), 274–281.

Keith, T. Z., Fine, J., Taub, G. E., Reynolds, M. R., & Kranzler, J. H. (2006). Short-term estimates of growth using curriculum-based measurement of oral reading fluency: Estimating standard error of the slope to construct confidence intervals. *School Psychology Review, 35*(1), 108–127.

Keith, T. Z., Kranzler, J. H., & Flanagan, D. P. (2001). What does the Cognitive Assessment System (CAS) measure?: Joint confirmatory factor analysis of the CAS and the Woodcock–Johnson Tests of Cognitive Ability (3rd edition). *School Psychology Review, 30,* 89–119.

Keith, T. Z., Low, J. A., Reynolds, M. R., Patel, P. G., & Ridley, K. P. (2010). Higher-order factor structure of the Differential Ability Scales–II: Consistency across ages 4 to 17. *Psychology in the Schools, 47*(7), 676–697.

Keith, T. Z., & Reynolds, M. R. (2018). Using confirmatory factor analysis to aid in understanding the constructs measured by intelligence tests. In D. P. Flanagan & E. M. McDonough (Eds.), *Contemporary intellectual assessment: Theories, tests, and issues* (4th ed., pp. 853–900). Guilford Press.

Keller, T. A., & Just, M. A. (2009). Altering cortical connectivity: Remediation-induced changes in the white matter of poor readers. *Neuron, 64,* 624–631.

Kelly, A. V. (2009). *The curriculum: Theory and practice.* Sage.

Kendall, P. C. (Ed.). (2011). *Child and adolescent therapy: Cognitive-behavioral procedures.* Guilford Press.

Kennard, M. A. (1938). Reorganization of motor function in the cerebral cortex of monkeys deprived of motor and premotor areas in infancy. *Journal of Neurophysiology, 1,* 477.

Kerns, C. M., & Kendall, P. C. (2014). Autism and anxiety: Overlap, similarities and differences. In T. E. Davis, S. W. White, & T. H. Ollendick

(Eds.), *Handbook of autism and anxiety* (pp. 75–89). Springer.

Kerns, C. M., Kendall, P. C., Berry, L., Souders, M. C., Franklin, M. E., Schultz, R. T., et al. (2014). Traditional and atypical presentations of anxiety in youth with autism spectrum disorder. *Journal of Autism and Developmental Disorders, 44,* 2851–2861.

Kerns, J. G., Cohen, J. D., MacDonald, A. W., Cho, R. Y., Stenger, V. A., & Carter, C. S. (2004). Anterior cingulate conflict monitoring and adjustments in control. *Science, 303*(5660), 1023–1026.

Kerr, Z. Y., Zuckerman, S. L., Wasserman, E. B., Vander Vegt, C. B., Yengo-Kahn, A., Buckley, T. A., et al. (2018). Factors associated with post-concussion syndrome in high school student-athletes. *Journal of Science and Medicine in Sport, 21*(5), 447–452.

Kessler, R. C., Avenevoli, S., Green, J., Gruber, M. J., Guyer, M., He, Y., et al. (2009). National Comorbidity Survey Replication Adolescent Supplement (NCS-A): III. Concordance of DSM-IV/CIDI diagnoses with clinical reassessments. *Journal of the American Academy of Child and Adolescent Psychiatry, 48,* 386–399.

Kibby, M. Y., & Cohen, M. J. (2008). Memory functioning in children with reading disabilities and/or attention deficit/hyperactivity disorder: A clinical investigation of their working memory and long-term memory functioning. *Child Neuropsychology, 14*(6), 525–546.

Kim, Y. S., Al Otaiba, S., Puranik, C., Folsom, J. S., Greulich, L., & Wagner, R. K. (2011). Componential skills of beginning writing: An exploratory study. *Learning and Individual Differences, 21*(5), 517–525.

Kimura, R., Swarup, V., Kiyotaka, T., Gandal, M. J., Parikshak, N. N., Funabiki, Y., et al. (2019). Integrative network analysis reveals biological pathways associated with Williams Syndrome. *The Journal of Child Psychology and Psychiatry, 60,* 585–598.

King, B. H., Holander, E., Kikich, L., McCracken, J. T., Scahill, L., Bregman, J. D., et al. (2009). Lack of efficacy of citalopram in children with autism spectrum disorders and high levels of repetitive behavior: Citalopram ineffective in children with autism. *Archives of General Psychiatry, 66,* 583–590.

Kinsbourne, M. (1997). Mechanisms and development of cerebral lateralization in children. In C. R. Reynolds & E. Fletcher-Janzen (Eds.), *Handbook of clinical child neuropsychology* (2nd ed., pp. 102–119). Plenum Press.

Kiyonaga, A., Scimeca, J. M., Bliss, D. P., & Whitney, D. (2017). Serial dependence across perception, attention, and memory. *Trends in Cognitive Sciences, 21*(7), 493–497.

Klaus, J., & Schutter, D. J. (2018). The role of left dorsolateral prefrontal cortex in language processing. *Neuroscience, 377,* 197–205.

Klin, A., & Volkmar, F. R. (2003). Asperger syndrome: Diagnosis and external validity. *Child and Adolescent Psychiatric Clinics of North America, 12,* 1–13.

Kløve, H. (1963). Clinical neuropsychology. In F. M. Forster (Ed.), *The medical clinics of North America.* Saunders.

Kluen, L. M., Dandolo, L. C., Jocham, G., & Schwabe, L. (2019). Dorsolateral prefrontal cortex enables updating of established memories. *Cerebral Cortex, 29*(10), 4154–4168.

Kluger, A., & Goldberg, E. (1990). IQ patterns in affective disorder, lateralized and diffuse brain damage. *Journal of Clinical and Experimental Neuropsychology, 12,* 182–194.

Kneen, R., & Solomon, T. (2008). Management and outcome of viral encephalitis in children. *Pediatrics and Child Health, 18,* 7–16.

Koegel, L., Matos-Freden, R., Lang, R., & Koegel, R. (2012). Interventions for children with autism spectrum disorder in inclusive school settings. *Cognitive and Behavioral Practice, 19,* 401–412.

Koelsch, S., Fritz, T., Schulze, K., Alsop, D., & Schlaug, G. (2005). Adults and children processing music: an fMRI study. *Neuroimage, 25*(4), 1068–1076.

Kolb, B., & Fantie, B. (1997). Development of the child's brain and behavior. In C. R. Reynolds & E. Fletcher-Janzen (Eds.), *Handbook of clinical child neuropsychology* (2nd ed., pp. 17–41). Plenum Press.

Kolb, B. & Whishaw, I. Q. (2021). *Fundamentals of human neuropsychology* (8th ed.). Worth Publishers.

Kolb, B., Whishaw, I. Q., & Teskey, G. (2023). *An introduction to brain and behavior.* Worth.

Konrad, K., & Eickhoff, S. (2010). Is the ADHD brain wired differently? A review on structural and functional connectivity in attention deficit hyperactivity disorder. *Human Brain Mapping, 31,* 904–916.

Konrad, K., Neufang, S., Hanisch, C., Fink, G. R., & Herpertz-Dahlmann, B. (2005). Dysfunctional attentional networks in children with attention deficit/hyperactivity disorder: Evidence from an event-related functional magnetic resonance imaging study. *Biological Psychiatry, 59,* 643–651.

Kontos, A. P., Covassin, T., Elbin, R. J., & Parker, T. (2012). Depression and neurocognitive performance after concussion among male and female high school and collegiate athletes. *Archives of Physical Medicine and Rehabilitation, 93,* 1751–1756.

Koomen, I., van Furth, A. M., Kraak, M. A. C., Grobbee, D. E., Roord, J. J., & Jennekens-Schinkel (2004). Neuropsychology of academic and behavioral limitations in school-age survivors of bacterial meningitis. *Developmental Medicine & Child Neurology, 46,* 724–732.

Kopelman, M. D., Stevens, T. G., Foli, S., & Grasby, P. (1998). PET activation of the medial temporal lobe in learning. *Brain, 121,* 875–887.

Korkman, M., Kirk, U., and Kemp, S. (2007). *NEPSY-II: A developmental neuropsychological assessment.* Psychological Corporation.

Kosslyn, S. M., Daly, P. F., McPeek, R. M., Alpert, N. M., Kennedy, D. N., & Caviness, V. S. (1993). Using locations to store shape: An indirect effect of a lesion. *Cerebral Cortex, 3,* 567–582.

Kovelman, I., Norton, E. S., Christodoulou, J. A., Gaab, N., Lieberman, D. A., Triantafyllou, C., et al. (2012). Brain basis of phonological awareness for spoken language in children and its disruption in dyslexia. *Cerebral Cortex, 22*(4), 754–764.

Kover, S. T., Pierpont, E. I., Kim, J-S., Brown, W. T., & Abbeduto, L. (2013). A neurodevelopmental perspective on the acquisition of nonverbal cognitive skills in adolescents with Fragile X syndrome. *Developmental Neuropsychology, 38,* 445–460.

Kowatch, R. A., Youngstrom, E. A., Horwitz, S., Demeter, C., Fristad, M. A., Birmaher, B., et al. (2013). Prescription of psychiatric medications and polypharmacy in the LAMS cohort. *Psychiatric Services, 64,* 1026–1034.

Koyama, M. S., Di Martino, A., Zuo, X. N., Kelly, C., Mennes, M., Jutagir, D. R., & Milham, M. P. (2011). Resting-state functional connectivity indexes reading competence in children and adults. *Journal of Neuroscience, 31,* 8617–8624.

Koziol, L. F., & Budding, D. E. (2009). *Subcortical structures in cognition.* Springer.

Koziol, L. F., & Budding, D. E. (2011). Pediatric neuropsychological testing: Theoretical models of test selection and interpretation. In A. S. Davis (Ed.), *Handbook of pediatric neuropsychology* (pp. 443–455). Springer.

Koziol, L. F., Budding, D. E., & Chidekel, D. (2010). Adaptation, expertise, and giftedness: Towards an understanding of cortical, subcortical, and cerebellar network contributions. *The Cerebellum, 9,* 499–529.

Koziol, L. F., Budding, D. E., & Chidekel, D. (2012). From movement to thought: Executive function, embodied cognition, and the cerebellum. *The Cerebellum, 11,* 505–525.

Koziol, L. F., Budding, D. E., & Hale, J. B. (2013). Understanding neuropsychopathology in the 21st century: Current status, clinical application, and future directions. In L. A. Reddy, A. S. Weissman, & J. B. Hale (Eds.), *Neuropsychological assessment and intervention for youth: An evidence-based approach to emotional and behavioral disorders* (pp. 327–345). American Psychological Association.

Kroesbergen, E. H., Huijsmans, M. D. E., & Friso-van den Bos, I. (2023). A meta-analysis on the differences in mathematical and cognitive skills between individuals with and without mathematical learning disabilities. *Review of Educational Research, 93*(5), 718–755.

Kronbichler, M., Hutzler, F., Staffen, W., Mair, A., Ladurner, G., & Wimmer, H. (2006). Evidence for a dysfunction of left posterior reading areas in German dyslexic readers. *Neuropsychologia, 44,* 1822–1832.

Kubas, B., Kułak, W., Sobaniec, W., Tarasow, E., Łebkowska, U., & Walecki, J. (2012). Metabolite alterations in autistic children: A 1H MR spectroscopy study. *Advances in Medical Sciences, 57*(1), 152–156.

Kubas, H. A., Schmid, A. D., Drefs, M. A., Poole, J. M., Holland, S., & Fiorello, C. A. (2014). Cognitive and academic profiles associated with math disability subtypes. *Learning Disabilities: A Multidisciplinary Journal, 20*(1), 31–44.

Kucian, K., Loenneker, T., Martin, E., & von Aster, M. (2011). Non-symbolic numerical distance effect in children with and without developmental dyscalculia: A parametric fMRI study. *Behavioral and Brain Function, 2,* 31.

Kyttala, M., Aunio, P., Lehto, J. E., Van Luit, J. E. H., & Hautamaki, J. (2003). Visuospatial working memory and early numeracy. *Educational and Child Psychology, 20,* 65–76.

Lachance, J. A., & Mazzocco, M. M. M. (2006). A longitudinal analysis of sex differences in math and spatial skills in primary school-age children. *Learning and Individual Differences, 16,* 195–216.

Lahey, B. B., Hart, E. L., Pliszka, S., Applegate, B., & McBurnett, K. (1993). Neurophysiological correlates of conduct disorder: A rationale and a review of research. *Journal of Clinical Child Psychology, 22*(2), 141–153.

Lahey, B. B., Hartung, C. M., Loney, J., Pelham, W. E., Chronis, A. M., & Lee, S. S. (2007). Are there sex differences in the predictive validity of DSM–IV ADHD among younger children? *Journal of Clinical Child and Adolescent Psychology, 36*(2), 113–126.

Lai, Y., Zhu, X., Chen, Y., & Li, Y. (2015). Effects of mathematics anxiety and mathematical metacognition on word problem solving in children with and without mathematical learning difficulties. *PLOS ONE, 10,* e0130570.

Laird, A. R., Fox, F. M., Eickhoff, S. B., Turner, J. A., Rey, K. L., McKay, D. R. et al. (2011). Behavioral interpretations of intrinsic connectivity networks. *Journal of Cognitive Neuroscience, 23,* 4022–4037.

Lajiness-O'Neill, R., Erdodi, L., & Bigler, E. D. (2010). Memory and learning in pediatric traumatic brain injury: A review and examination of moderators of outcome. *Applied Neuropsychology, 17*(2), 83–92.

Lajiness-O'Neill, R. R., Erdodi, L. A., Mansour, A., & Olszewski, A. (2013). Rehabilitation of memory deficits. In C. A. Noggle, R. S. Dean, & M. T. Barisa (Eds.), *Neuropsychological rehabilitation* (pp. 81–110). Springer.

Lam, C. G., Howard, S. C., Bouffet, E., & Pritchard Jones, K. (2019). Science and health for all children with cancer. *Science, 363*, 1182–1186.

Landerl, K., Gobel, S. M., & Moll, K. (2013). Core deficit and individual manifestations of developmental dyscalculia (DD): the role of comorbidity. *Trends in Neuroscience and Education, 2*, 38–42.

Landi, N., Frost, S. J., Mencl, W. E., Sandak, R., & Pugh, K. (2013). Neurobiological bases of reading comprehension: Insights from neuroimaging studies of word-level and text-level processing in skilled and impaired readers. *Reading and Writing Quarterly, 29*, 145–167.

Lange, S., Probst, C., Gmel, G., Rehm, J., Burd, L., & Popova, S. (2017). Global prevalence of fetal alcohol spectrum disorder among children and youth. *JAMA Pediatrics, 171*, 948–956.

Langfranchi, S. Cronoldi, C., Drigo, S., & Vianello, R. (2009). Working memory in individuals with fragile X syndrome. *Child Neuropsychology, 15*, 105–119.

Langlois, J. A., Rutland-Brown, W., & Wald, M. M. (2006). The epidemiology and impact of traumatic brain injury. *Journal of Head Trauma Rehabilitation, 21*, 375–378.

Larson, R. A. (2004). The U. S. trials in adult acute lymphoblastic leukemia (ALL). *Annals of Hematology, 83*(Suppl. 1), S127–S128.

Latzman, R. D., Elkovitch, N., Young, J., & Clark, L. A. (2010). The contribution of executive functioning to academic achievement among male adolescents. *Journal of Clinical and Experimental Neuropsychology, 32*(5), 455–462.

Latzman, R. D., & Markon, K. E. (2010). The factor structure and age-related factorial invariance of the Delis–Kaplan Executive Function System (D-KEFS). *Assessment, 17*(2), 172–184.

Laycock, R., Wilkinson, I. D., Wallis, L. I., Darwent, G., Wonders, S. H., Fawcett, A. J., & Nicolson, R. I. (2008). Cerebellar volume and cerebellar metabolic characteristics in adults with dyslexia. *Annals of the New York Academy of Sciences, 1145*, 222–236.

Leark, R. A., Greenberg, L. M., Kindschi, C. L., Dupuy, T. R., & Hughes, S. J. (2008). *TOVA professional manual*. TOVA Company, 9-0.

Lebel, C., Treit, S., & Beaulieu, C. (2019). A review of diffusion MRI of typical white matter development from early childhood to young adulthood. *NMR in Biomedicine, 32*(4), e3778.

Lebel, C., Walker, L., Leemans, A., Phillips, L., & Beaulieu, C. (2008). Microstructural maturation of the human brain from childhood to adulthood. *Neuroimage, 40*(3), 1044–1055.

Leddy, J. J., Sandhu, H., Sodhi, V., Baker, J. G., & Willer, B. (2012). Rehabilitation of concussion and post-concussion syndrome. *Sports Health, 4*, 147–154.

Lee, D., Riccio, C. A., D'Amato, R. C., Fletcher-Janzen, E., & Reynolds, C. R. (2005). Understanding and implementing cognitive neuropsychological retraining. In R. C. D'Amato, E. Fletcher-Janzen, & C. R. Reynolds (Eds.), *Handbook of school neuropsychology* (pp. 701–720). Wiley.

Lee, J. D., Kim, H. J., Lee, B. I., Kim, O. J., Jeon, T. J., & Kim, M. J. (2000). Evaluation of ictal brain SPET using statistical parametric mapping in temporal lobe epilepsy. *European Journal of Nuclear Medicine, 27*, 1658–1665.

Leech, S. L., Larkby, C. A., Day, R., & Day, N. L. (2006). Predictors and correlates of high levels of depression and anxiety symptoms among children at age 10. *Journal of the American Academy of Child & Adolescent Psychiatry, 45*, 223–230.

Leibenluft, E., & Stoddard, J. (2013). The developmental psychopathology of irritability. *Developmental Psychopathology, 325*, 1473–1487.

Leitão, S. & Fletcher, J. (2004). Literacy outcomes for students with speech impairment: Long-term follow-up. *International Journal of Language & Communication Disorders, 39*(2), 245–256.

Lenneberg, E. (1967). *Biological foundations of language*. Wiley.

Lerner, J. W., & Johns, B. W. (2015). *Learning disabilities and related disabilities: Strategies, for success* (13th ed.). Cengage.

Levisohn, L., Cronin-Golomb, A., & Schmahmann, J. D. (2000). Neuropsychological consequences of cerebellar tumor resection in children. *Brain, 13*, 1041–1050.

Lewis, M. H. (1996). Brief report: Psychopharmacology of autism spectrum disorders. *Journal of Autism and Developmental Disorders, 26*, 231–235.

Lewis, M. H., Aman, M. G., Gadow, K. D., Schroeder, S. R., & Thompson, T. (1996). Psychopharmacology. In J. W. Jacobson & J. A. Mulick (Eds.), *Marna of diagnosis and professional practice in mental retardation* (pp. 323–340). American Psychological Association.

Lezak, M. D. (1995). *Neuropsychological assessment* (3rd ed.). New York: Oxford University Press.

Lezak, M. D. (2009). Everything you wanted to know about clinical neuropsychology and now you can find it. *The Clinical Neuropsychologist, 23*(2), 363–367.

Lezak, M. D., Howieson, D. B., Bigler, E. D., & Tranel, D. (2012). *Neuropsychological assessment* (5th ed.). Oxford University Press.

Lezak, M. D., Howieson, D. B., Loring, D. W., Hannay, H. J., & Fischer, J. S. (2004). *Neuropsychological assessment* (4th ed.). Oxford University Press.

Li, W., Mai, X., & Liu, C. (2014). The default mode network and social understanding of others. What do brain connectivity studies tell us. *Frontiers in Human Neuroscience, 8,* 74.

Li, X., Liu, P., & Rayner, K. (2011). Eye movements guidance in Chinese reading: Is there a preferred viewing location? *Vision Research, 51,* 1146–1156.

Libertus, M. E., Felgenson, L., & Halberda, J. (2011). Preschool acuity of the approximate number system correlates with school math ability. *Developmental Science, 14,* 1292–1300.

Libon, D. J., Swenson, R., & Ashendorf, L. (2013). *Edith Kaplan and the Boston Process Approach: A tribute to an original thinker.* Oxford University Press.

Lichter, D. G., & Cummings, J. L. (Eds.). (2001). *Frontal–subcortical circuits in psychiatric and neurological disorders.* Guilford Press.

Lidzba, K., Küpper, H., Kluger, G., & Staudt, M. (2017). The time window for successful right-hemispheric language reorganization in children. *European Journal of Pediatric Neurology, 21*(5), 715–721.

Liepmann, H. (1908). *Die linke hemisphare und das handeln: Drei aufsatze aus dem apraxiegebiet.* Springer-Verlag.

Lin, C. K., Wu, H. M., Lin, C. H., Wu, Y. Y., Wu, P. F., Kuo, B. C., & Yeung, K. T. (2012). A small sample test of the factor structure of postural movement and bilateral motor integration using structural equation modeling. *Perceptual Motor Skills, 115,* 544–557.

Lindberg, R. & Brown, R. D. (2018). Mathematical difficulties and exceptionalities. In R. D. Brown (Ed.), *Neuroscience of mathematical cognitive development* (pp. 97–118). Springer International.

Liotti, M., & Mayberg, H. S. (2001). The role of functional neuroimaging in the neuropsychology of depression. *Journal of Clinical and Experimental Neuropsychology, 23,* 121–136.

Lipka, O., Siegel, L. S., & Vukovic, R. (2005). The literacy skills of English language learners in Canada. *Learning Disabilities Research & Practice, 20*(1), 39–49.

Lipsky, D. K., & Gartner, A. (1995). *The evaluation of inclusive education programs* (ERIC Document Reproduction Service No. ED385042). City University of New York, National Center on Educational Restructuring and Inclusion.

Llanes, E., Blacher, J., Stavropoulos, K., & Eisenhower, A. (2020). Parent and teacher reports of comorbid anxiety and ADHD symptoms in children with ASD. *Journal of Autism and Developmental Disorders, 50,* 1520–1531.

Loesch, D. Z., Bui, Q. M., Dissanayake, C., Clifford, S., Gould, E., Bulhak-Paterson, D., et al. (2007). Molecular and cognitive predictors of the continuum of autistic behaviours in fragile X. *Neuroscience and Biobehavioral Reviews, 31,* 315–326.

Longcamp, M., Anton, J.-L., Roth, M., & Velay, J.-L. (2003). Visual presentation of single letters activates a premotor area involved in writing. *NeuroImage, 19,* 1492–1500.

Lonigan, C. J., Anthony, J. L., Phillips, B. M., Purpura, D. J., Wilson, S. B., & McQueen, J. D. (2009). The nature of preschool phonological processing abilities and their relations to vocabulary, general cognitive abilities, and print knowledge. *Journal of Educational Psychology, 101*(2), 345.

Lorberg, B., Davico, C., Martsenkovskyi, D., & Vitiello, B. (2019). Principles in using psychotropic medication in children and adolescents. In J. M. Rey & A. Martin (Eds.), *IACAPAP e-Textbook of child and adolescent mental health* (pp. 1–25). International Association for Child and Adolescent Psychiatry and Allied Professions.

Lord, C., & Rutter, M. (2012). *Autism Diagnostic Observation Schedule–2.* Western Psychological Services.

Lorusso, M. L., Facoetti, A., & Bakker, D. J. (2011). Neuropsychological treatment of dyslexia: Does type of treatment matter? *Journal of Learning Disabilities, 44*(2), 136–149.

Lou, H. C., Henriksen, L., & Bruhn, P. (1984). Focal cerebral hypoperfusion in children with dysphasia and/or attention deficit disorder. *Archives of Neurology, 41*(8), 825–829.

Lou, H. C., Henriksen, L., Bruhn, P., Børner, H., & Nielsen, J. B. (1989). Striatal dysfunction in attention deficit and hyperkinetic disorder. *Archives of Neurology, 46*(1), 48–52.

Lourenco, S. F., & Longo, M. R. (2009). Multiple spatial representations of number: Evidence for co-existing compressive and linear scales. *Experimental Brain Research, 193,* 151–156.

Lovett, M. W., Steinbach, K. A., & Frijters, J. C. (2000). Remediating the core deficits of developmental reading disability: A double-deficit perspective. *Journal of Learning Disabilities, 33,* 334–358.

Lund, T. C., Miller, W. P., Nascene, D., Orchard, P., & Gupta, A. O. (2018). Repair of the blood brain barrier and neurotrophil recovery following HSCT in cerebral adrenoleukodystrophy. *Blood, 132*(Suppl. 1), 4628.

Luria, A. R. (1973a). The frontal lobes and the regulation of behavior. In K. H. Pribram & A. R. Luria (Eds.), *Psychophysiology of the frontal lobes* (pp. 3–26). Academic Press.

Luria, A. R. (1973b). *The working brain.* Basic Books.

Luria, A. R. (1980). Neuropsychology in the local diagnosis of brain damage. *International Journal of Clinical Neuropsychology, 2,* 1–7.

Luria, A. R., & Majovski, L. V. (1977). Basic approaches

used in American and Soviet clinical neuropsychology. *American Psychologist, 32*(11), 959.

Ma, X., & Xu, J. (2004). The causal ordering of mathematics anxiety and mathematics achievement: A longitudinal panel analysis. *Journal of Adolescence, 27,* 165–179.

Maccini, P., Mulcahy, C. A., & Wilson, M. G. (2007). A follow-up of mathematics interventions for secondary students with learning disabilities. *Learning Disabilities Practice, 22,* 58–74.

Machek, G. R., & Nelson, J. M. (2007). How should reading disabilities be operationalized?: A survey of practicing school psychologists. *Learning Disabilities Research & Practice, 22*(2), 147–157.

Mahone, E. M., & Denckla, M. B. (2017). Attention-deficit/hyperactivity disorder: a historical neuropsychological perspective. *Journal of the International Neuropsychological Society, 23*(9–10), 916–929.

Maisog, J. M., Einbinder, E. R., Flowers, D. L., Turkeltaub, P. E., & Eden, G. F. (2008). A meta-analysis of functional neuroimaging studies of dyslexia. *Annals of the New York Academy of Sciences, 1145,* 237–259.

Majerske, C. W., Mihalik, J. P., & Ren, D. (2008). Concussion in sports: Postconcussive activity levels, symptoms, and neurocognitive performance. *Journal of Athletic Trainers, 43,* 265–274.

Majovski, L. V. (1997). Development of higher brain functions in children: Neural, cognitive, and behavioral perspectives. In C. R. Reynolds & E. Fletcher-Janzen (Eds.), *Handbook of clinical child neuropsychology* (2nd ed., pp. 17–41). Plenum Press.

Makris, N., Hodge, S. M., Haselgrove, C., Kennedy, D. N., Dale, A., Fischl, B., et al. (2003). Human cerebellum: Surface-assisted cortical parcellation and volumetry with magnetic resonance imaging. *Journal of Cognitive Neuroscience, 15,* 584–599.

Male, A. G., & Gouldthorp, B. (2020). Hemispheric differences in perceptual integration during language comprehension: An ERP study. *Neuropsychologia, 139,* 107353.

Mammarella, I. C., & Cornoldi, C. (2014). An analysis of the criteria used to diagnose children with Nonverbal Learning Disability (NLD), *Child Neuropsychology, 20*(3), 255–280.

Mammarella, I. C., Ghisi, M., Bomba, M., Bottesi, G., Caviola, S., Broggi, F., & Nacinovich, R. (2016). Anxiety and depression in children with nonverbal learning disabilities, reading disabilities, and typical development. *Journal of Learning Disabilities, 49,* 130–139.

Mammarella, I. C., Giofrè, D., Ferrara, R., & Cornoldi, C. (2013). Intuitive geometry and visuospatial working memory in children showing symptoms of nonverbal learning disabilities. *Child Neuropsychology, 19*(3), 235–239.

Mansour, R., Dovi, A. T., Lane, D. M., Loveland, K. A., & Pearson, D. A. (2017). ADHD severity as it relates to ASD symptom severity as it relates to comorbid psychiatric symptomatology in children with ASD. *Research in Developmental Disabilities, 60,* 52–64.

Marcotte, T. D., & Grant, I. (Eds.). (2010), *Neuropsychology of everyday functioning* (1st ed.). Guilford Press.

Margolis, A. E., Bansal, R., Hao, X., Algermissen, M., Erickson, C., Klahr, K. W., et al. (2013). Using IQ discrepancy scores to examine the neural correlates of specific cognitive abilities. *Journal of Neuroscience, 33,* 14135–14145.

Margolis, A. E., Pagliaccio, D., Thomas, L., Banker, S., & Marsh, R. (2019). Salience network connectivity and social processing in children with nonverbal learning disability or autism spectrum disorder. *Neuropsychology, 33,* 135–143.

Mari, M., Castiello, U., Marks, D., Marraffa, C., & Prior, M. (2003). The reach-to-grasp movement in children with autism spectrum disorder. *Philosophical Transactions of the Royal Society of London. Series B: Biological Sciences, 358*(1430), 393–403.

Markey, A. M. (2010). The relationship between visual-spatial reasoning ability and math and geometry problem-solving. *Dissertation Abstracts International: Section B: The sciences and Engineering, 70,* 7874.

Marshall, D., Christo, C., & Davis, J. (2013). Performance of school age reading disabled students on the Phonological Awareness Subtests of the Comprehensive Test of Phonological Processing (CTOPP). *Contemporary School Psychology, 17,* 93–101.

Martinez, R., & Semrud-Clikeman, M. (2004). Emotional adjustment of young adolescents with different learning disability subtypes. *Journal of Learning Disabilities, 37,* 411–420.

Marzillier, S. L. (2009). What psychologists need to know about Lyme Disease. *Clinical Psychology Forum, 194,* 37–41.

Mascolo, J. T., Kaufman, N. L., & Hale, J. B. (2009). Illustrative case reports using the WISC-IV. In D. P. Flanagan & A. S. Kaufman, *Essentials of WISC-IV assessment* (2nd ed., pp. 468–515). Wiley.

Master, C. L., Gioia, G. A., Leddy, J. J., & Grady, M. F. (2012). Importance of "return to learn" in pediatric and adolescent concussion. *Pediatric Annals, 41,* 1–7.

Mastropieri, M. A., Scruggs, T. E., Guckert, M., Thompson, C. C., & Weiss, M. P. (2013). Inclusion and learning disabilities: Will the past be prologue? In J. P. Bakken, F. E. Obiakor & A. F. Rotatori (Eds.), *Advances in special education: Vol. 25. Learning disabilities: Practice concerns and students with LD* (pp. 1–17). Emerald Group.

Matchin, W., & Hickok, G. (2020). The cortical organization of syntax. *Cerebral Cortex, 30*(3), 1481–1498.

Mather, F. J., Tate, R. L., & Hannan, T. J. (2003). Post-traumatic stress disorder in children following road traffic accidents: A comparison of those with and without mild traumatic brain injury. *Brain Injury, 17,* 1077–1087.

Mather, N., & Jaffe, L. E. (2016). *Woodcock–Johnson IV: Reports, recommendations, and strategies* (3rd ed.). Wiley.

Mather, N., & Tanner, N. (2014). Introduction to the special issue on diagnosis and identification of individuals with specific learning disability: Pattern of strengths and weaknesses. *Learning Disabilities: A Multidisciplinary Journal, 20*(1), 1–7.

Matijasevich, A., Murray, J., Cooper, P. J., Anselmi, L., Barros, A. J., Barros, F. C., & Santos, I. S. (2015). Trajectories of maternal depression and offspring psychopathology at 6 years: 2004 Pelotas cohort study. *Journal of Affective Disorders, 174,* 424–431.

Mattis, S., Papolos, D., Luck, D., Cockerham, M., & Thode, H. C. (2011). Neuropsychological factors differentiating treated children with pediatric bipolar disorder from those with attention-deficit/hyperactivity disorder. *Journal of Clinical and Experimental Neuropsychology, 33,* 74–84.

Mattson, S. N., Crocker, N., & Nguyen, T. T. (2011). Fetal alcohol spectrum disorders: Neuropsychological and behavioral features. *Neuropsychology Review, 21,* 81–101.

Mauk, M. D., & Buonomano, D. V. (2004). The neural basis of temporal processing. *Annual Review of Neuroscience, 27,* 307–340.

Max, J. E. (2004). Effect of side of lesion on neuropsychological performance in childhood stroke. *Journal of the International Neuropsychological Society, 10,* 698–708.

Max, J. E., Fox, P. T., Lancaster, J. L., Kochunov, P., Mathews, K., Manes, F. F., et al. (2002). Putamen lesions and the development of attention-deficit/hyperactivity symptoms. *Journal of the American Academy of Child and Adolescent Psychiatry, 41,* 563–571.

May, P. A., Gossage, J. P., Kalberg, W. O., Robinson, L. K., Buckley, D., Manning, M., et al. (2009). Prevalence and epidemiological characteristics of FASD from various research methods with an emphasis on recent in-school studies. *Developmental Disabilities Research Reviews, 15,* 176–192.

Mayberg, H. (2001). Depression and frontal–subcortical circuits: Focus on prefrontal–limbic interactions. In D. G. Lichter & J. L. Cummings (Eds.), *Frontal–subcortical circuits in psychiatric and neurological disorders* (pp. 177–206). New York: Guilford Press.

Mayer, E. A., Padua, D., & Tillisch, K. (2014). Altered brain-gut axis in autism: Comorbidity or causative mechanisms? *BioEssays, 36,* 933–939.

Mayes, S. D., & Calhoun, S. L. (2006). Frequency of reading, math, writing disabilities in children with clinical disorders. *Learning and Individual Differences, 16,* 145–157.

Mayes, S. D., & Calhoun, S. L. (2007). Learning, attention, writing, and processing speed in typical children and children with ADHD, autism, anxiety, depression, and oppositional-defiant disorder. *Child Neuropsychology, 13*(6), 469–493.

Mazzocco, M. M. (2001). Math learning disability and math LD subtypes: evidence from studies of Turner syndrome, fragile X syndrome, and neurofibromatosis type 1. *Journal of learning disabilities, 34*(6), 520–533.

Mazzocco, M. M. M., Bhatia, N. S., & Lesniak-Karpiak, K. (2006). Visuospatial skills and their association with math performance in girls with fragile X or Turner syndrome. *Child Neuropsychology, 12*(2), 87–110.

Mazzocco, M. M. M., Feigenson, L., & Halberda, J. (2011). Impaired acuity of the approximate number system underlies mathematical learning disability (dyscalculia). *Child Development, 82,* 1224–1237.

Mazzocco, M. M. M., & Myers, G. F. (2003). Complexities in identifying and defining mathematics learning disability in the primary school-age years. *Annals of Dyslexia, 53,* 218–253.

Mazzocco, M. M. M., Myers, G. F., Lewis, K. E., Hanich, L. B., & Murphy, M. M. (2013). Limited knowledge of fraction representations differentiates middle school students with mathematics learning disability (Dyscalculia) versus low mathematics achievement. *Journal of Experimental Child Psychology, 115,* 371–387.

Mazzocco, M. M. M., & Thompson, R. E. (2005). Kindergarten predictors of math learning disability. *Learning Disabilities Research & Practice, 20,* 143–155.

McAuliffe, P., Brassard, M. R., & Fallon, B. (2008). Memory and executive functions in adolescents with posttreatment Lyme Disease. *Applied Neuropsychology, 15,* 208–219.

McClellan, J., Kowatch, R., & Findling, R. L. (2007). Work Group on Quality Issues. Practice parameter for the assessment and treatment of children and adolescents with bipolar disorder. *Journal of the American Academy of Child and Adolescent Psychiatry, 46,* 107–125.

McClure, E. B., Treland, J. E., Snow, J., Schamajuk, M., Dickstein, D. P., & Towbin, K. E. (2005). Deficits in social cognition and response flexibility in pediatric bipolar disorder. *American Journal of Psychiatry, 162,* 1644–1651.

McConaughy, S. H., & Achenbach, T. M. (2009).

Manual for the ASEBA Direct Observation Form. University of Vermont Research Center for Children, Youth, & Families.

McConaughy, S. H., Kay, P., Welkowitz, J. A., Hewitt, K., & Fitzgerald, M. D. (2013). *Collaborating with parents for early school success: The achieving–behaving–caring program.* Guilford Press.

McCrea, M. A. (2013). *Acute assessment and subacute management of sports concussion.* Paper presented at the 2013 International Sports Concussion Symposium, Minneapolis.

McCrea, M. A., Guskiewicz, K., Randolph, C., Barr, W. B., Hammeke, T. A., Marshal, S. W., et al. (2013). Incidence, clinical course, and predictors of prolonged recovery time following sport-related concussion in high school and college athletes. *Journal of the International Neuropsychological Society, 19,* 22–33.

McCrea, M. A., Prichep, L. S., Powell, M. R., Chabot, R., & Barr, W. B. (2010). Acute effects and recovery after sports-related concussion: A neurocognitive and quantitative brain electrical activity study. *Journal of Head Trauma Rehabilitation, 25,* 1–10.

McDermott, P. A., Fantuzzo, J. W., & Glutting, J. J. (1990). Just say no to subtest analysis: A critique on Wechsler theory and practice. *Journal of Psychoeducational Assessment, 8,* 290–302.

McDermott, P. A., Goldberg, M. M., Watkins, M. W., Stanley, J. L., & Glutting, J. J. (2006). A nationwide epidemiologic modeling study of LD: Risk, protection, and unintended impact. *Journal of Learning Disabilities, 39,* 230–251.

McDermott, P. A., Watkins, M. W., Rovine, M. J., & Rikoon, S. H. (2013). Assessing changes in socioemotional adjustment across early school transitions: New national scales for children at risk. *Journal of School Psychology, 51*(1), 97–115.

McGhee, R. L., Ehrler, D. J., & DiSimoni, F. (2007). *TTFC-2: Token Test for children* (2nd ed.). PRO-ED.

McGrath, L. M., Hutaff-Lee, C., Scott, A., Boada, R., Shriberg, L., & Pennington, B. F. (2008). Children with comorbid speech sound disorder and specific language impairment are at increased risk for attention deficit hyperactivity disorder. *Journal of Abnormal Child Psychology, 36,* 151–163.

McGrath, L. M., Pennington, B. F., Shanahan, M. A., Santerre-Lemmon, L. E., Barnard, H. D., Willcutt, E., et al. (2011). A multiple deficit model of reading disability and attention-deficit/hyperactivity disorder: Searching for shared cognitive deficits. *Journal of Child Psychology and Psychiatry, 52,* 547–557.

McGregor, M. L. (2014). Convergence insufficiency and vision therapy. *Pediatric Clinics of North America, 61*(3), 621–630.

McGrew, K. S. (2009). CHC theory and the human cognitive abilities project: Standing on the shoulders of the giants of psychometric intelligence research. *Intelligence, 37*(1), 1–10.

McGrew, K. S., Mather, N., LaForte, E. M., & Wendling, B. J. (2025). *Woodcock–Johnson V.* Riverside Assessments, LLC.

McGrew, K. S., & Wendling, B. J. (2010). Cattell–Horn–Carroll cognitive-achievement relations: What we have learned from the past 20 years of research. *Psychology in the Schools, 47*(7), 651–675.

McKean-Cowdin, R., Razavi, P., Barrington-Trimis, J., Baldwin, R. T., Agharzadeh, S., Cockburn, M., et al. (2013). Trends in childhood brain tumor incidence, 1973–2009. *Journal of Neuro-Oncology, 115,* 153–160.

McKnight, M. E., & Culotta, V. P. (2012). Comparing neuropsychological profiles between girls with Asperger's disorder and girls with learning disabilities. *Focus on Autism and Other Developmental Disabilities, 27*(4), 247–253.

McLeod, T. V., & Gioia, G. A. (2010). Cognitive rest: The often neglected aspect of concussion management. *Athletic Therapy Today, 15,* 1–3.

McMahon, K., Paciorkowski, A. R., Walters-Sen, L. C., Milunsky, J. M., Bassuk, A., Darbro, B., et al. (2017). Neurogenetics in the genome era. In K. Swaiman, S. Ashwayl, D. M. Ferriero, N. F. Schor, R. S. Finkel, A. L. Gropan, P. L., et al. (Eds.), *Swaiman's pediatric neurology* (6th ed., pp. 257–267). Elsevier.

McNorgan, C., Randazzo-Wagner, M., & Booth, J. R. (2013). Cross-modal integration in the brain is related to phonological awareness only in typical readers, not in those with reading difficulty. *Frontiers in Human Neuroscience, 7,* 388.

Meaden, H., & Halle, J. W. (2004). Social perceptions of students with learning disabilities who differ in social status. *Learning Disabilities Research and Practice, 19,* 71–82.

Meekes, J., Braams, O., Braun, K. P., Jennekens-Schinkel, A., van Nieuwenhuizen, O., & Dutch Collaborative Epilepsy Surgery Programme (DuCESP). (2013). Verbal memory after epilepsy surgery in childhood. *Epilepsy Research, 107*(1–2), 146–55.

Melby-Lervag, M., Lyster, S.-A.-H., & Hulme, C. (2012). Phonological skills and their role in learning to read: A meta-analytic review. *Psychological Bulletin, 138,* 322–352.

Mellet, E., Zago, L., Jobard, G., Crivello, F., Petit, L., Joliot, M., et al. (2014). Weak language lateralization affects both verbal and spatial skills: An fMRI study in 297 subjects. *Neuropsychologia, 65,* 56–62.

Melton, T. H., Croarkin, P. E., Strawn, J. R., & McClintock, S. M. (2016). Comorbid anxiety and depressive symptoms in children and adolescents: A systematic review and analysis. *Journal of Psychiatric Practice, 22,* 84–98.

Meltzer, L. (2010). *Promoting executive function in the classroom.* Guilford Press.

Meltzer, L. (Ed.). (2018). *Executive function in education: From theory to practice* (2nd ed.). Guilford Press.

Mendoza, J., & Foundas, A. (2007). *Clinical neuroanatomy: A neurobehavioral approach.* Springer Science & Business Media.

Menon, V. (2015a). Salience network. In A. W. Toga (Ed.), *Brain mapping: An encyclopedic reference* (pp. 597–611). Academic Press.

Menon, V. (2015b). *Arithmetic in the child and adult brain.* Oxford University Press.

Menon, V. (2016). Working memory in children's math learning and its disruption in dyscalculia. *Current Opinion in Behavioral Sciences, 10,* 125–132.

Mercer, C. D., & Mercer, A. R. (2001). *Teaching students with learning problems* (6th ed.). Merrill/Prentice-Hall.

Mercer, C. D., & Pullen, P. C. (2009). *Students with learning disabilities* (7th ed.). Pearson.

Mercer, N., & Howe, C. (2012). Explaining the dialogic processes of teaching and learning: The value and potential of sociocultural theory. *Learning, Culture and Social Interaction, 1*(1), 12–21.

Meredith, R. M. (2015). Sensitive and critical periods during neurotypical and aberrant neurodevelopment: A framework for neurodevelopmental disorders. *Neuroscience & Biobehavioral Reviews, 50,* 180–188.

Merikangas, K. R., He, J., Burstein, M., Swanson, S. A., Avenevoli, S., Cui, L., et al. (2010). Lifetime prevalence of mental disorders in U.S. adolescents: Results from the National Comorbidity Study—Adolescent Supplement (NCS-A). *Journal of the American Academy of Child and Adolescent Psychiatry, 49,* 980–989.

Merrell, K. W., Ervin, R. A., Gimpel Peacock, G., & Renshaw, T. (2022). *School psychology for the 21st century: Foundation and practices* (3rd ed.). Guilford Press.

Mervis, C. B., & John, A. E. (2010). Cognitive and behavioral characteristics of children with Williams syndrome: Implications for intervention approaches. *American Journal of Medical Genetics Part C: Seminars in Medical Genetics, 154C,* 229–248.

Meyer, M. L., Salimpor, V. M., Wu, S. S., Geary, D. C., & Menon, V. (2010). Differential contribution of specific working memory components to mathematics achievement in 2nd and 3rd graders. *Learning and Individual Differences, 20,* 101–109.

Meyer-Lindenberg, A., Mervis, C. B., & Berman, K. F. (2006). Neural mechanisms in Williams syndrome: A unique window to genetic influences on cognition and behavior. *Nature Reviews Neuroscience, 7,* 380–393.

Meyers, J., & Meyers, K. (1995). *The Meyers scoring system for the Rey–Osterrieth Complex Figure and Recognition trial.* Psychological Assessment Resources.

Meyler, A., Keller, T. A., Cherkassky, V. L., Lee, D., Hoeft, F., Whitfield-Gabrieli, S., & Just, M. A. (2007). Brain activation during sentence comprehension among good and poor readers. *Cerebral Cortex, 17,* 2780–2787.

Michael, E. B., Keller, T. A., Carpenter, P. A., & Just, M. A. (2001). fMRI investigation of sentence comprehension by eye and by ear: Modality fingerprints on cognitive processes. *Human Brain Mapping, 13,* 239–252.

Miciak, J., & Fletcher, J. M. (2020). The critical role of instructional response for identifying dyslexia and other learning disabilities. *Journal of Learning Disabilities, 53*(5), 343–353.

Miciak, J., Roberts, G., Taylor, W. P., Solis, M., Ahmed, Y., Vaughn, S., & Fletcher, J. M. (2018). The effects of one versus two years of intensive reading intervention implemented with late elementary struggling readers. *Learning Disabilities Research & Practice, 33*(1), 24–36.

Mick, E., Biederman, J., Prince, J., Fischer, M. J., & Faraone, S. V. (2002). Impact of low birth weight on attention deficit/hyperactivity disorder. *Journal of Developmental Behavioral Pediatrics, 23,* 16–22.

Middleton, F. A., & Strick, P. L. (2000). Basal ganglia output and cognition: Evidence from anatomical, behavioral, and clinical studies. *Brain and Cognition, 42,* 183–200.

Mikadze, Y. V., Ardila, A., & Akhutina, T. V. (2019). AR Luria's approach to neuropsychological assessment and rehabilitation. *Archives of Clinical Neuropsychology, 34*(6), 795–802.

Milberg, W. P., Hebben, N., & Kaplan, E. (2009). The Boston Process Approach to neuropsychological assessment. In I. Grant & K. Adams (Eds.), *Neuropsychological assessment of neuropsychiatric and nonmedical disorders* (3rd ed., pp. 42–63). Oxford University Press.

Miller, C. J., Hynd, G .W., & Miller, S. R. (2005). Children with dyslexia: Not necessarily at risk for elevated internalizing symptoms. *Reading and Writing, 18,* 425–436.

Miller, D. C. (2019). *Essentials of school neuropsychological assessment* (3rd ed.). Wiley.

Miller, F. G., Chafouleas, S. M., Welsh, M., Riley-Tillman, T. C., & Fabiano, G. A. (2019). Examining the stability of social, emotional, and behavioral risk status: Implications for screening frequency. *School Psychology, 34,* 43–53.

Miller, J. (2019). STEM education in the primary years to support mathematical thinking: Using coding to identify mathematical structures and patterns. *The International Journal on Mathematics Education, 51*(6), 915–927.

Miller, R. S., & Wang, M. T. (2019). Cultivating adolescents' academic identity: Ascertaining the mediating effects of motivational beliefs between classroom practices and mathematics identity. *Journal of Youth and Adolescence, 48,* 2038–2050.

Miller, S. A. (2013). *Writing in psychology.* Routledge.

Miller, S. L., & Tallal, P. (1995). A behavioral neuroscience approach to developmental language disorders: Evidence for a rapid temporal processing deficit. In D. Cicchetti & D. J. Cohen (Eds.), *Developmental psychopathology: Vol. 2. Risk, disorder, and adaptation* (pp. 274–298). Wiley.

Milner, A. D., & Goodale, M. A. (1995). *The visual brain in action.* Oxford University Press.

Minne, E., & Semrud-Clikeman, M. (2012). A social competence intervention for young children with high functioning autism and Asperger syndrome. *Autism, 16,* 586–602.

Mirsky, A. F., Pasculavaca, D. M., Duncan, C. C., & French, L. M. (1999). A model of attention and its relation to ADHD. *Mental Retardation and Developmental Disabilities Research Reviews, 5,* 169–176.

Mistry, S., Escott-Price, V., Florio, A. D., Smith, D. J., & Zammit, S. (2019). Investigating asociations between genetic risk for bipolar disorder and cognitive functioning in childhood. *Journal of Affective Disorders, 259,* 112–120.

Mitchell, J. R., & Nelson-Gray, R. O. (2006). Attention-deficit/hyperactivity disorder symptoms in adults: Relationship to Gray's behavioral approach system. *Personality and Individual Differences, 40,* 749–760.

Mitchison, G. M., & Njardvik, U. (2019). Prevalence and gender differences of ODD, anxiety, and depression in a sample of children with ADHD. *Journal of Attention Disorders, 23,* 1339–1345.

Mix, K. S., & Cheng, Y. L. (2012). The relation between space and math: developmental and educational implications. *Advances in Child Developmental Behavior, 42,* 197–243.

Moats, L. C. (2000). *Whole language lives on: The illusion of "balanced" reading instruction.* Diane Publishing.

Molfese, D. L. (2000). Predicting dyslexia at 8 years of age using neonatal brain responses. *Brain and Language, 72,* 238–245.

Molfese, D. L., Molfese, V. J., Garrod, K., & Molfese, D. L. (2012). Processing from imaging techniques: Implications for interventions for developmental disabilities. In Z. Breznitz (Ed.), *Reading, writing, mathematics and the developing brain: Listening to many voices* (pp. 5–24). Springer.

Molfese, D. L., Morse, P. A., & Peters, C. J. (1990). Auditory evoked responses to names for different objects: Cross-modal processing as a basis for infant language acquisition. *Developmental Psychology, 26,* 780–795.

Molfese, V. J., Molfese, P. J., Molfese, D. L., Rudasill, K. M., Armstrong, N., & Starkey, G. (2010). Executive function skills of 6–8 year olds: Brain and behavioral evidence and implications for school achievement. *Contemporary Educational Psychology, 35*(2), 116–125.

Molina, B. S. G., Hinshaw, S. P., Swanson, J. M., Arnold, L. E., Vitiello, B., Jensen, P. S., et al. (2009). The MTA at 8 years: Prospective follow-up of children treated for combined-type ADHD in a multi-site study. *Journal of the American Academy of Child and Adolescent Psychiatry, 48,* 484–500.

Molko, N., Cachia, A., Riviere, D., Mangin, J. F., Bruandet, M., Le Bihan, D., & Dehaene, S. (2002). Functional and structural alterations of the intraparietal sulcus in a developmental dyscalculia of genetic origin. *Neuron, 40,* 847–858.

Moll, J., de Oliveira-Souza, R., Passman, L. J., Cunha, F. C., Souza-Lima, F., & Andreiuolo, P. A. (2000). Functional MRI correlates of real and imagined tool use pantomimes. *Neurology, 54,* 1331–1336.

Moll, K., Göbel, S. M., & Snowling, M. J. (2015). Basic number processing in children with specific learning disorders: Comorbidity of reading and mathematics disorders. *Child Neuropsychology, 21*(3), 399–417.

Mong, M. D., & Mong, K. W. (2010). Efficacy of two mathematics interventions for enhancing fluency in elementary students. *Journal of Behavioral Education, 19,* 273–288.

Monuteaux, M. C., Faraone, S. V., Herzig, K., Navsaria, N., & Biederman, J. (2005). ADHD and dyscalculia: Evidence for independent familial transmission. *Journal of Learning Disabilities, 38*(1), 86–93.

Moss, J., Schunn, C. D., Schneider, W., & McNamara, D. S. (2011). *An fMRI study of zoning out during strategic reading comprehension.* Paper presented at the meeting of the Cognitive Science Society, Austin, TX.

Moss, J., Schunn, C. D., Schneider, W., McNamara, D. S., & VanLehn, K. (2011). The neural correlates of strategic reading comprehension: Cognitive control and discourse comprehension. *NeuroImage, 58,* 675–686.

Mueller, K. L., & Tomblin, J. B. (2012). Diagnosis of Attention-Deficit/hyperactivity disorder and its behavioral, neurological and genetic roots. *Topics in Language Disorders, 32,* 207–227.

Mula, M. (2018). Pharmacological treatment of anxiety disorders in adults with epilepsy. *Expert Opinion on Pharmacotherapy, 19*(17), 1867–1874.

Mulhern, R. K., & Butler, R. W. (2004). Neurocognitive sequelae of childhood cancers and their treatment. *Pediatric Rehabilitation, 7,* 1–14.

Muller, R., Kleinhans, N., Pierce, K., Kemmotsu, N., & Courchesne, E. (2002). Functional MRI of motor sequence acquisition effects of learning stage and performance. *Cognitive Brain Research, 14,* 277–293.

Muñoz-Sandoval, A. F., Woodcock, R. W., McGrew, K. S., & Mather, N. (2005). *Batería III Woodcock–Muñoz.* Riverside.

Murphy, M. M., Mazzocco, M. M., & McCloskey, M. (2010). Genetic disorders as models of mathematics learning disability: Fragile X and Turner syndromes. In M. A. Barnes (Ed.), *Genes, brain and development: The neurocognition of genetic disorders* (pp. 143–174). Cambridge University Press.

Murray, M. L., Hsia, Y., Glaser, K., Simonoff, E., Murphy, D. G. M., Asherson, P. J., et al. (2014). Pharmacological treatments prescribed to people with autism spectrum disorder (ASD) in primary health care. *Psychopharmacology, 231,* 1011–1021.

Mussolin, C., DeVolder, A., Grandin, C., Schlogel, X., Nassogne, M. C., & Noel, M. P. (2010). Neural correlates of symbolic number comparison in developmental dyscalculia. *Cognition, 115,* 10–25.

Mussolin, C., Meijas, S., & Noel, M. P. (2010). Symbolic and non-symbolic number comparison in developmental dyscalculia. *Journal of Cognitive Neuroscience, 22,* 860–874.

Nachev, P., Kennard, C., & Husain, M. (2008). Functional role of the supplementary and pre-supplementary motor areas. *Nature Reviews Neuroscience, 9*(11), 856–869.

Naglieri, J. A. (2002). Best Practices in Interventions for School Psychologists: A Cognitive Approach to Problem Solving. In A. Thomas & J. Grimes (Eds.), *Best practices in school psychology IV* (pp. 1373–1392). National Association of School Psychologists.

Naglieri, J. A., & Das, J. P. (1997). *Das–Naglieri Cognitive Assessment System administration and scoring manual.* Riverside.

Naglieri, J. A., Das, J. P., & Goldstein, S. (2014). *Cognitive assessment system* (2nd ed.). PAR.

Naglieri, J. A., & Goldstein, S. (Eds.). (2009). *Practitioner's guide to assessing intelligence and achievement.* Wiley.

Naglieri, J., & Johnson, D. (2000). Effectiveness of a cognitive strategy intervention in improving arithmetic computation based on the PASS theory. *Journal of Learning Disabilities, 33*(6), 591–597.

Naglieri, J. A., & Kaufman, A. S. (2008). IDEIA and specific learning disabilities: What role does intelligence play? In E. L. Grigorenko (Ed.), *Educating individuals with disabilities: IDEIA 2004 and beyond* (pp. 165–195). Springer.

Naglieri, J. A., & Otero, T. M. (2017). *Essentials of CAS2 assessment.* Wiley.

Naglieri, J. A., & Rohjahn, J. (2004). Construct validity of the PASS theory and CAS: Correlations with achievement. *Journal of Educational Psychology, 96,* 174–181.

Naidoo, R. B. (2006). *Fluid reasoning: Working memory and written expression in 9- to 14-year-old children with attention deficit hyperactivity disorder.* Unpublished doctoral dissertation, University of Texas at Austin, Austin, TX.

Nakamura, Y., Yashiro, M., Uehara, R., Sadakane, A., Tsuboi, S., Aoyama, Y., et al. (2012). Epidemiologic features of Kawasaki disease in Japan: results of the 2009–2010 nationwide survey. *Journal of Epidemiology, 22*(3), 216–221.

Nakao, T., Radua, J., Rubia, K., & Mataix-Cols, D. (2011). Gray matter volume abnormalities in ADHD: Voxel-based meta-analysis exploring the effects of age and stimulant medication. *American Journal of Psychiatry, 168,* 1154–1163.

Narhi, V., Lehto-Salo, P., Ahonen, T., & Marttunen, M. (2010). Neuropsychological subgroups of adolescents with conduct disorder. *Scandinavian Journal of Psychology, 51,* 278–284.

National Center for Health Statistics. (2006). *Health United States with chartbook on trends in The health of Americans (Table 58).* Author.

National Center on Response to Intervention. (2010, March). *Users guide to progress monitoring tools chart.* Retrieved from *www.rt4success.org/chart/progressMonitoring/progressmonitoringtoolschart.htm.*

National Institute of Child Health and Human Development (NICHD). (2000). *Report of the National Reading Panel. Teaching children to read: An evidence-based assessment of the scientific research literature on reading and its implications for reading instruction: Reports of the subgroups* (NIH Publication No. 00-4754). U.S. Government Printing Office.

Nelson, J. M., & Gregg, N. (2012). Depression and anxiety among transitioning adolescents and college students with ADHD, dyslexia, or comorbid ADHD/dyslexia. *Journal of Attention Disorders, 16,* 244–254.

Nelson, J. M., & Harwood, H. (2011). Learning disabilities and anxiety: A meta-analysis. *Journal of Learning Disabilities, 44,* 371–384.

Newcomer, P. L., & Hammill, D. D. (2019). *Test of Language Development—Intermediate: Fifth edition.* PRO-ED.

Newman, R. L., & Joanisse, M. F. (2011). Modulation of brain regions involved in word recognition by homophonous stimuli: An fMRI study. *Brain Research, 1367,* 250–264.

Newman, S. D., & Tweig, D. (2001). Differences in auditory processing of words and pseudowords: An fMRI study. *Human Brain Mapping, 14,* 39–47.

Newman, S. D., Willoughby, G., & Pruce, B. (2011). The effect of problem structure on problem-solving:

an fMRI study of word versus number problems. *Brain Research, 1410,* 77–88.

Ng, C.-T., Lung, T.-C., & Chang, T.-T. (2021). Operation-specific lexical consistency effect in fronto-insular-parietal network during word problem solving. *Frontiers in Human Neuroscience, 15,* 631438.

Nicholson, R. I., Fawcett, A. J., & Dean, P. (2001). Developmental dyslexia: The cerebellar deficit hypothesis. *Trends in Neuroscience, 24,* 508–511.

Nickerson, R. S. (1998). Confirmation bias: A ubiquitous phenomenon in many guises. *Review of General Psychology, 2*(2), 175–220.

Niedo, J., Lee, Y., Breznitz, B., & Berninger, V. (2013). Response to silent reading rate training at transition to silent reading for fourth graders with silent reading rate disabilities. *Journal of Learning Disabilities, 37*(2), 100–110.

Nielsen, K., Abbott, R., Griffin, W., Lott, J., Raskind, W., & Berninger, V. W. (2016). Evidence-based reading and writing assessment for dyslexia in adolescents and young adults. *Learning Disabilities, 21*(1), 38.

Nigg, J. T. (2005). Attention, task difficulty, and ADHD. *British Journal of Developmental Psychology, 23,* 513–516.

Niileksela C. R., & Reynolds, M. R. (2019). Enduring the tests of age and time: Wechsler construct across versions and revisions. *Intelligence, 77,* Article 101403.

Niklasson, L., Rasmussen, P., Okarsdottir, S., & Gillberg, C. (2001). Neuropsychiatric disorders in the 22q deletion syndrome. *Genetics in Medicine, 3,* 79–84.

Nilesen, T. S., Eisemann, M., & Kvernmo, S. (2013). Predictors and moderators of outcome in child and adolescent anxiety and depression: A systematic review of psychological treatment studies. *European Child and Adolescent Psychiatry, 22,* 69–87.

Noles, N. S., Scholl, B. K., & Mitroff, S. R. (2005). The persistence of object file representations. *Perception and Psychophysics, 67,* 324–334.

Noonan, M. P., Bolton, K. H., Chau, M., Rushworth, F. S., & Fellows, L. K. (2017). Contrasting effects of medial and lateral orbitofrontal cortex lesions on credit assignment and decision-making in humans. *Journal of Neuroscience, 37,* 7023–7035.

Norman, L. J., Carlisi, C. O., Christakou, A., Murphy, C. M., Chatiluke, K., Giampietro, V., et al. (2018). Frontostriatal dysfunction during decision making in Attention-deficit/hyperactivity disorder and obsessive–compulsive disorder. *Neuroimaging, 3,* 694–703.

Northcott, E., Connolly, A. M., Berroya, A., Sabaz, M., McIntyre, J., Christie, J., et al. (2005). The neuropsychological and language profile of children

with benign rolandic epilepsy. *Epilepsia, 46*(6), 924–930.

Norton, E. S., Kovelman, I., & Pettitto, L.-A. (2007). Are there separate neural systems for spelling? New insights into the role of rules and memory in spelling from functional magnetic resonance imaging. *Mind, Brain, and Education, 1,* 48–59.

Novak, G. P., Solanto, M., & Abikoff, H. (1995). Spatial orienting and focused attention in attention deficit hyperactivity disorder. *Psychophysiology, 32,* 546–559.

Nunes, T., & Bryant, P. E. (2006). *Improving literacy by teaching morphemes.* Routledge.

Nussbaum, N. L., & Bunner, M. R. (2009). Halstead–Reitan neuropsychological test batteries for children. In C. R. Reynolds & E. Fletcher-Janzen (Eds.), *Handbook of clinical child neuropsychology* (3rd ed., pp. 247–266). Springer Science + Business Media.

Nussbaum, R., McInnes, R. R., & Willard, H. F. (2015). *Thompson & Thompson genetics in medicine e-book.* Elsevier Health Sciences.

O'Brien, B. A., Wolf, M., & Lovett, M. (2013, April 4). *An examination of subtypes of developmental dyslexia and intervention effects.* Presented April 4, 2013 in Singapore at the Joint NIE, MOE and KKH Symposium on "Beyond the Mainstream: Exploring the Cognitive Development of Children with Special Needs and Children At-Risk of Academic Failure."

O'Connor, M. J., & Paley, B. (2009). Psychiatric conditions associated with prenatal alcohol exposure. *Developmental Disabilities Research Reviews, 15,* 225–234.

Odding, E., Roebroeck, M. E., & Stam, H. J. (2006). The epidemiology of cerebral palsy: Incidence, impairments, and risk factors. *Disability and Rehabilitation, 28,* 183–191.

Odegard, T. N., Ring, J., Smith, S., Biggan, J., & Black, J. (2008). Differentiating the neural response to intervention in children with developmental dyslexia. *Annals of Dyslexia, 58*(1), 1–14.

O'Driscoll, G. A., Wolff, A. V., Benkelfat, C., Florencio, P. S., Lal, S., & Evans, A. C. (2000). Functional neuroanatomy of smooth pursuit and predictive saccades. *NeuroReport, 11,* 1335–1340.

Ogbu, J. U. (2002). Cultural amplifiers of intelligence: IQ and minority status in cross-cultural perspective. In J. M. Fish (Ed.), *Race and intelligence: Separating science from myth* (pp. 241–278). Erlbaum.

Olson, I. R., Von Der Heide, R. J., Alm, K. H., & Vyas, G. (2015). Development of the uncinate fasciculus: Implications for theory and developmental disorders. *Developmental Cognitive Neuroscience, 14,* 50–61.

O'Neill, A. M. (1995). *Clinical inference: How to draw meaningful conclusions from tests.* Clinical Psychology.

O'Reilly, M., Rispoli, M., Davis, T., Machalicek, W., Lang, R., Sigafoos, J., & Didden, R. (2010). Functional analysis of challenging behavior in children with autism spectrum disorders: A summary of 10 cases. *Research in Autism Spectrum Disorders, 4*(1), 1–10.

Orengo, J. P., & Zoghbi, H. Y. (2025). The cerebellum and the hereditary ataxias. In S. Ashwal & P. L. Pearl (Eds.), *Pediatric neurology* (7th ed., pp. 998–1010). Elsevier.

Ortiz, S. O., Johnston, H. N., Wilcox, G., Francis, S. L., & Tomes, Y. I. (2014). The Primacy of IQ Subtest Analysis to Understand Reading Performance for Culturally Diverse Groups. *Learning Disabilities: A Multidisciplinary Journal, 20*(1), 45–54.

Ortiz, S. O., Piazza, N., Ochoa, S. H., & Dynda, A. M. (2018). Testing with culturally and linguistically diverse populations: New directions in fairness and validity. In D. P. Flanagan & E. M. McDonough (Eds.), *Contemporary intellectual assessment: Theories, tests, and issues* (4th ed., pp. 684–714). Guilford Press.

Oscar-Berman, M., & Fein, D. A. (2013). Edith Kaplan: Educational background and her impact on neuropsychology. In L. Ashendorf, R. Swenson, & D. J. Libon (Eds.), *The Boston process approach to neuropsychological assessment: A practitioner's guide* (pp. 18–22). Oxford University Press.

Ott, D., Caplan, R., Guthrie, D., Siddarth, P., Komo, S., Shields, D., et al. (2001). Measures of psychopathology in children with complex partial seizures and generalized epilepsy with absence. *Journal of the American Academy of Child and Adolescent Psychiatry, 40*, 907–914.

Ouellette, G., & Beers, A. (2010). A not-so-simple view of reading: How oral vocabulary and visual-word recognition complicate the story. *Reading and Writing, 23*, 189–208.

Owen, R., Sikich, L., Marcus, R. N., Corey-Lisle, P., Manos, G., McQuade, R. D., et al. (2009). Aripiprazole in the treatment of irritability in children and adolescents with autistic disorders. *Pediatrics, 124*, 1533–1540.

Owens, J. S., Allan, D. M., Hustus, C., & Erchul, W. P. (2018). Examining correlates of teacher receptivity to social influence strategies within a school consultation relationship. *Psychology in the Schools, 55*, 1041–1055.

Ozonoff, S., Gangi, D., Hanzel, E. P., Hill, A., Miller, M., Schwintenberg, A., et al. (2018). Onset patterns in autism: Variations across informants, methods, and timing. *Autism Research, 11*, 788–797.

Ozonoff, S., & Rogers, S. J. (2003). Autism spectrum disorders: A research review for practitioners. In S. Ozonoff, S. J. Rogers, & R. L. Hendren (Eds.), *Autism spectrum disorders: A research review for practitioners* (pp. 3–33). American Psychiatric Publishing.

Paciorkowski, A. R., Seltzer, L. E., & Neul, J. L. (2017). Developmental encephalopathies. In K. Swaiman, S. Ashwal, D. M. Ferriero, N. F. Schor, R. S. Finkel, A. L. Gropan, P. L. Pearl, & M. I. Shevell (Eds.), *Swaiman's pediatric neurology* (6th ed., pp. 242–248). Elsevier.

Pallier, G., Roberts, R. D., & Stankov, L. (2000). Biological versus psychometric intelligence: Halstead's (1947) distinction revisited. *Archives of Clinical Neuropsychology, 15*(3), 205–226.

Palomero-Gallagher, N., Vogt, B. A., Schleicher, A., Mayberg, H. S., & Zilles, K. (2009). Receptor architecture of human cingulate cortex: Evaluation of the four-region neurobiological model. *Human Brain Mapping, 30*, 2336–2355.

Papazoglou, A., King, T. Z., Morris, R. D., & Krawiecki, N. S. (2008). Cognitive predictors of adaptive functioning vary according to pediatric brain tumor location. *Developmental Neuropsychology, 33*, 505–520.

Park, H., & Lombardino, L. J. (2013). Relationships among cognitive deficits and component skills of reading in younger and older students with developmental dyslexia. *Research in Developmental Disabilities, 34*(9), 2946–2958.

Parola, A., Gabbatore, I., Bosco, F. M., Bara, B. G., Cossa, F. M., Gindri, P., & Sacco, K. (2016). Assessment of pragmatic impairment in right hemisphere damage. *Journal of Neurolinguistics, 39*, 10–25.

Parrilla, R., Kirby, J. R., & McQuarrie, L. (2004). Articular rate, naming speed, verbal short-term memory, and phonological awareness: Longitudinal predictors of early reading development? *Scientific Studies of Reading, 8*, 3–26.

Parry, P., Allison, S., & Bastiapalli, T. (2021). Pediatric bipolar disorder rates are still lower than claimed: A re-examination of eight epidemiological surveys used by an updated met analysis. *International Journal of Bipolar Disorder, 9*, https://doi.org/10.1186/s40345-021-00225-5.

Parush, S., Lifshitz, N., Yochman, A., & Weintraub, N. (2010). Relationships between handwriting components and underlying perceptual–motor functions among students during copying and dictation tasks. *Occupational Therapy Journal of Research, 30*, 39–48.

Passoulunghi, M. C., Marzocchi, G. M., & Fiorillo, F. (2005). Selective effect of inhibition of literal or numerical irrelevant information in children with attention-deficit hyperactivity disorder (ADHD) or arithmetic learning disorder. *Developmental Neuropsychology, 28*, 731–752.

Patel, S., Oishi, K., & Hillis, A. E. (2018). Right hemisphere regions critical for expression of emotion through prosody. *Frontiers in Neurology, 9*, 326904.

Pavuluri, M. N., Schenkel, L. S., Aryal, S., Harral, E. M., Hill, S. K., & Herbener, E. S. (2006). Neurocognitive function in unmedicated manic and medicated euthymic pediatric bipolar patients. *American Journal of Psychiatry, 163,* 286–293.

Pearson, J. M., Heilbronner, S. R., Barack, D. L., Hayden, B. Y., & Platt, M. L. (2011). Posterior cingulate cortex: Adapting behavior to a changing world. *Trends in Cognitive Sciences, 15*(4), 143–151.

Pedhazur, E. J. (1997). *Multiple regression in behavioral research: Explanation and prediction.* Thompson Learning.

Pelc, K., Cheron, G., & Dan. B. (2008). Behavior and neuropsychiatric manifestations in Angelman syndrome. *Neuropsychiatric Diseases and Treatment, 4,* 577–584.

Penner-Williams, J., Smith, T. E. C., & Gartin, B. (2009). Written language expression: Assessment instruments and teacher tools. *Assessment for Effective Intervention, 34,* 162–169.

Pennington, B. F. (2008). *Diagnosing learning disabilities.* Guilford Press.

Pennington, B. F., & Bishop, D. V. M. (2009). Relations among speech, language, and reading disorders. *Annual Review of Psychology, 60,* 283–306.

Pennington, B. F., Groisser, D., & Welsh, M. C. (1993). Contrasting cognitive deficits in attention deficit hyperactivity disorder versus reading disability. *Developmental Psychology, 29*(3), 511.

Pennington, B. F., McGrath, L. M., & Peterson, R. L. (2019). *Diagnosing learning disorders: From science to practice* (3rd ed.). Guilford Press.

Penny, A. M., Waschbusch, D. A., Carrey, N., & Drabman, R. S. (2005). Applying a psychoeducational perspective to ADHD. *Journal of Attention Disorders, 8,* 208–220.

Perepletchikova, F., Nathanson, D., Axelrod, S., Merrill, C., Walker, A., Grossman, M., et al. (2017). Randomized clinical trial of dialectiacal behavior therapy for pre-adolescent children with disruptive mood dysregulation disorder: Feasibility and outcomes. *Journal of the American Academy of Child and Adolescent Psychiatry, 56,* 832–840.

Peretz, I., & Zatorre, R. J. (2005). Brain organization for music processing. *Annual Review of Psychology, 56,* 89–114.

Perrin, J. M., Bloom, S. R., & Gortmaker, S. L. (2007). The increase of childhood chronic conditions in the United States. *JAMA, 297,* 2755–2759.

Petersen, S. E., Fox, P. T., Posner, M. I., Mintun, M., & Raichle, M. E. (1989). Positron emission tomographic studies of the processing of single words. *Journal of Cognitive Neuroscience, 1,* 153–170.

Peterson, R. L., Boada, R., McGrath, L. M., Willcutt, E. G., Olson, R. K., & Pennington, B. F. (2017). Cognitive prediction of reading, math, and attention: Shared and unique influences. *Journal of Learning Disabilities, 50,* 408–421.

Petrill, S., Logan, J., & Hart, S. (2012). Math fluency is etiologically distinct from untimed math performance, decoding fluency, and untimed reading performance: Evidence from a twin study. *Journal of Learning Disabilities, 45,* 371–381.

Pezzimenti, F., Han, G. T., Vasa, R. A., & Gotham, K. (2019). Depression in youth with autism spectrum disorder. *Child and Adolescent Psychiatric Clinics of North America, 28,* 397–409.

Pfeiffer, S. I., Reddy, L. A., Kletzel, J. E., Schmelzer, E. R., & Boyer, L. M. (2000). The practitioner's view of IQ testing and profile analysis. *School Psychology Quarterly, 15,* 376–385.

Pham, A., Fine, J. G., & Semrud-Clikeman, M. (2011). The influence of inattention and rapid automatized naming on reading performance. *Archives of Clinical Neuropsychology, 26,* 214–224.

Pham, A. V., & Riviere, A. (2015). Specific learning disorders and ADHD: Current issues in diagnosis across clinical and educational settings. *Current Psychiatry Reports, 38,* 38–45.

Phelps, L., Dempsey, M., Sapia, J., & Nelson, L. (2013). The efficacy of a school-based eating disorder prevention program: Building physical self-esteem and personal competencies. In N. Piran, M. Levine, & C. Steiner-Adair (Eds.), *Preventing eating disorders* (pp. 163–174). Routledge.

Piaget, J. (1965). *The child's conception of number.* Norton.

Piazza, M., Facoetti, A., Trussardi, A. N., Berteletti, I., Conte, S., Lucangeli, D., & Zorzi, M. (2010). Developmental trajectory of number acuity reveals a severe impairment in developmental dyscalculia. *Cognition, 116,* 33–41.

Pierpont, E. I., Tworog-Dube, E., & Roberts, A. E. (2013). Learning and memory in children with Noonan Syndrome. *American Journal of Medical Genetics, 161,* 2250–2257.

Pierpont, E. I., Tworog-Dube, E., & Roberts, A. E. (2015). Attention skills and executive functioning in children with Noonan syndrome and their unaffected siblings. *Developmental Medicine and Child Neurology, 57,* 385–392.

Pikulski, J. J., & Chard, D. J. (2005). Fluency: Bridge between decoding and reading comprehension. *The Reading Teacher, 58,* 510–519.

Pinel, P. J., & Edwards, M. (2007). *A colorful introduction to the anatomy of the brain.* Pearson.

Pisella, L., Havé, L., & Rossetti, Y. (2019). Body awareness disorders: Dissociations between body-related visual and somatosensory information. *Brain, 142*(8), 2170–2173.

Plante, E., Ramage, A. E., & Magloire, J. (2006). Processing narratives for verbatim and gist information by adults with language learning disabilities:

A functional neuroimaging study. *Learning Disabilities Research and Practice, 21,* 61–76.

Planton, S., Chanoine, V., Sein, J., Anton, J. L., Nazarian, B., Pallier, C., & Pattamadilok, C. (2019). Top-down activation of the visuo-orthographic system during spoken sentence processing. *Neuroimage, 202,* 116135.

Planton, S., Jucla, M., Roux, F-E., & Demonet, J.-F. (2013). The "handwriting brain": A meta-analysis of neuroimaging studies of motor vs orthographic processes. *Cortex, 49,* 2772–2787.

Plaza, M., & Cohen, H. (2007). The contribution of phonological awareness and visual attention in early reading and spelling. *Dyslexia, 13,* 67–76.

Pliszka, S. (2016). *Neuroscience for the mental health clinician* (2nd ed.). Guilford Press.

Poizner, H., & Battison, R. (2017). Cerebral asymmetry for sign language: Clinical and experimental evidence. In H. L. Lane & F. GrosJean (Eds.), *Recent perspectives on American Sign Language* (pp. 79–101). Psychology Press.

Polderman, T. J., Huizink, A. C., Verhulst, F. C., van Beijsterveldt, C. E., Boomsma, D. I., & Bartels, M. (2011). A genetic study on attention problems and academic skills: Results of a longitudinal study in twins. *Journal of the Canadian Academy of Child and Adolescent Psychiatry, 30,* 22–29.

Poldrack, R. A., Sabb, F. W., Foerde, K., Tom, S. M., Asarnow, R. F., Bookheimer, S. Y., & Knowlton, B. J. (2005). The neural correlates of motor skill automaticity. *Journal of Neuroscience, 25*(22), 5356–5364.

Pollitt, S., & Harrison, G. (2021). Does CBM maze assess reading comprehension in 8–9-year-olds at-risk for dyslexia? *Dyslexia, 27,* 265–274.

Ponsford, J., Cameron, P., Fitzgerald, M. D., Grant, M., Mikocka-Walus, A., & Schonberger, M. (2012). Predictors of postconcussive symptoms 3 months after mild traumatic brain injury. *Neuropsychology, 26,* 304–313.

Poeppel, D., Mangun, G. R., & Gazzaniga, M. S. (2020). *The cognitive neurosciences* (6th ed.). MIT Press.

Poreh, A. (2002). Neuropsychological and psychological issues associated with cross-cultural and minority assessment. In F. R. Ferraro (Ed.), *Minority and cross-cultural aspects of neuropsychological assessment* (pp. 329–343). Swets & Zeitlinger.

Poreh, A. M. (Ed.). (2012). *The quantified process approach to neuropsychological assessment*. Psychology Press.

Poretti, A., Meoded, A., Rossi, A., Raybaud, C., & Huisman, T. A. (2013). Diffusion tensor imaging and fiber tractography in brain malformations. *Pediatric Radiology, 43,* 28–54.

Porter M. A., & Coltheart, M. (2005). Cognitive heterogeneity in Williams syndrome. *Developmental Neuropsychology, 27,* 275–306.

Posner, M. I. (1994). Neglect and spatial attention. *Neuropsychological Rehabilitation, 4,* 183–187.

Posner, M. I., & Raichle, M. (1994). *Images of mind*. Scientific American Library.

Posner, M. I., Rothbart, M. K., & Voelker, P. (2016). Developing brain networks of attention. *Current Opinion in Pediatrics, 28*(6), 720.

Postal, K. S., & Armstrong, K. (2013). *Feedback that sticks: The art of effectively communicating neuropsychological assessment results*. Oxford University Press.

Potocki, A., & Laval, V. (2019). Comprehension and inference: Relationships between oral and written modalities in good and poor comprehenders during adolescence. *Journal of Speech, Language, and Hearing Research, 62,* 3431–3442.

Prabhakaran, V., Rypma, B., & Gabrieli, J. D. E. (2001). Neural substrates of mathematical reasoning: A functional magnetic resonance image study of neocortical activation during performance of the necessary arithmetic operations test. *Neuropsychology, 15,* 115–127.

Prabhakaran, V., Rypma, B., Narayanan, N. S., Meier, T. B., Austin, B. P., Nair, V. A., et al. (2011). Capacity-speed relationships in prefrontal cortex. *PLOS One, 6*(11), e27504.

Prado, J., Chadha, A., & Booth, J. R. (2011). The brain network for deductive reasoning: a quantitative meta-analysis of 28 neuroimaging studies. *Journal of Cognitive Neuroscience, 23*(11), 3483–3497.

Prayer, D., Kasprian, G., Krampl, E., Ulm, B., Witzani, L., Prayer, L., & Brugger, P. C. (2006). MRI of normal fetal brain development. *European Journal of Radiology, 57*(2), 199–216.

Preston, D., & Carter, M. (2009). A review of the efficacy of the picture exchange communication system intervention. *Journal of Autism and Developmental Disorders, 39,* 1471–1486.

Price, C. J. (2010). The anatomy of language: A review of 100 fMRI studies published in 2009. *Annals of the New York Academy of Sciences, 1191,* 62–88.

Price, C. J., & Devlin, J. T. (2011). The interactive account of ventral occipitotemporal contributions to reading. *Trends in Cognitive Sciences, 15*(6), 246–253.

Price, C. J., Wise, R. J. S., Watson, J. D. G., Patterson, K. E., Howard, D., & Frackowiak, R. S. J. (1994). Brain activity during reading: The effects of exposure duration and task. *Brain, 117,* 1255–1269.

Prifitera, A., Saklofske, D. H., & Weiss, L. G. (Eds.). (2008). *WISC-IV clinical assessment and intervention*. Elsevier.

Prins, M. L., & Giza, C. D. (2011). Repeat traumatic brain injury in the developing brain. *International Journal of Developmental Neuroscience, 30*(3), 185–190.

Pugh, K. R., Landi, N., Preston, J. L., Mencl, W. E.,

Austin, A. C., Sibley, D., et al. (2013). The relationship between phonological and auditory processing and brain organization in beginning readers. *Brain and Language, 125,* 173–183.

Pugh, K. R., Mencl, W. E., Jenner, A. R., Katz, L., Frost, S. J., Lee, J. R., et al. (2001). Neurobiological studies of reading and reading disability. *Journal of Communication Disorders, 34*(6), 479–492.

Pugh, K., Shaywitz, B., Shaywitz, S., Shakweiler, D., Katz, L., Fletcher, J., et al. (1997). Predicting reading performance through neuroimaging profiles: The cerebral basis of phonological effects in printed word identification. *Journal of Experimental Psychology: Human Perception and Performance, 23,* 299–318.

Pui, C.-H., & Evans, W. E. (2006). Treatment of acute lymphoblastic leukemia. *The New England Journal of Medicine, 354,* 166–178.

Pui, C.-H., Relling, M. V., Sandlund, J. T., Downing, J. R., Campana, D., & Evans, W. E. (2004). Rationale and design of Total Therapy Study XV for newly diagnosed childhood acute lymphoblastic leukemia (ALL). *Annals of Hematology, 83*(Suppl. 1), S124–S126.

Pui, C.-H., Sandlund, J. T., Pei, D., Campana, D., Rivera, G. K., Ribeiro, R. C., et al. (2004). Improved outcome for children with acute lymphoblastic leukemia: Results of Total Therapy Study XIIIB at St. Jude Children's Research Hospital. *Blood, 104,* 2690–2696.

Purcell, J. J., Napoliello, E. M., & Eden, G. (2011). A combined fMRI study of typed spelling and reading. *NeuroImage, 55,* 750–762.

Rabiner, D. L., & Malone, P. S. (2004). The impact of tutoring on early reading achievement for children with and without attention problems. *Journal of Abnormal Child Psychology, 32,* 273–284.

Racine, M. B., Majnemer, A., Shevell, M., & Snider, L. (2008). Handwriting performance in children with ADHD. *Journal of Child Neurology, 23,* 399–406.

Radel, R., Pelletier, L., Pjevac, D., & Cheval, B. (2017). The links between self-determined motivations and behavioral automaticity in a variety of real-life behaviors. *Motivation and Emotion, 41,* 443–454.

Rai, D., Culpin, I., Heuvelman, H., Magnusson, C. M., Carpenter, P., Jones, H. J., et al. (2018). Association of autistic traits with depression from childhood to age 18 years. *JAMA psychiatry, 75*(8), 835–843.

Rai, D., Lee, B. K., Dalman, C., Golding, J., Lewis, G., & Magnusson, C. (2013). Parental depression, maternal antidepressant use during pregnancy, and risk of autism spectrum disorders: population based case-control study. *BMJ, 346,* f2059.

Raichle, M. E., & Snyder, A. Z. (2007). A default mode of brain function: A brief history of an evolving idea. *Neuroimage, 37,* 1083–1090.

Raine, A., Park, S., Lencz, T., Bihrle, S., Lacasse, L., Widom, C. S., et al. (2001). Reduced right hemisphere activation in severely abused violent offenders during a working memory task as indicated by fMRI. *Aggressive Behavior, 27,* 111–129.

Raine, A., Yaralian, P. S., Reynolds, C., Venables, P. H., & Mednick, S. A. (2002). Spatial but not verbal cognitive deficits at age 3 years in persistently antisocial individuals. *Development and Psychopathology, 14,* 25–44.

Ramirz, G., & Beilock S. L. (2011). Writing about testing worries boosts exam performance in the classroom. *Science, 331,* 211–213.

Rammsayer, T. H., Hennig, J., Haag, A., & Lange, N. (2001). Effects of noradrenergic activation temporal information processing in humans. *Quarterly Journal of Experimental Psychology, 54B,* 247–258.

Ramos, B., Librenza-Garcia, D., Zortea, F., Watts, D., Zeni, C. P., Tramontina, S., & Passos, I. C. (2019). Clinical differences between patients with pediatric bipolar disorder with and without a parental history of bipolar disorder. *Psychiatry Research, 280,* 112501–112510.

Rapp, B., & Lipka, K. (2011). The literate brain: The relationship between spelling and reading. *Journal of Cognitive Neuroscience, 23,* 1180–1197.

Rasmussen, C., & Bisanz, J. (2005). Representation and working memory in early arithmetic. *Journal of Experimental Child Psychology, 91,* 137–157.

Rayner, K., Slattery, T. J., & Belanger, N. N. (2010). Eye movements, the perceptual span, and reading speed. *Psychonomic Bulletin and Review, 17,* 834–839.

Re, A. M., Pedron, M., & Cornoldi, C. (2007). Expressive writing difficulties in children described as exhibiting ADHD symptoms. *Journal of Learning Disabilities, 40,* 244–255.

Reber, J., & Tranel, D. (2019). Frontal lobe syndromes. In M. De Eposito & J. H. Grafman (Eds.), *The Frontal lobes* (pp. 147–164). Elsevier.

Reddy, L. A., Koziol, L. F., & Hale, J. B. (2013). Understanding neuropsychopathology in the 21st century: Current status, clinical application, and future directions. In L. A. Reddy, A. S. Weissman, & J. B. Hale (Eds.), *Neuropsychological assessment and intervention for youth: An evidence-based approach to emotional and behavioral disorders* (pp. 327–345). American Psychological Association.

Reddy, L. A., Weissman, A. S., & Hale, J. B. (2013). Neuropsychological assessment and intervention for emotion- and behavior-disordered youth: Opportunities for practice. In L. A. Reddy, A. S. Weissman, & J. B. Hale (Eds.), *Neuropsychological assessment and intervention for youth: An evidence-based approach to emotional and behavioral disorders* (pp. 3–10). American Psychological Association.

Rehabilitation Act (RA), 20 U.S.C. § 794 [statute] (1973a).

Rehabilitation Act (RA), 34 C.F.R. § 104 [regulations] (1973b).

Reilly, C., Senior, J., & Murtagh, L. (2015). A comparative study of educational provision for children with neurogenetic syndromes: Parent and teacher survey. *Journal of Intellectual Disability Research, 59*, 1094–1107.

Reitan, R. M. (1958). Validity of the Trail Making test as an indicator of organic brain damage. *Perceptual Motor Skills, 8*, 271–276.

Reitan, R. M. (1974). *Methodological problems in clinical neuropsychology.* Neuropsychology Press.

Reitan, R. M., & Wolfson, D. (1993). *The Halstead–Reitan Neuropsychological Test Battery: Theory and clinical interpretation* (2nd ed.). Neuropsychology Press.

Reynolds, C. R. (1997). Measurement and statistical problems in neuropsychological assessment of children. In C. R. Reynolds & E. Fletcher-Janzen (Eds.), *Handbook of clinical child neuropsychology* (2nd ed., pp. 180–203). Plenum Press.

Reynolds, C. R. (2010). Behavior Assessment System for Children. In I. B. Weiner & W. D. Craighead (Eds.), *The Corsini encyclopedia of psychology* (pp. 1–2). Wiley.

Reynolds, C. R. (2020). *Children's Trail Making Test–Second Edition* [CTMT–2] [Assessment instrument]. Psychological Assessment Resources.

Reynolds, C. R., & Fletcher-Janzen, E. (2009). *Handbook of clinical child neuropsychology* (3rd ed.). Springer.

Reynolds, C. R., & Kamphaus, R. W. (2003). *Reynolds Intellectual Assessment Scales (RIAS).* Psychological Assessment Resources.

Reynolds, C. R., Kamphaus, R. W., Rosenthal, B. L., & Hiemenz, J. R. (1997). Applications of the Kaufman Assessment Battery for Children (K-ABC) in neuropsychological assessment. In C. R. Reynolds & E. Fletcher-Janzen (Eds.), *Handbook of clinical child neuropsychology* (2nd ed., pp. 252–269). Plenum Press.

Reynolds, C. R., Kamphaus, R. W., & Vannest, K. J. (2015). *BASC3: Behavior Assessment System for Children.* PsychCorp.

Reynolds, C. R., & Mason, B. A. (2009). Measurement and statistical problems in neuropsychological assessment of children. In C. R. Reynolds & E. Fletcher-Janzen (Eds.), *Handbook of clinical child neuropsychology* (3rd ed., pp. 203–230). Springer Science + Business Media.

Reynolds, C. R., & Shaywitz, S. E. (2009). Response to Intervention: Ready or not? Or, from wait-to-fail to watch-them-fail. *School Psychology Quarterly, 24*(2), 130.

Reynolds, C. R., & Voress, J. K. (2007). *Test of Memory and Learning: Second edition.* PRO-ED.

Reynolds, C. R., & Voress, J. K. (2009). Clinical neuropsychological assessment with the Test of Memory and Learning. In C. R. Reynolds & E. Fletcher-Janzen (Eds.), *Handbook of clinical child neuropsychology* (3rd ed., pp. 297–319). Springer Science + Business Media.

Reynolds, M. R., Keith, T. Z., Fine, J. G., Fisher, M. E., & Low, J. A. (2007). Confirmatory factor structure of the Kaufman Assessment Battery for Children: Consistency with Cattell–Horn–Carroll theory. *School Psychology Quarterly, 22*(4), 511.

Riccio, C. A., Cash, D. L., & Cohen, M. J. (2007). Learning and memory performance of children with specific language impairment (SLI). *Applied Neuropsychology, 14*(4), 255–261.

Riccio, C. A., & Reynolds, C. R. (2013). Principles of neuropsychological assessment in children and adolescents. In D. H. Saklofske, C. R. Reynolds, & V. L. Schwean (Eds.), *The Oxford handbook of child psychological assessment* (pp. 286–330). Oxford University Press.

Riccio, C. A., Sullivan, J. R., & Cohen, M. J. (2010). *Neuropsychological assessment and intervention for childhood and adolescent disorders.* Wiley.

Rich, B. A., Carver, F. W., Holroyd, T., Rosen, H. R., Mendoza, J. K., Cornwell, B. R., et al. (2011). Different neural pathways to negative affect in youth with pediatric bipolar disorder and severe mood dysregulation. *Journal of Psychiatric Research, 45*, 1283–1294.

Richards, T. L., Aylward, E. H., Field, K. M., Grimme, A. C., Raskind, W., Richards, A. L., et al. (2006). Converging evidence for triple word form theory in children with dyslexia. *Developmental Neuropsychology, 30*, 547–589.

Richards, T. L., & Berninger, V. W. (2008). Abnormal fMRI connectivity in children with dyslexia during a phoneme task: Before but not after treatment. *Journal of Neurolinguistics, 21*(4), 294–304.

Richards, T. L., Berninger, V. W., Stock, P., Altemeier, L., Trivedi, P., & Maravilla, K. (2009). Functional magnetic resonance imaging sequential-finger movement activation differentiating good and poor writers. *Journal of Clinical and Experimental Neuropsychology, 31*(8), 967–983.

Richards, T. L., Berninger, V. W., Stock, P., Altemeier, L., Trivedi, P., & Maravilla, K. R. (2011). Differences between good and poor child writers on fMRI contrasts for writing newly taught and highly practiced letter forms. *Reading and Writing, 24*, 493–516.

Richlan, F., Kronbichler, M., & Wimmer, H. (2011). Meta-analyzing brain dysfunctions in dyslexic children and adults. *NeuroImage, 56*, 1735–1742.

Riddick, B. (2000). An examination of the relationship between labeling and stigmatization with special reference to dyslexia. *Disability and Society, 15*, 653–667.

Riegler, L. J., Neils-Strunjas, J., Boyce, S., Wade, S. L., & Scheifele, P. M. (2013). Cognitive intervention results in web-based videophone treatment adherence and improved cognitive scores. *Medical Science Monitor: International Medical Journal of Experimental and Clinical Research, 19*, 269.

Riley, C., DuPaul, G., Pipan, M., Kern, L., Van Brakle, J., & Blum, N. (2008). Combined Type Versus ADHD Predominantly Hyperactive-Impulsive Type: Is There a Difference in Functional Impairment? *Journal of Developmental and Behavioral Pediatrics, 29*, 270–275.

Rinaldi, C., & Samson, J. (2008). English language learners and response to intervention referral considerations. *Teaching Exceptional Children, 40*(5), 6–14.

Ripamonti, E., Aggujaro, S., Molteni, F., Zonca, G., Frustaci, M., & Luzzatti, C. (2014). The anatomical foundations of acquired reading disorders: A neuropsychological verification of the dual-route model of reading. *Brain and Language, 134*, 44–67.

Ris, M. D., Dietrich, K. N., Succop, P. A., Berger, O. G., & Bornschein, R. L. (2004). Early exposure to lead and neuropsychological outcome in adolescence. *Journal of the International Neuropsychological Society, 10*, 261–270.

Ritchey, K. D., & Coker Jr, D. L. (2013). An investigation of the validity and utility of two curriculum-based measurement writing tasks. *Reading & Writing Quarterly, 29*(1), 89–119.

Riva, D., Avanzini, G., Franceschetti, S., Nichelli, F., Saletti, V., Vago, C., & Pantaleoni, C. (2005). Unilateral frontal lobe epilepsy affects executive functioning in children. *Neurological Sciences, 26*, 263–270.

Riva-Posse, P., Holtzheimer, P. E., & Mayberg, H. S. (2019). Cingulate medicated dpressive symptoms in neurologica disease and therapeutics. *Handbook of Clinical Neurology, 166*, 371–379.

Roberts, B. W., & DelVecchio, W. E. (2000). The rank-order consistency of personality traits from childhood to old age: A quantitative review of longitudinal studies. *Psychological Bulletin, 126*, 3–25.

Robinson, R. G., Kubos, K. L., Starr, L. B., Rao, K., & Price, T. R. (1984). Mood disorders in stroke patients. Importance of location of lesion. *Brain, 107*, 81–93.

Roid, C. H. (2006). *Linking SB5 to instruction and intervention for children ages 2–16* (SB5 Technical Note #01-2006). Riverside.

Roid, G. (2003). *Stanford–Binet Intelligence Scale: Fifth Edition*. Riverside.

Roid, G. H., & Barram, R. A. (2004). *Essentials of Stanford–Binet Intelligence Scales (SB5) assessment*. Wiley.

Roid, G., Nellis, L., & McLellan, M. (2003). Assessment with the Leiter International Performance Scale—Revised and the S-BIT. In R. S. McCallum (Ed.), *Handbook of nonverbal assessment* (pp. 113–140). Kluwer Academic/Plenum.

Roid, G. H., Pomplun, M., & Martin, J. J. (2009). Nonverbal intellectual and cognitive assessment with the Leiter International Performance Scale—Revised (Leiter-R). In J. A. Naglieri & S. Goldstein (Eds.), *Practitioner's guide to assessing intelligence and achievement* (pp. 265–290). Wiley.

Rolls, E. T. (2015). Limbic systems for emotion and for memory, but no single limbic system. *Cortex, 62*, 119–157.

Rolls, E. T. (2019). *The orbitofrontal cortex*. Oxford University Press.

Romeo, R. R., Segaran, J., Leonard, J. A., Robinson, S. T., West, M. R., Mackey, A. P., et al. (2018). Language exposure relates to structural neural connectivity in childhood. *Journal of Neuroscience, 38*(36), 7870–7877.

Rommelse, N., Visser, J., & Hartman, C. (2018). Differentiating between ADHD and ASD in childhood: Some directions for practitioners. *European Child and Adolescent Psychiatry, 27*, 679–681.

Rosenberg-Lee, M., Barth, M., & Menon, V. (2011). What difference does a year of schooling make?: Maturation of brain response and connectivity between 2nd and 3rd grades during arithmetic problem solving. *Neuroimage, 57*(3), 796–808.

Rosenberg-Lee, M., Chang, T. T., Young, C. B., Wu, S., & Menon, V. (2011). Functional dissociations between four basic arithmetic operations in the human posterior parietal cortex: A cytoarchitectonic mapping study. *Neuropsychologia, 49*, 2592–2608.

Rosenthal, R., & Jacobson, L. (1968). *Pygmalion in the classroom*. Holt, Rinehart & Winston.

Rosqvist, H., Chown, N., & Stenning, A. (2020). *Neurodiversity studies: A new critical paradigm*. Routledge.

Ross, L., Johansen, C., Dalton, S. O., Mellemkjaer, L., Thomassen, L. H., Mortensen, P. B., et al. (2003). Psychiatric hospitalizations among survivors of cancer in childhood or adolescence. *The New England Journal of Medicine, 349*, 650–657.

Ross, S. A., Allen, D. N., & Goldstein, G. (2013). Factor structure of the Halstead–Reitan Neuropsychological Battery: A review and integration. *Applied Neuropsychology: Adult, 20*(2), 120–135.

Rossi, A. S. U., de Moura, L. M., de Mello, C. B., de Souza, A. A. L., Muszkat, M., & Bueno, O. F. A. (2015). Attentional profiles and white matter correlates in attention deficit/hyperactivity disorder predominantly inattentive type. *Frontiers of Psychiatry, 6*, 122.

Rossignoli-Palomeque, T., Perez-Hernandez, E., & Gonzalez-Marques, J. (2018). Brain training in children and adolescents: Is it scientifically valid? *Frontiers in Psychology*, 565.

Rotzer, S., Kucian, K., Martin, E., Von Aster, M., Klaver, P., & Loenneker, T. (2008). Optimized voxel-based morphometry in children with developmental dyscalculia. *NeuroImage, 39,* 417–422.

Rourke, B. P. (1994). Neuropsychological assessment of children with learning disabilities: Measurement issues. In G. R. Lyon (Ed.), *Frames of reference for the assessment of learning disabilities: New views on measurement issues* (pp. 475–514). Brookes.

Rourke, B. P. (2000). Neuropsychological and psychosocial subtyping: A review of investigations within the University of Windsor laboratory. *Canadian Psychology, 41,* 34–51.

Rourke, B. P., Ahmad, S. A., Collins, D. W., Hayman-Abello, B. A., & Warriner, E. M. (2002). Child clinical/pediatric neuropsychology: Some recent advances. *Review of Psychology, 53,* 309–339.

Rousselle, L., & Noel, M. P. (2007). Basic numerical skills in children with mathematics learning disabilities: A comparison of symbolic vs. non-symbolic number magnitude processing. *Cognition, 102,* 361–395.

Roux, F. E., Boetto, S., Sacko, O., Chollet, F., & Trémoulet, M. (2003). Writing, calculating, and finger recognition in the region of the angular gyrus: a cortical stimulation study of Gerstmann syndrome. *Journal of Neurosurgery, 99*(4), 716–727.

Ruan, J., Bludau, S., Palomero-Gallagher, N., Caspers, S., Mohlberg, H., Eickhoff, S. B., et al. (2018). Cytoarchitecture, probability maps, and functions of the human supplementary and pre-supplementary motor areas. *Brain Structure and Function, 223,* 4169–4186.

Rubia, K., Criaud, M., Wulff, M., Alegria, A., Brinson, H., Barker, G., et al. (2019). Functional connectivity changes associated with fMRI neurofeedback of right inferior frontal cortex in adolescent with ADHD. *Neurofeedback, 188,* 43–58.

Rubia, K., Halari, B., Cubillo, A., Mohammad, A. M., & Taylor, E. (2009). Methylphenidate normalises activation and functional connectivity deficits in attention and motivation networks in medication-naïve children with ADHD during a rewarded continuous performance task. *Neuropharmacology, 57,* 640–652.

Rubia, K., Halari, R., Smith, A. B., Mohammad, M., Scott, S., V., Giampietro., & Brammer, M. J. (2008). Dissociated functional brain abnormalities of inhibition in boys with pure conduct disorder and in boys with pure attention deficit hyperactivity disorder. *American Journal of Psychiatry, 165,* 889–897.

Rubia, K., Overmeyer, S., Taylor, E., Brammer, M., Williams, S. C., Simmons, A., & Bullmore, E. T. (1999). Hypofrontality in attention deficit hyperactivity disorder during higher-order motor control: a study with functional MRI. *American Journal of Psychiatry, 156*(6), 891–896.

Rubia, K., Overmeyer, S., Taylor, E., Brammer, M., Williams, S. C. R., Simmons, A., et al. (2000). Functional frontalisation with age: Mapping neurodevelopmental trajectories with fMRI. *Neuroscience & Biobehavioral Reviews, 24*(1), 13–19.

Rubia, K., Smith, A. B., Brammer, M. J., Toone, B., & Taylor, E. (2005). Abnormal brain activation during inhibition and error detection in medication-naive adolescents with ADHD. *American Journal of Psychiatry, 162,* 1067–1075.

Rubia, K., Smith, A. B., Mohammad, M., Taylor, E., & Brammer, M. E. (2009). Disorder-specific dissociation of orbitofrontal dysfunction in boys with pure conduct disorder during reward and ventrolateral prefrontal dysfunction in boys with pure attention-deficit/hyperactivity disorder during sustained attention. *American Journal of Psychiatry, 166,* 83–94.

Rubenstein, K., Matsushita, M., Berninger, V. W., Raskind, W., & Wijsman, E. (2011). Genome scan for spelling deficits: Effects of verbal IQ on models of transmission and trait gene localization. *Behavioral Genetics, 41,* 31–42.

Rubinsten, O., & Henik, A. (2006). Double dissociation of functions in developmental dyslexia and dyscalculia. *Journal of Educational Psychology, 98,* 854–867.

Ruffino, M., Trussardi, A. N., Gori, S., Finzi, A., Giovagnoli, S., Menghini, D., et al. (2010). Attentional engagement deficits in dyslexic children. *Neuropsychologia, 48,* 3793–3801.

Rushton, S., Juola-Rushton, A., & Larkin, E. (2010). Neuroscience, play and early childhood education: Connections, implications and assessment. *Early Childhood Education Journal, 37,* 351–361.

Russell, E. W., Russell, S. L., & Hill, B. D. (2005). The fundamental psychometric status of neuropsychological batteries. *Archives of Clinical Neuropsychology, 20*(6), 785–794.

Rykhlevskaia, E., Uddin, L. Q., Kondos, L., & Menon, V. (2009). Neuroanatomical correlates of developmental dyscalculia: Combined evidence from morphometry and tractography. *Frontiers in Human Neuroscience, 3,* 51.

Sackheim, H. A., Decina, P., & Malitz, S. (1982). Functional brain asymmetry and affective disorders. *Adolescent Psychiatry, 10,* 320–335.

Sady, M. D., Vaughan, C., & Gioia, G. A. (2011). School and the concussed youth: Recommendations for concussion education and management. *Physical Medical and Rehabilitation Clinics of North America, 22,* 701–719.

Salas, N. (2020). Nonphonological strategies in spelling development. *Frontiers in Psychology, 11,* https://doi.org/10.3389/fpsyg.2020.01071.

Saling, L. L., & Phillips, J. G. (2007). Automatic behaviour: Efficient not mindless. *Brain research bulletin, 73*(1–3), 1–20.

Sammler, D., Koelsch, S., & Friederici, A. D. (2011). Are left fronto-temporal brain areas a prerequisite for normal music-syntactic processing? *Cortex, 47*(6), 659–673.

Sanders, J. E., Im, H. J., Hoffmeister, P. A., Gooley, T. A., Woolfrey, A. E., Carpenter, P. A., et al. (2005). Allogeneic hematopoietic cell transplantation for infants with acute lymphoblastic leukemia. *Blood, 105,* 3749–3756.

Santoro, L. E., Chard, D. J., Howard, L., & Baker, S. K. (2008). Making the very most of classroom read-alouds to promote comprehension and vocabulary. *The Reading Teacher, 61,* 396–408.

Saricoban, H. E., Ozen, A., Harmanci, K., Razi, C., Zahmacioglu, O., & Cengizlier, M. R. (2011). Common behavioral problems among children with asthma: Is there a role of asthma treatment. *Annals of Allergy, Asthma, & Immunology, 106,* 200–204.

Sattler, J. (2008). *Assessment of children: Cognitive foundations* (5th ed.). Author.

Sattler, J. (2014). *Foundations of behavioral, social and clinical assessment of children* (6th ed.). Author.

Sattler, J. (2018). *Assessment of children.* Author.

Sattler, J. M. (2024). *Assessment of children: Cognitive foundations and applications* (7th ed.). Author.

Sattler, J. M., & Hoge, R. D. (2005). *Assessment of children: Behavioral, social, and clinical foundations* (5th ed.). Jerome M. Sattler.

Saygin, Z. M., Norton, E. S., Osher, D. E., Beach, S. D., Cyr, A. B., Ozernov-Palchik, O., et al. (2013). Tracking the roots of reading ability: White matter volume and integrity correlate with phonological awareness in prereading and early-reading kindergarten children. *Journal of Neuroscience, 33*(33), 13251–13258.

Scarborough, H. S. (2009). Connecting early language and literacy to later reading (dis)abilities: Evidence, theory, and practice. In S. B. Neuman & D. K. Dickinson (Eds.), *Handbook of early literacy research* (2nd ed., pp. 97–110). Guilford Press.

Schalock, R. L., Luckasson, R., & Tassé, M. J. (2021). *Intellectual disability: Definition, diagnosis, classification, and systems of supports* (12th ed.). AAIDD.

Scheeren, A., deRosnay, M., Koot, H. M., & Begeer, S. (2013). Rethinking theory of mind in high-functioning autism spectrum disorder. *Journal of Child Psychology and Psychiatry, 54,* 628–635.

Scheuermann, B., & Hall, J. A. (2008). *Positive behavioral supports for the classroom.* Pearson/Merrill Prentice Hall.

Scheuermann, B., Hall, J., & Billingsly, G. (2021). *Positive behavioral supports for the classroom* (4th ed.). Pearson.

Schiff, R., Ben-shushan, Y., & Ben-Artzi, E. (2017). Metacognitive strategies: A foundation for early word spelling and reading in kindergartners with SLI. *Journal of Learning Disabilities, 50,* 143–157.

Schlaggar, B. L., & McCandliss, B. (2007). Development of neural systems for reading. *Annual Review of Neuroscience, 30,* 475–503.

Schmacher, J., Hoffmann, P., Schmal, C., Schulte-Körne, G., & Nothen, M. M. (2007). Genetics of dyslexia: The evolving landscape. *Journal of Medical Genetics, 44,* 289–297.

Schneider, A. N., Parker, D. J., Crevier-Quintin, E., Kubas, H. A., & Hale, J. B. (2013). *Luria and learning: How neuropsychological theory translates into educational practice.* In B. J. Irby, G. Brown, R. Lara-Alecio, & S. Jackson (Eds.), *The handbook of educational theories* (pp. 751–759). IAP Information Age Publishing.

Schneider, W. J., Lichtenberger, E. O., Mather, N., & Kaufman, N. L. (2018). *Essentials of report writing* (2nd ed.). Wiley.

Schoemaker, M. M., Ketelaars, C. E. J., von Zonneveld, M., Mideraa, R. B., & Mulder, T. (2005). Deficits in motor control processes involved in the production of graphic movements of children with attention-deficit-hyperactivity-disorder. *Developmental Medicine & Child Neurology, 47,* 390–395.

Schonfeld, A. M., Paley, B., Frankel, F., & O'Conner, M. J. (2006). Executive functioning predicts social skills following prenatal alcohol exposure. *Child Neuropsychology, 12,* 439–452.

Schrank, F. A., McGrew, K. S., & Mather, N. (2014). *Woodcock–Johnson IV.* Riverside.

Schrappe, M., Reiter, A., Ludwig, W. D., Harbott, J., Zimmermann, M., Hiddemann, W., et al. (2000). Improved outcome in childhood acute lymphoblastic leukemia despite reduced use of anthracyclines and cranial radiotherapy: Results of trials ALL-BFM 90. *Blood, 95,* 3310–3322.

Schrieff, L., Donald, K., & Thomas, K. (2011). Cognitive and behavioural outcomes after traumatic brain injury in children. *Continuing Medical Education, 29,* 160–161.

Schubotz, R. I., & von Cramon, D. Y. (2001). Functional organization of the lateral premotor cortex: fMRI reveals different regions activated by anticipation of object properties, location and speed. *Cognitive Brain Research, 11,* 97–112.

Schulte-Körne, G., Ziegler, W., Deimel, W., Schumacher, E., Plume, C., Bachmann, A., et al. (2007). Interrelationship and familiality of dyslexia related quantitative measures. *Annals of Human Genetics, 71,* 160–175.

Schultz, R. T., Gauthier, I., Klin, A., Fulbright, R. K., Anderson, A. W., Volkmar, F., et al. (2000). Abnormal ventral temporal cortical activity during face discrimination among individuals with Autism and Asperger Syndrome. *Archives of General Psychiatry, 57,* 311–340.

Schwartz, D. L., Lin, X., Brophy, S., & Bransford, J. D. (2013). Toward the development of flexibly adaptive instructional designs. In C. M. Reigeluth (Ed.), *Instructional-design theories and models* (pp. 183–213). Erlbaum.

Schwartz, S., & Baldo, J. (2001). Distinct patterns of word retrieval in right and left frontal lobe patients: A multidimensional perspective. *Neuropsychologia, 39,* 1209–1217.

Schwartze, M., & Kotz, S. A. (2016). Contributions of cerebellar event-based temporal processing and preparatory function to speech perception. *Brain and Language, 161,* 28–32.

Sciberras, E., Efron, D., Patel, P., Mulraney, M., Lee, K. J., Mihalopoulos, C., et al. (2019). Does the treatment of anxiety in children with Attention-Deficit/Hyperactivity Disorder (ADHD) using cognitive behavior therapy improve child and family outcomes1 Protocol for a randomized controlled trial. *BMC Psychiatry, 19,* 359–368.

Scott, C. M. (2020). Language sample analysis of writing in children and adolescents: Assessment and intervention contributions. *Topics in Language Disorders 40,* 202–220.

Scott, J. G., & Schoenberg, M. R. (2011). Affect, emotions and mood. In M. R. Schoenberg & J. G. Scott (Eds.), *The little black book of neuropsychology: A syndrome-based approach* (pp. 249–265). Springer Science+ Business Media.

Sedky, K., Bennett, D., &Carvalho, K. (2013). The relationship between attention deficit hyperactivity disorder and sleep disordered breathing in pediatric populations: A meta-analysis. *Sleep, 36,* A310.

Segal, E., & Petrides, M. (2013). Functional activation during reading in relation to the sulci of the angular gyrus region. *European Journal of Neuroscience, 38,* 2793–2801.

Seghier, M. L., & Price, C. J. (2013). Dissociating frontal regions that co-lateralize with different ventral occipitotemporal regions during word processing. *Brain and Language, 126*(2), 133–140.

Selenius, E. N., Molero, Y., Lichenstein, P., Larson, T., Lundstrom, S., Ankarsater, H., & Gumpert, C. H. (2015). Childhood symptoms of ADHD overrule comorbidity in relation to psychosocial outcome at age 15: A longitudinal study. *PLOS ONE, 10,* e0137475.

Semrud-Clikeman, M. (2001). *Traumatic brain injury in children and adolescents.* Guilford Press.

Semrud-Clikeman, M. (2005). Neuropsychological aspects for evaluating LD. *Journal of Learning Disabilities, 38,* 563–568.

Semrud-Clikeman, M. (2007). *Social competence in children.* Springer.

Semrud-Clikeman, M. (2012). The role of inattention on academics, fluid reasoning, and visual-spatial functioning in two subtypes of ADHD. *Applied Neuropsychology: Child, 1,* 18–29.

Semrud-Clikeman, M. (2021). Understanding the development of the central nervous system and its relationship to clinical practice. In R. C. D'Amato, A. S. Davis, E. M. Power, & E. C. Eusebio (Eds.) *Understanding our biological basis of behavior: Developing evidence-based interventions for clinical, counseling and school psychologists* (pp. 31–52). Springer Nature.

Semrud-Clikeman, M., Bledsoe, J., & Vroman, L. (2013). System and family support. In C. A. Noggle, R. S. Dean, & M. T. Barisa (Eds.), *Neuropsychological rehabilitation* (pp. 257–273). Springer.

Semrud-Clikeman, M., Bledsoe, J., & Vroman, L. (in press). Medical, school, and family systems in neurorehabilitation. In C. A. Noggle & R. Ball (Eds.), *Contemporary neuropsychology.* Springer.

Semrud-Clikeman, M., & Ellison, P. A. (2009). *Child neuropsychology: assessment and interventions for neurodevelopmental disorders.* Springer Science Business Media, LLC.

Semrud-Clikeman, M., Fine, J. G., Bledsoe, J., & Zhu, D. C. (2012). Gender differences in brain activation on a mental rotation task. *International Journal of Neuroscience, 122*(10), 590–597.

Semrud-Clikeman, M., Fine, J. G., Bledsoe, J., & Zhu, D. C. (2013). Volumetric differences among children with Asperger Disorder, nonverbal learning disabilities, and controls on MRI. *Journal of Clinical and Experimental Neuropsychology, 5,* 540–550.

Semrud-Clikeman, M., & Glass, K. (2010). The relation of humor and child development: Social, adaptive, and emotional aspects. *Journal of Child Neurology, 25*(10), 1248–1260.

Semrud-Clikeman, M., Guy, K., Griffin, J. D., & Hynd, G. W. (2000). Rapid naming deficits in children and adolescents with reading disabilities and attention deficit hyperactivity disorder. *Brain and Language, 74,* 70–83.

Semrud-Clikeman, M., & Harder, L. (2011). The relation between executive functions and written expression in college students with ADHD. *Journal of Attention Disorders, 15,* 215–223.

Semrud-Clikeman, M., LaFavor, T., & Gross, A. C. (2017). Evidence-based interventions for traumatic brain injury (TBI) and concussions in children and adolescents. In L. Theodore (Ed.), *Handbook of applied interventions for children and adolescents* (pp. 483–494). Springer.

Semrud-Clikeman, M., Pliszka, S. R., Lancaster, J., & Liotti, M. (2006). Volumetric MRI differences in treatment-naïve vs chronically treated children with ADHD. *Neurology, 67,* 1023–1027.

Semrud-Clikeman, M., Steingard, R. J., Filipek,

P., Biederman, J., Bekken, K., & Renshaw, P. F. (2000). Using MRI to examine brain–behavior relationships in males with attention deficit disorder with hyperactivity. *Journal of the American Academy of Child and Adolescent Psychiatry, 39*, 477–484.

Semrud-Clikeman, M., & Teeter Ellison, P. A. (2009). *Child neuropsychology: Assessment and interventions for neurodevelopmental disorders* (2nd ed.). Springer.

Semrud-Clikeman, M., & Trauner, D. (2017). Nonverbal learning disability and associated disorders. In K. Swaiman, S. Ashwayl, D. M. Ferriero, N. F. Schor, R. S. Finkel, A. L. Gropan, P. L. Pearl, & M. I. Shevell (Eds.), *Swaiman's pediatric neurology* (6th ed., pp. 437–441). Elsevier.

Semrud-Clikeman, M., Walkowiak, J., Wilkinson, A., & Butcher, B. (2010). Differences on direct and indirect executive function measures among children with Asperger's Syndrome, ADHD: combined type, ADHD: predominately inattentive type, and controls. *Journal of Autism and Developmental Disorders, 40*, 1017–1027.

Semrud-Clikeman, M., Walkowiak, J., Wilkinson, A., & Christopher, G. (2010). Neuropsychological findings in nonverbal learning disabilities. *Developmental Neuropsychology, 35*, 582–600.

Semrud-Clikeman, M., Walkowiak, J., Wilkinson, A., & Minne, E. (2010). Behavior and social perception in children with Asperger's Disorder, nonverbal learning disability, or ADHD. *Journal of Abnormal Child Psychology, 38*, 509–519.

Sen, H. S. (2009). The relationship between the use of metacognitive strategies and reading comprehension. *Procedia Social and Behavioral Sciences, 1*, 2301–2305.

Sencibaugh, J. M. (2007). Meta-analysis of reading comprehension interventions for students with learning disabilities: Strategies and implications. *Reading Improvement, 44*(1), 6–22.

Serdaroglu, E., Konuskan, B., Oguz, K. K., Gurler, G., Yalnizoglu, D., & Anlar, B. (2019). Epilepsy in neurofibromatosis type 1: Diffuse cerebral dysfunction? *Epilepsy & Behavior, 98*, 6–9.

Sergeant, J. A. (2005). Modeling attention-deficit/hyperactivity disorder: a critical appraisal of the cognitive-energetic model. *Biological Psychiatry, 57*(11), 1248–1255.

Sergent, J., Zuck, E., Terriah, S., & MacDonald, B. (1992). Distributed neural network underlying musical sight-reading and keyboard performance. *Science, 257*, 106–109.

Sesma, H. W., Mahone, E. M., Levine, T. M., Eason, S. H., & Cutting, L. E. (2009). The contribution of executive skills to reading comprehension. *Child Neuropsychology, 15*, 232–246.

Sethi, A., Aber, J. L., Shoda, Y., Rodriguez, M. L. &

Mischel, W. (2000). The role of strategic attention deployment in development of self-regulation: Predicting preschooler's delay of gratification from mother–toddler interactions. *Developmental Psychology, 36*, 767–777.

Sethi, A., Gregory, S., Dell'Acqua, F., Thomas, E. P., Simmons, A, Murphy, D. G. M., Hodgins, S., Blackwood, N. J., & Craig, M. C. (2015). Emotional detachment in psychopathy: Involvement of the dorsal default-mode connections. *Cortex, 62*, 11–19.

Sevadjian, C., Canas, A., Fournier, A., Miller, D., & Maricle, D. (2011, September). Multivariate analyses of variance between a mixed clinical sample of children ages 8–19 and a comparable age group from the standardization sample of the Delis–Kaplan Executive Function System (D-KEFS). *Archives of Clinical Neuropsychology, 26*(6), 532.

Seymour, K. E., & Miller, L. (2017). ADHD and depression: The role of poor frustration tolerance. *Current Developments in Disorders Report, 4*, 14–18.

Shaffer, D., Schonfeld, L. O'Conner, P. A., Stokman, C., Trautman, P., Shafer, S., et al. (1985). Neurological soft signs. *Archives of General Psychology, 42*, 342–351.

Shalev, N., Stelle, A., Nobre, A. C., Karmiloff-Smith, A., Cornish, & Scerif, G. (2019). Dynamic sustained attention markers differentiate atypical development: The case of Williams syndrome and Down's syndrome. *Neuropsychologia, 132*, 07148.

Shalev, R. S. (2004). Developmental Dyslcalculia. *Journal of Child Neurology, 19*, 765–771.

Shallice, T. (1982). Specific impairment in planning. *Philosophical Transactions of the Royal Society of London, 298*, 199–209.

Shapiro, E., Jones, S. A., & Esolar, M. L. (2017). Developmental and behavioral aspects of mucopolysaccharidoses with brain manifestations—Neurological signs and symptoms. *Molecular Genetics and Metabolism, 122*, 1–7.

Shapiro, E., King, K., Ahmed, A., Rudser, K., Rumsey, R., Yund, B., et al. (2016). The neurobehavioral phenotype in mucopolysaccharidosis type IIIB: An exploratory study. *Molecular Genetics and Metabolism, 6*, 41–47.

Shaw, S. R., Glaser, S. E., & Ouimet, T. (2010). Developing the medical liaison role in school settings. *Journal of Educational and Psychological Consultation, 2*, 106–117.

Shaywitz, S. E. (2003). *Overcoming dyslexia: A new and complete science-based program for reading problems at any level.* Alfred A. Knopf.

Shaywitz, S. E., Mody, M., & Shaywitz, B. A. (2006). Neural mechanisms in dyslexia. *Current Directions in Psychological Science, 15*(6), 278–281.

Shaywitz, S. E., & Shaywitz, B. A. (2016). Reading disability and the brain. In M. Scherer (Ed.), *On developing readers: Readings from educational leadership* (pp. 146–151). ASCD.

Shaywitz, B. A., Shaywitz, S. E., Blachman, B. A., Pugh, K. R., Fulbright, R. K., Skudlarski, P., et al. (2004). Development of left occipitotemporal systems for skilled reading in children after a phonologically-based intervention. *Biological Psychiatry, 55*, 926–933.

Shaywitz, S. E., Shaywitz, B. A., Fulbright, R. K., Skudlarski, P., Mencl, W. E., Constable, R. T., et al. (2003). Neural systems for compensation and persistence: Young adult outcome of childhood reading disability. *Biological Psychiatry, 54*, 25–33.

Shenal, B. V., Harrison, D. W., & Demaree, H. A. (2003). The neuropsychology of depression: A literature review and preliminary model. *Neuropsychology Review, 13*, 33–42.

Shenhav, A., Cohen, J. D., & Botvinick, M. M. (2016). Dorsal anterior cingulate cortex and the value of control. *Nature Neuroscience, 19*(10), 1286–1291.

Shephard, E., Tye, C., Ashwood, K. L., Azadi, B., Asherson, P., Bolton, P. F., & McLoughlin, G. (2017). Resting state neurophysiology patterns in children with ADHD, ASD, and ADHD+ASD. *Journal of Autism and Developmental Disorders, 48*, 110–128.

Sheridan, S. M., Kratochwill, T. R., & Bergan, J. R. (2013). *Conjoint behavioral consultation: A procedural manual*. Springer Science + Business Media.

Shilyansky, C., Karlsgodt, K. H., Cummings, D. M., Sidiropoulou, K., Hardt, M., James, A. S., et al. (2010). Neurofibomin regulates corticostriatal inhibitory networks during working memory performance. *Proceedings of the National Academy of Science USA, 107*, 13141–13146.

Shimamura, A. P. (2000). The role of the prefrontal cortex in dynamic filtering. *Psychobiology, 28*, 207–218.

Shinn, M., Brown-Chidsey, R., & Andren, K. J. (2013). Identifying and validating academic problems in a multi-tiered system of services and supports model in a time of shifting paradigms. In R. Brown-Chidsey (Ed.), *Assessment for intervention: A problem-solving approach* (pp. 199–228). Guilford Press.

Shinn, M. M., & Shinn, M. R. (2002). *AIMSweb training workbook: Administration and scoring of reading curriculum-based measurement (R-CBM) for use in general outcome measurement*. Edformation.

Shinn, M., & Yoshikawa, H. (Eds.). (2008). *Toward positive youth development: Transforming schools and community programs*. Oxford University Press.

Siegal, M., & Blades, M. (2003). Language and auditory processing in autism. *Trends in cognitive sciences, 7*(9), 378–380.

Siegel, L. S., & Mazabel, S. (2014). Basic cognitive

processes and reading disabilities. In H. L. Swanson, K. R. Harris, & S. Graham (Eds.), *Handbook of learning disabilities* (2nd ed., pp. 186–213). Guilford Press.

Sihvonen, A. J., Teppo Särkämö, T., Rodríguez-Fornells A., Ripollés P., Münte, T. F., & Soinila, S. (2019). Neural architectures of music—Insights from acquired amusia. *Neuroscience & Biobehavioral Reviews, 107*, 104–114.

Silani, G., Frith, U., Demonet, J-F., Fazio, F., Perani, D., Price, C., & Paulescu, E. (2005). Brain abnormalities underlying altered activation in dyslexia: A voxel based morphometry study. *Brain, 128*, 2453–2461.

Sillanpaa, M., Haataja, L., & Shinnar, S. (2004). Perceived impact of childhood-onset epilepsy on quality of life as an adult. *Epilepsia, 45*, 971–977.

Silver, L. B. (1990). Attention deficit-hyperactivity disorder: is it a learning disability or a related disorder? *Journal of Learning Disabilities, 23*(7), 394–397.

Silverberg, N. D., & Millis, S. R. (2009). Impairment versus deficiency in neuropsychological assessment: Implications for ecological validity. *Journal of the International Neuropsychological Society, 15*(1), 94–102.

Simos, P. G., Fletcher, J. M., Sarkari, S., Billingsley, R. L., Denton, C., & Papanicolaou, A. C. (2007). Altering the brain circuits for reading through intervention: A magnetic source imaging study. *Neuropsychology, 21*, 485–496.

Sijtsema, J. J., & Ojanen, T. J. (2018). Social networks and aggression. In T. Malti & K. H. Rubin (Eds.), *Handbook of child and adolescent aggression* (pp. 230–248). Guilford Press.

Sipal, R. F., Schuengel, C., Voorman, J. M., Van Eck, M., & Becher, J. G. (2009). Course of behavioural problems of children with cerebral palsy: The role of parental stress and support. *Child: Care, Health, and Development, 36*, 74–84.

Skirbekk, B., Hansen, B. H., Oerbeck, B., & Kristensen, H. (2011). The relationship between sluggish cognitive tempo subtypes of attention-deficit/hyperactivity disorder, and anxiety disorders. *Journal of Abnormal Child Psychology, 39*, 513–525.

Skogli, E. W., Teicher, M. H., Andersen, P. N., Hovik, K. T., & Oie, M. (2013). ADHD in girls and boys—Gender difference in co-existing symptoms and executive function measures. *BMC Psychiatry, 13*, 298.

Skottun, B. C. (2000). The magnocellular deficit theory of dyslexia: The evidence from contrast sensitivity. *Vision Research, 40*, 111–127.

Skranes, J., Vangberg, T. R., Kulseng, S., Indredavik, M. S., Evensen, K. A. I., Martinussen, M., et al. (2007). Clinical findings and white matter abnormalities seen on diffusion tensor imaging in adolescents with very low birth weight. *Brain, 130,* 654–666.

Slavin, R. E., Lake, C., Chambers, B., Cheung, A., & Davis, C. (2009). Effective reading programs for elementary grades: A best-evidence synthesis. *Review of Educational Research, 79,* 1391–1466.

Smith, D. D. (1981). *Teaching the learning disabled.* Prentice-Hall.

Snowden, J. (2017). The neuropsychology of Huntington's Disease. *Archives of Clinical Neuropsychology, 32,* 876–887.

Snowling, M. J. (2012). Changing concepts of dyslexia: Nature, treatment, and comorbidity. *Journal of Psychology and Psychiatry, 53,* e1–e3.

Snowling, M. J., Hulme, C., & Nation, K. (Eds.). (2022). *The science of reading: A handbook.* Wiley.

Snowling, M. J., Moll, K., & Hulme, C. (2021). Language difficulties are a shared risk factor for both reading disorder and mathematics disorder. *Journal of Experimental Child Psychology, 202,* 105009.

Sobanski, E., Banaschewski, T., Asherson, P., Buitelaar, J., Chen, W., Franke, B., et al. (2010). Emotional lability in children and adolescents with attention deficit/hyperactivity disorder (ADHD): Clinical correlates and familial prevalence. *Journal of Child Psychology and Psychiatry, 51,* 915–923.

Sousa, D. A., & Tomlinson, C. A. (2011). *Differentiation and the brain: How neuroscience supports the learner-friendly classroom.* Solution Tree Press.

South, M., & Rodgers, J. (2017). Sensory, emotional, and cognitive contributions to anxiety in autism spectrum disorders. *Frontiers in Human Neuroscience, 11,* 1–10.

Sowell, E. R., Thompson, P. M., Welcome, S. E., Henkenius, A. L., Toga, A. W., & Peterson, B. S. (2003). Cortical abnormalities in children and adolescents with attention-deficit hyperactivity disorder. *The Lancet, 362*(9397), 1699–1707.

Spearman, C. (1904). "General intelligence," objectively determined and measured. *American Journal of Psychology, 15,* 201–293.

Speece, D. L. (1990). Aptitude–treatment interactions: Bad rap or bad idea? *Journal of Special Education, 24,* 139–149.

Speece, D. L., & Ritchey, K. D. (2005). A longitudinal study of the development of oral reading fluency in young children at risk for reading failure. *Journal of Learning Disabilities, 38*(5), 387–399.

Spek, A. A., van Ham, N. C., & Nyklicek, I. (2013). Mindfulness-based therapy in adults with an autism spectrum disorder: A randomized controlled trial. *Research in Developmental Disabilities, 34,* 246–253.

Spencer, T. J., Biederman, J., & Mick, E. (2007). Attention-deficit/hyperactivity disorder: Diagnosis, lifespan, comorbidities, and neurobiology. *Journal of Pediatric Psychology, 32,* 631–642.

Spencer, T., & Peterson, D. B. (2018). Bridging oral and written language: An oral narrative language intervention study with writing outcomes. *Language, Speech, and Hearing Services in Schools, 49,* 569–581.

Spittle, A. J., Treyvaud, K., Doyle, L. W., Roberts, G., Lee, K. J., Inder, T. E., et al. (2009). Early emergence of behavior and social-emotional problems in very preterm infants. *Journal of the American Academy of Child and Adolescent Psychiatry, 48,* 909–918.

Spitz, G., Maller, J. J., O'Sullivan, R., & Ponsford, J. L. (2013). White matter integrity following traumatic brain injury: The association with severity of injury and cognitive functioning. *Brain Topography, 26,* 648–660.

Spooner, D. M., & Pachana, N. A. (2006). Ecological validity in neuropsychological assessment: A case for greater consideration in research with neurologically intact populations. *Archives of Clinical Neuropsychology, 21*(4), 327–337.

Spottiswoode, B. S., Meintjes, E. M., Anderson, A. W., Molteno, C. D., Stanton, M. E., Dodge, N. C., et al. (2011). Diffusion tensor imaging of the cerebellum and eyeblink conditioning in fetal alcohol spectrum disorder. *Alcoholism: Clinical and Experimental Research, 35,* 2174–2183.

Spreen, O., & Benton, A. L. (1977). *Neurosensory Center Comprehensive Examination for Aphasia (NCCEA).* University of Victoria Neuropsychology Laboratory.

Springer, S. P., & Deutsch, G. (1998). *Left brain, right brain: Perspectives from cognitive neuroscience* (5th ed.). Freeman.

Squire, L. R. (2004). Memory systems of the brain: a brief history and current perspective. *Neurobiology of Learning and Memory, 82*(3), 171–177.

Staines, W. R., Padilla, M., & Knight, R. T. (2002). Frontal–parietal event-related potential changes associated with practicing a novel visuomotor task. *Cognitive Brain Research, 13,* 195–202.

Standage, D., Blohm, G., & Dorris, M. C. (2014). On the neural implementation of the speed-accuracy trade-off. *Frontiers in Neuroscience, 8,* 88630.

Stark, K. D., Arora, P., & Funk, C. L. (2011). Training school psychologists to conduct evidence-based treatments for depression. *Psychology in the Schools, 48,* 272–282.

Stark, K. D., Banneyer, K. N., Wang, L. A., & Arora, P. (2012). Child and adolescent depression in the family. *Couple and Family Psychology: Research and Practice, 1*(3), 161.

Starkstein, S. E., & Kremer, J. L. (2001). Cerebral aging: neuropsychological, neuroradiological, and neurometabolic correlates. *Dialogues in Clinical Neuroscience, 3*(3), 217–228.

Starza-Smith, A., Talbot, E., & Grant, C. (2007). Encephalitis in children: A clinical neuropsychology perspective. *Neuropsychological Rehabilitation, 17,* 506–527.

Steege, M. W., Pratt, J. L., & Watson, T. S. (2009). *Conducting school-based functional behavioral assessments: A practitioner's guide* (2nd ed.). Guilford Press.

Steege, M. W., Pratt, J. L., Wickerd, G., Guare, R., & Watson, T. S. (2019). *Conducting school-based functional behavioral assessments: A practitioner's guide* (3rd ed.). Guilford Press.

Stein, J. F. (2001). The neurobiology of reading difficulties. In M. Wolf (Ed.), *Dyslexia, fluency, and the brain* (pp. 3–22). York Press.

Stein, M. I. (2014). *Stimulating creativity: Individual procedures.* Academic Press.

Sternberg, R. J. (2018). The triarchic theory of successful intelligence. In D. P. Flanagan & E. M. McDonough (Eds.), *Contemporary intellectual assessment: Theories, tests, and issues* (4th ed., pp. 174–194). Guilford Press.

Stiles, J. (2008). *The fundamentals of brain development: Integrating nature and nurture.* Harvard University Press.

Stone, W. L., Klopfenstein, K. J., Hajianpour, M. J., Popescu, M. I., Cook, C. M., & Krishnan, K. (2017). Childhood cancers and systems medicine. *Frontiers in Bioscience, 22,* 1148–1161.

Stoodley, C. J., & Schmahmann, J. D. (2010). Evidence for topographic organization in the cerebellum of motor control versus cognitive and affective processing. *Cortex, 46*(7), 831–844.

Straub, K., & Obrzut, J. E. (2009). Effects of cerebral palsy on neuropsychological function. *Journal of Developmental and Physical Disability, 21,* 153–167.

Strauss, E., Semenza, C., Hunter, M., Hermann, B., Barr, W., Chelune, G., et al. (2000). Left anterior lobectomy and category-specific naming. *Brain and Cognition, 43,* 403–406.

Strauss, E., Sherman, E. M. S., & Spreen, O. (2006). *A compendium of neuropsychological tests: Administration, norms, and commentary* (3rd ed.). Oxford University Press.

Strong, C. A. H., Tiesma, D., & Donders, J. (2010). Criterion validity of the Delis–Kaplan Executive Function System (D-KEFS) fluency subtests after traumatic brain injury. *Journal of the International Neuropsychological Society, 17*(2), 230–237.

Stuebing, K. K., Barth, A. E., Molfese, P. J., Weiss, B., & Fletcher, J. M. (2009). IQ is not strongly related to response to reading instruction: A meta-analytic interpretation. *Exceptional Children, 76*(1), 31–51.

Stuss, D. T. (2011). Functions of the frontal lobes: Relation to executive functions. *Journal of the International Neuropsychological Society, 17*(5), 759–765.

Stuss, D. T., & Alexander, M. P. (2005). Does damage to the frontal lobes produce impairment in memory? *Current Directions in Psychological Science, 14*(2), 84–88.

Stuss, D. T., & Benson, D. F. (2019). The frontal lobes and control of cognition and memory. In E. Perecman (Ed.), *The frontal lobes revisited* (pp. 141–158). Psychology Press.

Stuss, D. T., Gallup, G. G., Jr., & Alexander, M. P. (2001). The frontal lobes are necessary for theory of mind. *Brain, 124*(2), 279–286.

Stuss, D. T., & Knight, R. T. (2013). *Principles of frontal lobe function* (2nd ed.) Oxford University Press.

Suchan, B., Yagliez, L., Wunderlich, G., Canavan, A. G. M., Herzog, H., Tellmann, L., et al. (2002). Hemispheric dissociation of visual-pattern processing and visual rotation. *Behavioral Brain Research, 136,* 533–544.

Sulkowski, M. L., Wingfield, R. J., Jones, D., & Coulter, W. A. (2010). Response to intervention and interdisciplinary collaboration: Joining hands to support children's healthy development. *Journal of Applied School Psychology, 2,* 118–133.

Sumner, E., Connelly, V., & Barnett, A. L. (2013). Children with dyslexia are slow writers because they pause more often and not because they are slow at handwriting execution. *Reading and Writing, 26,* 991–1008.

Surian, L., & Siegal, M. (2001). Sources of performance on theory of the mind tasks in right hemisphere damaged patients. *Brain and Language, 78,* 224–232.

Sutton, G. P., Barchard, K. A., Bello, D. T., Thaler, N. S., Ringdahl, E., Mayfield, J., & Allen, D. N. (2011). Beery–Buktenica Developmental Test of Visual–Motor Integration performance in children with traumatic brain injury and attention-deficit/hyperactivity disorder. *Psychological Assessment, 23*(3), 805.

Svátková, A., Mandl, R. C., Scheewe, T. W., Kahn, R. S., Cahn, W., & Pol, H. H. (2014). EPA–1717: Effects of exercise therapy on white matter integrity in patients with schizophrenia and healthy controls-a longitudinal DTI study. *European Psychiatry, 29*(S1), 1–1.

Svatkova, A., Nestrasil, I., Rudser, K., Fine, J. G., Bledsoe, J., & Semrud-Clikeman, M. (2016). Unique white matter microstructural patterns in ADHD presentations—A diffusion tensor imaging study. *Human Brain Mapping, 37,* 3323–3336.

Swanson, E., Wanzek, J., Haring, C., Ciullo, S., & McCulley, L. (2013). Intervention fidelity in special and general education research journals. *The Journal of Special Education, 47*(1), 3–13.

Swanson, H. L. (2012). Cognitive profile of adolescents with math disabilities: Are the profiles different from those with reading disabilities. *Child Neuropsychology, 18,* 125–143.

Swanson, H. L., Howard, C. B., & Saez, L. (2006). Do different components of working memory underlie different subgroups of reading disabilities. *Journal of Learning Disabilities, 39*(3), 252–269.

Swanson, H. L., Jerman, O., & Zheng, X. (2009). Math disabilities and reading disabilities: Can they be separated? *Journal of Psychoeducational Assessment, 27,* 175–196.

Swanson, H. L., Mink, J., & Bocian, K. M. (1999). Cognitive processing deficits in poor readers with symptoms of reading disabilities and ADHD: More alike than different? *Journal of Educational Psychology, 91,* 321–333.

Swanson, H. L., Olide, A. G., & Kong, J. E. (2018). Latent class analysis of children with math difficulties and/or math learning disabilities: Are there cognitive differences? *Journal of Educational Psychology, 110,* 931–951.

Swanson, J., Castellanos, F. X., Murias, M., LaHoste, G., & Kennedy, J. (1998). Cognitive neuroscience of attention deficit hyperactivity disorder and hyperkinetic disorder. *Current Opinion in Neurobiology, 8*(2), 263–271.

Szekely, A., Silton, R. L., Heller, W., Miller, G. A., & Mohanty, A. (2017). Differential functional connectivity of rostral anterior cingulate cortex during emotional interference. *Social Cognitive and Affective Neuroscience, 12,* 476–486.

Szucs, D., Devine, A., Soltesz, F., Nobes, A., & Gabriel, F. (2013). Developmental dyscalculia is related to visuo-spatial memory and inhibition impairment. *Cortex, 49,* 2674–2688.

Szwed, M., Dehaene, S., Kleinschmidt, A., Eger, E., Valabregue, R., Amadon, A., & Cohen, L. (2011). Specialization for written words over objects in the visual cortex. *NeuroImage, 56,* 330–344.

Talairach, J., & Tournoux, P. (1988). *Co-planar stereotaxic atlas of the human brain: 3-dimensional proportional system: An approach to cerebral imaging.* Thieme Medical Publishers.

Tamm, L., Nakonezny, P. A., & Hughes, C. W. (2012). An open trial of a metacognitive executive function training for young children with ADHD. *Journal of Attention Disorders, 18,* 551–559.

Tarbox, J., Szabo, T. G., & Aclan, M. (2020). Acceptance and commitment training within the scope of practice of applied behavior analysis. *Behavior Analysis Practice, 15,* 11–32.

Taubitz, L. E., Pedersen, W. S., & Larson, C. L. (2015). BAS reward responsiveness: A unique predictor of positive psychological functioning. *Personality and Individual Differences, 80,* 107–112.

Taylor, H. G., Drotar, D., Schluchter, M., & Hack, M. (2006). Consequences and risks of <1000g birth weight for neuropsychological skills, achievement, and adaptive functioning. *Developmental and Behavioral Pediatrics, 27,* 459–469.

Teichner, G., & Golden, C. J. (2000). The relationship of neuropsychological impairment to conduct disorder in adolescence: A conceptual review. *Aggression and Violent Behavior, 5,* 509–528.

Temple, E., Poldrack, R. A., Salidis, J., Deutsch, G. K., Tallal, P., Merzenich, M. M., & Gabrieli, J. D. (2001). Disrupted neural responses to phonological and orthographic processing in dyslexic children: an fMRI study. *Neuroreport, 12*(2), 299–307.

Terman, L. M. (1916). *The measurement of intelligence.* Houghton Mifflin.

Teuber, H. L. (1975, January). Recovery of function after brain injury in man. In *Ciba Foundation Symposium 3: Outcome of severe damage to the central nervous system* (pp. 159–190). Wiley.

Thaler, N. S., Allen, D. N., McMurray, J. C., & Mayfield, J. (2010). Sensitivity of the test of memory and learning to attention and memory deficits in children with ADHD. *The Clinical Neuropsychologist, 24*(2), 246–264.

Thibert, K. A., Raymond, G. V., Tolar J., Miller, W. P., Orchard, P., & Lund, T. C. (2016). Cerebral spinal fluid levels of Cytokines are elevated in patients with metachromatic leukodystrophy. *Science Reports, 6,* 24579.

Thiele, E. A., & Korf, B. R. (2017). Phakomatoses and allied conditions. In K. Swaiman, S. Ashwayl, D. M. Ferriero, N. F. Schor, R. S. Finkel, A. L. Gropan, P. L. Pearl, & M. I. Shevell (Eds.), *Swaiman's pediatric neurology* (6th ed., pp. 362–372). Elsevier.

Thom, R. P., Pereira, J. A., Sipsock, D., & McDougle, C. J. (2021). Recent updates in psychopharmacology for the core and associated symptoms of Autism Spectrum Disorder. *Current Psychiatry Reports, 23,* https://doi.org/10.1007/s11920-021-01292-2.

Thomas-Sohl, K. A., Vasquez, D. F., & Maria, B. L. (2004). Sturge-Weber syndrome: A review. *Pediatric Neurology, 30,* 303–310.

Thompson-Schill, S. L., Jonides, J., Marshuetz, C., Smith, E. E., D'Esposito, M., Kan, I. P., et al. (2002). Effects of frontal lobe damage on interference effects in working memory. *Cognitive, Affective, & Behavioral Neuroscience, 2*(2), 109–120.

Thomson, J. M., Leong, V., & Goswami, U. (2013). Auditory processing interventions and developmental dyslexia: A comparison of phonemic and rhythmic approaches. *Reading and Writing, 26,* 139–145.

Thorndike, R. L., Hagen, E. P., & Sattler, J. M. (1986). *The Stanford–Binet Intelligence Scale: Fourth Edition. Guide for administration and scoring.* Riverside.

Thurman, D. J. (2014). The epidemiology of traumatic brain injury in children and youths: A review of research since 1990. *Journal of Child Neurology, 31,* 20–27.

Thurstone, L. L. (1938). *Primary mental abilities*. University of Chicago Press.

Tiffin, J., & Asher, E. J. (1948). The Purdue Pegboard: Norms and studies of reliability and validity. *Journal of Applied Psychology, 32*(3), 234–247.

Tikellis, G., Dwyer, T., Paltiel, O., Phillips, G. S., Lemeshow, S., Golding, J., et al. (2018). The International Childhood Cancer Cohort Consortium (I4C): A research platform of prospective cohorts for studying the aetiology of childhood cancers. *Pediatric and Perinatal Epidemiology, 32,* 568–583.

Till, C., Racine, N., Araujo, D., Narayanan, S., Collins, D. L., Aubert-Broche, B., et al. (2013). Changes in cognitive performance over a 1-year period in children and adolescents with multiple sclerosis. *Neuropsychology, 27*(2), 210.

Tolar, T. D., Fuchs, L., Fletcher, J. M., Fuchs, D., & Hamlett, C. L. (2016). Cognitive profiles of mathematical problem solving learning disability for different definitions of disability. *Journal of Learning Disabilities, 49*(3), 240–256.

Toll, S. W., Kroesbergen, E. H., & Van Luit, J. E. (2016). Visual working memory and number sense: Testing the double deficit hypothesis in mathematics. *British Journal of Educational Psychology, 86*(3), 429–445.

Toll, S. W. M., Van der Ven, S. H. G., Kroesbergen, E. H., & Van Luit, J. E. H. (2011). Executive functions as predictors of math learning disabilities. *Journal of Learning Disabilities, 44,* 521–532.

Toll, S. W. M., & Van Luit, J. E. H. (2012). Early numeracy intervention for low-performing kindergartners. *Journal of Early Intervention, 34,* 243–264.

Tomporowski, P. D., Davis, C. L., Miller, P. H., & Naglieri, J. A. (2008). Exercise and children's intelligence, cognition, and academic achievement. *Educational Psychology Review, 20,* 111–131.

Toste, J. R., Didion, L., Peng, P., Filderman, M. J., & McClelland, A. M. (2020). A Meta-Analytic Review of the Relations Between Motivation and Reading Achievement for K–12 Students. *Review of Educational Research, 90*(3), 420–456.

Tourian, L., LeBeouf, A. Breton, J. J., Cohen, D., Gignac, M., Labelle, R., et al. (2015). Treatment options for the cardinal symptoms of disruptive mood dysregulation disorder. *Journal of the Canadian Academy of Child and Adolescent Psychiatry, 24,* 41–54.

Tucha, L., Tucha, O., Walitza, S., Sontag, T. A., Laufkötter, R., Linder, M., & Lange, K. W. (2009). Vigilance and sustained attention in children and adults with ADHD. *Journal of Attention Disorders, 12,* 410–421.

Tucha, O., Mecklinger, L., Laufkötter, R., Klein, H. E., Walitza, S., & Lange, K. W. (2006). Methylphenidate-induced improvements of various measures of attention in adults with attention deficit hyperactivity disorder. *Journal of Neural Transmission, 113,* 1575–1592.

Tuller, B., Jantzen, K. J., Olvera, D., Steinberg, F., & Scott Kelso, J. A. (2007). The influence of instruction modality on brain activation in teenagers with nonverbal learning disabilities: Two case histories. *Journal of Learning Disabilities, 40,* 348–359.

Tulving, E., & Markowitsch, H. J. (1997). Memory beyond the hippocampus. *Current Opinion in Neurobiology, 7,* 209–216.

Turken, U., Whitfield-Gabrieli, S., Bammer, R., Baldo, J. V., Dronkers, N. F., & Gabrieli, J. D. (2008). Cognitive processing speed and the structure of white matter pathways: convergent evidence from normal variation and lesion studies. *Neuroimage, 42*(2), 1032–1044.

Tyler, L. K., Russell, R., Fadili, J., & Moss, H. E. (2001). The neural representation of nouns and verbs: PET studies. *Brain, 124*(8), 1619–1634.

Uddin, L. Q., Supekar, K., & Menon, V. (2010). Typical and atypical development of functional human brain networks: insights from resting-state FMRI. *Frontiers in Systems Neuroscience, 4,* 1447.

Uhry, J. K., & Clark, D. B. (2005). *Dyslexia: theory and practice of instruction*. York Press.

Uljarevic, M., Lane, A., Kelly, A., & Leekam, S. (2016). Sensory subtypes and anxiety in older children and adolescents with autism spectrum disorder. *Autism Research, 9,* 1073–1078.

Umilta, C. K., Priftis, & Zorzi, M. (2009). The spatial representation of numbers: Evidence from neglect and pseudoneglect. *Experimental Brain Research, 192,* 561–569.

Undheim, A. M., & Sund, A. M. (2008). Psychosocial factors and reading disabilities: Students with reading difficulties drawn from a representative population sample. *Scandinavian Journal of Psychology, 49,* 377–384.

Ungerleider, L. G., & Mishkin, M. (1982). Two cortical visual systems. In D. J. Engle, M. A. Goodale, & R. J. Mansfield (Eds.), *Analysis of visual behavior* (pp. 549–586). MIT Press.

Utianski, R. L., Clark, H. M., Duffy, J. R., Botha, H., Whitwell, J. L., & Josephs, K. A. (2020). Communication limitations in patients with progressive apraxia of speech and aphasia. *American Journal of Speech–Language Pathology, 29*(4), 1976–1986.

Vaidya, C. J., Austin, G., Kirkorian, G., Ridlehuber, H. W., Desmond, J. E., Glover, G. H., & Gabrieli, J. D. (1998). Selective effects of methylphenidate in attention deficit hyperactivity disorder: A functional magnetic resonance study. *Proceedings of the National Academy of Sciences, 95*(24), 14494–14499.

Valera, E. M., Faraone, S. V., Biederman, J., Poldrack,

R. A., & Seidman, L. J. (2005). Functional neuroanatomy of working memory in adults with attention-deficit/hyperactivity disorder. *Biological Psychiatry, 57,* 439–447.

Valera, E. M., Faraone, S. V., Murray, K. E., & Seidman, L. J. (2007). Meta-analysis of structural imaging findings in Attention Deficit/Hyperactivity Disorder. *Biological Psychiatry, 61,* 1361–1369.

Vandenberghe, R., Price, C., Wise, R., Josephs, O., & Frackowiak, R. S. (1996). Functional anatomy of a common semantic system for words and pictures. *Nature, 383,* 254–256.

VanDerHeyden, A., McLaughlin, T., Algina, J., & Synder, P. (2012). Randomized evaluation of a supplemental grade-wide mathematics intervention. *Review of Research in Education, 6,* 1251–1284.

VanDerHeyden, A. M., Witt, J. C., & Gilbertson, D. A. (2007). Multi-year evaluation of the effects of a Response to Intervention (RTI) model on identification of children for special education. *Journal of School Psychology, 45,* 225–256.

Van der Knaap, M., Schiffman, R., Mochel, F., & Wolf, N. I. (2019). Diagnosis, prognosis, and treatment of leukodystrophies. *Lancet, 18,* 962–972.

van der Meer, J., Oelermans, A., van Steijin, D. J., Lappenschaar, M. G., de Sonneville, L. M., Buitelaar, J. K., & Rommelse, N. N. (2017). Are Autism Spectrum Disorder and ADHD different manifestations of one overarching disorder? Cognitive and symptom evidence from a clinical and population sample. *Journal of the American Academy of Child and Adolescent Psychiatry, 11,* 1160–1172.

Van der Plas, E., Erdman, L., Nieman, B. J., Weksberg, R., Butcher, D. T., O'Connor, D. L., et al. (2018). Characterizing neurocognitive late effects in childhood leukemia survivors using a combination of neuropsychological and cognitive neuroscience measures. *Child Neuropsychology, 24,* 999–1014.

Vanderver, A. Wolff, N. I. (2017). Genetic and metabolic disorders of the white matter. In K. Swaiman, S. Ashwayl, D. M. Ferriero, N. F. Schor, R. S. Finkel, A. L. Gropan, P. L. Pearl, & M. I. Shevell (Eds.), *Swaiman's pediatric neurology* (6th ed., pp. 747–758). Elsevier.

Van Herwegen, J., Ashworth, M., & Palikara, O. (2019). Views of professionals about the educational needs of children with neurodevelopmental disorders. *Research in Developmental Disabilities, 91,* 103422.

van Lieshout, M., Luman, M., Twisk, J. W. R., van Ewijk, H., Groenman, A. P., Thissen, A. J., et al. (2016). A 6-year follow-up of a large Europena cohort of children with attention deficit hyperactivity disorder-combined subtype: Outcomes in late adolescence and young adulthood. *European Child and Adolescent Psychiatry, 25,* 1007–1017.

Van Meter, A. R., Burke, C., Youngstrom, E. A., Faedda, G. L., & Correll, C. U. (2016). The bipolar prodome: Meta-analysis of symptom prevalence prior to initial or recurrent mood episodes. *Journal of the American Academy of Child and Adolescent Psychiatry, 55,* 543–555.

Van Meter, A. R., Moreira, A. L., & Youngstrom, E. A. (2011). Meta-analysis of epidemiologic studies of pediatric bipolar disorder. *Journal of Clinical Psychiatry, 72,* 1250–1256.

Vasilopoulos, T., Franz, C. E., Panizzon, M. S., Xian, H., Grant, M. D., Lyons, M. J., et al. (2012). Genetic architecture of the Delis–Kaplan Executive Function System Trail Making Test: Evidence for distinct genetic influences on executive function. *Neuropsychology, 26*(2), 238.

Vaughn, S., Miciak, J., Clemens, N., & Fletcher, J. M. (2024). The critical role of instructional response in defining and identifying students with dyslexia: A case of updating existing definitions. *Annals of Dyslexia, 74,* 325–336.

Vega, C., Vestal, M., DeSalvo, M., Berman, R., Chung, M., Blumenfeld, H., & Spann, M. N. (2010). Differentiation of attention-related problems in childhood absence epilepsy. *Epilepsy & Behavior, 19,* 82–85.

Vellutino, F. R., Fletcher, J. M., Snowling, M. J., & Scanlon, D. M. (2004). Specific reading disability (dyslexia): What have we learned in the past four decades? *Journal of Child Psychology and Psychiatry, 45*(1), 2–40.

Vigliocco, G., Vinson, D. P., Druks, J., Barber, H., & Cappa, S. F. (2011). Nouns and verbs in the brain: A review of behavioural, electrophysiological, neuropsychological and imaging studies. *Neuroscience & Biobehavioral Reviews, 35*(3), 407–426.

Vigneau, M., Beaucousin, V., Herve, P. Y., Duffau, H., Crivello, F., Houde, O., & Tzourio-Mazoyer, N. (2006). Meta-analyzing left hemisphere language areas: Phonology, semantics, and sentence processing. *NeuroImage, 30,* 1414–1432.

Vizard, T., Pearce, N., Davis, J., Sadler, K., Ford, T., Goodman, A., et al. (2018). Mental health of children and young people in England, 2017: Emotional disorders. *NHS Digital.*

Voeller, K. S. (2001). Attention-deficit/hyperactivity disorder as a frontal–subcortical disorder. In D. G. Lichter & J. L. Cummings (Eds.), *Frontal–subcortical circuits in psychiatric and neurological disorders* (pp. 334–371). Guilford Press.

Vogelstein, B., & Kinzler, K. W. (2015). The path to cancer: Three strikes and you're out. *New England Journal of Medicine, 373,* 1895–1898.

Volkmer, S., Galuschka, K., & Schulte-Körne, G. (2019). Early identification and intervention for children with initial signs of reading deficits—A blinded randomized controlled trial. *Learning and Instruction, 59*, 1–12.

von Aster, M., & Shalev, R. S. (2007). Number development and developmental dyscalculia. *Developmental Medicine & Child Neurology, 49*, 868–873.

Vourkas, M., Michelyannis, S., Simos, P. G., Rezaie, R., Fletcher, J. M., Cirino, P. T., & Papanicolaou, A. C. (2011). Dynamic task-specific brain network connectivity in children with severe reading difficulties. *Neuroscience Letters, 488*, 123–128.

Vukovic, R. K., & Siegel, L. S. (2006). The double-deficit hypothesis: A comprehensive analysis of the evidence. *Journal of Learning Disabilities, 39*, 25–47.

Waber, D. P., De Moor, C., Forbes, P. W., Almli, C. R., Botteron, K. N., Leonard, G., et al. (2007). The NIH MRI study of normal brain development: performance of a population based sample of healthy children aged 6 to 18 years on a neuropsychological battery. *Journal of the International Neuropsychological Society, 13*(5), 729–746.

Waber, D. P., Forbes, P. W., Almli, C. R., Blood, E. A., & Brain Development Cooperative Group. (2012). Four-year longitudinal performance of a population-based sample of healthy children on a neuropsychological battery: The NIH MRI study of normal brain development. *Journal of the International Neuropsychological Society, 18*(2), 179–190.

Wagner, R. K., Puranik, C. S., Foorman, B., Foster, E., Wilson, L. G., Tschinkel, E., et al. (2011). Modelling the development of written language. *Reading and Writing, 24*, 203–220.

Wagner, R. K., Torgesen, J. K., Rashotte, C. A., & Pearson, N. A. (2013). Comprehensive test of phonological processing–second edition. *Canadian Journal of School Psychology, 302*, 155–162.

Wakely, M. B., Hooper, S. R., de Kruif, R. E., & Swartz, C. (2006). Subtypes of written expression in elementary school children: A linguistic-based model. *Developmental Neuropsychology, 29*(1), 125–159.

Walker, S., Henderson, L. M., Fletcher, F. E., Knowland, V. C. P., Cairney, S. A., & Gaskell, M. G. (2019). Learning to live with interfering neighbours: the influence of time of learning and level of encoding on word learning. *Royal Society Open Science, 6*(4), 181842.

Wandell, B. A., Rauschecker, A. M., & Yeatman, J. D. (2012). Learning to see words. *Annual Review of Psychology, 63*, 31–53.

Wanzek, J., & Vaughn, S. (2011). Is a three-tier reading intervention model associated with reduced placement in special education? *Remedial and Special Education, 32*(2), 167–175.

Ward, E., DeSantis, C., Robbins, A., Kohler, B., & Jemal, A. (2014). Childhood and adolescent cancer statistics. *Cancer Journal for Clinicians, 64*, 83–103.

Watkins, M. W., & Canivez, G. L. (2022). Assessing the psychometric utility of IQ Scores: A tutorial using the Wechsler Intelligence Scale for Children—Fifth Edition. *School Psychology Review, 51*(5), 619–633.

Watkins, M. W., Glutting, J. J., & Youngstrom, E. A. (2005). Issues in Subtest Profile Analysis. In D. P. Flanagan & P. L. Harrison (Eds.), *Contemporary intellectual assessment: Theories, tests, and issues* (pp. 251–268). Guilford Press.

Watson, S. M. R., & Gable, R. A. (2012). Unraveling the complex nature of mathematics learning disability: Implications for research and practice. *Learning Disability Quarterly, 36*, 178–187.

Watts, S. J., Rodgers, J., & Riby, D. (2016). A systematic review of the evidence for hyporesponsivity in ASD. *Review Journal of Autism Developmental Disorders, 3*, 286–301.

Webb, N. M., Franke, M. L., Ing, M., Wong, J., Fernandez, C. H., Shin, N., & Turrou, A. C. (2014). Engaging with others' mathematical ideas: Interrelationships among student participation, teachers' instructional practices, and learning. *International Journal of Educational Research, 63*, 79–93.

Wechsler, D. (1939). *Measurement of adult intelligence.* Williams & Wilkins.

Wechsler, D. (2014). *Wechsler Intelligence Scale for Children—Fifth Edition.* Pearson Assessment.

Wegbreit, E., Cushman, G. K., Puzia, M. E., Weissman, A. B., Kim, K. L., Laird, A. R., & Dickstein, D. P. (2014). Developmental meta-analyses of the functional neural correlates of bipolar disorder. *JAMA Psychiatry, 71*, 926–935.

Wegrzyn, M., Riehle, M., Labudda, K., Woermann, F., Baumgartner, F., Pollmann, S., et al. (2015). Investigating the brain basis of facial expression perception using multi-voxel pattern analysis. *Cortex, 69*, 131–140.

Weisenberg, T. H., & McBride, K. E. (1935). *Aphasia: A clinical and psychological study.* Commonwealth Fund.

Weissman, D. H., & Woldorff, M. G. (2005). Hemispheric asymmetries for different components of global/local attention occur in distinct temporoparietal loci. *Cerebral Cortex, 15*(6), 870–876.

Weissman, M., Wickramaratne, P., Gameroof, M., Warner, V., Pilowsky, D., Kohad, R. G., et al. (2016). Offspring of depressed parents: 30 years later. *American Journal of Psychiatry, 173*, 1024–1032.

Weller, M. D., Holmes Bernstein, J., Bellinger, D. C., & Waber, D. P. (2000). Processing speed in children with Attention Deficit Hyperactivity Disorder, Inattentive type. *Child Neuropsychology, 6*, 218–234.

Wepman, J. M., & Reynolds, W. M. (1987). *Wepman*

Auditory Discrimination Test—Second Edition. Western Psychological Services.

Wetherwill, L., Foroud, T., & Goodlett, C. (2018). Meta-analyses of externalizing disorders: Genetics or prenatal alcohol exposure. *Alcoholism: Clinical Experimental Research, 42,* 162–172.

Wheaton, M. G., Fitzgerald, D. A., Phan, K. L., & Klumpp, H. (2014). Perceptual load modulates anterior cingulate cortex response to threat distractors in generalized social anxiety disorder. *Biological Psychology, 101,* 13–17.

Wheeler, M. A., Stuss, D. T., & Tulving, E. (1995). Frontal damage produces episodic memory impairment. *Journal of the International Neuropsychological Society, 1,* 525–536.

Whitaker, H. A., Bub, D., & Leventer, S. (1981). Neurolinguistic aspects of language acquisition and bilingualism. *Annals of the New York Academy of Sciences, 379,* 59–74.

White, J. L., & Kratochwill, T. R. (2005). Practice guidelines in school psychology: Issues and directions for evidence-based interventions in practice and training. *Journal of School Psychology, 43*(2), 99–115.

Whiteside, S. P. H., Sim, L. A., Morrow, A. S., Farah, W. H., Hilliker, D. R., Murad, M. H., & Wang, Z. (2020). A meta-anslysis to guide the enhancement of CBT for childhood anxiety: Exposure of anxiety management. *Clinical Child and Family Psychology Review, 23,* 102–121.

Wiig E. H., Semel E., & Secord W. A. (2013). *Clinical evaluation of language fundamentals–Fifth edition* (CELF-5). Pearson.

Wiggins, J. L., Brotmann, M. A., Adelma, N. E., Kim, P., Oakes, A. H., Reynolds, R. C., et al. (2016). Neural correlates of irritability in disruptive mood dysregulation and bipolar disorders. *American Journal of Psychiatry, 173,* 722–730.

Wiggs, C. L., Weisberg, J., & Martin, A. (1999). Neural correlates of semantic and episodic memory retrieval. *Neuropsychologia, 37,* 103–118.

Wilens, T., Biederman, J., Brown, S., Tanguay, S., Monuteaux, M. C., Blake, C., & Spencer, T. J. (2002). Clinically referred preschool children and youths with ADHD. *Journal of the American Academy of Child and Adolescent Psychiatry, 41,* 262–268.

Wilens, T. E., & Kaminski, T. A. (2020). Stimulants: Friend or foe? *Journal of the American Academy of Child and Adolescent Psychiatry, 59,* 36–37.

Willcutt, E. G., Betjemann, R. S., McGrath, L. M., Chhabildas, N., Olson, R. K., & Defries, J. C. (2010). Etiology and neuropsychology of comorbidity between RD and ADHD: The case for multiple-deficit models. *Cortex, 46,* 1345–1361.

Willcutt, E. G., DeFries, J. C., Pennington, B. F., Smith, S., Cardon, L. R., & Olson, R. K. (2003). Genetic etiology of comorbid reading difficulties and attention deficit/hyperactivity disorder. In R. Plomin, J. C. DeFries, I. W. Craig & P. McGuffin (Eds.), *Behavioral genetics in the postgenomic era* (pp. 227–246). American Psychological Association.

Willcutt, E. G., Doyle, A. E., Nigg, J. T., Faraone, S. V., & Pennington, B. F. (2005). Validity of the executive function theory of attention-deficit/hyperactivity disorder: A meta-analytic view. *Biological Psychiatry, 57,* 1336–1346.

Willcutt, E. G., & Pennington, B. F. (2000). Psychiatric comorbidity in children and adolescents with reading disability. *The Journal of Child Psychology and Psychiatry and Allied Disciplines, 41*(8), 1039–1048.

Willcutt, E. G., Petrill, S. A., Wu, S., Boada, R., DeFries, J. C., Olson, R. K., & Pennington, B. F. (2013). Comorbidity between reading disability and math disability: Concurrent psychopathology, functional impairment, and neuropsychological functioning. *Journal of Learning Disabilities, 46,* 500–516.

Williams, K. J., Austin, C. R., & Vaughn, S. (2017). A synthesis of spelling interventions for secondary students with learning disabilities. *Journal of Special Education, 52,* 3–15.

Williams, K. T. (2018). *Expressive Vocabulary Test—Third Edition.* Pearson.

Willis, W. G. (1986). Actuarial and clinical approaches to neuropsychological diagnosis: Applied considerations. In J. E. Obrzut & G. W. Hynd (Eds.), *Child neuropsychology: Vol. 2. Clinical practice* (pp. 245–262). Academic Press.

Wilson, B. A. (2011). *Wilson reading system.* Wilson Language Training Corporation.

Wilson, C. E., Palermo, R., Schmalzl, L., & Brock, J. (2010). Specificity of impaired facial identity recognition in children with suspected developmental prosopagnosia. *Cognitive Neuropsychology, 27*(1), 30–45.

Wilson, C. J., Liu, L. J., Yang, J. J., Kang, G., Ojha, R. P., Neale, G. A., et al. (2015). Genetic and clinical factors associated with obesity among adult survivors of childhood cancer: A report from the St. Jude Lifetime Cohort. *Cancer, 121,* 2262–2270.

Wilson, K. R., Hansen, D. J., & Li, M. (2011). The traumatic stress response in child maltreatment and resultant neuropsychological effects. *Aggression and Violent Behavior, 16,* 87–97.

Wise, J. C., Sevcik, R. A., Morris, R. D., Lovett, M. W., & Wolf, M. (2007). The relationship among receptive and expressive vocabulary, listening comprehension, pre-reading skills, word identification skills, and reading comprehension by children with reading disabilities. *Journal of Speech, Language and Hearing Research, 50,* 1093–1109.

Witsken, D. E., D'Amato, R. C., & Hartlage, L. C. (2008). Understanding the past, present, and future of clinical neuropsychology. In R. C. D'Amato & L. C. Hartlage (Eds.), *Essentials of neuropsychological assessment: Treatment planning for rehabilitation* (2nd ed., pp. 3–29). Springer.

Witt, J. C., & VanDerHeyden, A. M. (2007). The System to Enhance Educational Performance (STEEP): Using Science to Improve Achievement. In S. R. Jimerson, M. K. Burns, & A. M. VanDer-Heyden (Eds.), *Handbook of response to intervention: The science and practice of assessment and intervention* (pp. 343–353). Springer.

Wiznitzer, M., & Scheffel, D. L. (2009). Learning disabilities. In R. B. David, J. B. Bodensteiner, D. E. Mandelbaum & B. Olson (Eds.), *Clinical pediatric neurology* (pp. 479–492). Demos.

Wodrich, D. L., Spencer, M. L. S., & Daley, K. B. (2006). Combining RTI and psychoeducational assessment: What we must assume to do otherwise. *Psychology in the Schools, 43*(7), 797–806.

Wolf, M. (Ed.). (2001). *Dyslexia, fluency, and the brain.* York Press.

Wolf, M., O'Rourke, A. G., Gidney, C., Lovett, M., Cirino, P., & Morris, R. (2002). The second deficit: An investigation of the independence of phonological and naming-speed deficits in developmental dyslexia. *Reading and Writing, 15,* 43–72.

Wolf, U., Rapoport, M. J., & Schweizer, T. A. (2009). Evaluating the affective component of the cerebellar cognitive affective syndrome. *Journal of Neuropsychiatry and Clinical Neurosciences, 21,* 245–253.

Wood, S. M., Shah, S. S., Steenhoff, A. P., & Rustein, R. M. (2009). The impact of AIDS diagnoses on long-term neurocognitive and psychiatric outcomes of surviving adolescents with perinatally acquired HIV. *AIDS, 23,* 1859–1865.

Woodcock, R. W. (1993). An information processing view of *Gf–Gc* theory. *Journal of Psychoeducational Assessment (WJ-R Monograph),* 80–102.

Woodcock, R. W., McGrew, K. S., & Mather, N. (2001). *Woodcock–Johnson III Test of Cognitive Abilities.* Riverside.

Woodcock, R., McGrew, K. S., Schrank, F. A., & Mather, N. (2014). *Woodcock–Johnson Test of Cognitive Abilities.* Houghton Mifflin, Harcourt-Riverside.

World Health Organization. (2022). *International Classification of Diseases* (11th rev.). Author. (Original work published 1993)

Wozniak, J. R., Mueller, B. A., Bell, C. J., Muetzel, R. L., Hoecker, H. L., Boys, C. J., & Lim, K. O. (2013). Global functional connectivity abnormalities in children with fetal alcohol spectrum disorders. *Alcoholism: Clinical and Experimental Research, 37,* 748–756.

Wozniak, J. R., Mueller, B. A., Muetzel, R. L., Bell, C. J., Hocker, H. L., Nelson, M. L., et al. (2011). Interhemispheric functional connectivity disruption in children with prenatal alcohol exposure.

Alcoholism: Clinical Experimental Research, 35, 849–861.

Wozniak, J. R., Muetzel, R. L., Mueller, B. A., McGee, C. L., Hoecker, H. L., Nelson, M. L., et al. (2009). Microstructural corpus callosum anomalies in children with prenatal alcohol exposure: An extension of previous diffusion tensor imaging findings. *Alcoholism: Clinical Experimental Research, 33,* 1825–1835.

Wright, P. W., Hale, J. B., Backenson, E. M., Eusebio, E. C., & Dixon, S. G. (2013). Forest Grove v. TA. Rejoinder to Zirkel: An attempt to profit from malfeasance? *Journal of Psychoeducational Assessment, 31*(3), 318–325.

Wyczesany, M., Capotosto, P., Zappasodi, F., & Prete, G. (2018). Hemispheric asymmetries and emotions: Evidence from effective connectivity. *Neuropsychologia, 121,* 98–105.

Xiang, T., Lohrenz, T., & Montague, P. R. (2013). Computations substrates of norms and their violations during social exchange. *The Journal of Neuroscience, 33,* 1099–1108.

Xiao, C., Bledsoe, J., Wang, S., Chaovalitwongse, W. A., Mehta, S., Semrud-Clikeman, M., & Grabowski, T. (2016). An integrated feature ranking and selection framework for ADHD characterization. *Brain Informatics, 3,* 145–155.

Xu, J., Kemeny, S., Park, G., Frattali, C., & Braun, A. (2005). Language in context: Emergent features of word, sentence, and narrative comprehension. *NeuroImage, 25,* 1002–1015.

Yarkoni, T., Speer, N. K., & Zacks, J. M. (2008). Neural substrates of narrative comprehension and memory. *NeuroImage, 41,* 1408–1425.

Yeates, K. O., Armstrong, K., Janusz, J., Taylor, H. G., Wade, S., Stancin, T., & Drotar, D. (2005). Long-term attention problems in children with traumatic brain injury. *Journal of the American Academy of Child & Adolescent Psychiatry, 44*(6), 574–584.

Yeates, K. O., Ris, M. D., Taylor, H. G., & Pennington, B. F. (Eds.). (2009). *Pediatric neuropsychology: Research, theory, and practice.* Guilford Press.

Yin, H. H., & Knowlton, B. J. (2006). The role of the basal ganglia in habit formation. *Nature Reviews Neuroscience, 7,* 464–476.

Yoshimasu, K., Barbaresi, W. J., Colligan, R. C., Killian, J. M., Voigt, R. G., Weaver, A. L., & Katusic, S. K. (2011). Written-language disorder among children with and without ADHD in a population-based birth cohort. *Pediatrics, 128,* e605–e612.

Young, G. S., Rogers, S. J., Hutman, T., Rozga, A., Sigman, M., & Ozonoff, S. (2011). Imitation from 12 to 24 months in autism and typical development: a longitudinal Rasch analysis. *Developmental Psychology, 47*(6), 1565.

Young, J. R., Yanagihara, A., Dew, R., & Kollins, S. H. (2021). Pharmacotherapy for preschool children with Attention Deficit Hyperactivity Disorder (ADHD): Current status and future directions. *CNS Drugs, 35,* 403–424.

Ysseldyke, J. E., & Reschly, D. J. (2014). The evolution of school psychology: Origins, contemporary status, and future directions. In P. Harrison & A. Thomas (Eds.), *Best practices in school psychology: Data-based and collaborative decision making* (Vol. I, pp. 71–86). National Association of School Psychologists.

Ysseldyke, J. E., & Sabatino, D. A. (1973). Toward validation of the diagnostic–prescriptive model. *Academic Therapy, 8,* 415–422.

Ysseldyke, J. E., & Salvia, J. (1974). Diagnostic–prescriptive teaching: Two models. *Exceptional Children, 41*(3), 181–185.

Zago, L., Petit, L., Turbelin, M. R., Andersson, F., Vigneau, M., & Tzourio-Mazoyer, N. (2008). How verbal and spatial manipulation networks contribute to calculation: An fMRI study. *Neuropsychologia, 46,* 2403–2414.

Zametkin, A. J., Liebenauer, L. L., Fitzgerald, G. A.,

King, A. C., Minkunas, D. V., Herscovitch, P., et al. (1993). Brain metabolism in teenagers with attention-deficit hyperactivity disorder. *Archives of General Psychiatry, 50*(5), 333–340.

Zang, Y. F., Jin, Z., Weng, X., Zhang, L., Zeng, Y. W., & Yang, L. (2005). Functional MRI in attention-deficit hyperactivity disorder: Evidence for hypofrontality. *Brain Development, 27,* 544–550.

Zhao, C., Yuang, L., Xie, S., Zhang, Z., Pan, H., & Gong, G. (2019). Hemispheric module-specific influence of the X chromosome on white matter connectivity: Evidence from girls with Turner Syndrome. *Cerebral Cortex, 29,* 4580–4594.

Zhou, H.-X., Chen, X., Shen, Y.-Q., Li, L., Chen, N.-X., Zhu, Z.-C., et al. (2020). Rumination and the default mode network: Meta-analysis of brain imaging studies and implications for depression. *NeuroImage, 206,* 116287.

Ziegler, J. C., & Goswami, U. (2005). Reading acquisition, developmental dyslexia, and skilled reading across languages: A psycholinguistic grain size theory. *Psychological Bulletin, 131,* 3–29.

Index

Note. f or *t* following a page number indicates a figure or table.